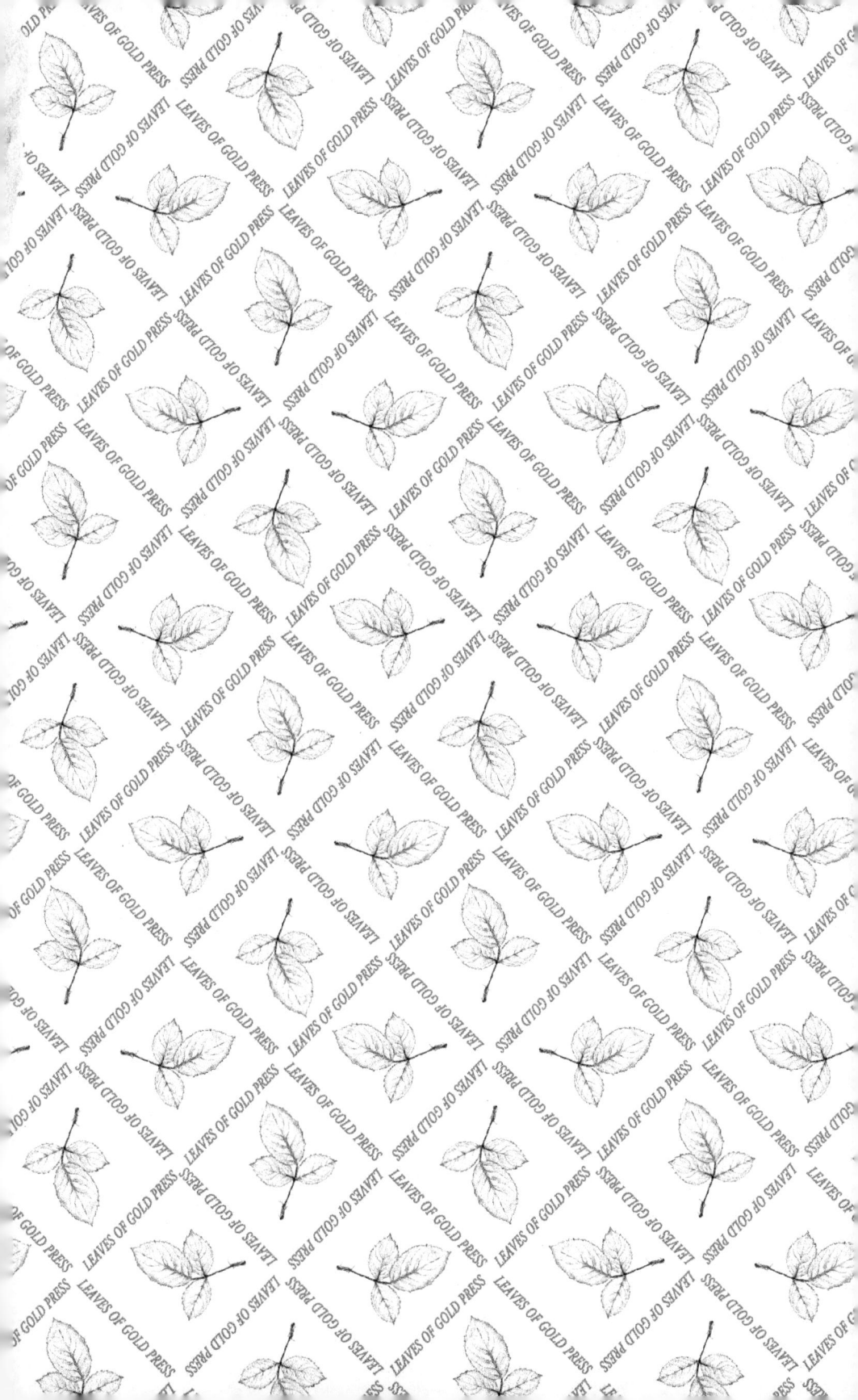

HOW TO LOSE WEIGHT

The Satiety Diet

Authors: Chris Clark
James L. Gibb,
Editor: C. Egan
Title: How to lose weight: the satiety diet / Chris Clark and James L. Gibb

BISAC code: HEA019000
HEALTH & FITNESS / Diet & Nutrition / Weight Loss

ISBN: 978-0-9875754-7-0 (hardcover)
ISBN: 978-0-9875754-8-7 (paperback)

LEAVES of GOLD
PRESS

Leaves of Gold Press
ABN 67 099 575 078
PO Box 3092, Brighton, 3186, Victoria, Australia
www.leavesofgoldpress.com

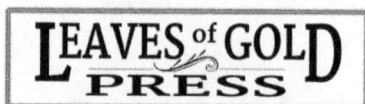

HOW TO LOSE WEIGHT

The Satiety Diet

BOOK #1 IN THE SATIETY DIET SERIES

Chris Clark, B. A.,
and James L. Gibb, B.A. Dip. Ed.

"Satiety is the key to weight loss."

CONTENTS

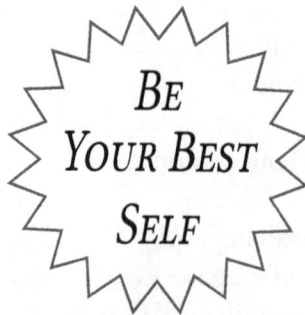

BE
YOUR BEST
SELF

FOREWORD

The Satiety Diet is a healthy, weight-control lifestyle. This book, and its companion volumes, took many years to research and write. Far from being ordinary "diet books", they include science-based data about a vast range of lifestyle factors beyond diet, all of which are powerful tools for weight control.

When the first draft of the original manuscript was finished, it was realised that the authors had gathered more information than could fit into a single volume. The draft exceeded the maximum number of pages available from the printers for a book of its dimensions. Additionally, the publishers were hesitant to offer readers a book that was too bulky, heavy and hard to manage.

Every subject that had been researched was important to successful weight loss. The content was too valuable to leave anything out. What could be done?

The answer was to split the book into two parts.

Book #1: *How to Lose Weight: The Satiety Diet*

Book #2: *The Satiety Diet Weight Loss Toolkit*

In anticipation of readers' requests for recipes, a cookbook was also added to the series—

Book #3: *Crispy, Creamy, Chewy: The Satiety Diet Cookbook*

The authors found it challenging to choose which information to take out of Book #1 for inclusion in Book #2, while doing full justice to readers of the first volume. After much revising, planning and brain-storming, they ended up successfully dividing the manuscript in the manner they deemed most appropriate.

If space had permitted, they would have included in Book #1 the topics, "Sleep Tools" (how to get a better night's sleep) and "Children and Obesity" (decreasing your child's obesity risk). The former section gives effective and thrifty tips for getting that sound sleep which is such an essential element of weight control, mood enhancement and all-round better health. Parents and caregivers are strongly urged to read the latter section in Book #2. Many well-meaning parents are making mistakes they are unaware of, and may be inadvertently contributing to their child's future struggles with body-weight.

The Satiety Diet Weight Loss Toolkit also contains chapters on such topics as "Weight Loss Mind Tricks," "Dining Out Tools" and "Sweetness and Sweeteners."

For more information on the contents of Book #2: *The Satiety Diet Weight Loss Toolkit*, turn to the afterword at the end of this book.

We hope that the Satiety Diet will help you live your best life.

Chris Clark and James L. Gibb
2019

BACKGROUND

Losing weight can be hard. If it was not hard, we'd all be slim and there would be no "obesity crisis".

At first glance, everything seems straightforward; if we simply ate less and exercised more we would all lose weight. Right?

If only it were that simple! In real life, it's more complicated than that.

A SCIENCE-BASED GUIDE

The Satiety Diet guide to weight loss is grounded in scientific research. This research proves what we all know—that losing weight is a complex business with many interconnecting factors. There is no single "magic bullet" that provides the answer.

Some weight loss gurus advocate simply cutting out one food group or another, such as sugar, or fat, or carbs. Others claim that consuming certain foods, supplements or beverages (such as cider vinegar or buttered coffee) will make the pounds drop away.

The Satiety Diet looks at recent research into the myriad ways not only your food, but also your thoughts, habits, environment and almost every aspect of your life can profoundly affect your body-weight. Science is the foundation for this comprehensive guide.

The Satiety Diet is the science-based way to lose weight and keep it off forever.

ALL DIETS WORK. SO WHY DON'T THEY WORK?

"Lose 14 pounds in 4 weeks!" "Drop 3 dress sizes in eight weeks!" We've all heard claims like these. Rapid loss of large amounts of weight loss is possible, of course, if you just stop eating, or eat barely anything, and start exercising rigorously. But in reality, who can sustain such a tortuous regime? Drastic weight-loss diets work—but only if you stick to them.

It's sticking to them that is the problem!

People fail at losing weight because it's so difficult to keep going, over a sufficient period of time, on most diets.

If you can't lose weight through diet and exercise, it's probably not your fault. It's more likely to be the diet's fault. The diet that works is the diet that you can stick to. At long last, you have found a diet that's easier to stay with—

The Satiety Diet.[1]

To lose weight you don't have to be ravenous half the time, you don't have to exercise way more than you think is reasonable, and you don't have to tie your self-worth to the number on the bathroom scales.

In fact, if you do any of those things, you're likely to sabotage your weight loss.

LONG-TERM SUCCESS

Why does the Satiety Diet work in the long-term, when others fail?

It works because it doesn't rely on a handful of basic, simplistic guidelines. It is a comprehensive, holistic, multi-faceted approach. This is the only approach that makes sense when addressing complex problems with as many contributing factors as overweight and obesity.

At the end of the day, weight loss or gain depends on how much energy the body has consumed and how much energy the body has expended. Obesity and overweight, however, are not necessarily the

---

1   Satiety is pronounced sa-TIE-e-tee.

result of greediness, laziness or lack of willpower. Your eating patterns are influenced by powerful biochemical, emotional, behavioral, environmental and psychosocial factors.

Why do people give up on weight-loss diets?

Some of the factors that hinder weight loss include:
- Hunger
- Cravings
- Food "addiction"
- Lack of motivation
- Struggling to break old habits (such as WHAT you eat and HOW you eat)
- Emotional needs (e.g. "comfort eating")

The Satiety Diet provides science-based solutions to these problems.

THE SATIETY DIET IS A POSITIVE APPROACH

What if we told you that to lose weight you have to:
- Starve yourself
- Go without your favorite foods and drinks
- Exercise vigorously in the gym for several hours every day
- Feel guilty if you don't do all the above?

Well, we're not going to tell you that!
Some of the things you'll do to lose weight on the Satiety Diet are:
- Satisfy your appetite and cravings
- Spend more time eating
- Spend more time planning and preparing meals (or get someone else to do it for you!)
- Do some gentle physical activities you enjoy
- Sleep better
- Be kind to yourself

To lose weight, give yourself more, not less!

As living creatures, we are highly motivated to seek the energy we need to survive. We get this energy from food and store it as fat on our bodies. Acquiring energy is a primeval need, hard-wired into us. That's one reason it's hard to lose weight.

It's not just energy/food we are "programmed" to seek.

Most of us have an innate drive to gather and accumulate things in general, rather than to "give away" and "let go". We tend to yearn for more money, more health, more power, more possessions, more love, more respect.

"Weight loss" sounds negative. Think of it more positively, as:

* becoming slimmer
* turning back into the real you
* feeling better
* looking better
* achieving your healthy goal
* relieving your body of a burden of unwanted fat

More! Not less!

Most weight-loss diets deny us our natural desire for MORE. We are told we must aim for LESS. Eat less food. Drink less alcohol. Consume fewer Calories. Limit food variety—cut out this food, or that food, or entire food groups.

No wonder we find those regimes hard to stick to!

The Satiety Diet is all about giving yourself MORE—more variety, more flavor, more delicious recipes, more vegetables, more enjoyment of food, more time to eat, more colorful dining, more calm and happiness, more satisfaction and enjoyment of living, more pleasure in movement, improved fitness, better health, and more delight in simply being the best you can be.

4

SATIETY DIET OR SATIETY LIFESTYLE?

The Satiety Diet is more than a "diet" in the popular sense of the word. It is an easygoing, healthy lifestyle. Why, then don't we call it the "Satiety Lifestyle"? Because most people view the word "diet" as referring to weight control, and that's what we're all about. Besides, this is a lifestyle based on a way of eating, and "a way of eating" is one definition of a diet.

THE BEST DIET IS THE ONE YOU STICK TO . . .

Researchers regularly compare the latest weight loss diets to find out which ones work better than others. A study published in 2014 reviewed the clinical diet trials of more than 7200 adults.

The popular diets they compared were Atkins®, Weight Watchers®, Zone®, Jenny Craig®, LEARN®, Nutrisystem®, Ornish®, Volumetrics®, Rosemary Conley®, Slimming World® and South Beach®. [Johnston et al. (2014)]

Their conclusion?

That there was no significant difference in the amount of weight lost on any of these diets.

Broadly, they all worked as well as each other.

"Overall, the differences between the different diets regarding their impact on weight loss were relatively small," said co-author Associate Professor Geoff Ball of the University of Alberta.

The researchers concluded that, "This supports the practice of recommending any diet that a patient will adhere to in order to lose weight."

Associate Professor Amanda Salis of the Boden Institute of Obesity, Nutrition, Exercise and Eating Disorders commented that the "strength of the findings is very robust".

The fact cannot be over-emphasized—*any diet will work, as long as you stick to it for long enough.* It's sticking to it that's the key.

And the Satiety Diet makes this a lot easier!

SATIETY BOOSTS WEIGHT LOSS

Satiety can be defined as "the feeling or state of being sated, satisfied and replete . . . the absence of hunger and the feeling of having eaten enough food."

The diet you stick to is likely to be the diet that provides satiety. If you've chosen a way of eating that leaves you hungry and dissatisfied and battling against cravings, you're unlikely to tolerate it for long enough to lose significant amounts of weight.

For many reasons, the Satiety Diet is easier to stick to than other diets. It's a mode of living that's healthier, slimmer, calmer, and happier. As a way of life, it can be maintained over the long-term— for months, or years, or for the rest of your days, because:

- It is based on a wide range of proven, powerful psychological techniques for weight loss.
- It teaches you to understand and communicate with your body.
- It does not limit the types of foods that can be eaten.
- It focuses on food variety, with emphasis on a combination of low GI foods and moderate amounts of protein; particularly plant-protein, with its numerous added nutritional benefits.
- It promotes satiety, which in turn lowers the risk of over-eating.
- It addresses the problems at the root of obesity, such as cravings, bad eating habits and self-limited food choices.
- It's not a program you have to sign up to and pay for.
- It's an approach that is easy to follow.
- It does not require any special equipment, or demand that you endure long bouts of painful, rigorous, exhausting exercise.
- It encourages you to use free social support networks, available 24/7 to anyone who has access to the Internet. Social support has been shown to sustain motivation and encourage adherence to long-term goals.
- The Satiety Diet is as kind to you as you should be to yourself.

MINIMAL REBOUND WEIGHT-GAIN

The best diet is also the one that doesn't lead to rebound weight-gain afterwards. A large majority of dieters regain their lost weight within a few months or years of ceasing the diet. Some end up weighing even more than before they started the diet.

There doesn't have to be an "afterwards" with the Satiety Diet. As a pleasant, sustainable lifestyle, it can continue indefinitely.

"The issue is about adherence, and it's how closely and how long can you keep sticking to the plan over time that matters," says Professor Susan Jebb from the University of Oxford, a UK government adviser on obesity.

A maintainable approach to weight loss is just as important as the diet, and the Satiety Diet provides this.

YOUR NEW, REWARDING CAREER!

Treat your weight loss journey as if it's your job.

Successful weight loss depends largely on your state of mind. If you view your weight loss journey as an inconvenience, or a penance, or a difficult task you would like to be finished with as soon as possible, you're less likely to stick with it.

Think of your weight loss journey as your new, agreeable, part-time job. It's a job with very good pay. The payment is a fitter, leaner, healthier body. And while the job does occupy some of your time, it is not very difficult—basically, it involves planning, eating, sleeping, moving, de-stressing and getting happy.

As with any job, you do it every day.

And as with every job, you sometimes get time off.

With this job, however, if you don't turn up for work, you might have to pay a fine. That fine may be weight gain.

Simply stick to your new part-time job for as long as you want to get paid.

7

OBESITY AND OVERWEIGHT ARE HEALTH RISKS

When people become obese their swollen fat cells can burst, allowing fat to leak into the bloodstream and causing low-grade inflammation. Over time, this inflammation can cause damage to any and every one of their internal organs, leading to diseases such as heart problems, fatty liver, diabetes and insulin resistance. [ABC Catalyst (2015)] If you can lose weight, you can stop the inflammation.

Overweight/obesity can negatively affect your life in many ways:

- It places extra stress on your joints which can exacerbate arthritis and lead to joint pain.
- It makes it harder for you to move around, leading to lethargy and lack of exercise.
- It can generate emotional issues, such as depression, that stem from low self-esteem and an unhealthy body image.
- There is an increased risk of cardiovascular disease, stroke, cancer, high blood pressure, Type 2 diabetes, sleep apnea, and gallstones.

OBESITY CREEPS UP STEALTHILY

Very few people would say "I want to be obese" and then proceed to work towards that goal.

Excess body-fat creeps up on you, stealthily, a little at a time. Day by day, if you consume just a few more Calories than you expend, your body stores a tiny bit more fat. At the end of a year, at the end of two years, or ten, those tiny increments have added up to a lot of extra weight. . .

. . . until one day you might look in the mirror, or see a photograph of yourself, and be shocked to note the change in your body-shape.

WHY DOES YOUR BODY STORE FAT?

Fat cells are where the body stores most of its fuel.

The primary fuels for the cells of your body are glucose (a simple sugar) and fatty acids (compounds produced by the breakdown of fats). When you put food into your digestive system, your body breaks it down, absorbs the nutrients into your blood and uses them to nourish your cells.

Your digestive tract, however, is not constantly full of food supplying your cells with nutrients and energy. Your body stores these resources in two "reservoirs", to be used during the periods your digestive tract is empty, such as when you wake up after a night's sleep. Your short-term reservoir stores carbohydrates for immediate use, and your long-term reservoir stores fat, to supply energy over a longer period.

The short term reservoir is located in the cells of the liver and the muscles, and it is filled with a complex carbohydrate called glycogen, which is a molecule for storing glucose. The long-term reservoir is your fat cells.

Research indicates that when people are making split-second decisions about what food to choose, they are more likely to choose healthful food over Calorie-loaded "junk" food if they already have sound knowledge about food and nutrition. One of the missions of this book is to help you learn about which foods will help weight loss, and which foods are likely to make you fat and unhealthy.

ARE YOU REALLY OVERWEIGHT?

You've started reading this book, so there's a good chance you want to lose weight. Our image of our own bodies, however, is often at odds with reality. People can be tiny and think they are overweight (e.g. anorexics) or huge and believe they are slim. Frequent stories of overweight people who began a weight loss regime only after seeing a photo or video of themselves corroborates this. They believed they were of a normal weight until they saw themselves through the eyes of others.

Body mass index (BMI).

For a long time we've all been measuring how fat or thin we are using the standard of the Body Mass Index, or BMI. The basis of this system was devised in the middle of the 19th century.

The modern term "Body Mass Index" for the ratio of human body weight to squared height was coined in a paper published in the July 1972 edition of the *Journal of Chronic Diseases*, by Ancel Keys. In this paper, Keys argued that what he termed the BMI was ". . . if not fully satisfactory, at least as good as any other relative weight index as an indicator of relative obesity".

The definition of overweight is a BMI over 25–30 kg/m2

The definition of obesity is a BMI over 30 kg/m2

Scientists are now questioning whether Body Mass Index is really the best indicator of a person's fat level. The system fails to take into account the positioning of fat stores (adipose tissue) in the body. Furthermore, with the BMI system, all body fat is considered equal, but in reality we have more than kind of fat, including brown, beige and white. Brown is the "good" fat that burns Calories, helping your body generate heat to insulate you against the cold. By contrast, white fat stores energy, and too much of it leads to obesity.

White fat is chiefly found in two places in the body. Subcutaneous white fat lies just beneath the skin and can be thought of as 'neutral' fat. Subcutaneous fat is what makes people look lumpy when they have too much of it.

10

Visceral white fat, furthermore, is really bad for your health. It's the deep fat that wraps itself around your vital inner organs. Its presence increases the risk of such problems as:

- cardiovascular disease
- insulin resistance
- chronic inflammation

(Fortunately visceral fat is the first to go when you start exercising and eating well. It burns off before subcutaneous fat.)

A piece of string.

Instead of measuring your BMI to find out whether you need to lose weight, you could take a piece of string and measure your waist-to-height ratio (WHtR).

Researchers from Oxford Brookes University decided to use the string method to indicate whether people were overweight. First they measured someone's height with the string, then they folded the string in half. If the folded string fitted easily around the person's waist, they judged that the person was not overweight.

The reasoning behind the string measurement is that the abdomen (the waist) is where white fat usually accumulates, while brown fat is distributed in other parts of the body. [Rivas (2015)]

Researchers Ashwell & Gibson (2015) agreed that WHtR is superior to BMI as a measurement of overweight and obesity. [Ashwell & Gibson (2015).]

For people under the age of forty, a WHtR of over 0.5 is a cause for concern, and indicates an increased risk of ill health.

- For people under forty, the critical value is 0.5
- For people aged 40–50 the critical value is between 0.5 and 0.6
- For people over 50 the critical values start at 0.6.

THE MULTI-FACETED APPROACH TO WEIGHT LOSS

Like other serious health issues such as cancer, diabetes and heart disease, obesity can have a wide range of causes.

Diabetes, for example, can be triggered by genetic makeup, ethnicity, health, diet, lifestyle and other environmental factors. Similarly, overweight and obesity can be attributed to such elements as food "addictions", your genotype, stress, shift work, consumption of sodas/soft drinks, eating processed foods, lack of sleep, too much fatty, sugary fast food, poor nutrition, rarely experiencing satiation or satiety, eating while watching TV, over-indulgence in alcohol, or the community of microbiota that inhabits your gut.

If you fix only one or two of these causes by say, cutting out all carbohydrates or just avoiding sugar, you could be setting yourself up for failure in the long term. Eating and weight loss are complex matters; too complex to be addressed by simply banning whole food groups or cutting down food portions.

Some examples of relatively simplistic approaches to weight loss include:
- Avoiding carbohydrates
- Counting Calories
- Eating only salads or soups
- Intermittent fasting
- Limiting portion sizes

These regimes, which focus primarily on one weight-loss technique, overlook the large number of factors contributing to overweight and obesity. They fail to cater for the fact that the human body is intricately complex, and so is the process of eating.

There is not one single reason why people don't stick to diets. There are many causes of obesity, and so we need multiple ways to address it.

There's more to digestion and weight control that simply adding or subtracting Calories. An intricate, elaborate interaction of chemicals in your body is what manipulates how much food you eat, and how much you want to eat. Hormonal messages are generated in your fat cells, gut and pancreas, and your thoughts and emotions modify these messages. It takes more than just willpower and counting Calories to ensure that your daily food intake enables you to achieve both good health and your ideal body weight.

The Satiety Diet helps you regulate your appetite by informing you about the messages your body receives, both internally and externally, regarding hunger and satiety.

Many keys to the lock.

Imagine that the treasure chest containing your healthy weight is currently closed and locked. Its lid is not held down by one single padlock; it is securely fastened by numerous locks, chains, padlocks, latches, rivets, screws, nails, ropes, wire and other means of preventing you from opening it.

Someone hands you a key. That key may be a fad diet, or advice about avoiding certain foods, or encouragement to exercise more, or a subscription to some food-delivery service that promises weight loss. You use the key and it opens one of the locks.

All the other locks, chains etc. remain intact.

The lid, therefore, remains shut. Long-term, permanent weight loss remains inaccessible.

The path to healthy, lasting weight loss can't be accessed by way of one method alone. One key is not enough. The Satiety Diet gives you a vast, jingling bundle of keys and wire-cutters and combination-codes and saws and metal-cutters, so that you have everything you need to break open that treasure chest and achieve your healthy weight.

While satiety is the most important key to weight loss, other factors are at play. As one researcher said, "Overall, it is clear that, although the processes of satiation and satiety have the potential to control energy intake, many individuals override the signals generated. Hence, in such people, satiation and satiety alone are not sufficient to prevent weight gain in the current obesogenic environment.

"Knowledge about foods, ingredients and dietary patterns that can enhance satiation and satiety is potentially useful for controlling bodyweight.

"This, however, must be coupled with an understanding of the myriad of other factors that influence eating behavior, in order to help people to control their energy intake." [Benelam (2009)]

THE "FATTEST COUNTRIES"

In 2007 Forbes Magazine published a list of the world's fattest and leanest populations. The "fattest countries" have this in common; the staple diet includes large amounts of cooked or canned meat, fast foods and other highly processed salty, sugary, fatty foods with low nutritional value.

AVOIDING APPETITE TRIGGERS

Pictures of food can act as appetite triggers. For this reason, the authors of this book have kept food images to a minimum—in fact, there is only one black-and-white picture of food in these pages, and it's drawn in a stylized manner so as not to look too realistic.

The Satiety Diet's 3-point approach to weight loss is all about:

Food: Nutrition, colors, portion sizes, textures etc.

Mind: Your mindset, mind tricks, meditation etc.

Movement: Exercises you love, incidental exercise etc.

PART ONE

YOUR INNER GUARDIAN & APPETITE

YOUR INNER GUARDIAN

Every body has an Inner Guardian.

You have one.

Inner Guardians exist in every normal, healthy animal, including human beings.

Your Inner Guardian can be thought of as a silent, invisible force inside your body, or your "internal hard-wiring". You're born with it, and one of its primary jobs is to ensure that you go on living.

Of course the Inner Guardian is not an actual entity. It doesn't really have a mind of its own. It doesn't make its own decisions and act like an individual, conscious being, but for the purposes of discussion we are treating it as if it does.

Your Inner Guardian might be described as your operating manual, or your guide to survival.

Your Inner Guardian's purpose is to keep you alive.

But why?

Not because you are intrinsically valuable as an individual, but because you are a member of the human race, and the Guardian's ultimate purpose is to keep our species existing in perpetuity.

Your Inner Guardian's aim is to gauge how useful you are to the tribe/clan/population and, depending on this, to extend or curtail your life accordingly.

Preserving the human race vs. the individual.

For your Inner Guardian, ensuring your survival as an individual is second in importance only to ensuring the survival of the human race.

Associated with the fundamental need for each human being to stay alive is a wider story-arc; the need for each person to contribute to the welfare of the human tribe.

Inner Guardians are installed in us before birth, while we're still in the womb. They take part in a story that is greater than simply self-preservation. More than that—they exist to ensure that each of us is

16

able to contribute to the welfare of our family, to our tribe, and thus to the human species.

The task of your body's Inner Guardian is to preserve your life, until such time as it receives the signals that tell it to commence winding down and preparing for death. Your Inner Guardian, while primarily concerned with keeping you vital and breathing, is also able to abandon that task under certain circumstances. Those circumstances may include:

- The internal lifespan clock, indicating that it's time to wind down when you get old.
- Signals gauged from your lifestyle, by which the Guardian may deduce that you are no longer needed by your tribe.

Your Inner Guardian protects your Tribe.

Why does the Inner Guardian care about your tribe?

Our Guardians evolved long ago, in prehistoric times. They remain attuned to a prehistoric, tribal way of living, and have not adapted to the 21st century. Every individual human being is part of a genetic or social family or tribe, and tribes are what comprise the human species. Human beings cannot survive alone. We are social animals.

Complex physiological survival mechanisms evolved in our ancestors a few million years ago. Under their influence, the species homo sapiens sapiens flourished. For 99% of the time human beings have walked this planet, it's been "humans versus the environment", and Inner Guardians have been our protection.

So the Inner Guardian is not only an analogy for the individual body's inbuilt survival mechanisms, it is also a driving force that works for the good of the species.

That's why, when the chips are down, your own Inner Guardian will work to preserve the human race, rather than you, the individual. If your Inner Guardian thinks you're not useful to your tribe (and therefore to humans as a species), it may cease keeping you healthy. It's on your side as long as it thinks there's a chance you are making a useful contribution to the continuation of humankind.

17

Inner Guardians are ancient systems.

In developed nations where obesity is a problem, all the requirements for staying alive are easily accessible. Calorie-dense food is abundant and people's bodies don't need to store extra fat.

The primeval Inner Guardian, however, evolved in a very different environment—the harsher world of our hunter-gatherer ancestors. Inner Guardians have barely altered since then. They haven't kept pace with the rapidly changing technology that can deliver Calorie-dense food at the touch of a button. They're not configured to "understand" this new situation. That's why they keep insisting that we eat more high-energy foods, even when we are overweight.

Many people think of dieting as an extreme, inflexible way of eating. This kind of diet carries a high risk of rebound weight gain after the dieter abandons the regime and returns to "normal" eating.

Weight loss is much more successful and sustainable, in the long term, if people make gradual changes.

The power of the Inner Guardian.

Your Inner Guardian is supremely powerful. It drives the biochemicals in your body, making its demands very difficult for willpower to defeat. You may resist that chocolate cream pie, but you might pay the price by feeling deprived, becoming obsessed with the thought of what you missed, and possibly even food-bingeing later on, to compensate.

For most people, the Inner Guardian is strong enough to triumph over potent directives issued by the conscious mind. Very few people can hold out against its demands in the long term.

These drives are incredibly potent. Few measures can stop them. Possibly drugs, illness (mental or physical), or hypnotherapy may do so, or extremely dedicated meditation, a form of self-hypnosis. People who try to fight them may end up with obesity, anorexia, bulimia or other eating disorders.

How much easier it is to lose weight when you know how to use body-speech to communicate with that powerful internal force! We'll discuss more about body-speech later.

The reason your Inner Guardian strives to be stronger than your mind is because your mind may become disabled, partially disabled or misled. Your mind's thoughts are what determines your actions and behaviors, and therefore what you eat and drink, and whether you put yourself at risk or seek shelter from a storm. Your thoughts, therefore, can exert a powerful influence on whether or not you survive. At worst, the human mind can even become infused with notions which can lead to suicide.

Your conscious mind has little chance of winning in a battle against your Inner Guardian. "I must not eat cake because I will get fat" means nothing to the Guardian, who steamrolls such thoughts with the command, EAT CAKE.

So you end up in a painful struggle. "Want it," says Guardian. "Eat it!"

"Don't eat it", says your conscious mind.

"WANT IT," says your Inner Guardian. "EAT IT!"

"Don't eat…"

"WANT IT. EAT IT. NOW!"

More than just survival.

The Inner Guardian is concerned with both life and death.

Your body is programmed to stay alive, but it is also programmed to die if certain signals tell your Inner Guardian that, for whatever reason, it's time. Our Inner Guardians have more control over death than we realize. Without delving too deeply into this topic, it's worth mentioning that:

- People can perish from "self-willed death," or "bone-pointing syndrome", engendered by ostracization from a social group.
- There is an indisputable relationship between loneliness and early death. Yet loneliness is a state of mind, not a physical illness.

- Statistically significant numbers of people die on, or close to, a day that is significant in their lives, such as their birthday, a religious festival or some other biographical event. [Phillips et al. (1992)]

How can the physiological workings of your body "know" what the date is? Or what the significance of that date is? How can the inner chemistry of your body "know" if people in your social group have shunned you?

It happens by means of a powerful language we can call "body-speech"—an interplay of environmental inputs, biochemicals and the electro-chemical reactions we call thoughts.

Inner Guardians and fat stores.

Your Inner Guardian does its utmost to preserve your fat stores, which contain most of the energy (Calories) your body needs to move and function. Its prime motive is to defend your life for as long as it thinks you are helping the tribe to survive.

Your Inner Guardian stores fat in your cells as a survival insurance policy in case something energy-draining happens in the future, such as famine, or pregnancy, or arduous work.

It knows exactly how much energy you have stored in your body in the form of fat, and deduces from that whether you must be living either in a land of plenty, or a land of scarcity and famine. You might be surrounded by shelves groaning under the weight of baked goods every day of your life, but if you eat nothing but a lettuce leaf a day, your Inner Guardian will register a world of famine.

This is how it reads the evidence of the body.

And this is an example of body-speech.

Because the Inner Guardian protects the body's fat stores, fat is extraordinarily difficult to shed. [Brown (1991)]

Your Inner Guardian "remembers" how much fat has been stored in your body at any given moment, over the history of your lifetime. It remembers unfailingly, forgetting nothing. It preserves memories of old famines (i.e. long-term, severely Calorie-restricted diets) from your past. And it reasons that if there has been a famine once, then it

20

can happen again. It becomes vigilant, ready to act at the first sign of famine and lock down your fat stores.

Famine is "bad" in the opinion of your Inner Guardian. Its duty is to protect you against energy loss, using powerful measures. It wants to protect your body's fat stores so that you have sufficient energy to allow you to find food for yourself and for your tribe or, in the case of young women, to form a baby in the womb and make milk to nourish new offspring.[2]

Women in particular are predisposed to store fat. Throughout human evolution, "Females with greater energy reserves in fat would have a selective advantage over their lean counterparts in terms of withstanding the stress of food shortage, not only for themselves but for their fetuses or nursing children as well. Humans have evolved the ability to 'save up' food energy for inevitable food shortages through the synthesis and storage of fat." [Huss-Ashmore (1980)]

When you begin a new diet and severely deprive yourself of Calories you are telling your Inner Guardian that food is scarce. It doesn't matter if you can see food all around you; it doesn't matter that in your conscious mind you know you can get food at any time because the fridge is full, the shops are well stocked and you have some money in your pocket. If you feel hungry for a prolonged period of time (more than a few days) you are signaling to your body in that silent language of "body-speech" that *food is scarce*. Your Inner Guardian receives this information and takes measures to protect you. It is trying to be your friend. It wants you to live.

This is why, when you embark on a weight-loss diet for the first time, or even after a long period of not dieting, you will be most successful. The all-powerful "save the fat" imperative hasn't yet kicked in.

As soon as it kicks in, you may start wanting to eat even when you're not really hungry.

---

2   In cases of extreme Calorie restriction, the Inner Guardian switches off ovulation to protect women against the energy-drain of child-bearing.

If you've dieted in the past, your Inner Guardian may compel you to store up fat for the future, by driving you to seek the most Calorie-dense foods, loaded with fat and sugar.

If you are too hungry for too long (we're talking days, not hours), "starvation mode" sets in and your Inner Guardian takes a firmer hold on your energy stores. It begins to conserve energy, so that you feel weak and tired. It may boost hunger signals, so that you develop cravings.

Experts disagree on how many days of starvation it takes for your metabolism to start slowing down, but it does happen eventually.

A slow metabolism is your body's way of latching onto your energy (fat) stores to protect you from the perceived famine. As your metabolism slows, lethargy sets in and you expend less energy.

Your Inner Guardian's primitive drives are stronger than your conscious mind. In healthy people, hunger and cravings nearly always win any battle with willpower.

It's not only about protecting fat stores

Weight loss is about more than just working with the Inner Guardian's famine-fighting prowess.

We have discussed the way normal, healthy human bodies are genetically programmed to store fat, in case of famine. Your body's Inner Guardian is stronger than conscious thought. It makes you prefer high-energy foods, and if it receives signals that appear to threaten starvation, it takes steps to hang on to fat stores.

Many people cannot hold out against these natural survival drives for long enough to lose significant amounts of fat. And if they do, those drives often cause rebound weight gain after the diet has finished.

There is, however, more to the story than that. Recent scientific research suggests that our primeval famine-proofing DNA is not the only factor contributing to the obesity epidemic. [Beil (2014)]

"The remarkable failure of diet therapies has made some researchers rethink their commonsensical theory of obesity as being caused by overeating; the clinical evidence of the past 40 years simply does not support this simplistic notion." [Bennett (1987)]

Such procedures as metabolism, digestion, assimilation, appetite, cravings and satiety involve a wide variety of subtle and not so subtle interactions between a wide range of factors such as the formulation of the food itself, its sensory attributes, the dining environment, the time of day, the hormones and other biochemicals produced by our bodies, and even our mental processes.

The Satiety Diet is the multi-faceted approach that takes into account these other factors that are vital for successful weight loss.

Body-speech.

Healthy young children are tuned in to their bodies. They know when they are really hungry, they know which foods will fulfil their nutritional needs, and they know when they've had enough to eat. They understood their own body-speech.

"Body-speech" is a useful concept. It can help you understand and implement the multi-faceted approach to weight loss. Body-speech is a language that is neither spoken, written nor coded in hand-signs. It is the language of biochemical signals, and it affects you profoundly, on conscious and subconscious levels. It is the code of survival used by your invisible Inner Guardian to communicate and interact with you and the processes/systems inside your body, as well as with the environment outside your body.

Deep down, so deep that you may not even be aware of it, your body is programmed to learn, through "body-speech" cues, how useful you are to the human species. For millennia, our bodies have communicated with our changing environment using this silent, prehistoric language that has kept the human race going. This language is intended to help us survive as hunters and gatherers. Your body's internal language is subtler, yet way more powerful than spoken language or body language.

Body-speech vs. languages of the conscious mind.

Body-speech is your body's own inherent, native language, as distinct from the languages used by the conscious mind. It is a system of communication that's common to all living creatures, for it was not invented by human beings.

The conscious mind can communicate through:

- your "mother tongue",
- whatever other spoken languages you've learned,
- body language (e.g. gestures and facial expressions),
- the language of your conscious thoughts,
- sign language.

There is a significant difference between body-speech and those languages of the conscious mind.

For example, you might think, "My body has excess fat stores, which I want to lose. I have just eaten a healthful garden salad, and my body has received all the nutrients I need. I really want to eat fewer Calories, and lose weight. Therefore, logically, I will have no desire to eat that slice of chocolate cream pie for dessert."

Those are statements made by the conscious mind. The Inner Guardian cannot hear such statements, because they are not made in body-speech. The Inner Guardian is deaf to all that. It perceives the pie as a desirable energy source and sends out hormonal hunger signals that are almost impossible for willpower to override. Which is why the pie ends up being eaten in spite of all the logical reasons why it shouldn't.

You may try to tell yourself to avoid high Calorie foods, or to eat less food, by consciously using willpower.

You could say aloud to your body, "Body, there is no need for you to store fat. I am surrounded by plentiful food at all times. You do not need to carry energy reserves."

You could stand in front of a mirror and tell this to your reflection. You could record it as an audio file and replay it repeatedly to yourself through headphones.

This can do no harm (and in fact it might help a little!).

But no matter whether you speak to your body in Abaza, Chinese, English, Zuri'retan or any other code, you are still speaking to your body in a language that's not its native tongue; a language that the ancient, primeval Inner Guardian cannot properly understand.

Your Inner Guardian cannot hear your commands if you are not using body-speech.

Body-speech vs body language.

It is important to distinguish between "body-speech" and "body language".

Body language is a separate kind of non-verbal communication system. It is generally used to convey feelings, intentions, thoughts and attitudes. People and other animals use it for communication between each other and between species. It comprises conscious and unconscious physical behaviors, such as:

- facial expressions
- body posture
- gestures
- eye movement
- touch
- movement through space.

Body language refers to such gestures as crossing ones arms, or shaking ones head to signal negativity, or jumping for joy, or smiling to signify happiness.

Body-speech, on the other hand, is not used to convey meaning between individual entities.

Body-speech refers to the way each Inner Guardian communicates with its environment and with the body's own internal processes. It is a language that's not made up of sounds. It's not even made up of hand signs or gestures.

Its an ancient system that predates the spoken word; a language of hormones and chemicals, of pain and pleasure, of mental images and sensory experiences, and more.

25

Mental imagery.

You can translate words into body-speech via mental imagery.

We've said that body-speech isn't a spoken language and that's true. However, verbal cues can be translated into body-speech.

There are some instances in which your Inner Guardian responds indirectly to spoken or written words. This is because your brain acts as an interpreter, decoding those words into images/feelings which can be understood in body-speech.

Take for example the words "hungry" and "hunger". When you read or hear these words, your brain interprets them and your Inner Guardian, in response, may actually arouse your appetite. Food advertisers know this—for example the companies who create the ads for Snickers®[3] and Hungry Jack's®.

Many people, on hearing the word "chocolate", begin longing for chocolate, the food. Words like "creamy", "silky", "crunchy", "crispy" and "nutty" can make the foods listed on a menu seem more appetizing. [Preston (2014)]

Body-speech responds to sensory inputs.

Your body's internal dialogue also responds to sensory inputs from everything you eat, smell, think, feel, see, hear and touch. What you see with your eyes is one type of sensory input. The sounds of spoken language that enter your ears are sensory input too. Your mind decodes this input, translating it into mental imagery or emotional states.

In response, silent signals flash up and down internal pathways of your body, such as your nervous system and circulatory system. For example, your body might respond to a sweet taste in your mouth by delivering a shot of insulin into your bloodstream. It might send signals to your salivary glands in response to your mental pictures when you imagine eating a lemon.

Your whole body-speech signaling system is supervised your Inner Guardian.

---

3   Slogan: "You're not you when you're hungry."®

This is how body-speech works on appetite:

- Things happen (input) such as social interactions, the sight of food, thoughts of food, words that conjure food-related images in the brain, certain smells, familiar routines, an emotion which may or may not even be related to food, (such as love or fear), stressful situations, vigorous movement, lack of movement, stress and so on.
- The input triggers the body's release of chemicals and hormones, electrical impulses and other substances, and physiological events.
- The Inner Guardian translates/decodes these physiological messages. (It does not necessarily do this accurately. For example, sometimes thirst is mistaken for hunger.)
- The Guardian reacts by sending out commands which, in most cases, drive the body's owner to obtain food and eat it.

This is the way the Inner Guardian reads and interprets the environment—not through conscious thoughts and reasoning, and not necessarily by direct observation with the eyes and ears, but by what movements the body makes, what it feeds itself, what images and feelings are formed by the brain, what hormones and chemicals are stimulated by events and emotions.

Learning to understand and speak body-speech, your body's own essential language, can help you to live well.

Losing touch with your body-speech

You're born with an innate ability to understand body-speech, but external influences can make you lose your sensitivity to it. Why do so many of us lose touch with this important, innate knowledge as we grow up? There could be several reasons, such as:

- Your parents/caregivers might have believed it was their responsibility to cram as much food into you as possible, possibly resorting to cajoling, bribery or even punishment.
- You may not have been offered a wide range of fresh, nutrient-dense foods to choose from.

27

- You might have been taught that sweet foods such as candy and desserts are "treats" or "rewards", which makes Calorie-dense, fatty, sugary foods seem more desirable.
- You were probably subjected to a barrage of junk food advertising on billboards, radio and TV.
- You were probably exposed to the brightly colored, alluring pictures on the wrappers of junk foods.
- You might have learned to eat when you're not hungry, because it's officially "meal-time" or because it's a habit.
- You might have started eating "junk" food because of peer pressure.
- Dieting can interfere with your body-speech feedback mechanisms.

All of these messages, and more, can subvert your body's natural instincts. By the time you became an adult you may have completely lost touch with them, and forgotten how to listen to your body.

Getting back in touch with your body-speech

To counteract this:

- Become aware of your own natural biorhythms, your "body-clock".
- Become aware of what makes you want food—your blood sugar levels, your emotions, seeing or smelling food, your food habits, whether you eat according to your appetite's demands, or according to triggers of time and place.
- Don't eat when you don't really want to eat, just because it's breakfast time or lunchtime or dinnertime, or someone offers food.
- Don't allow your real hunger become desperate ravenousness. Always have next meal planned and ready to be accessed quickly and easily. Keep emergency Satiety Diet snacks on hand.
- Be aware of all the food you eat. Concentrate on it and make eating a special occasion. Never, for example, eat while walking around, reading or watching a movie!

The Inner Guardian measures your tribal usefulness.

Social connection is vitally important to human beings. In order to survive, we need to live and work in groups. All by ourselves, we are comparatively weak and slow. We cannot run as fast as many other land-animals, our sense of smell is minimal and we lack the physical strength of other predators. It is our cooperation in groups that gives us an advantage.

What your Inner Guardian wants to know is,
- How well is your tribe thriving, and
- How important to it are you?

If your tribe is doing well and you're actively involved in that success, this reflects on you, and your Inner Guardian sees benefit in helping you to stay healthy. When you are an essential part of a thriving tribe—working hard, reproducing, being good at social interaction—then you are important to that wider group of tribes called the human species.

Tell your body you're useful to your tribe.

Your Inner Guardian wants what is best for you—or rather, for your species. It wants you to be a lean, mean, fighting machine who can contribute to the continuation of the human species. If you use body-speech to tell your Inner Guardian you're not useful to your species any more, your Inner Guardian will cease to look after you properly. For example, by sitting down and not moving, you could be telling your I.G. that your tribe is getting along fine without your input. The tribe does not need your hunting or gathering or child-minding or weaving skills. It follows that you must be redundant. You might even be a liability to the tribe. As you exercise less and store up excess fat, the Inner Guardian ceases to be so vigilant on your behalf, and you risk developing degenerative diseases, arthritis, cancers etc.

Body-speech inputs and longevity.

Through body-speech inputs, your Inner Guardian learns many things about you and about how useful you are to the tribe. It can, for example, find out whether you are sociable, or physically active, or mentally agile. It could be argued that your Inner Guardian "deduces" your levels of sociability and activity and intellectual resourcefulness to discover whether you are worthy of living longer.

All healthy human bodies receive many forms of body-speech input. These inputs—which involve nuanced and complicated interplays of hormones, other biochemicals, electro-chemical reactions etc.—can signify conditions such as:

* Whether you have someone to care for and nurture (oxytocin)
* Happiness levels (serotonin)
* Whether you are married or in a long term, reasonably satisfactory relationship (serotonin and oxytocin)
* How much sleep you get (melatonin)
* How much stress you are subjected to, and how we deal with it (cortisol)
* How much food you get and when (insulin, ghrelin etc.)

Longevity (long life) is associated with such factors as:
* Having plenty of social connections [Holt-Lunstad et al. (2010), TED (2017)]
* Being married or in a stable de facto relationship [Lillard & Panis (1996), McDonald (2008)]
* Having children [Doheny,(2012), Modig et al. (2017)]
* Nurturing and loving a companion dog [BVA (2007), Motooka (2006), BBC News (2007), DeNoon (2013)][4]
* Being physically active [Reimers et al. (2012)]
* Using your brain to learn new things. [Lager & Torssander (2012)]

---

4   Note that people who don't really care about their pets don't get any health benefit. It's the caring that stimulates oxytocin and other beneficial body-speech signals.

The primeval Inner Guardian interprets these inputs as meaning that people are deeply connected with their tribe and working for its benefit.

If you have companionship, respect and esteem, this input "tells" your body that you must be needed by the tribe. When women have given birth, their bodies "know" that they need to stay around to care for their progeny. Women who give birth later in life are likely to live longer. Their Inner Guardians give them more time to bring up their children.

If you don't appear to be useful to the tribe, your Inner Guardian doesn't see much point in keeping you around for a long time. In fact, you might be a drain on the tribe's resources.

Furthermore, when you're part of a tribe that is doing badly, your Guardian "thinks" that some of the fault must be yours, because you are responsible for the tribe's functioning, just like every other member. Again—your Inner Guardian suspects you may not deserve help.

It could be argued that when people become ill due to lifestyle choices such as over-eating or under-exercising, they have, in a sense, failed to convince their Inner Guardian that they play an essential role in the welfare of the tribe, and thus in the perpetuation of the human race.

Numerous body speech inputs are linked not only with longevity, but also with appetite regulation. Many inputs that contribute to a longer life can also have an effect on appetite and body-weight. This is why it's useful to learn about them.

In no particular order, here are some broad illustrations of body-speech inputs.

Physical activity.

For most of us, slothfulness comes naturally—particularly as we age. Over time, people develop a tendency to conserve body energy rather than expend it. Those who stay fit generally live longer than those who do not. Let's look at this in the context of the Inner Guardian.

31

The biochemicals that are released throughout your body when you move tell your Inner Guardian how intensely you are exercising and kind of exercise it is—whether resistance training, weight lifting, walking, aerobic exercise and so on.

In the view of the Inner Guardian, if you are regularly active when young, you are probably healthy and fit. You are therefore worthy of preservation so that you can procreate, and work for the tribe.

If you're regularly active when older, your Inner Guardian deduces that you're sufficiently motivated (probably by your desire to nurture and protect the tribe) to deny your natural inclination to sit around conserving energy, and instead go and make yourself useful by food-foraging, fuel-gathering, child-minding etc.

At any age, regular exercise indicates that you could be either running away from danger or helping to fight it off. And that means the tribe probably needs you.

Your Inner Guardian achieves this extension of life by many mechanisms, such as giving you improved blood flow and heart health, increased muscle tone and bone strength etc. By way of these gifts, the Inner Guardian bestows a better chance of living longer. The end result is that in general, regular exercise leads to better health and a longer life.

Relaxation.

If your Inner Guardian learns that you have leisure to relax and a safe environment in which do do it, it deduces that you and the tribe must be enjoying a season of plenty and living in a well-guarded, secure place. After all, you can only relax if you are not required to always be looking for food. When there is plenty of food available, you can feel calm and serene. You can sit back and take it easy for a while. A secure, bounteous environment spells success for the tribe. In such conditions the tribe can thrive and multiply. When you spend some time chilling out (but not too much time), you are signaling to your Inner Guardian via body-speech that you and your tribe are thriving. Conversely if you spend all your time relaxing, you are signaling that you are not needed by the tribe; you are superfluous. Balance between exercise and relaxation is the key.

Mental agility.

Using your brain to solve problems, learn new skills and adapt to new scenarios tells your Inner Guardian that you are good for the tribe; you are helping it function in an ever-changing world that is always throwing up new challenges. You might be useful at inventing new tools, for example, or figuring out a new way to cross a river, or how to heal the sick.

Keep your mind active by learning new things as often as possible. Research published in the *British Medical Journal* shows that learning new things challenges the brain and keeps cognitive function from declining. In turn, this promotes a longer, healthier life.

Familiar faces.

If the people around you are largely unfamiliar to you, it signifies in body-speech that you may not be good at long-term relationships. In turn this can indicate that you may not be a useful member of the tribe. Alternatively, it might mean that you have become separated from your tribe.

Such separation could be because you have been cast out, or because the tribe has been wiped out. Either way, in the language of your Inner Guardian, your measure of worthiness to live decreases.

In traditional tribal societies, young women may leave the social group of their childhood when they marry, and join their husband's group. However this is only likely to happen once in their lives, and the people of husband's tribe would not be entirely unfamiliar to them. Stable partnerships and friendships contribute to longevity.

Love and friendship.

Being frequently in touch with people you care for, and who care about you, signifies to your Inner Guardian that you must be making a helpful contribution to the tribe in some way. Note that your contribution does not have to be a physical one. A good storyteller, for example, or a joker who can make everyone laugh— these are valuable tribe members. Body-speech inputs inform your Inner Guardian whether you are loved and liked and socially supported. Having an active social life shows that you are good for the tribe; you are helping it function.

As mentioned earlier, affection stimulates the release of oxytocin. When you hug a person you like or love, your body releases oxytocin, a biochemical sometimes called "the love hormone". Oxytocin has a dampening effect on the "stress hormone" cortisol, which is associated with increased appetite, high blood pressure and heart disease. [McQuaid et al., (2016)]

Marital status.

Your Inner Guardian knows whether you are married (or in a stable de facto relationship), and this is not all about sex. Various other body-speech clues communicate your "primary personal relationship" to your body. Perhaps you are getting regular home cooked meals. Perhaps you are getting lots of hugs, or maybe you have a confidante to whom you can unload your worries. Married men live longer than unmarried men. This makes sense in terms of body-speech—if a man is are married, he is more likely to be needed by the tribe to support a wife and children.

Fertility and child-rearing.

If you have borne or raised children you are a useful member of your tribe, because you are helping to perpetuate it.

Your status as a parent is another type of body-speech input. This is most obviously true for women, whose body chemistry undergoes massive changes during pregnancy. By way of hormonal and neuronal changes, however, men's Inner Guardians can usually be informed whether men are fathers. [Gholipour (2014)]

Inner Guardians "want" to prolong the lives of parents. Parents, who generally have a huge emotional investment in their offspring, are needed to bring up the tribe's next generation.

For women, the risk of breast cancer declines with the number of children borne. Mothers are more valuable to the tribe. They have proved their fertility and they need to stay around to care for their children.

In body-speech, breastfeeding signals that a woman's baby (or an adopted baby) is surviving, and therefore the breastfeeding mother is useful to the continuation of the tribe.

Body-speech input includes the oxytocin that flows through a parent. The Inner Guardian has no language for cans of factory-produced infant formula, but even if a mother is bottle feeding, the Inner Guardian learns about this nurturing act from the oxytocin that the mother's body releases when she holds and feeds her child.

"Many parents might good-naturedly scoff at the notion, but a new study shows that being a parent may help you live longer. Danish researchers compared men and women who had children with those who did not to see if the childless were more likely to die early. They were." [Doheny (2012)]

"Childless couples are at increased risk of dying early of all causes," says researcher Esben Agerbo, PhD, associate professor at Aarhus University in Aarhus, Denmark. Professor Agerbo notes that the benefit of parenthood on longevity was stronger for women than for men. The study findings echo those of previous research. It is published in the *Journal of Epidemiology and Community Health*.

For the rest of her life, a woman's Inner Guardian remembers whether she has had children. It remembers whether she breastfed them and for how long. Her body is also imprinted with all the details of her menstrual cycle. Through oxytocin levels, the Inner Guardian learns the depth of her attachment to her children or, in fact, to anyone else's children; maternal love is not limited by blood-ties. Deep, personal attachments to the younger generation are signals that indicate usefulness to the tribe and its continuation.

"Historically, women have lived longer than men in almost every country in the world. . . Women do not live longer than men because they age more slowly, but because they are more robust at every age." [Austad (2006)]. In terms of body-speech and the Inner Guardian, the theory is that as hunters get older they get slower and less able to bring in food. For the tribe, child-rearing is easier and more efficient when older women are available to help care for the young ones. Older men, on the other hand, may not still be fit to actively hunt.

Having sex.

Having sex more often is associated with healthier, longer life. [Persson (1981)]. Your Inner Guardian would interpret frequent sex as meaning:

- You have companionship, which indicates that you are accepted by the tribe
- You must be reasonably fit, which means you are useful to the tribe
- You probably have fairly good social skills
- You might be quite physically attractive, or at least acceptable, which infers that you possess desirable genes, to be passed on to a new generation.

Emotions.

Your emotions, such as happiness and sadness, inform your Inner Guardian. Laughter, for example, is a body-speech input. It has been shown to lower cortisol levels, burn Calories, enhance memory and protect against heart disease. If you're laughing, things must be going well for you and the tribe. Laughter tells your Inner Guardian that you are relaxed and happy, and that your current situation is beneficial to the survival of both you and your tribe.

Stress.

Stress is another part of the body-speech vocabulary. Incoming signals from the body's environment (such as extreme heat, continuous loud noises, physical pain), or even just thoughts in your head, can cause anxiety.

Your Inner Guardian assumes that if you're generally in a positive frame of mind then it's likely that either—

- Things are going well for you, in which case things are likely to be going well for the people around you. This indicates you are a cog in a successful tribal machine. Or—
- Things are going badly for you but you are coping well, which in turn is helpful and supportive for the people around you.

Everyone experiences stressful situations at times. It's how we react to that stress that's important. It has been shown that "… it is our reactions to our stressful situations that can predict health problems later in our lives, regardless of present health and the stressors themselves." [NYR (2013)]

Cortisol is the primary stress hormone. Elevated cortisol levels can:
- Interfere with learning and memory,
- Lower immune function and bone density,
- Contribute to increased weight gain, blood pressure, cholesterol and susceptibility to heart disease.

Chronic stress and elevated cortisol levels are linked with increased risk for depression, mental illness, lowered resilience and decreased life expectancy.

The Inner Guardian interprets prolonged stress as a signal that you can't get away from the adverse conditions causing the stress. It reasons that surely you would escape from it if you could! Your Guardian can deal more easily with transient stress—a passing scare from a mountain lion, or perhaps a loud electrical storm or a heated argument with a ferocious member of the tribe. But ongoing stress indicates that you are in a dangerous place and not escaping from it. Your current environment, it assumes, is a bad place to procreate; a bad place to try to survive. This may signal to your Inner Guardian, "this body has a limited future". Alternatively, if you're feeling stressed for no good reason, you're probably not much use to the tribe.

You can remove yourself from stressful situations either physically or mentally. If you cannot physically escape from stress, use such methods as meditation or calming self-talk, or distractions, or counseling, to help you deal with it.

Sleep.

Poor sleep can lead to adverse health effects including obesity, diabetes, decreased immune function, cardiovascular disease and hypertension. " . . . insufficient sleep can ultimately affect life expectancy and day-to-day well-being." [Harvard (2008)]

Several studies have linked insufficient sleep and weight gain. For example, one study found that people who slept fewer than six hours per night on a regular basis were much more likely to have excess body weight, while people who slept an average of eight hours per night had the lowest relative body fat of the study group. [Kohatsu et al. (2006)]

Another study found that babies who are "short sleepers" are much more likely to develop obesity later in childhood than those who sleep the recommended amount. [Taveras et al. (2008)]

Sleep problems can be due to such factors as physical ill-health, mental ill-health, stress and poor nutrition. Your Inner Guardian deduces that if you're not getting enough sleep, your mind or body— or both—are not fit and healthy. Or perhaps your tribe is not secure at nights; it does not have enough fit and alert sentinels posted on the lookout for danger in the darkness, or a safe sleeping-place. Lack of sleep could mean problems with you or your tribe. Perhaps that is why your Inner Guardian increases your appetite when you're getting insufficient sleep—it thinks you're going to need more energy to survive!

Generosity towards others.

When you are helping other people or animals, your stress levels subside and this can actually prolong life. [Poulin et al. (2012)] This is another example of the tribe's importance to body-speech input.

Eating a wide variety of foods.

Consuming a range of different foods is another kind of body-speech input. Physiologically speaking, the consumption of a large variety of foods provides a wide range of macronutrients and micronutrients.

When you eat diverse foods (and get plenty of exercise[5]), your Inner Guardian reads the influx of nutrients and hormones as a signal that you or your social group are fit, strong and competent enough to exploit large parts of the countryside.

Different food plants and food animals inhabit different environmental niches and micro-climates. For example if you always ate only one type of tuber and two types of leaves, this would indicate that you have access to only a limited patch of ground. Only a bunch of fit, healthy humans would have the energy to range widely, so food variety indicates that you and your tribe must be thriving and living in a beneficial environment. You, who are a cog in this successful machine, deserve to survive and live longer.

Feasting and fasting

Feasting indicates (in body-speech) that there is a wide variety of food available in plentiful supply, ergo the tribe is in a situation where it can thrive. Allowing yourself to experience hunger—though not ravenous hunger—between feasts indicates to your Inner Guardian that when you're not sitting down to a decent meal you are probably out looking for food or otherwise actively helping the tribe survive. In between meals you are so busy and active that you don't have time to sit around snacking.

When reacting to hunger, your Guardian also sharpens your senses, keeps you alert, tends to make you sleepless—because you need to be on the alert and awake to find food.

While hunger is desirable, chronic hunger and ravenousness are not. Lack of good sleep caused by chronic hunger can cause other health problems—including increased appetite!

Become hungry between meals, but when you do eat, eat well!

---

5   Exercise releases endorphins and other hormones throughout the body.

Satiety.

Satiety is the feeling of being full and satisfied between meals. It indicates to your Inner Guardian whether you have had "enough to eat". If you're always hungry—thus reasons your Inner Guardian—then food must be scarce. The Guardian interprets this and acts upon it, locking down your fat stores.

Signals of a successful member of a successful tribe

If your Inner Guardian is receiving signals that your tribe's environment abounds with easily-obtained energy-dense foods (you're eating lots of sugar and fat) and that there is no need for you to go hunting or gathering (you don't exercise much), it deduces that you're probably not necessary for the tribe's survival.

When you lead a sedentary life, your body-speech inputs tell your Inner Guardian that your tribe doesn't need you to move around and find food, or cook, or compete, or play games and sports, or look after children, or defend it from enemies, or do other things that are good for the community.

If you're just sitting around most of the time it "thinks" you are probably redundant, and might even be hampering the tribe. The diseases that spring from a sedentary lifestyle may now arise . . .

Oxytocin as a body-speech input

We've already mentioned oxytocin, the "love hormone". Here's another example of a body-speech input; when your mind forms an image of someone you love—such as a partner, a child, a pet—your body may release a burst of oxytocin. The mental image might be triggered by actually setting eyes on the loved one, or by speaking of them, or thinking of them. Either way, oxytocin begins to course through the blood, and this is a body-speech input.

The Inner Guardian interprets the presence of oxytocin as proof that:

• It's likely that you are useful to at least one other member of the community/tribe, because you care about them.

- You are capable of compassion and love and therefore (presumably) nurturing behavior. Again, this makes you useful to the tribe.

The presence of oxytocin in your body can cause your Guardian to think you're worthy of living longer. If your Inner Guardian "learns" from body-speech inputs that you care about lots of friends/family/social connections, it infers that you must be useful to your tribe. As a result, it uses its resources to increase your longevity.

In summary:

All these stimuli—exercise, stress, laughter, hunger, loneliness, companionship, maternity, paternity etc., trigger the release of complex hormones and other chemicals throughout your body and brain. Your Inner Guardian uses them to interpret what is happening in your body's surroundings.

We live in a world that has changed drastically in the last few centuries. Our body's ancient hard-wiring and primeval language evolved to protect us. In the modern world, however, it can do the opposite. It can sabotage our efforts at weight loss.

The Inner Guardian ensured the survival of our ancestors throughout thousands of years and thousands of human generations. Has it now turned against us? Are its efforts to guard us killing us instead?

Fortunately, if you understand what is going on with body-speech, you can make your Inner Guardian your ally once more.

How to communicate with your body.
Work with your Inner Guardian, not against it.

For most healthy people, their Inner Guardian's drive to ensure their survival is an overwhelming imperative. Your Inner Guardian exists solely for the purpose of preserving *you* (as long as you're useful to your tribe). It drives you to seek energy to consume, and it does its best to hang on to your existing stores of energy (body fat).

Many dieters who want to lose weight try to directly oppose and defeat these imperatives. This is a losing battle. Denying hunger usually leads to cravings and bingeing, and the vicious cycle begins again.

Your Inner Guardian is stuck in the past. It is hard-wired to help you survive in an ancient environment that has long since vanished; an environment that existed before the technological revolutions that made food so easy to come by. For millennia, this adaption has served humanity well. Now it's having the opposite effect. In the 21st century many of us are surrounded by *too much* food, too easily acquired, containing *too much* energy.

When you try to fight *against* your Inner Guardian's energy-seeking drives, you are likely to either:
• Lose the battle and gain weight
• Yo-yo diet, gaining and losing weight on the carousel of dieting
• Develop an eating disorder such as anorexia nervosa and/or bulimia, in which you battling obsessively and constantly to stay thin
• Die of starvation

So . . . what's the answer?

You cannot re-wire your Inner Guardian, but fortunately you *can* communicate with it, if you learn to speak its ancient, silent language, "body-speech".

By talking to it in its own language you can make it "know" that you are surrounded by ample food containing ample energy. And when it understands that, it can cease driving you with hunger and cravings to eat more, more, more, and pile on more and more weight.

42

You can actually use your Inner Guardian's motivations to your advantage, if you recognise them and work with them.

If instead of fighting against your Inner Guardian you work with it, cooperating with it, you're more likely to achieve your goal of weight loss. After all, your Guardian really does want what's best for you.

These are the messages you need to send to your Inner Guardian:

- There is no danger of famine, so it's okay for the Guardian to loosen its hold on your fat stores.
- Your body needs to utilise fat stores for activity, so your Guardian should free up that energy by burning the fat.

Signaling "no-famine".

Tell your Inner Guardian, "There is no famine" by reaching satiety at every meal.

Your Inner Guardian reads what's happening outside your body by the signals it receives through your senses and emotions. It can only know that there is no famine in the outside world if you give it the right messages.

In ancient days, if there was no famine, if food was abundant, then most people could eat whenever they felt hungry. People rarely felt ravenously hungry in times of food abundance, and if for some reason they did get to that point, there was enough food for them to feast on until they reached satiety. The opposite of feeling hungry is regular satiety.

Imagine: One of your nomadic, stone-age ancestors feels hungry in a season of abundance. There is plenty of food available, so he or she sits down with a tribal group (it makes sense, efficiency-wise, for food to be prepared in large batches), with a meal spread out in front of them. Everyone eats until their body's mechanisms signal satiety. Then they rest awhile (thus aiding digestion), before continuing their daily activities.

A few hours later, they feel hungry again. There is plenty of food at hand, so the tribe repeats the process for the next meal.

On the other hand, in times of famine, the people of the tribe would have constantly felt hungry. In order to survive they had to keep moving; travelling and seeking for food, eating a berry here, a nut there; catching small animals or fish, "grazing" where possible, but never filling up and reaching satiety.

Not just hunter-gatherers, but also ancient farmers who lived in settlements had to keep active—plowing and reaping, tending the land. And if there was not much food to go around, they too would have eaten small amounts at each meal, never quite reaching satiety.

Constant grazing on small amounts of food but never reaching satiety is one of the body-speech *famine signals*. The trick is to reach satiety *at every meal*, so that your Inner Guardian thinks there's no famine and therefore is willing to release fat stores.

It will, however, never be willing to release all your fat stores in one go! It is too prudent for that. To lose weight you must work with your Inner Guardian and accept the fact that that fat loss is a gradual process. The Guardian protects those energy stores vigilantly, and at the first sign that large amounts are being taken away, it clamps down, shuts the storehouse door and locks it.

The Inner Guardian is wary!

Remember that it is perfectly okay, and even essential, to feel hungry before each meal. Your Inner Guardian is not going to panic and think there's a famine if you're simply hungry. Mild hunger is normal and desirable. It's ravenous hunger that is is not so desirable when you want to lose weight.

Signaling "Release fat stores".

Tell your Inner Guardian, "You need to release stored energy" by being active.

To help convince the Guardian to let go of your stored energy reserves, *keep moving*. Here's the theory: In the ancient code of body-speech if you're moving and you're hungry, your Inner Guardian assumes that you are probably looking for food. Movement uses precious energy, and your Inner Guardian deduces that when you're hungry you are unlikely to be using up precious energy unless you are seeking for that vital resource, food. Therefore your Guardian will release a small amount of stored fat, allowing you to use energy in this good cause.

If body-speech signals tell your Inner Guardian that food is not plentiful, it will clamp down and protect your fat stores. It will still release energy but in smaller amounts; enough to keep your body functioning. Your metabolism will slow down. You will feel lethargic, and you may also feel cold. You will gain weight easily and find it hard to lose. Exercise is the perfect signal to your Inner Guardian that it needs to use up fat stores.

In summary: Speak to your Inner Guardian by sending it body-speech signals of both satiety and exercise.

It is important to use *both* these signals—satiety *and* exercise. If your Inner Guardian is getting the satiety message that that food is plentiful and you do *not* need to move to look for it (e.g. fruit simply drops into your outstretched hand without your having to budge!) then it deduces that there is no need to release stored energy reserves. On the contrary, it will "think" that the important thing is to make the body store more energy and get fatter, ready for the next famine!

Understand the way your body works.

Causes of "hunger" (i.e. triggers that make you want to eat) may include thirst, stress, lack of sleep, the sight of food, (either in reality or by way of media) reading about food, talking about food, the smell of food (we recommend having a separate, closed-off kitchen in your home!) negative emotions, your daily and monthly biorhythms, and so on.

Your Inner Guardian's drive to help you survive is what you are pitting yourself against when you diet. Because of this, right from the beginning of a weight-loss diet you are automatically at a disadvantage. On most diets, if you lose weight it's likely you will eventually gain it back—and possibly gain even more. Your Inner Guardian thinks there's been a famine and says, "I had better get hold of more fat stores in case that famine happens again".

45

In the long term, you cannot beat Mother Nature at her own game. Find out how she functions, and work with her—for she is *powerful*.

Identify your own patterns and work *with* them not against them, because if you work against your Inner Guardian you can never truly win. You may win temporarily, or you may win at huge cost, by ending up with an eating disorder.

Tell your body it doesn't need to hold on to fat.

To re-learn the language of body-speech, it helps to understand how it works. For example, when you sit down at a table and your eyes behold a set of assorted dinner plates all filled to the edges with colorful food, all intended for you to eat, your Inner Guardian tells you in body-speech, "There are plenty of nutritious, variously-colored foods within easy reach. You can relax. You don't have to hold onto your fat stores because clearly there's no famine right now."

At the sight and smell of all this food served up to you, powerful biochemical signals are transmitted through your body. Cortisol levels fall as you relax. Ghrelin levels fall as you "eat with your eyes" and mindfully savor the food entering your mouth. Leptin and dopamine levels rise.

That's putting it simply. The process is a lot more complex than that—it's a finely tuned dance of thoughts and biochemicals that science has only just begun to understand.

Satiation and satiety—those are strong body-speech signals your Inner Guardian understands. When you achieve satiation and satiety, you are signaling to your Inner Guardian that you are surrounded by enough food and variety of nutrition that you don't need to hold onto fat stores.

The Inner Guardian and hunger.

Hunger is the physiological need for food (as distinct from appetite, which is the desire for food).

You can think of physical hunger as being regulated by your Inner Guardian, your built in life preserver. Your Guardian receives signals from the interactions of biochemical substances within your body, including ghrelin, sometimes called the "hunger hormone", and leptin, also known as the "satiety hormone".

Ghrelin and leptin communicate in a language that's non-verbal; body-speech. If you can learn to communicate in body-speech, you and your hunger hormones may not have to forever live at odds with each other.

Eating disorders.

Some people are constantly at war with their Inner Guardian. They are engaged in a seemingly endless weight loss battle.

The mental turmoil associated with this can result in "yo-yo dieting", or eating disorders such as anorexia nervosa, bulimia, binge eating, avoidant/restrictive food intake disorder etc. With such psychological illnesses, the struggle to disobey the Inner Guardian's hunger imperatives is so arduous that it can occupy the sufferer's mind all the time. Patients may obsess about food night and day, struggling against that tireless, potent, inner defender; their Inner Guardian.

Whenever a patient's Guardian wins a battle, that person may surrender to a bout of feasting and gorging. Afterwards their conscious mind tells them that they must purge, and they become caught in the harrowing cycle of their eating disorder.

Many sufferers of eating disorders are driven by a powerful motivator—the desire to be loved and accepted. This is, in fact, a primordial drive that's "hard-wired" into us because, as discussed earlier, human beings cannot survive alone. We need a group, a tribe. And to belong to a tribe we must be accepted. The Inner Guardian knows this.

When the conscious mind is somehow taught to believe the fallacy that thinness means attractiveness and acceptability, eating disorders can emerge.

The modern media bombard us with images of slim models (male and female) who are supposed to represent the epitome of beauty and acceptability. For some people, their conscious mind learns to equate

47

social acceptability with slimness, and the painful cycle of conflict begins. The deluded inner voices argue,

"To survive, you must be socially accepted.

"To be socially accepted you must be thin (this is the fallacy).

"To be thin you must stop eating.

"But to survive, you must eat . . . "

With eating disorders, the Inner Guardian is actually turning against itself. Here are two opposing survival directives fighting a psychological battle. Patients suffer terrible distress, and if they do not recover their health can seriously deteriorate. Eating disorders can be life-threatening.

It may sometimes be possible to override the Inner Guardian's control using only willpower, but this is a hard task and can come at a terrible cost. People with eating disorders are forever fighting to override the inner compulsion to eat. They pay dearly, suffering from mental and physical illness.

If you think you have an eating disorder, consult your doctor.

In this book we are focussing on healthy people who are overweight or obese, and who want to lose weight.

Body-speech that regulates appetite.

The Inner Guardian, by comparison with the mind's conscious workings, is unsophisticated and primitive. Unlike the conscious mind it does not directly receive information through the eyes and ears and other senses.[6]

When you do battle against your Inner Guardian, weight loss is extremely difficult. The trick is to work with your Guardian, not against it—that is, to lose weight "by stealth", by "sneaking" fat off your body in a way that doesn't make the Guardian think there's a famine.

You can learn to communicate with your Inner Guardian using body-speech. Most of us would like to be able to speak that silent,

---

6   Our senses can be deceived, which is perhaps why the Inner Guardian does not depend on them.

potent language of the body; to communicate with our Inner Guardians. We would like to tell them to help us live long and prosper, to stay healthy and NOT to store excessive fat.

Your Inner Guardian receives input from the world around your body by way of signals. With regard to appetite, these signals include (but are not limited to):

- What you eat
- How much energy, nutrition or variety exists in what you eat
- How you eat
- When you eat
- Who you eat with
- What you eat off
- How your brain interprets what your eyes see
- How your brain interprets what your mouth feels
- How your brain interprets tastes
- How your brain interprets smells
- What your teeth crunch
- How long and how thoroughly your jaws chew (and whether they chew at all)

- What hormones and other chemicals are coursing through your body as a result of stress or happiness or any other emotion
- What temperature your skin is
- How your brain interprets what your ears hear
- How much food your stomach receives
- How much exercise your body has undertaken
- Your level of blood sugar
- Your level of hydration

Your Inner Guardian is engineered to understand and react to incoming communications like these. They are complex, and the way the Inner Guardian responds to them is also complex.

APPETITE

Appetite is the desire to consume food. It may or may not be driven by hunger.

Eating triggers.

Certain things trigger physiological signals that tell your body to get ready for eating. These triggers may be psychological, chemical, cultural, the result of habit etc. Factors such as the smell or sight of food, sounds associated with food such as clinking tableware, and even mental images and thoughts of food stimulate your cerebral cortex. Your brain then sends messages via the vagus nerve to your stomach, telling it to secrete gastric juices in readiness for receiving food.

The process of eating.

The introduction of food into your body involves such step by step processes as:

- Experiencing the texture and taste of the food. This is called the orosensory response. After you take a mouthful of food, your mouth senses that food in many ways, including through your taste-buds, and the act of chewing and using your tongue.
- Signals are sent from your mouth to your brain. Depending on your past experiences with tasting that particular food, these messages tell you whether to keep eating or spit it out!
- After the act of swallowing comes the expansion of your stomach. This activates the stomach's stretch receptors, which send more signals to your brain.
- When the food passes further along your digestive tract, natural chemicals it contains stimulate other physiological mechanisms.
- Your body releases hormones and other substances in response to fats, proteins, caffeine etc. appearing in your digestive tract.
- After food is absorbed into your body there will usually be a rise in your blood sugar.

The "tube" of your body is that open-ended digestive tract which stretches from the mouth to the anus (and which therefore could be construed as technically still 'outside' the body). When you eat, you bring food not simply inside this "tube" but deeper still; into your blood, your bones, your very cells. What you eat invades your body to the fullest extent.

No wonder so many of us have complicated relationships with food!

Hunger and Appetite.

What drives us to eat?

People usually call the sensation of desiring or needing food "hunger", but that feeling may not be true hunger at all. The desire for food—which is called "appetite"—can be triggered by many things other than true hunger.

Often, the terms "hunger" and "appetite" are used interchangeably, but their meanings are, in fact, different.

Hunger is a motivational state; the physiological need for food. Its purpose is to regulate energy intake, ensuring that it's adequate for maintaining the body's metabolism. It is modulated by complex interactions between the digestive tract, the adipose tissue (fat stores) and the brain. Physical hunger generally arises after an extended period without food. Normally, this occurs around three to six hours after a meal.

Appetite, on the other hand, is the desire for food. It may or may not be driven by hunger. Delicious-looking foods can stimulate your appetite even when you're not feeling hungry.

Hunger and appetite share some traits in common. They can be boosted by psychological stress, or by a reduction of the body's store of nutrients.

For people living modern lifestyles, hunger and appetite can lead to obesity.

Hunger is " . . . your body's built-in mechanism for food intake regulation. Its job is to drive you to eat enough to meet your body's energy and micronutrient needs, and no more. The [hunger] mechanism works very well under normal circumstances. Obviously, it never would have survived millions of years of evolutionary testing if it did not work to the benefit of our health. But our modern lifestyle does not constitute 'normal circumstances' in relation to the environment in which most of our evolution took place. Consequently, [hunger and] appetite cannot be entirely relied upon to ensure that we don't overeat." [Pacific Health Laboratories (2008)]

Regulation of hunger and appetite.

Your body regulates appetite via the neuroendocrine system.

Together the endocrine system and nervous system can be called the "neuroendocrine system". It's the endocrine system that detects changes in your body, such as those that happen when food enters your mouth. It reacts to these changes by releasing hormonal messengers. These appetite-regulating hormones include leptin, ghrelin, insulin and cholecystokinin (CCK). They play a role in hunger, satiation/satiety and energy balance.

Meanwhile your nervous system sends out electrical impulses and biochemicals called neurotransmitters. These direct the various parts of your digestive system to churn and process the food, and keep pushing it through your body.

In other words when you eat food, your body responds in numerous ways. Signals are transmitted back and forth between your brain and your body's other organs.

"Various physiologic feedback mechanisms involving the mouth, stomach, intestines, and brain all work together to increase or decrease your hunger. Many hormones play a role." [Blake (nd)]

In human beings, the part of the brain called the hypothalamus is the chief regulator of appetite. "The hypothalamus senses external stimuli mainly through a number of hormones such as leptin (and) ghrelin . . . They are produced by the digestive tract and by adipose tissue (fat)." [Wikipedia (Oct. 2017)]

Here are some other "external stimuli" involved in the control of hunger and appetite:

The stretching of the stomach signals fullness.

Your brain and stomach start to register feelings of fullness about 20 minutes after you begin eating a meal.

When you eat, food passes into the bag-like stomach, which stretches to accommodate the food. The stretching of your stomach triggers the appetite control switch in your brain. This tells you to stop eating (satiation) and dampens your hunger for a while, until your body requires more energy and nutrients.

TIP: To make good use of this appetite-reducing trigger, eat foods that occupy a lot of room in your stomach, but contain few Calories. Examples include vegetable soups, which contain quite a lot of water, and fresh garden salads.

When your stomach is chronically over-stretched by overeating, your body's sensors lose their sensitivity. That appetite control switch in your brain becomes confused and the "stop eating" signals don't work properly.

TIP: The solution to this problem—eat smaller portions.

Nutrient signals.

Blood levels of glucose, amino acids, and fatty acids provide a constant flow of information to the brain that may be linked to regulating hunger and energy intake. Nutrient signals that indicate fullness, and thereby inhibit hunger, include rising blood glucose levels, elevated blood levels of amino acids and blood concentrations of fatty acids. [Bernstein & Nash (2006)]

CCK helps reduce appetite.

When food enters your stomach it also triggers off the release of cholecystokinin, or CCK. This is a protein that helps reduce appetite and prolong satiety. One of CCK's actions is to close the valve that leads from your stomach into the lower GI tract, temporarily trapping the food so that the stomach can do its work of grinding and breaking down the food into smaller particles. The longer food remains in your stomach, the longer you feel full and satisfied.

CCK works best with real food.

So why isn't everyone's CCK working to prevent the global obesity crisis? Has the mechanism broken down?

It's not the mechanism that's the problem—it's the food we're eating. Our appetite control switches were designed to respond to the natural, whole foods our ancestors consumed throughout most of human history. Those foods were generally a lot lower in Calories than the processed, high-sugar, high-fat foods we eat these days. Our appetite control switches still become active when we have eaten a certain amount of processed food, but that amount of food will have contained a greater number of Calories than "real" food. It's now much easier to consume more Calories than we need, before the appetite control switches kick in (which is about 20 minutes after we begin a meal). When you're eating processed food, it's easy to consume loads of Calories before CCK tells your brain that you're full.

> TIP: In order to keep your natural appetite-regulating mechanisms in good working order, base your diet on real foods with fewer Calories—such as unprocessed vegetables, legumes, whole grains, fruits and lean meats.

CCK release is best stimulated by certain nutrients.

The greatest stimulator of CCK release is the presence of fatty acids and/or certain amino acids in the churned-up food passing out of the stomach into the the first part of the small intestine immediately beyond the stomach. [Chaudhri et al. (2006)]

> TIP: This suggests that if you begin a meal with some foods rich in protein and fatty acids, such as soy foods, walnuts, hemp seeds, chia seeds, or oily fish, it's more likely your appetite switch will be working properly.

Leptin.

As mentioned, leptin is often referred to as the "satiety hormone".

"The fluctuation of leptin and ghrelin hormone levels results in the motivation of an organism to consume food. When an organism eats, adipocytes (fat cells) trigger the release of leptin into the body. Increasing levels of leptin result in a reduction of one's motivation to eat. After hours of non-consumption, leptin levels drop significantly. These low levels of leptin cause the release of a secondary hormone, ghrelin, which in turn reinitiates (brings back) the feeling of hunger." [Wikipedia (29th May 2016)]

Leptin is chiefly produced by your fat cells. Its main job appears to be sending signals to the brain to regulate your appetite and control your energy intake.

There are other places in your body where leptin is produced, and leptin plays other roles besides appetite control. But as a general rule, the more fat cells you have, the more "satiety hormone" will be produced; while the leaner you are, the less leptin will be released. This is your Inner Guardian's way of trying to ensure that you don't get too fat or too thin.

Nonetheless, we humans have found many ways to ignore the natural signaling of our leptin so that we can overeat.

The bodies of people with more adipose tissue produce more leptin. In overweight or obese people, this overproduction of leptin can cause the hypothalamus to become resistant to leptin. The satiety signals to the brain are disrupted, which means that although the pancreas is still producing the "satiety hormone", people don't get the message that they have eaten enough and should stop. They keep eating, resulting in weight gain.

This can set up a perpetual cycle. It helps explain why dieting alone is ineffective in most obese adults—and why even obese adults who successfully lose weight through dieting overwhelmingly put weight back on afterwards.

Ghrelin

Ghrelin stimulates appetite, and is sometimes called the "hunger hormone". It is produced by cells in the gastrointestinal tract.

"Besides regulating appetite, ghrelin also plays a significant role in regulating the distribution and rate of use of energy." [Wikipedia (Oct. 2017)]

The discovery of ghrelin's action was accidental. When performing gastric bypass surgery to help obese patients lose weight, surgeons remove the part of the stomach that secretes ghrelin. It was first thought that it was the smaller stomach size that reduced the patient's appetite. Later it was found that it was not simply the smaller stomachs, but the decreased ghrelin production that helped patients reduce their food intake.

Any changes in the normal production levels of ghrelin or leptin can lead to obesity. When you diet by depriving yourself of food to the point of hunger, the increased ghrelin secretion sends your brain even stronger signals to drive you to eat, overriding your willpower. This is an example of your helpful Inner Guardian in action!

People suffering from anorexia nervosa can have high levels of ghrelin. They may feel extreme hunger and continually battle to suppress their desire to eat.

Cultural and social influences.

Over the past few decades several factors have combined to increase our "cultural and social appetite", which can override our "physical appetite", leading to an increase in the number of Calories we consume. These factors include larger portion sizes of fast foods, packaged foods and restaurant menu items, the ready availability of high-Calorie foods that are cheap and palatable, and the constant bombardment of commercial advertising for food.

Studies suggest that the amount you eat is greatly influenced by how easy it is for you to get food, how much food is served up to you (portion sizes), packaging design and commercial advertisements for food. [Wansink (2004), Chandon & Wansink (2012)]

"Social rituals of eating, such as eating while distracted (e.g. while driving or watching TV), eating too rapidly (e.g. while rushing to do errands), or always having dessert may also affect our desire to override natural hunger and fullness cues." [Andrews (2016)]

How can you counteract the effects of these social and cultural pressures?

TIPS:

- Learn to recognize the physical signs of your own hunger and satiety. Eat only when you are truly hungry and stop eating when you feel satiated but not over-full.
- Learn to order, buy, prepare and serve smaller food portions.
- Learn to eat mindfully.
- Learn to override habits that may make you overeat (such as always having dessert).

Your biological clock.

The circadian rhythms of your body—which are regulated by the hypothalamus region of your brain—act to stimulate or inhibit hunger.

Your emotional state.

Some people gain weight when they are feeling anxious or depressed. Others lose weight.

It is thought that when you experience an increase in stress, your body's production of ghrelin may be affected. This would explain why you can feel hungry even in stressful situations.

The Second Brain.

Your appetite is not only regulated by hormonal and neural messages passing between your digestive system and your brain, but also by your body's enteric nervous system. Sometimes referred to as "the second brain" or "the mini-brain", this is located in the gut. It produces neurotransmitters which transmit, intensify and modify various signals passing between the body's cells.

"Although we've all been aware of the effect our brain can have on our digestive system (there's nothing like a deadline or presentation to trigger a trip to the bathroom), few understand the power our gut is having over our brain and its likely connection to mental health and general wellbeing." [Moore (2012)]

Some neurotransmitters involved in appetite regulation include gamma aminobutyric acid (GABA), serotonin, histamine and dopamine. That's why low serotonin levels, low dopamine levels some antihistamine drugs can cause an increase in appetite.

And it is also why increasing your levels of dopamine and serotonin may have the effect of curbing your appetite. In this book and others in this series, we suggest ways to boost your serotonin and dopamine.

This second brain is capable of far more than simply processing the food you eat. It can also influence your mood and psychological well-being. It mainly communicates with the microbes that live in your gut—the "microbiota". These are the tiny organisms that make up the vitally important "microbiome". More about that later!

Yes, there are "fat genes".

Satiation and satiety signals within the body vary from person to person. In some people, the desire to stop eating happens quite quickly after food is consumed. They have strong satiation and satiety signals, and for them it is easier to stay at a healthy weight. In others, it takes longer for these signals to develop, so they eat more and are more likely to become overweight.

People who have weak or delayed satiety signals need to eat more food to reach satiety. Their "satiety threshold" is raised, and they tend to feel hungry for much of the time. This can lead to excess weight gain.

Sometimes a high satiety threshold is induced by prolonged, drastic dieting. The body goes into "starvation mode", and hunger hormone levels skyrocket.

Sometimes the satiety threshold is raised due to damage to, or malformation of the areas of the brain associated with appetite regulation.

People with weak satiation and satiety signals find it very hard to deny their insistent hunger signals. Hunger is a powerful drive. This susceptibility to hunger can also be genetic.

MC4R deficiency.

An inherited disadvantage called "melanocortin 4 receptor deficiency" (MC4R) can prevent the brain from receiving satiety signals. Methods of testing for this "fat gene" are currently being developed.

The FTO gene—a genetic reason for obesity.

Recent research has uncovered a number of other genes that are linked with a high satiety threshold and increased risk of obesity. Prominent among these is one called the FTO gene.

"It seems that certain variants of the FTO gene are associated with obesity in humans." [Loos & Yeo (2014)]

"One variant of the FTO gene has been associated with weight gain in 42% of Caucasians, another with weight gain in about 5% of Africans, and another with weight gain in about 21% of Asians. People with this FTO gene variant tend to overeat and prefer high-sugar and high-fat foods. . . FTO risk variants are a double threat; they cause weight gain by making carriers eat more and eat badly." [GB HealthWatch (2016)]

The FTO gene variants helped our ancestors survive food shortages, but in modern times we are suffering from an over-abundance of food rather than a dearth of it. Now many of us have the opposite problem—not how to find as much high Calorie food as possible and store it on our bodies, but how to *avoid* those foods and remove fat from our too-heavy bodies. So the FTO gene variant, once a valuable survival tool, has become a health liability.

Does this mean that people with "obesity gene" variants are doomed to a life of obesity? Not at all. The weight loss methods outlined in this book will work for everyone.

Obesity researchers disagree about the exact year in which the "obesity epidemic" began, and the factors that triggered it.

This goes to show how complex the problem is. Solving it will involve more than simply telling people to eat less and move more.

PART TWO

SATIETY

WHAT IS SATIETY?

SATIATION VS SATIETY

People use the terms "satiation" and "satiety" interchangeably, to mean "satisfying hunger". Technically, however, the two terms mean different things.

Satiation.

Satiation is what happens when you're consuming a meal and you get the feeling that you've had enough to eat. It's a sensation of fullness and repleteness; the sense that you really don't want to eat any more of that meal. When you feel full enough to want to stop eating, you've reached satiation.

Your brain reads signals from your body that tell it when satiation has been reached.

". . . when food is eaten, it interacts with receptors lining the stomach and intestine, causing the release of peptides and other factors that coordinate the process of dige stion with the particular food being consumed. Some of the peptides provide a signal to the nervous system, and as the integrated signal accumulates, it ultimately creates the sensation of fullness and contributes to cessation of eating." [Woods (2004)]

One factor that determines how much you eat at one meal is how much food and drink it takes for you to reach satiation. The less food it takes, the better your weight loss will be. That is why highly satisfying, Calorie-sparse foods are so helpful for weight loss.

Satiation is more than just feeling full. It refers to your feeling of being satisfied by the amount and type of food you have just eaten. It is possible to feel unsatisfied even if your stomach is full. For example, if you drank a great deal of water or ate a whole head of iceberg lettuce at one sitting your stomach might be fully distended, but it's unlikely you would feel satisfied. You would probably feel the urge to seek foods with higher Calorie content.

Satiety.

Satiety, by contrast, refers to what happens between meals. It is to do with the length of time before you begin feeling hungry again. It's like "long-term satiation".

Like satiation, satiety is the feeling or state of being sated, satisfied and replete. It is the absence of hunger and the feeling of having eaten enough food. This feeling springs from a complex interaction of blood sugar levels, biochemicals, fullness and psychological factors.

Satiety's role is to regulate how much you eat throughout the day. "Ideally, satiety dwindles as nutrients diminish. When nutrients diminish, hunger returns." [Anthony (2014)]

To lose weight, you need to consume fewer Calories. It is, however, hard to do this if you have to battle constantly against hunger. To relieve your body once and for all from the burden of being overweight, it is important to consistently achieve both satiation and satiety, while eating fewer Calories.

For example, you might reach satiation after eating a Calorie-sparse salad, but feel hungry again soon afterwards. To help with between-meal satiety, that Calorie-sparse salad could:

- be mixed with some other satisfying ingredients (without adding too many extra Calories)
- be visually presented in a way that enhances satiety
- be eaten mindfully, in a way that enhances satiety

Clearly, when you feel utterly satisfied between meals, you won't feel the need to eat. (You may still feel a desire for the taste or texture of foods, but that desire will not be the result of hunger.) When you lack the drive to consume Calories, it's easier to lose weight.

In summary; satiation is the point at which you've eaten enough to feel full. But when it comes to managing your Calorie intake, satiation is only half the story. You might feel pleasantly full after a meal and be perfectly happy to stop eating. But if you're hungry just 45 minutes later, you haven't completely solved the problem. Satiety is what keeps hunger at bay between meals.

These days, scientists are busy developing drugs to enhance satiety, so that people will eat less and lose weight. Increasing satiety while eating lower-Calories foods helps you lose weight by making it easier for you to consume less energy.

How long does satiety last?

Once satiety is reached, the sensation of satisfaction and lack of hunger should remain with you for at least an hour or two. Depending on numerous variables, some people may not start to feel hungry for many hours after a meal. Everyone is different, and certain situations can also influence how long your satiety lasts.

This book provides tips on how to extend the period of satiety.

SATIATION IS IMPORTANT FOR SATIETY

To achieve satiety (long-term absence of hunger) between meals, it's useful to reach satiation (a feeling of repleteness) at each meal. But never go beyond "satiation" to "overfull"!

It's just as important to avoid undereating as overeating. If you leave the dinner-table feeling slightly peckish and dissatisfied, you're more likely to experience real hunger sooner after the meal. And then you'll be tempted to reach for the nearest snack...

There are many benefits of reaching satiation at each meal.

- You will feel better than before you started the meal.
- You will feel satisfied.
- You can stop thinking about food for a while.
- You're more likely to experience satiety between meals. Your appetite will take longer to be aroused.
- There is less chance that you'll respond readily to appetite-triggers in your environment.
- You're less likely to get the urge to graze on snacks between meals.
- You're less likely to want to consume a lot of food at your next meal.
- There's less chance of your developing 'cravings'.

An important key to losing weight is controlling how much energy you consume. This can be regulated by allowing your body to achieve satiation and satiety in a healthy way, without gorging on energy-dense foods.

WHY DO WE OVERRIDE SATIATION AND SATIETY SIGNALS?

Dr. Paul Biegler of Monash University's Centre for Human Bioethics writes, "The body is generally good at homoeostasis, keeping variations in things such as temperature to a minimum. A set point for weight makes evolutionary sense; too thin and we risk starvation, too fat and our sluggish bulk runs the gauntlet of predation. Yet adult obesity rates have nearly tripled in developed countries, from 25% in 1980 to over 68% in 2012. So what might be loosening the firm grip of energy homoeostasis?" [Biegler (2016)]

Even though our bodies possess complex techniques to regulate the amount of energy we consume, many people still keep eating after they feel full. Other than satiety signals, a host of other factors can cause you to ignore and overrule your body's internal satiation and satiety signals.

We discuss this further in the section "Hunger and Overeating".

STAVING OFF HUNGER VS REACHING SATIETY

Dieters trying to lose weight will often snack on small amounts of low Calorie foods through the day. This method of eating may *stave off* hunger but it does not allow satiety to be reached. The Inner Guardian thinks, "There must be a food shortage, because I am receiving only enough food to barely keep me going. I will respond to the food shortage by protecting the energy stores and hanging on to the fat."

The idea is to convince the Inner Guardian that there is *not* a food shortage, so that it will more willingly let go of those fat stores.

THE PROCESS OF DIGESTION

Together, the stomach and intestines are known as the gastrointestinal (GI) tract. The food you eat passes into this digestive system, where it is processed both mechanically and chemically until it is broken down into small, easily-absorbed fragments.

It is here that carbohydrates are disassembled into simple sugars such as glucose and fructose, most fats are dismantled into fatty acids and monoacylglycerols, and proteins are pulled apart to become amino acids.

Your body then absorbs these basic nutritional units, along with any micronutrients that are present, such as vitamins and minerals.

The whole operation of digestion is regulated by signals passing to and fro along the pathways of your enteric nervous system, as well as various hormonal and other chemical signals produced by cells lodged in the lining of your gastrointestinal tract.

Gastrointestinal satiety signals.

Gastrointestinal peptides are synthesized in certain areas of your brain, as well as being manufactured in your GI tract.

Steven Woods, doctor of Physiology, Biophysics and Experimental Psychology in the USA writes, ". . . when food is eaten, it interacts with receptors lining the stomach and intestine, causing the release of peptides and other factors that coordinate the process of digestion with the particular food being consumed. Some of the peptides provide a signal to the nervous system, and as the integrated signal accumulates, it ultimately creates the sensation of fullness and contributes to cessation of eating.

"Although dozens of enzymes, hormones, and other factors are secreted by the GI tract in response to food [inside the GI tract], only a handful are able to influence food intake directly. Most of these cause meals to terminate and hence are called satiety signals..." [Woods (2004)]

Satiety signals create a sensation of fullness and reduce your desire to eat.

Inside your gut, an intricate network of biological substances generates signals that are sent to your brain when you eat or drink. In conjunction with the signals from your other senses (such as sight and taste) and the rest of your digestive tract, they interact with your central nervous system to forge the sense of satiety.

"Satiety signals are relayed to the brain, either indirectly via nerves such as the vagus [nerve] from the gastrointestinal tract, or else directly via the blood[stream]. Most factors that influence how much food is eaten during individual meals act by changing the sensitivity to satiety signals. These include adiposity signals [i.e. body-speech signals giving information about how much fat mass is already stored in the body] as well as habits and learning, the social situation, and stressors." [Woods (2004)]

These satiety-signal inducing, hunger-suppressing substances include cholecystokinin (CCK) and leptin.

There are also GI signals that have the opposite effect to the satiety signals, and actually promote sensations of hunger and appetite. One of these hunger-stimulating substances is ghrelin.

Satiety signals are produced in your GI tract during meals. They transmit information about mechanical properties of your food (e.g., how much it stretches your stomach stretch) and chemical properties of the food (as signaled by the release of certain hormones).

Having a range of different satiety signals enables species that are omnivores, such as humans, to eat a wide range of whatever foods are available.

It means that your body produces a medley of gut peptides, each of which is tailored to digest the particular food passing through your GI tract, while simultaneously telling your brain exactly what foods you have eaten. Your body produces different signals in response to particular macronutrients (carbohydrates, fats, proteins), or combinations of these macronutrients.

By keeping account of signals that convey information about how much energy is in the food you've eaten, your brain is able to make you want to stop eating when you have consumed sufficient Calories, even before you have absorbed those Calories in significant quantities.

If this did not happen, then any time you ate a meal that was too large, your body could become overwhelmed by a deluge of carbs and fat.

TWO TYPES OF SATIETY

Satiety and satiation are produced by the hunger-suppressing signals that are triggered by eating. As mentioned earlier, satiation develops during a meal and makes the diner want to stop eating. Satiety, on the other hand, develops after a meal and suppresses hunger between meals.

There are two types of satiety: short-term and long-term.

The short-term satiety system.

This system notes how full your stomach is, and which nutrients have arrived in your gut. Its job is to send hunger signals (such as ghrelin) to your brain when it's time for another meal.

In the short term, your brain receives satiety signals by means of hormones and nutrient signals. It's when the nutrients and other products of your food are absorbed that your body sends messages to your brain telling it, 'We have enough building and maintenance materials to be going on with for now, thank you very much, and we don't need to order any more for a while. In fact, eating more right now, is going to give us a work overload because we're busy processing the last meal. So stop sending out hunger signals and send out satiety signals instead, until we run low on building and maintenance materials. When that happens, we'll notify you."

Hormone signals: The hormones insulin and cholecystokinin (CCK) are released from the GI tract during food absorption. They act to suppress feeling of hunger.

Nutrient signals: Signals triggered in the digestive system by food's nutrients tell your brain that you have consumed sufficient vitamins, minerals, protein etc. and you don't need any more in the immediate future. They include the following:
- Rising blood glucose levels
- Elevated blood levels of amino acids
- Blood concentrations of fatty acids

In other words, if your meal contains a range of nutrients such as sugars[7], proteins and fatty acids, it is more likely to give you satiety.

> TIP: This is why, for short-term satiety, it's so important for you to eat a diverse array of foods containing a wide variety of nutrients.

The long-term satiety system.

This system calculates how much fat is stored in your body. Under normal circumstances, when your long-term satiety system senses that you have plenty of well-filled fat cells, it releases various hormones and biochemicals to inform the energy-intake regulating parts of your brain. In turn, your brain sends signals to dampen hunger and make you eat less food. When your fat stores diminish, it increases your hunger.

This is meant to act as a balancing mechanism. As mentioned earlier, fat cells produce the "satiety hormone", leptin. It's leptin that lets your brain know the total amount of energy that is stored in your body. The more fat (energy) you store, the more leptin your fat cells produce. People with large fat stores release more leptin and therefore should, theoretically, eat less in the longer term.

---

7   Not necessarily processed table sugar; sugars occur naturally in many whole foods.

The long-term satiety system can be disrupted by dieting.
In that case, why doesn't leptin do its job properly and make us all slim?

Leptin is not simply "the satiety hormone". Its role is more complex. High blood levels of leptin do help with weight loss, but this hormone's main function is to protect your body against weight loss when nutrition is scarce.

Leptin "thinks" that its main job when you are on a restricted diet is to plummet to low levels. Leptin is still living in the past. It has not yet updated itself to recognise the overabundance of food that surrounds many people in the 21st century.

COMPONENTS OF SATIETY

"Satiety is moderated by a combination of cognitive, sensory and physiological signals . . . Sensory and cognitive signals generated during consumption [of food] are important for satiety . . . " [Chambers et al. (2015)]

" . . . satiation and satiety are not intrinsic but are instead the result of a complex interaction between culture, the organism and food." [Blundell & Bellisle (2012)]

Satiety is regulated not only by the type of food you eat, but also by events that take place even before you eat or drink, and which continue as food passes through your GI tract, being digested and absorbed.

Many of the components necessary for satiety are also necessary for satiation. There is considerable overlap, because satiation after meals is important for satiety between meals.

Andrew Hill, Professor of Medical Psychology at Leeds University, says: "Hunger and satiety rely on a whole constellation of psychological and physical factors that most people are unaware of."

Some of them are described below.

You need as many as possible of these components to reach satiety when eating a meal. Otherwise you are likely to leave the table feeling vaguely dissatisfied. You will feel hungry sooner after the meal, and will probably be bothered by a constant desire to snack.

And if you snack, it's likely that you will end up consuming more Calories in one day than you would have, if you'd simply reached satiation and satiety at every meal.

Fullness and emptiness.

The part of the brain which is responsible for controlling your energy intake receives satiety signals in response to such factors as:

* Feelings of fullness.

When the stomach is comfortably expanded, its stretch receptors send fullness signals to the brain. Note that for weight loss, the stomach should not be over-stretched.

For people who eat relatively quickly, the first satiety signal their brains receive may be the sense of the stomach's fullness.

Fullness, however, is not the equivalent of satiety. Your stomach could be full of water, for example, but you could still feel hungry.

It may take 15-20 minutes after a mouthful of food has been swallowed for the entire gamut of satiety signals from that food to reach the brain. These signals tell the brain a lot about the food, such as the precise macronutrients and micronutrients that are beginning to be absorbed.

* Lack of the feeling of fullness.

Or you could eat a small savory muffin loaded with carbs, protein and Calories. Such a small snack would not stretch your stomach enough to give you a feeling of fullness. Lack of fullness can sometimes hamper satiety, although it is not essential for satiety.

Satiety is not the same as fullness.

You can feel "full" after a meal even if your stomach is not stretched to the limit. This is because your brain registers a feeling of fullness, or satiety, in response not only to the amount of food consumed, but also to the food's nutrients. Cells in your gut record the nutrient content of the food you have swallowed. Then they release appetite-suppressing compounds that are sent to your brain, resulting in that sense of satiety.

71

If the volume or bulk of a meal were the only thing that triggered satiety, then you would feel satiety after eating, say, a whole head of lettuce and a bunch of celery in one sitting. Your stomach would bulge—but you would be unlikely to feel satisfied. Fullness does not necessarily equal satiety.

That is not to say that food volume does not play a role in satiety—it does. Satiety, however, is complex. In fact, you experience satiety for each food/macronutrient/texture. If you eat mainly protein, for example, you might find yourself craving for fruit and vegetables, and losing interest in protein foods. If you eat nothing but huge amounts of fresh salads you might end up craving for bread and despising the thought of salads. Live on a lot of slurpy soups and you could end up craving crunchy foods. Chew on nothing but hard, crunchy victuals and you might find yourself yearning for creamy textures.

This "per food" satiety system seems to be nature's method of ensuring that you eat a nutritionally balanced diet.

Blood sugar levels.

A gentle elevation of blood sugars is important for satiety. When you eat a meal, your blood sugars should rise a little—not too much. This rise signals to your Inner Guardian that you have consumed energy, so it doesn't need to make you want to eat more.

When blood sugars fail to rise much, satiety is hard to reach. For example, you could eat an enormous bowl of multicolored salad (for fullness) containing crunchy, creamy and other textures, with a wide range of flavors (for sensory enjoyment) and rich in all sorts of nutrients (for nutrition), yet if this bowl of salad failed to make your blood sugars rise sufficiently, you would be unlikely to achieve satiety.

Sensory enjoyment.

Appetite-regulating signals begin to be generated even before food or drink is consumed. Your senses play a huge role here—the sight and smell of food, food-related sounds, objects and places associated with food in your memory; all act together to awaken your appetite and begin the process of satiety. A medley of bright food colors including, for example, reds and purples, might send the signal, "nutritious anthocyanins are on the way!" The process continues when food or drink enters your mouth, then travels through your digestive system to be assimilated.

When you have eaten mindfully, taking pleasure in the sight, sound, texture, flavor etc. of the food, your Inner Guardian feels certain that you have had a proper meal. It gets the message that it doesn't have to release hunger hormones to make you eat more.

Lack of sensory enjoyment makes it hard to reach satiety. For example you could eat an entire head of cabbage (for fullness), along with some multivitamin and mineral supplements (for nutrition) and some sugar syrup (to raise your blood sugars) but you would be very unlikely to reach satiety, because you'd be missing the sensory enjoyment.

Nutritional satiety.

The variety of food and drinks offered at a meal can affect satiety. Nutritional satiety is reached when your body detects that you have consumed the range and proportion of nutrients it needs for optimum functioning.

When your diet is lacking in good nutrition, it is hard to reach satiety. To take an extreme example, let us imagine that you eat nothing but foods made with sugar, fat and refined flour. Crunchy bread croutons. Creamy cheese sauces. Cakes and ice-creams artificially colored with every hue of the rainbow, artificially flavored with every edible chemical known to man. You're getting all the textures, the colors and the flavors (sensory enjoyment). You're eating until you're full. Your blood sugars are rising at every meal. But you are suffering from malnutrition and you cannot reach satiety, so all through the day you find yourself reaching for more food… sound familiar?

Note that processed foods can be "nutrition decoys". They closely resemble foods that contain the nutrients for which your body craves. Yet no matter how much of them you consume of these decoys, you'll always want more—because they contain few or none of the needed nutrients.

For example, artificially colored and flavored orange drinks resemble the actual juice of oranges. Real oranges are rich in vitamin C and also contain vitamin A, thiamin, folate, potassium, fiber, copper, magnesium, flavonoids, hesperidin, and a variety of other trace vitamins and minerals. Your body needs these nutrients, and your senses tell you that the orange-colored liquid *smells* like oranges and *tastes* like oranges. Therefore you swig down the mixture of water, sugar, synthetic coloring agents, orange flavoring agents, acidity regulators, stabilizers, preservatives and so on.

Your senses might be fooled into thinking it's real orange juice but your digestive processes know exactly what is going on. They are not getting the building blocks they need for your body's good health! So they keep sending insistent signals to the brain... More orange juice! More! And the vicious cycle continues.

The same goes for "protein decoys" like salty, fatty potato fries/chips/crisps, which have sensory characteristics that are similar to protein, but contain very little of it.

Thoughts can influence satiety.

The way you think about your food is important. Mindful eating involves being aware of your emotions and physical sensations, and focusing on the characteristics of your meal while you eat. This technique can give you positive feelings about food, and enhance satiety. Moreover, your personal perceptions of the food and drink you consume—such as how many Calories it contains—can influence how much satiety you get from that food.

Portion size and the size of tableware can have a significant effect on satiety too. The color of tableware also has a psychological impact.

Your emotional state can affect satiety

When you feel anxious, angry, upset, sad etc. your digestive system is not working at its best. Nutrients may not be properly absorbed. Furthermore, your body could be releasing large quantities of cortisol, which can increase appetite. The combination of heightened hunger and malabsorption of nutrients is a sure way to defeat satiety. Feeling relaxed before, during and after eating can help boost satiety.

Your body-fat stores can influence satiety.

A mentioned already, there are two types of satiety. With the long-term satiety system, the Inner Guardian knows how much fat is already present in the body, ready to use as energy for survival. If you have plenty of stored fat, you're likely to reach satiety more easily than people with very little fat. This, however, is subject to a clause: Obese people can also struggle to achieve satiety, depending on a range of other factors.

Your microbiome and satiety.

We discuss the microbiome at greater length later in this book. Suffice to say, the tiny organisms that live in your intestines play an important role in the regulation of your energy balance, satiety and weight. It is thought that they may influence the development of obesity, and scientists think that manipulating the composition of the microbiome might be a useful tool in the fight against obesity.

Other components of satiety.

Other factors interact with your body's digestive function to influence how much food you eat. These include:

- things you have learned (such as what is an acceptable portion size)
- habits (such as always adding extra salt to our food)
- the social situation (such as dining out)

SATIETY HELPS YOU LOSE WEIGHT MORE EASILY

Excess body-fat is hard to lose for a range of reasons including external stimuli, obesogens, easy access to cheap high-energy foods, emotions, habits, lack of sleep, circadian rhythms, food additives and food "addictions".

However it's mainly hunger, cravings, and feeling deprived that so often derail people's attempts to lose weight. Losing weight is hard to do when you're hungry. Here's where satiety plays a role. Satiety means not getting hungry until it's time for the next meal in a few hours' time.

One of the downfalls for people who want to lose weight is lack of satiety. When a meal does not provide real satiety you become hungry sooner after you've eaten, and you tend to eat more at the next meal.

When a meal gives you feelings of both satiation and satiety, you are likely to eat less food and feel fuller for longer after the meal is over. If you continue eating less food and feeling less hungry over a given period of time, you are more likely to lose weight.

One of the secrets to losing weight is to achieve prolonged satiety while eating a wider range of nutritious, Calorie-sparse foods. In this way you can reduce your energy intake without having to feel deprived, without having to exert tremendous willpower, and while boosting your general health.

Satiety often seems hard to achieve. You might eat a Calorie-dense meal which you'd expect would provide satiety because it's so packed with energy, only to find your appetite returning not long afterwards.

If you frequently feel hungry you're more likely to seek out snacks, and those snacks are likely to be high in Calories.

Knowing how to achieve satiety is critical for weight loss.

HUNGER IS NOT YOUR ENEMY

Hunger is your body's way of ensuring that you get the Calories you need for survival. Yet for people who want to lose weight, hunger seems to be the worst enemy.

We all know that we could lose weight simply by eating less food, or eating low Calorie food, but the more we try to deny ourselves, the hungrier we get. What's more, the hungrier we get, the more our bodies drive us to overeat, which in turn causes weight gain.

It appears that trying to lose weight by avoiding food just has the opposite effect.

Of course, the best way to stop feeling hungry is to eat. The trick for weight loss is to learn how to assuage hunger and reach satiety while consuming as few Calories as possible, and that's what this book is about.

THE SATIETY DIET CAN HELP YOU ACHIEVE SATIETY

There are many factors that can boost satiety and help weight loss. Researchers have found that our sensitivity to satiety signals can actually be changed, not only by physical substances such as the hormones insulin and leptin, but by social, learned, and environmental factors as well. In this book we provide tips for reaching and prolonging satiety, using science-based methods.

Your body sends internal signals and also communicates with your environment using the silent language of body-speech. You can use these signals to help you reach satiety.

Most human beings were born with their satiety signals functioning normally. People whose lives are shaped by western culture and who eat according to the Western Dietary Pattern have been exposed, over time, to certain foods, ingredients, food additives, commercial advertising and a host of other elements which may have desensitized, overridden and invalidated their natural satiety signals, making them lose touch with their body's internal language. This has led to a health crisis on a grand scale.

Despite the fact that there are so many complex mechanisms regulating our energy intake, many of us continue to eat even after we feel satiated, or stop ourselves from eating even when we feel hungry. This is because the other elements that affect our eating behavior are so numerous, complex, nuanced and interactive.

Sometimes people become deaf to their body's satiety signals. That's when they are in danger of gaining an unhealthy amount of weight.

Hunger and appetite triggers can cause you to ignore satiety signals. They include such factors as your emotional condition, portion size, food variety, and social situations.

You can communicate with your Inner Guardians to reverse this desensitization and invalidation. By recognizing your satiety signals you can reset them to their normal configuration. Using the vast resources of this book and the tips in *The Satiety Diet Weight Loss Toolkit* (book #2 in the Satiety Diet series), you can stay on track, continuing to use your knowledge of satiety signals to help you lose weight and stay slim.

SATIETY: HOW TO GET IT!

FACTORS THAT INFLUENCE SATIETY

The feeling of satiety is not simply produced by the physiological effects of nutrients in the digestive system. It's not only the characteristics of the food you eat that play a part. It's also your environment, your thoughts and beliefs, your mindset and your senses of sight, taste, smell, touch and hearing.

In other words, satiety is regulated by a mixture of psychological processes, sensory experiences and signals generated by your body.

The way these factors interact with each other can determine how satiating a food will be.

". . . contextual cues from cognitive and sensory signals generated at the time of consumption influence the consumer's experience of satiety and also, critically, moderate nutrient-based satiety." [Chambers et al. (2015)]

The nutrients in foods have a huge impact on how much satiety they provide. Whether or not a particular food produces feelings of satiety depends on many things, such as the amount of protein, carbohydrate, fat and fiber it contains. Foods rich in protein and fiber produce better satiety.

Even before you ingest food, however, other things can affect how well that food will satisfy your appetite. These things are all interconnected. If one is neglected, the others may be thrown out of balance.

Factors that influence satiety can include the following:

PSYCHOLOGICAL FACTORS

Satiety begins before the first bite.

Even before you start eating a meal, your body is receiving signals that affect satiety. Everything you see, smell, hear, taste, think and feel before, during and even after a meal can affect how much satiety that meal will give you after the meal is over. It can also influence how much food you eat before you reach satiation.

" . . . These early satiety signals will integrate with post-ingestive and post-absorptive signals to determine satiety." [Chambers et el. (2015)] [Halford & Harrold (2012)]

When you sit down in front of a meal, ready to eat, your Inner Guardian receives signals about food through your senses and thoughts. These signals, passing back and forth between your brain and the rest of your body, tell your digestive system to expect the arrival of nutrients.

Before you even take the first bite, your body has already registered the sensory characteristics of the food in front of you—its shape and color, its smell, its probable texture and so on. Your brain will already have taken note of the environment in which you are going to eat this food, and retrieved any existing knowledge and memories about how wonderful or awful that food tastes, and how good for you or bad for you it is.

With all this input flooding in, your digestive system responds by preparing itself to receive the food. Your Inner Guardian wants you to process the forthcoming nutrients as efficiently as possible. It wants to prime your body to get the maximum benefit out of your food. Therefore, it begins to release various digestive hormones and secretions, and tells your stomach to make ready to start churning and various muscles of your digestive system to get ready to open and close.

Research suggests that the body's responses to food even before you eat intensifies the after-meal feelings of satiety by increasing the efficiency of digestion and ensuring that the body absorbs and metabolizes nutrients as best it can.

This is why your pre-eating experience is one of the key elements for weight loss!

Tip: Use positive pre-meal experiences to prolong satiety.
Before you eat, admire your food; smell it, enjoy the colors and the arrangements of the table and the plate. Think about how nutritious and filling and tasty your food will be. Imprint the memory of this meal on your mind, even before you take the first bite.
This will help you enjoy the meal more.
Preserving the pleasant sensory memory of your meal both before you eat it and while you are eating it, may also help you say satiated for longer after the meal is over.

Expectations of food can change your satiety response.

Why do marketing researchers ask people about their expectations of a food product? Because the mind is so powerful that it can influence and even override physiological processes. As part of a study published in *The American Journal of Clinical Nutrition*, people were given, over a period of four days,

- a cherry-flavored drink that they were told would form a gel in their stomachs
- a cherry-flavored drink
- cherry-flavored firm gelatin cubes that they were told would stay in their solid form in their stomachs
- cherry-flavored firm gelatin cubes that they were told would turn to liquid in their stomachs [Cassady et al. (2012)]

None of these drinks and foods really *would* turn to a gel in their stomachs. That was a falsehood told to the subjects of the experiment to see whether their thoughts alone could influence their experience of the comestibles. The gelatin cubes, however, would turn to liquid when they reached the stomach.

The drink and the gelatin cubes contained the same amount of Calories, nutrients and flavor. Only the texture was different (and the people's expectations). The researchers also used other techniques to make sure there were no other variables in the study.

The results?

When people ate the solid food (the gelatin cubes):
- they reported feeling less hungry
- the food passed through their digestive system more slowly
- they had lower levels of the hunger hormone, ghrelin
- their levels of satiety hormones and neurotransmitters also changed
- on that day, they ate less food afterwards

But more remarkably, when they believed that the gelatin cubes would stay solid in their stomachs, all those satiety responses listed above were heightened!

Their thoughts powerfully influenced their satiety levels.

This result supports the concept that even before you start to eat, your satiety response is influenced by:
- the way you think about the food (cognitive information)
- the way the food looks and its texture etc. (sensory information)

Knowledge about food.

You now know that your perception of foods while you are eating them, and even before and after you eat them, can influence satiety. Satisfaction can also be enhanced by what you know about the food's nutrients, composition, characteristics etc., whether learned from the food's labeling or by other means. The appetite-reducing characteristics of lower Calorie foods can actually be boosted by giving people reasons to believe the food is satiating. Before you eat a particular food, you instinctively judge how satiating it will be, based on how it looks. Before you swallow it, you form beliefs about how satiating it will be based on how it feels in the mouth. These appraisals, made even before the food arrives in your stomach, actually play a hugely important part in appetite control.

The diner's state of mind.

Your general state of mind when you eat a meal plays a role in how much satiety you might get from your food.

Factors that can influence your state of mind include:
- your previous sleep quality
- your stress levels
- any cravings you might be experiencing
- your past dietary habits

Characteristics of meals.

Certain other variables affect how much satiety a meal will provide. These include:
- meal timing
- meal composition
- meal duration
- the quality of the dining environment
- the diner's expectations
- lighting
- sound
- characteristics of the tableware (if any)
- food quantity
- food presentation

Food labels: Perceptions of food.

Your perception of food can influence how much you eat, and how much satiety you get from that food. Food manufacturers use the labels on processed foods to influence the way consumers think about the food and even the way it looks. They employ words and images to moderate our cognitive and sensory perception of the food.

"The labels on foods and the beliefs that individuals have about the satisfaction derived from particular foods can affect food intake." [Rolls (1995)]

If belief alone can change people's satiety responses, as shown by the cherry-flavored food study published in *The American Journal of Clinical Nutrition*, then it's worthwhile for food manufacturers to make us believe good things about their products.

Labels also have a stronger effect on our satiety expectations when they provide nutritional information about the food.

Food labels usually provide a list of nutrients as well as a short blurb or catch-phrase stating something positive indicating how you should feel after eating the product, such as "really satisfying," "fuels your body," or "keeps you going". There may be some blurb about food characteristics that are associated with satiety, such a "high protein," or "high fiber".

It's been shown that this kind of food labeling really can influence not only how much of the food product people will eat, but also whether they eat more or less of other foods later the same day.

"For example, lunch intake was higher after consuming a high Calorie yoghurt labeled low-fat compared to when no information was presented on the yoghurt; after consuming a beverage presented as a high Calorie milkshake, participants reported feeling fuller and eating less at a test meal than when this information was not present; and branding a fruit 'smoothie' beverage with a high satiety message enhanced subjective reports of fullness and reduced hunger." [Chambers et al. (2015)]

It's not just people's eating behavior and their reporting of hunger levels that support the idea that food labels can influence the satiety response.

A 2011 study entitled "Mind over milkshakes: mindsets, not just nutrients, determine ghrelin response" found that when a milkshake was labeled as "620-Calorie indulgent", the hunger hormone levels of the people who drank it plummeted. When people drank a milkshake made to exactly the same recipe but labeled "120-Calorie sensible", their hunger hormone levels still dropped, but not as sharply. [Crum et al. (2011)]

A 1992 study tested the hypothesis that the way people perceive the fat content of foods might influence how much they eat. Just before lunch, people were given one of two containers of yoghurt, both the same volume. Both the yoghurts contained the same number of Calories, but one was labeled "low-fat" and the other labeled "high-fat."

The people who ate the yogurt labeled "low-fat" ate a lot more for lunch than the people who ate the "high fat" yogurt. [Rolls et al. (1992)]

Other research [Marriott (1995)] has looked at people's opinion of pudding packaged in three different ways:

- Commercial (with many bright colors and attractive, realistic images)
- Military (with printed text, in only two or three colors such as brown, black and khaki)
- Neutral (functionally designed, few-color packaging with some text and small, simple images)

The pudding inside the packaging was all the same, but people rated the pudding in the military packaging as tasting worse than the others, and they ate less of it.

Neuroimaging techniques using machines called fMRI scanners can show researchers what's going on inside the living brain.

Based on previous studies that showed how intensely people's expectations and beliefs could affect their brain's response to food, scientists at the John B. Pierce Laboratory in Connecticut scanned the brains of people who were looking at food labels. They found that ". . . descriptions creating beliefs about the healthy or hedonic [pleasurable] properties of a beverage can strongly influence neural [brain] response. Labeling a low-Calorie drink as a 'treat' produces brain response resembling those elicited by an actual treat". [Veldhuizen et al. (2013)]

The power of your senses is stronger than the power of food labels.

Food labels, however, don't have as much power to influence you as food's sensory characteristics. Even if the labels on two beverages both tell you "this drink reduces appetite", you are going to feel more satiated after consuming the thick and creamy beverage than the thin, less creamy one. [Chambers et al., (2013)].

Food manufacturers know that while food labels can have some influence on boosting satiety, making foods more nutritious and manipulating their sensory characteristics can make them even more satiety-inducing.

Get happy for satiety.
Serotonin promotes satiety.

Serotonin, like dopamine, is a neurotransmitter that plays a role in satiety. This biological compound chiefly abounds in the gastro-intestinal tract, the blood-stream, and the central nervous system. It has several important functions, including the regulation of mood, appetite, and sleep. It also affects some cognitive functions such as memory and the ability to learn. [de Matos Feijó et al., (2011)]

Serotonin can promote satiety. Studies have shown that when people are dosed with drugs that enhance their serotonin levels, they tend to eat more slowly and consume less food, which suggests that the extra serotonin in their systems "specifically enhanced" satiation and satiety. [Simansky (1995)]

So effective is serotonin at helping weight loss that serotonergic appetite suppressants such as fenfluramine (Pondimin) and chlor-phentermine were once prescribed to treat obese patients. They gave the patients a feeling of satiety and reduced appetite. However these drugs are no longer licensed as weight loss aids, chiefly because:
- Some people were using them as recreational drugs.
- The artificial surge of serotonin had unwanted side effects.
- Some people were overdosing, and seriously damaging their health.

The antidepressant properties of serotonin can help with weight loss.

Boosting your serotonin levels may do more than merely enhance your feelings of satiety. When serotonin is circulating in the brain, it also works as an antidepressant. Drugs that act on brain serotonin levels are used in the treatment of depression, raising levels of happiness and reducing anxiety. Being in a good mood can protect you from both mental *and* physical disorders. Positive feelings and geniality encourage cordial relationships with other people, which can boost your social network and increase your support from friends and relatives. All of these side-benefits of serotonin can function to boost weight loss.

When people feel happy, they are more likely to:
- eat well
- exercise more
- have lower levels of anxiety, and thus lower levels of the stress hormone, cortisol
- experience fewer cravings for fattening "comfort foods"
- experience fewer cravings for sugary, high-energy foods

How to boost your serotonin levels without drugs.

95% of the body's serotonin exists in the gut, and it's this serotonin that can influence appetite and satiety. Meanwhile, it's the serotonin in the brain that can influence mood, and boost happiness. It's harder to get serotonin into the brain than it is to get it into your bowels, because of the "blood-brain barrier" that protects the brain.

For the best chance of weight loss, it's in our interests to boost serotonin in both the gut and the brain.

Neuroscientist Dr. Alex Korb says, " . . . four ways to boost serotonin activity are sunlight, massage, exercise, and remembering happy events." [Korb (2011)]

Certain foods may also boost serotonin levels, and your microbiome also plays an important role. This is why kefir and prebiotics can make a difference.

86

1. Be exposed to bright sunlight.

The brain produces more serotonin on sunny days than on overcast days. [Lancet (2002)]

This does not mean you have to put in a swimsuit and lie on a beach! It simply means that exposed to intense sunshine is a powerful way to elevate your serotonin levels and improve your mood. The sunlight does not even have to touch your skin—when bright (not direct[8]) daylight enters your eyes, it triggers a serotonin response in your body. So potent is this effect that bright sunlight can be as effective as antidepressants.

Sunlight shining through a window into a room is not as really bright enough to make a difference, so ideally you should get your daily dose of sunlight outdoors. Care should be taken not to overdo sun exposure, because when the skin absorbs too much ultraviolet radiation, there is a risk of skin cancer.

[Golden et al., (2005); Epperson et al., (2004); Lambert et al., (2002)]

2. Indulge in massage therapy.

The mechanism behind the value of massage therapy is not fully explained, but study after study has reported on the positive, measurable effect of massage on serotonin (and dopamine) levels. Massage can also improve the quality of sleep and reduce pain and anxiety. [Field et al., (2005)]

Can't afford a masseur, or your friends and family are not into giving you a free massage? You can easily practice self-massage using your hands or a foam roller. Use a little sweet almond oil or lavender oil to help your hands glide across your body. Or if you have access to a spa-bath, the jets of water can have a wonderful massaging effect on your muscles.

---

8   Never look directly at the sun.

3. Exercise aerobically.

Numerous studies over several years have suggested that exercise, particularly vigorous physical "aerobic" exercise, improves mood and reduces anxiety by raising serotonin levels. [Salmon (2001)]

So effective does exercise seem to be at reducing depression that government institutions recommend it as a treatment for patients who are depressed. [NIHCE (2007)]

It is thought that the mood-lifting effect happens because exercise boosts serotonin levels in the brain. [Post et al., (1973); Chaouloff et al., (1985); Wilson & Marsden (1996); Béquet et al., (2001); Meeusen et al., (2001)]

4. Think happy thoughts and remember happy events.

It might sound far-fetched, but your thoughts can actually change your brain. Your thoughts affect the chemical and electrical processes in your brain and, if you continue to have the same thoughts repeatedly, they can even affect the structure of your brain. Positive thoughts can help raise your levels of serotonin. [Perreau-Linck et al., (2007)]

" . . . alterations in thought, either self-induced or due to psychotherapy, can alter brain metabolism . . . " [Young (2007)]

It may not be easy, however, to just switch on happy thoughts at will. To encourage happy thoughts, try watching a humorous movie or TV show, listening to a comedy radio show or podcast, or reading a funny book, or socializing with people who like to have a good laugh.

Photographs can help you remember joyful events, as can talking about happy times with people who shared those times with you.

5. Keep your population of gut microbes healthy and diverse.

The microbial inhabitants of your gut provide a strong barrier to defend the walls of your intestines, preventing toxins and pathogens from getting into your bloodstream. In addition, they break down your food to help you absorb nutrients. And they do even more than that—they stimulate the neural pathways linking your gut and your brain.

The billions of microorganisms living in your gut have a powerful impact on the way your neurons and neurotransmitters work. Almost all of your serotonin is produced in your gastrointestinal tract. The walls of your gut are covered with millions of neurons (nerve cells), which pass messages back and forth to your brain, so it follows that your gut neurons can influence your mood.

When you populate your GI tract with a wide range of beneficial bacteria, you give it the best chance of producing higher levels of neurotransmitters, including serotonin. And how do you create a healthy, diverse microbiome?

- Eat plenty of all kinds of fiber. This provides the environment in which microbes thrive.
- Enjoy a widely varied diet, to encourage a widely varied microbe population.
- Consume prebiotic kefir and probiotics, which may enhance the microbiome.
- Try eating small amounts of protein in combination with carbohydrates.

6. Consume foods containing tryptophan.

Serotonin is also known as 5-hydroxytryptamine, or 5-HT.[9] For your body to manufacture serotonin, it needs to obtain molecules of 5-HTP, which is a chemical by-product of the amino acid called tryptophan. Amino acids are found within proteins. So when you eat any form of protein—such as chia seeds, chickpeas or pepitas, for

---

9   It's important to distinguish 5-HT from 5-HTP, which is 5-Hydroxytryptophan. The two abbreviations look very similar, but the compound 5-HTP is a serotonin "precursor", which means that it participates in a chemical reaction that produces serotonin.

example—it's very likely that you are getting some tryptophan.

Your body converts tryptophan into 5-HTP, and then converts 5-HTP into serotonin (in addition to another neurotransmitter, melatonin, which regulates sleep).

You can get tryptophan into your body by eating foods that contain it, such as walnuts, spirulina, roasted soybeans, sesame seeds and chick peas. Consuming these foods can raise your gut's serotonin levels quite readily.

Eating tryptophan-rich foods, however, may *not* immediately and directly raise your brain's serotonin levels. And it's the serotonin in your brain that can work as an antidepressant.

Beware of the turkey myth!

There's a popular myth that turkey has high levels of tryptophan and that eating it will make you feel sleepy. The truth is that turkey does not contain any more tryptophan than any other protein source. In fact, eating turkey may actually lower the tryptophan available to your brain. This is due to the fact that all the amino acids use the same method to get through your blood-brain barrier, a protective membrane that stops undesirable stuff from entering your brain and only allows the beneficial stuff through. Tryptophan has to jostle with all the other amino acids, competing with them to get through this barrier. Yet tryptophan is the scarcest amino acid, generally outnumbered by the others, and the more of the other amino acids that are entering the brain, the less tryptophan manages to get through. Turkey and other meats contain the full range of amino acids, so any tryptophan they contain doesn't have a very good chance of making it into your brain to be converted to serotonin. It's the same with many other foods that contain tryptophan, such as warm milk and salmon.

7. Eat carbs with small portions of protein

Eating carbs with small portions of protein can boost tryptophan. While eating large amounts of protein can *decrease* the amount of tryptophan available to the brain, studies suggest that combining carbohydrates with small amounts of protein can *boost* it. When you eat carbohydrates your body responds by releasing insulin, which redirects the more common amino acids into your muscles without affecting tryptophan. This means that tryptophan has less competition and is more easily able to enter the brain to begin the conversion to serotonin.

"To some extent, tryptophan availability to the brain can be enhanced by ingestion of carbohydrates and reduced by ingestion of proteins." [Richard et al., (2009)]

Simon Young, Ph.D., research psychologist at McGill University, says that to achieve this effect the amount of protein has to be pretty small. "When you eat a mixture of protein and carbohydrate, you don't need very much protein in there to counteract the carbohydrate effect," he says. "In any real meal that you'll take in, the effects of protein will predominate, and you'll get a decrease in the ratio of tryptophan to other amino acids." [Strand (2003)]

"Consuming tryptophan or a carbohydrate-rich, protein-poor meal increases brain levels of tryptophan and serotonin," concludes researcher B.J. Spring, Professor of Preventive Medicine, Psychology, Psychiatry and Behavioral Sciences, based at Northwestern University in the USA. [Spring (1984)]

Can you have too much tryptophan and serotonin?

Some people take tryptophan supplements in an effort to boost their levels of brain serotonin. We don't recommend the use of supplements. If you do take them, make sure the tryptophan supplements are pure, and manufactured by a reputable company.

Taking tryptophan supplements can lead to the risk of overdosing. Studies have shown that a constant elevated level of serotonin in the bones is linked to osteoporosis. Having too much serotonin in your system is also dangerous, as it can cause "serotonin syndrome".

It would be virtually impossible to overdose on tryptophan by eating tryptophan-rich foods.

And why spend money on manufactured substances when you can raise your brain and gut serotonin levels simply by going outside into the sunshine, exercising, thinking happy thoughts, having a massage or eating a carbohydrate-rich, low-protein meal?

Gorge on happiness instead of Calories.

Pleasure is one of the keys to satiety. Low levels of the so-called "happiness hormone" dopamine (the neurotransmitter that helps regulate your brain's reward and pleasure centers) have been associated with increased appetite.

To help explain how this mechanism works, we must first discuss leptin, the "satiety hormone".

When leptin was first purified in 1995 by geneticist Jeffrey Friedman, scientists became excited at the prospect of administering it to obese patients to help them lose weight.

The treatment, however, didn't work.

Despite high leptin levels, some laboratory animals (and humans) continued to eat and gain weight. They were "leptin resistant". [Myers (2015)] (Interestingly, when leptin-resistant rats who were gaining weight on a high-fat diet were given some moderate exercise, their leptin became more active and their weight and food consumption stabilized.)

So-called leptin resistance can be generated by:
- obesity
- a high-fat diet
- the process of aging (beginning in middle age)

Research is now beginning to suggest that the leptin does much more than just regulate appetite by giving you the sensation of fullness. It may also affect the reward centers in your brain, increasing or decreasing your desire for food and heightening or reducing the pleasurability of eating. [Berthoud (2011)]

Professor Christopher D. Morrison, co-author of a 2016 study, says that scientists are turning to the study of the way appetite is affected by not just homeostatic mechanisms (the body's attempts to balance energy expended with Calories consumed) but also by hedonic mechanisms (the body's search for pleasure).

"The brain doesn't just tell us whether we're hungry or full," he says. "We eat for other reasons, including pleasure, and in obesity that may play an important role." [Berthoud et al., (2016)]

Morrison's study suggests that many of the physiological reasons we over-eat are outside of our awareness, which is why trying to use "self-restraint" so often fails.

A 2009 study published in the journal *Cell Metabolism* supports the hypothesis that one of the ways leptin governs appetite is by making us perceive food as being more or less desirable. [Leinninger et al., (2009)]

Dopamine.

And here's where the "happiness hormone" dopamine[10] enters the picture. Leptin can increase dopamine levels, which in turn can decrease appetite. When researchers injected leptin into the brains of mice, it led to an increase in the amount of dopamine in the brain's reward system. The mice ate less food and quickly lost weight.

Professor Martin Myers, one of the researchers, notes that addictive drugs such as cocaine and amphetamines, which drastically elevate dopamine levels, also act as powerful appetite-suppressants.

The administration of leptin to the brain also appears to have an anti-depressant effect on laboratory mice. [Sherman (2009)]

Myers says, "The problem in obesity isn't a lack of satiety signaling, but over-response to the rewarding foods that continually surround us." In other words, we are surrounded by foods that, when eaten, stimulate elevated levels of feel-good dopamine. And we tend to chase that good feeling by overeating.

---

10   Dopamine can act as both a hormone and a neurotransmitter.

For ethical reasons the same experiment hasn't been performed on humans, but what if we could flood our own brains with dopamine, raising its base-line level just as injected leptin does to mice? What if we could help suppress our appetite by doing things to make us feel happy?

For suggestions on "how to increase dopamine naturally," see Book #2 in the Satiety Diet series, *The Satiety Diet Weight Loss Toolkit.*

SENSORY CHARACTERISTICS OF FOOD

Definitions.

We've added some definitions in this section, to help readers better understand the terminology.

1. Orosensory.

This is a word that describes the mouth's experience of food— its taste, texture, temperature etc. How well a food suppresses your appetite after you eat it depends largely on the orosensory experience of eating. [Cecil et al., (1998)]

In fact, food's palatability (i.e. how good it tastes) isn't as important to satiety as its orosensory characteristics. [Sorensen et al., (1999), de Graaf et al., (1999)]

2. The difference between taste and flavor.

Taste is the sensation produced when a substance in your mouth reacts chemically with taste receptor cells located on your taste buds. Taste happens mostly on your tongue, but also in other parts of your mouth where taste buds are located. Your taste buds are sensitive to at least five tastes— sweet, sour, salt, bitter, and umami. (Umami has been described as "savory", or "meaty".)

". . . the sense of taste is a nutrient sensor which informs the brain and the gut about the inflow of nutrients. The sense of taste has an important contribution to the satiating effect of foods." [de Graaf (2019)]

Flavor, on the other hand, is a "hedonic" sense, meaning a sense that relates to pleasure. It is is the pleasurable (or unpleasant) sensation you get when you experience a substance in your mouth. Flavor is your brain's final analysis of the food in your mouth, based mainly on the inputs of taste and aroma.

Your perception of flavor involves not only taste but also mouthfeel (texture and consistency), smell, temperature and your expectations.

Perhaps you are wondering, *can my expectations really affect flavor?* Indeed they can, and significantly! One study found that adding more red coloring to a drink made of sugar and water increased people's perception of the drink's sweetness. The volunteers participating in the study also rated darker colored drinks as being 2–10% sweeter than lighter ones, even though their concentration of sugar was 1% less. [Johnson & Clydesdale (2006)]

The flavors of food are determined by a mingling of:
- Taste
- Smell—if you've lost your sense of smell, you might notice that food flavors seem bland.
- Trigeminal nerve stimulation—The trigeminal nerve is responsible for functions such as biting and chewing. It's this nerve that registers food texture and temperature.

3. Neurogastronomy.

This is the name given to a field of science that studies the way people's brains perceive food. Research in this field examines, among other things, the part our senses play in eating, dining and general food appreciation.

4. Eating vs Dining.

Note that "eating" is considered to be the process of merely feeding your body, while "dining" is the experience of eating. Dining can include social elements, food appreciation, the setting, how the food is presented, its colors and textures, how it makes you feel and even how the food is grown. All these elements can contribute to the way you experience food.

Food's sensory characteristics.

Food comes from diverse sources, in an assortment of shapes and colors, and provides a wide range of nutrients. It's not just the nutrients in food, but food's sensory characteristics that are thought to be even more important, psychologically, for achieving satiety. These characteristics include taste intensity, flavor profile, texture, consistency, smell and appearance.

Most people would say that we humans have five senses—sight, hearing, taste touch and smell. These days, neuroscientists say we have many more than that—between 22 and 33. For the purposes of this book, we'll limit the discussion to the well-known five.

Your brain's neurological links between taste, smell, touch, hearing and sight all make an impact on your experiences of food and dining.

The act of eating is more than simply shoveling food into your mouth in order to keep yourself alive. There is a whole lot more going on, involving interactions between your senses—which receive the sounds and feelings and tastes and smells of food—and your brain, which interprets those sensations.

When you eat, signals travel from your nose, your teeth, the roots of your teeth, your tongue, the muscles and bones of your jaws, your nerves, your sensors, and all other parts of your mouth to your brain. Your Inner Guardian receives reports on taste, texture, smell, and a huge range of subtle clues regarding the foreign substances (food) entering your body.

For example, if sweetness is detected in your mouth, your Inner Guardian tells your body to produce the hormone insulin. A sweet taste indicates that sugar is entering your body, and it's insulin that regulates blood sugar.[11]

For satiety and weight loss, it is important to vary the flavors, smells, shapes, colors, temperatures and textures of your food. Eating should be a pleasant, multi-sensory experience.

11　The Inner Guardian's ancient language has no signal to differentiate between artificial sweeteners and natural ones such as sugar and honey. Therefore insulin may be released in any case.

In this section we will discuss the sensory characteristics of food and how you can exploit these characteristics to get the best satiety from healthful, Calorie-sparse foods. When low energy-density foods satisfy you and keep hunger at bay, it is easier to lose weight.

Why food's sensory characteristics are important.

Why is it that the sensory characteristics of a meal can be more important for satiety than the food's nutrients?

Research shows that when you truly believe super-healthful foods will give you the best feelings of satiety, that's exactly what happens!

And by the same reasoning, if you eat super-healthful foods in a way that makes you feel the food won't satisfy you, then you're unlikely to reach satiety.

Here's a good example: Sometimes patients in hospitals are unable to eat normally, so doctors insert a "nasogastric tube" to feed them. This is a plastic tube that passes through one of the nostrils and runs down the esophagus into the stomach. Specially formulated runny food, packed with vitamins, minerals and macronutrients, can then be pumped into the patient's stomach. The patient, however, never chews the food, never feels the food in his or her mouth, never tastes the food and generally doesn't smell it, either. There is no plate involved, no knife or fork or spoon; none of the accoutrements of a normal meal. The liquidized food looks like slush.

It's easy to understand that people who are fed this way have weak satiety responses to food. It's hard for them to feel satisfied after one of these meals, despite the fact that their stomachs are stretching as the food fills them up, and the food is rich in a wide variety of nutrients.

Sense #1: Sight.
Experiencing food through the eyes.

Most people would probably say that it's the taste of food that determines whether they eat a lot of it or not. However taste is not our first sensory contact with food. Before we taste it, we see it.

Just the sight of food alone can make people want to eat that food, because it activates parts of the brain and neural pathways that are linked with "reward". [Bajaj (2013)]

The Chinese have a saying: "You eat first with your eyes, then your nose, then your mouth." The Japanese, too, strongly believe in the value of food's visual presentation.

"We eat with our eyes" because the way food looks gives us cues as to how it probably tastes and feels in the mouth. If the food looks appetizing, we expect it to taste good. If the food looks unappealing, we expect it to taste bad.

These prejudices actually influence your brain. When you take a bite of the food, your senses are affected by your thoughts. Good-looking food (and drink) is likely to taste better; bad-looking food is likely to taste worse. The way food looks can even influence the way you perceive its flavor and mouthfeel.

Many things can affect food's appearance, including color, texture, presentation (e.g. tableware) and different methods of preparation.

Several studies have involved participants wearing virtual reality headsets while eating. Using this technology the participants ate one food while simultaneously looking at another. They then reported on their experience, and the results showed that "changing the visual appearance of the food was shown to dramatically modify the taste, as well as the perceived texture, of foods . . . " [Choi et al., (2014), Narumi et al., (2012), Okajima & Spence (2011), Okajima et al., (2013), Schöning et al., (2012), Swerdloff (2015), Victor(2015a]

The sight and smell of food.

The sight (and smell) of food can trigger digestive processes. Even before any food has touched your lips, even without the presence of actual food, your body physically responds to the sight or smell of food in a variety of complex ways. Hormones such as insulin and ghrelin can be released in response to the sight or smell of food. [Wadhera & Capaldi-Phillips (2014), Bossert-Zaudig et al., (2016)]

"Visual exposure to food elicits the physiological release of saliva and other regulatory peptides required for digestion," says Devina Bajaj, author of the 2013 Arizona State University dissertation "Effect of Number of Food Pieces on Food Selection and Consumption in Animals and Humans".

In other words, as soon as you set eyes on food—or even images of food—your eyes send signals to your brain, which in turn sends signals to your digestive system to "Get ready for incoming nutrition!" Your body begins to secrete the substances necessary for digestion. These substances include saliva, which contains enzymes that begin the process of breaking down the food. [Pedersen et al., (2001), Keesman et al., (2016)].

Images of food.

Seeing pictures of food has the same effect on the brain as seeing real food.

It doesn't matter to your Inner Guardian whether your eyes are seeing genuine food, a colorful plastic model of food, or a picture of food. Its ancient language evolved long before the advent of magazines TV, movies, photographs, video, books, newspapers, illustrations, paintings, billboards and other media that can convey vibrant, realistic pictures of food. In fact the pictures don't even have to be all that realistic… they can be black and white engravings, or semi-abstract sketches. If your brain interprets a picture as being about food, your Inner Guardian may awaken hunger in response.

Hunger makes food look better.

Our brains are wired to seek food when we are hungry and to be less enthusiastic about it when we've reached satiety.

This means that when you are hungry, not only does actually food taste better and smell better, it also looks better to you. [Critchley & Rolls (1996)]

Using sight for satiety

Here are some tips on using the sight of food to your advantage:

1. Visual presentation and mindfulness.

To achieve the best satiety, make your meals look as interesting and satisfying as possible, and really notice the food you're eating.

2. Look at your entire meal before you eat.

When you sit down to begin a meal it is important to take in the sight of all your courses simultaneously displayed in front of you. This manner of dining is called "*service à la Française*," that is, "service in the French style". It contrasts with "*service à la Russe*," which means "service in the Russian style", a format of food presentation in which courses are brought to the table one by one, in sequence.

Absorb the sight of the food you are about to eat. Your Inner Guardian can read your mind's reaction to what your eyes see. When you look at your entire meal you are seeing the sight of food abundance. You are seeing food's various colors and shapes. Look at the condiments, the dishes and side-dishes and accoutrements such as table settings; table napkins, perhaps a vase of flowers, the tablecloth. Make an occasion of every meal, so that the Guardian *knows* you've eaten and knows you've eaten *well*. In body-speech, this is reassurance that there is *plenty* of food available in the environment.

3. Eat beautiful food.

The Satiety Diet gives you many weight loss tools. Eating good-looking meals helps you reach satiety. It also helps you to remember the last meal you ate, by making it easier and pleasanter to recall a visual image of it, which is one of our weight-loss strategies. Furthermore, eating beautiful food may help you to eat more slowly and mindfully—another powerful weight loss tactic.

You can make food look its best in your own home kitchen.

Beautiful food

When chefs arrange food artistically on a plate they refer to their actions as "plating". They know that the way food is plated has a profound impact on how much diners enjoy the food.

Some of the elements important to attractive plating are:

- The way we perceive the association between color and flavor
- Other uses of color
- Whether to arrange the food on the plate centrally or off to one side
- The orientation of foods on the plate
- The number of foods on the plate (odd or even numbers)
- The number of colors on the plate

Beautiful food: The way you associate color and flavor.

In 2014, researchers asked 452 participants from various countries and cultures around the world to look at images of color patches, shapes and textures, and to select the flavor/taste adjective that best described the image. They reported that most people strongly associated white with "salty", red with "sweet", green with "sour" and black with "bitter". Other studies have shown that people may also associate yellow with "sour", possibly due to the color and taste of lemons. [Wan et al., (2014)]

Find out more about food colors in the section "Colorful Foods".

Beautiful food: Arrangement on the plate.

Many chefs favour artistically placing food towards one side of the plate, and leaving a space on the other side empty. Jozef Youssef founder of the gastronomic project "Kitchen Theory", tested 600 diners to find out whether they preferred their food to be served in the middle of the plate or over to one side. They found that "respondents did indeed have a clear preference, and it was towards central plating."

Beautiful food: The orientation of foods on the plate.

A 2014 study looked at whether positioning food artistically on a plate would influence the diner's expectations and thereby change their experience of the food.

A salad was positioned on a plate in one of three different arrangements:

- Just served onto the plate in no particular way, with all the ingredients jumbled together.
- With all the ingredients placed in ways that made them resemble a painting by the Russian abstract artist Kandinsky.
- With the ingredients set out on the plate in an orderly but inartistic arrangement (imagine a military-style line-up of ingredients).

Before they ate the food, the study's participants said they liked the look of the food on the artistic plates better than the food on the other plates. They also said they'd be willing to pay more for it if they were eating out! After they'd eaten, the participants said they liked the flavor of the artistic food better than that of the other plated foods.

The researchers concluded that, in support of earlier findings, these results showed that displaying food attractively could improve people's enjoyment of it. "… In particular, the use of artistic (visual) influences can enhance a diner's rating of the flavor of a dish." Beautifully presented food can affect your expectations, which in turn affects your experience of eating the food. [Michel et al., (2014)]

What—you're not a Russian abstract artist? You failed Art in high school? Don't despair. We all possess artistic intuition. In the home kitchen, just arrange food on plates in a way that appeals to your eye. Have confidence in your own aesthetic taste. With practice, you'll get better at it.

Here's a tip: Use contrasting colors in your plating arrangement. Colors can help make your plateful of food more beautiful. Contrasting colors such as the pink of strawberries and the purple of blueberries, or the scarlet of tomatoes and the vibrant greens of salad leaves will add to the attractiveness of a dish.

Beautiful food: Odd or even numbers.

Most people find odd numbers of food elements on their plate more attractive than even numbers. So, for example, put 1, 3 or 5 cherry tomatoes in your artistic salad. [Woods et al., (2016)]

Beautiful food: Table decoration and layout

A beautifully laid out table, attractively decorated, can greatly add to your enjoyment of a meal.

Beautiful food: Use a variety of interesting tablewares. [12]

The shape, color, size and style of tableware (also called dinnerware or crockery) also affect the way diners perceive and enjoy meals. Professional chefs take great care in choosing tableware that enhances the appearance and the "feeling" of their dishes. As Jozef Youssef says, "Just think about it; would sushi taste as appealing when served on a plain white circular plate? Would Irish stew taste the same if served from a tagine?" [Youssef (2015)]

Colorful foods

Eat colorful foods. Color is closely associated with the attractiveness of different foods. The mere sight of food activates neurons in the hypothalamus of the brain. People who eat in the dark, or who eat blindfolded, lose much of the pleasure in their food.

Food of varied colors and rich, vibrant colors can make your meal look more appealing, taste better and have more satiety-power. Monotone meals comprising, say, beige-colored potatoes, beige cauliflower, beige fish and beige sauce tend to look unappealing. These days a lot of colorful vegetable alternatives are available—for example, purple broccoli, green, purple or orange cauliflower, yellow carrots, purple potatoes and sweet potatoes (yams), red lettuce.

---

12   For more on this topic, see "Tableware" in the book *The Satiety Diet Weight Loss Toolkit.*

One study found that color in the food industry can be used
". . . to increase or decrease appetite, enhance mood, [and] calm
down customers…" [Singh (2006)]

In that case, which colors increase appetite and which ones
decrease it?

Warm colors make food seem more attractive.

Studies have shown that warm colors like reds, yellows and oranges
are more likely than cool colors (such as blues) to stimulate activate
your hunger and attract your attention. [Spence (2015)]

Fast food companies' branding prominently features the color red.
People in the fast food industry know that we associate reds and
yellows with appetizing foods. They prefer to use these colors in their
logos, on their packaging, in their advertising and in the decoration
of their retail outlets.

Other color associations

Color can influence you not only on the conscious level but also
subconsciously. Green may be associated with a sour taste, but it is
also associated with freshness and optimum nutrition.

As mentioned elsewhere, putting three food items of three different
colors on your plate is more likely to satisfy you on a subconscious
level, if you're an adult, while children seem to prefer seven different
items and six colors. [Zampollo (2012)]

* *Blue Foods.*

The color blue, in foods, is said to be an appetite suppressant.
Imagine a food that's the color of a clear summer sky. That's a color
rarely found in anything that's edible! Borage petals and cornflower
petals come to mind, but people rarely eat these.

Why is blue considered an unappetizing color?[13] Perhaps because

---

13 That said, the Japanese are famous for their artistic use of food colorings,
including blue! And in tropical equatorial Asia Thailand and Malaysia, a bright blue food
coloring derived from the flower of the "blue butterfly pea" has been used for centuries.

naturally-colored sky-blue food is uncommon. Meat doesn't come in shades of blue and neither do leafy vegetables. Most of the foods we think of as blue, such as blueberries, are actually purple.

Research from around the world shows that as a general rule it is hard to persuade people to taste blue-colored foods. In one study, people sat down to a delicious meal on a plate, comprising colorful foods in yellows, reds, and greens etc. Before they started eating, the lighting in the room was changed to blue. The meal and the surroundings all took on a blue tinge. Under these conditions, the study's participants consumed the meal that they knew—cognitively—was really composed of multi-colored ingredients. However their eyes told them a different story, and they struggled to finish the meal. Some of them even felt sick afterwards.

Based on the premise that the color blue suppresses appetite, some weight loss gurus suggest strategies such as eating off blue tableware, installing a blue light in the dining room or kitchen, dyeing your food blue or wearing blue-tinted sunglasses.

That's rather missing the point.

The idea is to choose food colors and lighting that increase appetite (and satiety) when you're eating Calorie-sparse foods, and switch to food colors and lighting that suppress appetite when eating foods that are Calorie-dense. The increase in appetite can be regulated by mindful eating, and offset by improved satiety.

Satiety is inextricably associated with satisfaction. If you're presented with a meal that's all one bland color, for example, or if you're offered a meal in which everything is dyed a repulsive bright blue, you're not going to get as much satisfaction from that meal.

We recommend that you do not eat healthful, home cooked, low Calorie meals in a blue-lit room. After the meal is over, you will go about your daily activities in a modern world which is saturated with warm-colored images of fatty, sugary foods. Your Inner Guardian is probably going to be on the lookout for foods of the colors it missed. You're likely to glimpse images of more appetizing-looking foods, or to conjure mental images of them. That kind of thinking leads to cravings.

* Black foods.

Black is also said to make food look repellent, but this is debatable. In Vietnamese cuisine for example the plant ramie (*Boehmeria nivea*), is used for its black food dye. The Western palate delights in black rice, black beans, black sesame seeds, black corn chips, foods colored with squid ink and other "black" foods.

* Purple foods.

Blue is a "cold" color, but purple is a blend of blue and red, which makes it "warmer". This is probably why most of us enjoy eating purple foods such as blueberries, grapes, aubergines, plums and purple carrots.

The purple coloring in plant-based foods is bestowed by a natural pigment called an anthocyanin. Anthocyanins may appear red, purple, or blue depending on their pH. The more acidic the pH, the redder the hue of the anthocyanin. The more alkaline (basic) the pH, the more the color shifts through purple toward blue. This would indicate that purple foods have a fairly neutral pH.

Plants use anthocyanins to keep themselves in good health. These compounds can do the same for people.

While psychologists and researchers tell us that we find warm-colored foods most attractive, it's vibrantly-colored foods—in particular purple foods—that can bring us a host of health benefits, including weight loss!

Professor Lindsay Brown of the University of Southern Queensland has been conducting research into whether purple fruits and vegetables can actually help obese people to lose weight, so that their levels of inflammation will subside and their overall health will improve.

Professor Brown and his team fed rats a high-carbohydrate, high-fat diet. They became obese, and developed high blood pressure, fatty liver, poor heart function and arthritis. Then, without changing anything else, the researchers added purple plum juice to the unhealthful diet of the obese, unwell rats.

The rats lost weight. Not only that but their blood pressure, fat levels, liver function and heart function all returned to normal.

Professor Brown was surprised by the spectacular results. "… the anthocyanins in purple carrots, in Queen Garnet® plums … completely reverse all of those [obesity-related ill-health] changes, so we haven't changed the diet—they're still getting this high-carbo-hydrate, high-fat diet—and yet with that intervention, all of those parameters that characterize obesity are back to normal," he said.

Can eating purple carrots help with weight loss?

The next step is human trials, but until they are completed, it might be worthwhile to incorporate dark purple plums into your diet. Queen Garnet® plums may have the highest anthocyanin content of any fruit, but purple carrots have the highest anthocyanin content of any vegetable, so if you can't get hold of those plums you could eat some raw purple carrots each day.

Sense #2: Taste (and flavor).

Having discussed the sense of *sight* as it relates to food, let's turn our attention to *taste*. We are capable of sensing five tastes—sweet, sour, salt, bitter, and umami. What we often think of as the flavor of food is actually a combination of the food's taste, smell and texture, and our expectations.

The main reason people choose to eat particular foods is because they like the flavor.

Intense flavors help satiety.

Body-speech is working for you, sending signals back and forth before your food even hits your stomach, telling your body to produce hormones, digestive juices and other substances in certain quantities.

When your tongue senses strong flavors, signals tell the Inner Guardian that yes, it is definitely food that has entered your mouth. It's not just something tasteless and devoid of nutrition, like sawdust! With strong flavors your Inner Guardian is likely to file the information: "Sufficient food has been received. Therefore I don't need to release any more hunger signals."

The important thing to remember is that stronger flavors are more likely to fuel satiety. When you eat foods with intense flavors, you tend to remember those foods more vividly. You have clearer and more lasting memories that you have had something to eat, and this knowledge helps to keep hunger at bay for longer.

Pleasant flavors help satiety

It's important, when on a weight loss journey, to make every meal as delicious as possible. Depriving yourself of foods that make your taste buds happy can be self-defeating and even dangerous.

Keri Glassman, R.D., a member of *Women's Health Magazine's* advisory board and author of "The New You and Improved Diet", says that depriving yourself of delicious foods, "… can be really disruptive to four things: your metabolism, your overall health, your workout, and your emotional relationship with food."

When you stop eating foods that taste good because you think they are fattening, you put yourself at risk of ultimately giving in to binge-eating and gaining back all the weight you lost, plus possibly more. Trying to convince your brain to perceive foods that taste good as "bad" and bland, or unpalatable foods as "good" can end up damaging your healthy relationship with food. You could put yourself in danger of developing an eating disorder.

Balancing palatability with portion size.

Pleasant flavors may prompt you to eat more, but there are ways to mitigate this.

Scientists have a name for deliciousness. It's "palatability".

Palatability depends very much on your thoughts and beliefs. You can learn to perceive foods as palatable or unpalatable. This can lead to you having a desire/hunger/craving for foods that simply give you pleasure, rather than simply wanting foods that contain the nutrition your body needs for survival.

Your appetite is controlled in four ways—of which, usually, you are not consciously aware:

- A direct loop with a positive feedback mechanism. When food is very palatable (delicious) you want to eat more of it.
- A direct loop with a negative feedback mechanism. After you consume food and feel full, your body sends satiation signals to you brain, telling you to stop eating.
- An indirect loop with both positive and negative feedback mechanisms that can modify the strength of the direct loops. Cues telling you to to eat more food or less food can be things like the size of the dinner plate, and the visibility of food within reach.

Serving smaller food portions can help you enjoy palatable foods while losing weight. Use other tips in this book, such as mindful eating and serving food on smaller plates, to help you eat less food without having to exert huge amounts of willpower.

For more tips to help you avoid the temptation to overeat delicious food that is Calorie-dense, and create delicious high-satiety dishes that are lower in Calories, take a look at the companion books in the Satiety Diet series:

The Satiety Diet Weight Loss Toolkit (book #2 in the series) and *Crispy, Creamy, Chewy: The Satiety Diet Cookbook* (book #3).

Sense #3: Smell.

We've looked at Sight and Taste; now it's Smell's turn. The smell of a food is a property that can be detected by your nose, with its olfactory organs.

The smell of food can be good or bad. Generally words like "aroma", "fragrance", "scent", perfume" or "bouquet" are used to describe pleasant smells. The words "stink", "stench" or "odor" are usually applied to bad smells.

Smell plays a vital role in the way you perceive the flavor of food and drink. So important is this role, that some chemosensory scientists believe it is responsible for as much as 80% of the way people perceive flavor, compared to only 20% for taste.

When food manufacturers talk about the smell of food, they generally employ the tern "aroma". After all, their aim is to produce foods that smell pleasant!

Mark Anthony, technical editor of the magazine *Food Processing: the information source for food and beverage manufacturers*, writes about the importance of aroma to taste and flavor.

" . . . much of what we call taste is an intricately entwined matrix of flavor, aroma chemicals and texture or mouthfeel. It's no wonder food manufacturers are very picky about how their products smell." [Anthony (2014)]

When food manufacturers begin to formulate a new food or beverage product they pour millions of dollars into developing the flavor. There are even companies that specialize in creating and manufacturing edible flavors that can be added to food products. Their researchers have to take into account not only taste but also smell, texture (mouthfeel) and appearance. Of all these attributes, smell is the most strongly linked to flavor.

Professor Barry Smith, founder of the Center for the Study of the Senses, suggests trying a simple experiment to show how inextricably entwined are flavor and smell. Place a number of assorted jellybeans into a jar, then close your eyes so that you can't see the color of the jellybeans. Pinch your nostrils between your forefinger and thumb so that you can't smell anything. With those two senses blocked off, take a bean out of the jar, at random, and put it in your mouth. Lightly chew it and roll it on your tongue. Think about it—what can you taste?

It's probable that you experience sweetness and a slight acid "tingle", but it's unlikely that you could you identify the flavor of that jellybean.

The second part of the experiment is easy. Simply release the pressure on your nose and breathe in. What a difference! Suddenly the full flavor of the jellybean hits you!

How does smell affect flavor?

"Of the three chemical senses,[14] smell is the main determinant of a food item's flavor. While the taste of food is limited ... the smells of a food are potentially limitless. A food's flavor, therefore, can be easily altered by changing its smell while keeping its taste similar. Nowhere is this better exemplified than in artificially flavored jellies, soft drinks and candies, which, while made of bases with a similar taste, have dramatically different flavors due to the use of different scents or fragrances." [Wikipedia (26th Jul. 2016)]

Because smell is so closely connected to flavor, if your sense of smell is diminished or impaired (for example, by smoking, stress or illness) you might choose to change your diet by seeking stronger-tasting foods, or you might add to your food strong-flavored sauces, or condiments such as salt, to enhance the flavor.

Breathing in and breathing out.

What is the difference between smelling something, and sensing food's flavor in the mouth by way of its smell?

We have two ways of detecting smells. When we breathe in, we sense external smells (orthonasal smell perception), and when we breathe out, we perceive the smell of food in the mouth (retronasal smell perception).

When you smell a flower, for example, you sense its perfume when you breathe in to sniff it. On the other hand, when you are experiencing the flavor of a bite of food you are already chewing, you detect the smell when you breathe out.

This means that the same food can smell quite different, depending on whether it's sitting in front of you as yet untasted, or whether you've taken a bite.

---

14 The three chemical senses are smell, taste and the trigeminal chemosensory system, which detects chemical irritants such as air pollution.

When food enters your mouth, your saliva changes the configuration of its molecules, and thus alters the chemistry of the food's smell, which you detect when you breathe out. This explains why some foods, such as durian fruit or Gorgonzola cheese, hard-boiled eggs, dim sims or asafoetida, can smell very different, even disgusting, before you taste them and release the deliciousness.

External smells and food appreciation.

In restaurants, some well-known chefs use external smells as a way of enhancing the flavor of their dishes. Staff carry atomizers around the dining room, spraying evocative food aromas such as "smoke", "tarragon", "matcha tea" or "wet earth", to compliment the particular dish the diners are consuming.

French designer Eric Gormand even invented the first "culinary hookah", by which one can inhale various flavors while dining, to enhance the flavor of each dish.

Smells and emotions.

Not only is food's smell inextricably tied to its flavor, but your sense of smell is also closely tied to your memories and emotions. The parts of the brain that process smells are closely linked to the parts that process emotion and memory. Unpleasant smells can send pain signals to your brain to warn you of impending danger, while pleasant smells can lull, relax and comfort you.

Smell is the *only one* of our senses that affects the memory and emotion sectors of the brain, which is why your brain ties the flavor of food to intense emotional memories.

Certain smells can awaken buried memories, such as the smell of baking cookies reminding people of their grandma. Or they can trigger emotions associated with that smell, such as a sense of security and comfort.

Chris Clark says: "The smell of newly-cut grass makes me feel calm, because my dad used to mow the lawns every Saturday morning. When I was a child I associated that smell with the beginning of the weekend—no school for two whole days!"

Because of the emotional aspect of aroma, we can come to like or dislike the flavor of certain foods on the basis of some past emotional experience.

Strong smelling food gives better satiety.

Strong, pleasant food aromas are highly satisfying and can boost satiety. Give your meals more satiety-power by adding aromatic seasonings such as freshly grated ginger, lemon zest, sprigs of fresh mint, cinnamon, grated nutmeg, rosemary, cilantro (coriander) or basil.

Strong smelling food also makes you take smaller bites.

While the texture and ingredients of the food on your plate affect how much you load onto your fork or spoon, the smell also plays an important part. People tend to eat smaller mouthfuls of strongly smelling foods. This applies whether those foods smell strongly appealing or (externally) strongly disagreeable. As mentioned, examples of foods that can smell disagreeable but taste good include Gorgonzola cheese and durian fruits.

In a 2012 study, volunteers were all shown the same bland food. They could press a button to choose how much of this food would be placed onto their spoon. Just before they pressed the button, the researchers secretly released a pleasant aroma, close to the participants' noses. The more intense the aroma, the smaller the amount that was loaded onto the spoons. The weaker the aroma, the more food the participants piled on to the cutlery.

It appeared that the participants were instinctively seeking to experience a certain level of flavor; not too much, and not too little.

"Higher aroma intensities resulted in significantly smaller [bite] sizes," wrote the researchers. [de Wijk (2012)]

Eating smaller bites of your food is useful for weight loss. It slows down your eating, makes you eat more mindfully, and in the end, it may help you eat less. When you shovel large amounts of food into your mouth, you're more likely to have overeaten before your natural satiety signals kick in. When you eat more slowly, you give your satiety signals a chance to work before you consume too much.

Judging by the results of de Wijk's study, it's worthwhile adding strong, pleasant smells to your meals, or eating food that naturally has a strong and delicious smell. With fragrant, aromatic, spicy and even hot-spicy foods, not only will your meal taste better, you could be taking smaller bites without even thinking about it. Taking smaller bites means taking longer to eat a meal—a proven weight loss strategy that can lead you to eat a little less and still feel satisfied.

Just make sure you listen to your body's satiety signals!

Sense #4: Touch (mouthfeel, texture, consistency).

Food texture is more accurately called "mouthfeel". It refers to the physical sensations in the mouth induced by food or drink.

Custards and purées, for example, have a smooth and creamy mouthfeel. They look smooth and swirly, and flow across the tongue like silk. If you drew your fingertips through custard, it would feel soft and velvety.

So important is texture, that we humans often rate it more highly than flavor. A tender cut of meat is more expensive than a tough cut, even if the tough cut is more flavorsome.

Of all food's characteristics, it's the texture/consistency/mouthfeel that could be even more important for satiety than flavor.

In fact, it is so important to consumers that food manufacturers spend billions of dollars each year researching it. The science of food structure is called "food rheology". Scientists who work in this field have coined the terms "mouthfeel", or "oral haptics". Mouthfeel is defined as "a food's physical and chemical interaction in the mouth". It includes characteristics such as graininess, fracturability, gumminess, moisture release, smoothness, viscosity and hardness.

Textural awareness is usually subconscious. When you think of the sensory characteristics of food you tend to think of flavor first, followed by look and smell. Yet texture is extremely important. If the texture of a food is "wrong" you will reject it completely. In fact, when a food's texture is changed (for example by puréeing it to the consistency of soup) people who taste it find it hard to identify exactly what that food is! Flavor alone is not sufficient for you to identify a food.

Our mouths are amazingly sensitive. After all, they are the gateway between our bodies and the environment, so they have to be on guard against anything harmful, such as poisonous or sharp substances.

Your perception of texture is so finely-honed that, for example, when you eat ice cream, your mouth can feel crystals of ice so tiny that they measure only 40 microns (0.04 mm or 0.001inch) in diameter. These interfere with your sense of smoothness, which is why food manufacturers spend huge amounts of money working out ways to discourage these miniature crystals from growing. So far, one of the best methods researchers have discovered is to freeze ice cream using liquid nitrogen. The freezing process happens so quickly that crystals have barely any time to form. Any that do form measure less than 40 microns, which means that the ice cream's texture feels super-creamy.

For better satiety, include a wide range of textures in your meals. When your mouth senses a variety of textures, your Inner Guardian receives signals that you are consuming a variety of foods, which suggests that a variety of hunger-satisfying nutrients is flooding into your digestive system.

Texture.

The texture of food usually refers to mouthfeel, but it can also refer to the way food looks. For example, Danish rye bread (or rugbrød, as it is called in Danish), has a rough texture and looks rough-textured. It is densely packed with seeds and cracked grains. If you ran your fingertips over a slice of rugbrød, it would feel slightly knobbly, rugged and coarse.

Consistency/Viscosity.

Consistency is linked with mouthfeel. The consistency of food alludes to its degree of density, firmness, thickness, runniness or viscosity. For food scientists, consistency and viscosity have their own separate definitions. A liquid with higher viscosity usually has a firmer consistency, however, so for the purposes of this book we won't go into the finer distinctions.

If a food is too dense and firm to flow at all, it's considered to be solid, not viscous. Viscosity applies to foods that are not solid, and can be defined as "a measure of the resistance of a fluid to flow". You can think of viscosity as "thickness".

Water, for example, has a thin consistency, and flows very easily when you pour it. It has a low viscosity.

Milk is slightly more viscous than water, but not as viscous as sugar syrup or honey. Tomato paste and peanut butter are comparatively dense and firm, with high viscosity. They are quite resistant to flow and you have to squeeze them out of the tube or scoop them out of the container. They are considered to be "semi-solids".

Texture/mouthfeel and food dislikes.

It's texture, too, that can be at the root of people's greatest aversions to certain foods. As we discuss in the section on learning to love more foods, it's the perceived "sliminess" of some foods that is repugnant to Western palates.

Texture even trumps nutrients for satiety-power.

So important is the effect of a food's texture on its satiating power, that texture even outperforms nutrients! Even protein, the macronutrient that's known to be the most satiating, cannot compete with texture.

Researchers wanted to know whether it was the particular sensory characteristics of high protein foods that made those foods more satiating, or whether it was the actual protein itself, regardless of the texture, mouthfeel etc. They gave people a high-carbohydrate drink that had been processed in a way that made it feel and taste exactly like a high-protein drink. They also gave people a high-protein drink that had been processed to make it *lose* the sensory characteristics of protein.

The high-carb "fake protein" drink was rated as more satiating than the high-protein drink that didn't taste high-protein! [Bertenshaw et al., (2009), Bertenshaw et al., (2013)]

Texture is vital to the food manufacturing industry.

"Food texture design and optimization is increasingly a key area of focus in food formulation and development," says Yadunandan Lal Dar, a director of ingredient applications at Ingredion, Inc., during a presentation at the 2014 Institute of Food Technologists' annual meeting and food exposition in New Orleans, USA.

The food manufacturing industry relies greatly on chemical additives called "texturants". Texturants are included in many processed food formulae for many reasons, such as:

- to act as a stabilizer for the food
- to provide a textural structure
- to improve a food's "mouthfeel"
- to reduce the cost of ingredients (e.g. "creamy mouthfeel" texturants can be cheaper than real dairy products)

Crispy, creamy, chewy (and crunchy).

There are numerous words we use to describe food mouthfeel/ textures, such as gooey, runny, flaky, smooth, silky, fluffy, spongy, hard, brittle, crispy, crusty, creamy and crunchy. The list is long!

Mouthfeel is an important concept, because it influences how much we eat. Malcolm Bourne, Emeritus Professor in Food Science and Technology at Cornell University, is a consultant for the food industry and the author of "Food Texture and Viscosity, Concept and Measurement". He says the three texture notes that people enjoy most are crispiness, creaminess and chewiness.

To that list, we would add "crunchy". Crunchy is different from crispy in that crispy foods give you one brisk, snapping sound at the first bite; they are brittle, yet tender. Crunchy foods, on the other hand, are harder. They continue to provide not only a satisfying coarse, gravelly sound as you chew on them, but also a resistance, which can pulse vibrations through your teeth and jaws.

For the best chance of satiety, try to include all four of these textures in your meals.

Tip: Many crispy foods are notoriously energy-dense and high in fat—for example, potato crisps/chips. Crispy foods with fewer Calories include some crispbreads (especially oven-baked), dried vegetable chips, celery, apples, crispy noodles, pretzels and baked bagel crisps.

1. Creamy

Creaminess means "having the consistency of cream", and cream's consistency is generally thick, slow-flowing and viscous. Creamy, viscous foods have better satiety power than thin, watery foods. Furthermore, fibers categorized as viscous have more satiating power than less viscous fibers. [Vuksan (2009)]

* Thickness, creaminess and, satiety.

The food manufacturing industry has spent a lot of time and effort finding out what makes foods more satiating. They have found that thickening runny food products to make them more viscous and creamy than they were before makes people:
- expect to feel more satiated after eating the food product
- eat more slowly
- report that they felt more satiated by the food
- feel less hungry after eating

* Creaminess, the power of the mind and the satiety response.

Your expectations of how satiating a food or drink will be, even before you swallow it, depend on certain properties of its taste and texture. Researchers who published a study in the journal *Appetite* wanted to know whether people's expectations of satiation and satiety would influence how much of a drink they consumed. [McCrickerd et al., (2014)]

The researchers gave people four different versions of the same low-Calorie fruit yoghurt beverage. They manipulated the characteristics of the yogurt drinks to make them thicker and more viscous, or thinner and runnier. They also manipulated the "mouth feel" of the drinks, making them feel smoother, silkier and creamier in the mouth, or less creamy.

The extra viscosity of the beverage was achieved by adding increasing concentrations of tara gum, an indigestible, almost odorless natural thickening substance.

They ended up with four drinks identical in Calorie and nutrient value that possessed four different sensory characteristics:

1) A thin consistency with not a very creamy taste
2) A thin consistency with a very creamy taste
3) A thick consistency with not a very creamy taste
4) A thick consistency with a very creamy taste

Even before tasting the drinks, participants said they thought the drinks with the thick, viscous consistency would give them the best feelings of satiety.

They also felt that *both* the drinks with thicker consistency had a creamier mouth-feel, despite the fact that only one of them had its creaminess enhanced.

The two thin, runny drinks were considered to have a less creamy mouth-feel, even though one of them had its creaminess amplified!

Both men and women reported greater satiation when they consumed drinks that were thicker and creamier.

Men did not appear to choose to consume less of the drink when consistency and texture suggested higher satiety, but the study found that "…women will select smaller portions of a drink when its sensory characteristics indicate that it will be satiating." So maybe the women were more weight-conscious than the men!

The intensified thickness and creaminess of the fourth drink led people to expect that it would give them greater satiety when they consumed it. Not only that, but it really *did* give them better satiety!

119

When you expect a food or drink to provide greater satiety, you're more likely to choose to consume less of it. The researchers hoped that ". . . enhancing the thick and creamy characteristics of a drink might also result in smaller portion size selection." [Hogenkamp et al., (2011)]

* Consistency has more impact than mouthfeel.
The results of these studies suggest that when it comes to your expectations of how satiated you will feel after you consume a food or drink, it is thick, viscous food textures that influence you, more than creamy mouth-feel. Other research supports this, adding that chewiness, too, gives people the expectation that a food will be satiating. [Forde et al., (2013)]

* The effect of texture.
The texture of food can affect how Calorie-dense and satisfying you think it is.

Most of us are more attracted to creamy, viscous, soft, smooth foods such as custard, cooked oatmeal, whipped cream and mashed potatoes than to harder, drier foods such as celery or dry crackers.

The results of a study published in *The Journal of Consumer Research* suggest that people are likely to view soft, smooth, creamy foods as being fattier and higher in Calories than rough, hard foods that need more chewing. The sensation of the food in their mouths (mouthfeel) affected their perception of how many Calories that food contained.

For the study's participants, their estimation of Calories influenced their subsequent food choices and the amount of food they ate in total. When they ate a food they thought was loaded with Calories, they afterwards chose to eat a food that was low in Calories, to compensate. They also ate less food, in total, after eating the soft, creamy food. [Biswas et al., (2014)]

Scientists think we prefer creamy-textured foods because that's the texture naturally associated with a high fat content. [Montmayeur & le Coutre (2010)]

This discovery could be a great weight loss tool! Eating creamy, viscous, slippery foods that are low in Calories may "trick" your brain into thinking you've consumed more energy than you really have. This could influence how much food—and what kind of food—you end up eating.

* Thick and creamy foods.
Expectations play a huge role in satiety!

As we've discussed, thick, creamy foods provide better satiety than thin, runny foods. Beginning in early childhood, without realizing it, you learn about different foods as you sample each one. It's another method your body uses to help you survive. You learn instinctively that particular characteristics of foods can indicate how nutritious that food is. This would have been useful knowledge long ago when humans were hunter-gatherers. People could tell—just by biting or sipping a potential food to find out how chewy it was, or even just by looking at how runny or thick it was—whether it was likely to provide plenty of much-needed energy.

As you grew up, you gathered a store of information about food, including facts about its texture, such as:

- Viscous foods are more likely to be highly nutritious and satiating than thin liquids. (Think honey, cream, gravy.)
- Thin liquids are more likely to quench thirst than viscous foods and fluids, but they are likely to have fewer nutrients. (Think water, tea, clear soups.)

In the story of *Goldilocks and the Three Bears*, the best porridge was not too hot and not too cold, but just right.

Similarly, when food texture is not to hard/dry and not too thin/wet, but thick and creamy, it is just right for promoting satiety.

For example, the ingredients in a granola bar (also called a cereal bar or muesli bar) are less satiating than those same ingredients mixed with water and served as porridge, because viscous, creamy foods trigger satiety signals better than hard, dry foods.

As well as satiation, thick and creamy foods also provide more satiety than thin-textured, runny foods such as fruit juices, energy drinks and clear soups. Watery, low-viscosity drinks cannot provide as much satiety as thicker foods because they pass through the mouth very quickly. The brain doesn't recognize the Calories in fast-pouring liquids in the same way as the Calories in more viscous or solid foods, such as tough, chewy breads or creamy porridges and soups.

Studies confirm that when you consume Calories in a semi-solid (viscous) or solid form you are much more likely to feel satiated than if you consume the same number of Calories in liquid form. And if you don't feel satiated, you are likely to want to eat more. [Almiron-Roig et al., (2013)]

In fact, researchers have found that there is a significant link between weight gain and Calories consumed in thin, runny, liquid form, such as soft drinks, sodas and other sugar-laden beverages. [Malik et al., (2006), Vartanian et al., (2007)]

* The power of the mind.

Your mind has the power to change your physiological responses.

The results of the aforementioned studies support the idea that when your expectations of satiety are boosted while you are eating a food, either by the texture of the food or by other means, your body is more satiated by the food's nutrients at a physiological level. That is, even your hormones and neurotransmitters tend to agree that the food was more satiating (although they're never 100% fooled!).

Your thoughts and expectations powerfully influence the release of biochemicals in your body. Therefore the satiating creaminess and viscosity of foods may encourage you to eat or drink smaller portions without feeling deprived.

2. Creamy plus crispy/crunchy.

Creamy, viscous foods mixed with crispy, crunchy foods tend to have even greater satiety-power. Think crispy nachos with smooth dips, or velvety chocolate bars studded with roasted almonds, or creamy Satiety Porridge sprinkled through with crunchy chopped nuts and seeds.

3. Chewy.

Gnawing is a gratifying experience. More than that, it is integral to our good health and our experience of satiety—and thus it is an excellent weight-loss tool.

* Chewy foods help boost satiety.

Foods with a chewy texture need to remain in your mouth for longer, as you break them down with our jaws and teeth to make them easy to swallow. This means that you enjoy the food's taste, smell and texture for longer, and your body has more time to prepare itself to receive and digest the food. Increased enjoyment and efficient digestion lead to better satiety.

Therefore, as you learn about food during childhood, you come to expect that the foods with a chewy texture will be more satiating than foods with a thin, runny, liquid texture.

Hard foods such as carrots, apples, nuts, French breads such as baguettes, and leathery, tough, stringy, fibrous foods such as fruit leathers (not recommended for weight loss) or jerky all promote chewing.

The chewiness of foods is so important to satiety that it is discussed at greater length later in this book.

4. Crunchy

Crunchiness and chewiness are different, but they go hand in hand. Crunchy foods include nuts, rusks, hard toast, raw carrots and oven-baked croutons.

Swap textures for better satiety

Swapping solid, dry foods for viscous foods with similar Calorie levels that contain more moisture and bulk can provide a better sense of fullness and satiety. Some examples include:

- Fresh fruit in place of dried fruits
- Dry-popped popcorn in place of crackers (popcorn contains a lot of air!)

Exploiting food's sensory characteristics.

Can you use sensory characteristics to trick your body into being satiated on lower Calorie foods? Is it possible to make any food satiating simply by making it thicker or chewier, and sticking a label on it claiming that it provides excellent satiety? Can you use these tricks to make low Calorie foods so satiating that you can lose weight easily and without hunger, just by eating them?

Our bodies are cleverer than that. Yes, they can be tricked to a certain extent, but nature has hard-wired us with survival instincts. There are numerous physiological processes working deep inside our digestive systems to prevent us from being fooled into, say, chowing down on thickened, artificially sweetened, creamy-mouthfeel cucumber purée and feeling as satiated as we would if we were eating a deep-fried chocolate bar.

The satiating power of protein-rich, high-Calorie drinks is increased by making them thicker and creamier. However with low-protein, low-Calorie versions of the same drink, which are still equally thick and creamy, the satiating power is *not* increased. In spite of the protein-poor, low-Calorie drink's sensory characteristics indicating that it ought to be satiating, the body is not tricked.

Nonetheless, when protein-rich, high-Calorie drinks are thin, runny and lacking in that creamy mouth-feel, our bodies *can* be tricked into feeling less satiated. [Yeomans & Chambers (2011)]

To summarize: the extent to which drinks (and foods) give us feelings of satiety and suppresses appetite depends on the food or drink's sensory characteristics, such as thickness or chewiness, being fairly accurate indicators of the nutrients it contains.

The lesson for weight loss? If you're going to consume high Calorie foods and drinks, make sure you consume those that have satiety-promoting sensory characteristics. For example, avoid sugary sodas and energy drinks. Don't add sugar to coffee and tea. Choose chewy biscuits and crackers instead of those that just "melt" in your mouth. If you're making porridge, make it thick and creamy and add crunchy, chewy bits.

* Use this body-trick wisely.

The appetite-reducing characteristics of low-Calorie foods can be boosted by making them thicker, creamier and/or chewier. Remember to use this body-trick wisely. Make sure the low-Calorie foods you eat are rich in nutrients. Some foods are low in nutrients—e.g. pasta, pretzels, candy, French fries, ice-cream, and foods made with refined, white flour. When manufacturers give these foods sensory characteristics that are normally associated with satiety (e.g. creaminess or chewiness), the foods are likely to trigger "rebound appetite" and make you want to eat more. Those enticing sensory characteristics tell your Inner Guardian to prepare the body for an influx of Calories. When the Calories don't arrive, your Inner Guardian boosts your desire for food and demands them!

Rebound appetite

Additionally, there's something important to remember when you want to lose weight. It's this—

> When the genuine satiating power of a food is low but its sensory characteristics indicate that it should be high, eating that food can actually make you feel hungrier!

For example, if you eat a fat-free, artificially-sweetened, low-Calorie tub of yoghurt that's thick and sweet-tasting, with a very creamy mouth-feel, you'll probably feel extra-hungry shortly afterwards.

It is thought that this is because the thickness and creaminess must trigger the release of hormones and other substances in the body, sending signals to the digestive system to get ready for a load of incoming nutrients such as sugars, fats and proteins. And then, when that expected load of nutrients fails to arrive, the body responds by sending out hunger signals. Your Inner Guardian virtually says to you, "Hey, I know there are some good nutrients nearby, because we felt them in your mouth a moment ago. Now I'll make you feel hungry so that you'll feel driven to go and get them!"

Sense #5: Hearing.

Sound is probably not a sensory characteristic that you'd usually associate with food, but it's an important element in your appreciation of the things you eat.

You might not realize how well your body is attuned to sounds in your environment because human brains have worked out ways to block out sounds when we need to concentrate on something else, such as reading this book. Right at this moment, if you allow yourself to "tune in" to the sounds that are within your hearing, you may become aware of just how many sounds you are processing unconsciously, during the course of your daily life.

We are so sensitive to sound that by the time we are adults, many of us can even tell the difference between the sound of hot water being poured and the sound of cold water being poured, just by listening. Some people can even tell the difference between the sound of Champagne and tonic water being poured.

Sound can influence your perception of food to make it appear more or less appealing. The sounds of food can include mouth sounds such as "crunch" and "slurp", but they also include sounds associated with dining, such as clinking cutlery and crockery, the pouring of liquids, the hum of conversation, and even background music and the relaying of orders to the kitchen staff in an eatery.

Freshness.

Take for example the crisp "snap!" you hear when you break a raw carrot or a stalk of fresh celery. That sounds tells you the vegetable is fresh. Limp, stale celery and carrots do not make that sound. Your Inner Guardian wants you to eat fresh food because it is more nutritious and less likely to harbor pathogens, so your mind associates crisp, crunchy, snapping sounds with freshness and desirability.

In a study conducted in Oxford, UK, participants wore headphones while eating potato chips (crisps). These chips that were all identical in shape, size, curvature, flavor etc. The researchers played back, through the headphones, the sound made when the participants bit into each chip and chewed it.

They then altered these crunching sounds, making them louder or softer, higher or lower, more or less muffled etc., snd asked the participants their opinion of the food they were eating. When they could clearly hear the loud, crunching sounds they were making, they perceived the chips as being fresher than when the sounds were softer. [Zampini & Spence (2004)]

Loud ambient noise decreases flavor perception.

The noise levels that surround you when you are eating can have a significant effect on your enjoyment of food. This is one reason why airline food generally seems to lack flavor—operating jet engines are quite noisy, and their steady, loud drone dampens the sounds you unconsciously associate with eating. At these levels, noise can diminish your aptitude for registering tastes—especially "sweet" and "salty". Noise levels in eateries can climb to very high levels too, depending on the acoustics of the building's interior, the soft furnishings or lack thereof, the proximity of the kitchen to the dining area and a number of other factors. No matter whether you are surrounded by engine noises, shrieking coffee machines or blaring music, hearing any loud sounds while you are eating can decrease your enjoyment of food.

Tip: To increase your chances of deriving satiety from your meals, eat them in quiet surroundings. Don't eat in a loud, stressful environment, e.g. a noisy household with people running around. Eating out in a restaurant or cafe environment is fine as long as there's not a lot of crashing and yelling coming from the kitchen! In fact, a gentle murmur of conversation from other patrons may help you achieve better satiety.

Be wary of background music during meals. One study found that when people listened to pleasant music while they were eating, they were likely to stay longer at the dinner table and eat more food. [Stroebele & de Castro (2006)]

Background music can influence taste perception.

Speaking of music, research has found that people associate certain sounds with certain tastes/flavors. "Synaesthesia" is the word used to describe what happens when the brain produces an impression relating to one of the senses (such as sight) during stimulation of another sense (such as smell). Examples of synasthesia include "hearing a color" or "tasting a sound". Few people are fully blown synaesthetes, but most of us do have the tendency to connect sounds and tastes. [Crisinel & Spence (2010a); Crisinel & Spence (2009); Crisinel & Spence (2010b); Simner et al., (2010)]

Participants in many of these studies associated high-pitched sounds with sour-tasting or sweet-tasting foods, and low-pitched brass instrument notes with bitter foods. Harsh-sounding music also seemed to enhance the bitter (e.g. chocolate and coffee), sour (e.g. passionfruit) or even crunchy characteristics of food, while more dulcet and harmonious pieces, especially played on a piano, heightened people's perception of creaminess and sweetness.

Some innovative restaurants serve certain dishes accompanied by "soundscapes" designed to go with the dish—for example recordings of crashing waves and seagulls to accompany a seafood dish.

Oxford University psychologist Charles Spence design ed a study in which participants ate pieces of identically-flavored bittersweet toffee while listening to soundscapes. One soundscape was "sweet" while the other was "bitter".

When asked to report on the taste of the toffee, the participants said that it was either sweeter or more bitter, depending the sounds they had been listening to. [Crisinel et al., (2012)]

For more about the association between sweet sounds and sweet tastes, see *The Satiety Diet Weight Loss Toolkit* (# 2 in the Satiety Diet series).

MACRONUTRIENTS

What are macronutrients?

In the field of nutrition, a macronutrient is defined as any of the nutritional components of the diet that are required in relatively large amounts. It is generally agreed that the three major macronutrients are:

- protein
- carbohydrates (starches and sugars)
- lipids (fat).

Some authorities argue that there are actually three more macronutrients:

- Dietary fiber. "Fiber is a complex and varied macronutrient encompassing a range of non-starch polysaccharides (carbohydrates) and lignin ... which are either soluble or insoluble and fermentable or non-fermentable." [Burton-Freeman (2000)]
- Water. Occasionally even this is counted as a macronutrient, because it is essential for life.
- Macrominerals. These are minerals your body needs in larger amounts than trace minerals. They include calcium, phosphorus, magnesium, sodium, potassium, chloride and sulfur.

Micronutrients

Micronutrients are nutrients our bodies need in small quantities, in order to function properly. They include vitamins, minerals and phytonutrients. Phytonutrients differ from vitamins in that the former are found only in plant-based foods.[15]

Your body needs 13 vitamins for normal growth and development. Throughout your life you must regularly consume enough vitamins to support normal body functions. A deficiency in any one of these 13 vitamins can cause ill-health.

---

15 Some of the phytonutrients are also vitamins, such as vitamins A, C, E, K and folate.

Macronutrients affect satiety.

Macronutrient intake is important for satiety and weight loss, because appetite isn't just a general desire for food. People (and other animals) have separate appetites for each of the macronutrients. For example, if you ate as much protein and fat as you wanted, in vast quantities, you would probably still have a "carb appetite". You would be hankering for carbohydrates despite having gorged on protein and fat.

"The macronutrient composition of the diet can influence hunger, satiety, food intake, body weight, and body composition." [Rolls (1995)]

Meals containing carbohydrate, protein and fat generate feelings of satiety and fullness. When these three macronutrients enter your small intestine, your body produces a substance called GLP-1, which promotes satiety and suppresses appetite. [Flint et al., (1998)]

This indicates that people need carbohydrates, protein and fat in each meal to achieve satiety. A satiating diet for weight loss should contain some slowly-digested carbs, some protein and a very small amount of fat.

Nutrients rated in order of satiety value.

1. Protein gives you the fastest, most prolonged satiety. (It also contains Calories, so count them. Choose protein sources that are high in fiber.)
2. Complex carbohydrates—that is, fiber-rich, whole foods high in carbohydrates.
3. Refined carbohydrates.
4. Sugar—it may be satisfying in the short term but it doesn't provide long term satiety.
5. Fat—this exerts the weakest effect on satiety compared to carbohydrates and protein. It is, nonetheless, still necessary.

[Blundell & Macdiarmid (1997)]

The effect of macronutrients.

Not all Calories have the same effect on satiety. Two meals containing the same number of Calories can have different effects on your satiety, depending on their proportions of macronutrients. For instance, people whose diet is high in protein and carbohydrate generally experience greater satiety than people whose diet is high in fat, even when the two diets contain exactly the same number of Calories. [Westerterp-Plantenga (1999)]

Including a large proportion of fat in a meal also has another drawback for people who want to lose weight. It contains more than twice the Calories per unit of weight (grams, pounds etc.) than carbohydrate and protein. This means that a food rich in fat is usually lighter and smaller than a carbohydrate-rich or protein-rich food with the same number of Calories. Food that looks smaller and weighs less sends signals to the Inner Guardian that say: "You're not getting very much to eat—it won't be enough to stop you from feeling hungry! You need to eat more!"

Foods rich in carbs, fiber and protein are best for satiety

Let's add fiber into the equation. Chambers et al., in their 2015 article "Optimizing Foods for Satiety", wrote that when meals are abundant in protein and fiber and include more carbohydrate than fat, they are better able to satisfy the appetite. (Note that fat in very small portions is also recommended for satiety.) A great way to get protein combined with dietary fiber is to eat plant-based foods.

High protein foods may also contain carbs and fat.

Whole foods rich in protein include not only animal-based foods, but also a wide range of plant-based foods such as grains, seeds and beans.

When you eat a high-protein whole food, you're not just eating pure protein. Food is more complex than that. High protein whole foods, whether animal or plant-based, contain other macronutrients, such as carbohydrates and fat. So if you're aiming to eat a certain percentage of protein at every meal, for example, you should take into account the carbohydrates and fat that already exist in your high-protein food.

131

How many Calories are in the different macronutrients?
As an approximate measure:
* Protein = 4 Calories per gram,
* Carbohydrates = 4 Calories per gram
* Fat = 9 Calories per gram
* Soluble fiber = 2 Calories per gram
* Insoluble fiber = virtually zero Calories

Macronutrients: Fats.
When you want to lose weight, it's your body's stored fat you want to get rid of—not bone or lean muscle! All fats and oils are high in Calories. They are nature's energy stores. Some people might be tempted to say, "If I want to lose fat I shouldn't eat fat." But the way the body works is not that simple!

Why do people eat too much fat?
It's easy to eat too much fat because:
* Fat makes food taste better. Fat's deliciousness can override your natural satiety signals.
* Fat is not as satiating as the other macronutrients.

Fat exists in most animal-based foods, oils, nuts, and seeds. It's also in some fruits. Fatty foods are delicious. And when you want a burst of delicious high-energy food, fat-laden dishes such as ice-creams, French fries, chocolate or cheese seem most desirable.

For weight loss, eat a little "healthful" fat.
You need small amounts of fat in your diet in order to remain healthy. Dietary fats are essential to provide you with energy, maintain proper functioning of nerves and brain and support cell growth in your skin and other tissues. Fats help your body absorb some nutrients, such as fat-soluble vitamins A, D, E and K.

132

According to the American Heart Association, fats: ". . . also help protect your organs and help keep your body warm. . . They produce important hormones, too. Your body definitely needs fat." [AHA (2016)]

Not only does a little of the right kind of dietary fat keep you healthy, it can also help you lose weight.

* Fat helps dampen hunger.

While fat is lowest on the satiety-producing list, trying to completely eliminate all fat from your diet can increase your hunger levels. Fat can have a significant effect on appetite.

In a 2010 technical book called *Fat Detection* the author says that fats ". . . appear to regulate appetite through several mechanisms including the release of appetite hormones and inhibition of gastric emptying and intestinal transit." [Samra (2010)]

Of the three main macronutrients, fat produces the weakest effects on both satiation and satiety. It also contains more Calories per gram than protein or carbohydrates. Despite this, a little fat is necessary for satiety, and necessary for losing weight and keeping it off.

* Very low-fat diets are hard to stick to.

Fat adds flavor and texture to foods. It's hard to pass that up, day after day! A diet that contains a little fat is far more satisfying, and can dampen food cravings.

* Zealously cutting fat from your diet may lead to rebound weight gain.

As mentioned, people have a natural appetite for all the macronutrients. Our bodies need all of them in a balanced ratio. Those who lose weight on a zero-fat or very-low-fat diet often compensate after they cease the diet, by over-indulging in the fatty foods they missed.

* For weight loss, choose "low-fat".

A low-fat diet is better for weight loss than "no fat" or "too much fat". Recent research indicates that it is fat, not carbohydrate, that is linked to overeating and obesity. Two studies undertaken at Cornell University (USA) suggested that it is hard *not* to lose weight when consuming a diet composed only of low-fat foods. [Prewitt et al., (1991), Rolls (1995)]

* Cutting out fat is not the same as cutting out Calories.

Even if you completely banished fat from your diet, you could still become fat by consuming Calories from other sources. Fat doesn't directly make you "fat"—consuming too many Calories makes you "fat". Your body stores any excess energy from food as fat, no matter whether that energy is derived from carbohydrates, fat or protein. In order to lose weight it's important to track and limit both how much fat you are eating every day, and how many Calories you're eating each day.

* Choose your dietary fat wisely.

As discussed, a little bit of the right kind fat is better than too much fat or no fat at all. For weight loss and optimum health, it's desirable to eat small amounts of healthful fats.

People who live in some of the "leanest" countries in the world include moderate amounts of mainly polyunsaturated and mono-unsaturated dietary fats in their diet. The Mediterranean Diet, for example, contains plenty of olive oil and nuts. [Brimelow(2014)]

Different types of fat.

All dietary fats are a combination of different fatty acids—saturated and unsaturated. Unsaturated fats can be divided into two categories; polyunsaturated and monounsaturated.

* Saturated fats

Your body can manufacture its own saturated fatty acids, so they are not essential in your diet. Besides, eating too much saturated fat can raise your blood cholesterol levels, in addition to making you put on weight.

It's not feasible to attempt cutting out all saturated fatty acids from your diet, because all fats contain at least a small amount. However for optimum health and weight loss, avoid consuming large portions of foods rich in saturated fatty acids, such as fatty meat, chicken, butter and cream. [Noakes (2018)]

Certain saturated fats called medium-chain triglycerides (MCTs) are said to be more satiating than others, but some studies suggest that MCT oil consumption can raise the risk of cardiovascular disease.

* Unsaturated fats

Choose foods that contain the more healthful fatty acids (polyunsaturated and monounsaturated). Polyunsaturated fats include omega-3 and omega-6 fatty acids, which are known as essential fatty acids because your body cannot produce them, so you have to get them from food.

More than 75% of the fat in avocados is beneficial. Every 50 grams contains 5 grams of monounsaturated fat and 1 gram of polyunsaturated fat. Avocados are also a good source of dietary fiber. For weight loss eat them in very small portions, as they are relatively Calorie-dense.

These "good" types of fat have beneficial effects on your health and may also help with weight loss. A 2016 study found that the fats consumed as part of a typical Mediterranean diet (e.g. the fats in olive oil, eggs, nuts, seeds and fatty fish) may decrease the risk of heart disease, breast cancer and type 2 diabetes. [Bloomfield et al., (2016)]

Unsaturated fats: Trans fats.

Not all unsaturated foods are healthful, however. Since the middle of the 20th century, food manufacturers have been using a process called hydrogenation to change liquid unsaturated fats into solids. During this processing, a form of fat called "trans fat" is produced. Eating artificially made trans fats rases your levels of harmful LDL cholesterol and increases the risk of heart disease. The main source of trans fats in processed food is "partially hydrogenated oil", so check food labels and avoid it!

Keep your intake of trans fats (hydrogenated fats) as low as possible.

Unsaturated fats: Polyunsaturated fats Omega-3 and Omega-6.

Omega-6 fats have a pro-inflammatory effect, while Omega-3 fats are anti-inflammatory. [Calder (2006)] As research indicates, diets that include large amounts of Omega-6 fats but few Omega-3 fats can increase inflammation in your body. A diet in which the amounts of both types or fat is balanced in a 1:1 ratio reduces inflammation.

Omega-3 fats are found in foods such as fatty fish and flaxseed oil. These fats play a part in appetite regulation, although opinion is divided on whether they stimulate or curb appetite. One thing is for sure: they are good for you. In fact, they are essential for good health!

Beware of the fat + sugar combination!

Fat eaten together with sugar can be addictive, and sabotage weight loss.

If it's weight loss you want, it appears you can try a diet that lets you eat fat without sugar, or one that allows sugar without fat. When fat is eaten in combination with refined carbohydrates such as sugar, it seems to increase your appetite. (Both diets are likely to result in rebound weight gain afterwards.)

The twin Van Tulleken brothers, both doctors in the UK, tried an experiment in which one of them went on a low-fat diet but kept eating sugary foods, and the other gave up sugar but ate fatty foods. Both of them lost weight! [Van Tulleken (2014)]

136

These results suggest that following a relatively fat-rich diet with zero sugar (in any form) could help you lose weight. They also suggest that you could lose weight if you eat a sugary diet with zero fat. But eat fat and sugar together, and you'll probably *gain* weight.

Note that the Satiety Diet does *not* recommend cutting out entire macronutrient groups. It's not good for your health, and it can trigger cravings, not to mention rebound weight gain.

Paul Kenny, an associate professor in the Department of Molecular Therapeutics at The Scripps Research Institute in Florida, USA, is a co-author of a 2010 study, published in *Nature Neuroscience*. The study suggests that high-Calorie food can be just as addictive as smoking or substance abuse. All of these factors produce both neurochemical changes in the body, and behavioral changes. In particular, Kenny remarks that these changes could actually be caused by "a combination of both sugar and fat."

In Kenny's study, rats preferred cheesecake—the food that contained the largest amounts of both fat and sugar. [Kenny (2010)]

Nicole Avena, a visiting research associate at Princeton University's Department of Psychology has also been studying food addiction. She and her colleagues discovered that very different physiological effects result from binge-eating fats than from binge-eating sugars. "Sugar and fat affect the brain in very different ways," Avena says. [Avena et al., (2008)]

It's when the physiological effects of both sugar and fat hit the brain simultaneously that the brain's pleasure centers go into overdrive. So gratifying is the experience that it can become truly addictive.

137

Fat is hidden in many foods.

You don't have to add a dollop of olive oil, butter or cheese to your meal to ensure you're getting some fat in your diet.

Fat is a natural component of all whole foods that come from animal sources. It can also be found in grains, legumes, avocados, nuts and edible oils, so for example just because you are eating a slice of bread without butter or margarine, it doesn't mean you are not eating any fat.

If you are calculating your daily fat intake, the fat hidden in foods should be taken into consideration.

Complex carbs + protein + low-fat = a satiety boost.

As mentioned earlier, the proportion of macronutrients you include in your diet can affect your appetite, your satiety threshold, how much food you eat, how much you weigh and how much fat your body stores. As a result, "… currently the best dietary advice for weight maintenance and for controlling hunger is to consume a low-fat, high-carbohydrate diet with a high fiber content." [Rolls (1995a)]

It is easier to lose weight on a high fiber diet than on a high fat diet.

"Daily energy intake is lower on low-energy density, high-fiber diets than on high-fat, energy-dense diets," wrote researcher Barbara Rolls when trying to find out why soldiers in the US army were losing weight while eating military rations. [Rolls (1995)]

Carbohydrates help weight loss better than fats.

Gram for gram, there are more Calories in fat than in carbs. More than twice as many, in fact. People who consume more of their energy from carbohydrate than fat have less risk of being overweight or obese. It is thought that this is because carbohydrate-rich foods are more satiating than fatty foods. [Astrup et al., (2000); Gaesser (2007)]

In a 1994 study called "Carbohydrates and Human Appetite", participants were allowed to eat as much food as they wanted. When they were offered a variety of high fat foods they ended up consuming more Calories than when they were presented with carbohydrate-rich foods. They did this without being conscious of it, which shows how easy it is to consume more Calories than you need. [Blundell et al., (1994)]

Even more alarmingly, a study called "Fat as a Risk Factor for Overconsumption" suggested that when people eat fatty foods, their increased consumption of Calories does not give them better feelings of satiety. [Blundell & Macdiarmid (1997)]

Swap, swap, swap!

Swapping high fat foods for low-fat foods can help to reduce fat intake. As mentioned, fat is not as good at providing satiety as carbs and protein, but you need to include a small amount of it in your diet to achieve weight loss. One way to enjoy the sensory pleasure and health benefits of dietary fat without putting on excess weight is to eat low-fat foods.

A study published in *The American Journal of Clinical Nutrition* found that when obese men were given high-carbohydrate yogurts before a meal, they ate less food during the meal than they did after a pre-meal serving of high-fat yoghurt. The researchers concluded that: "Both the amount of fat in the diet and total energy intake should be managed in weight-loss regimens. Low-fat foods and fat substitutes can help to reduce fat intake. . . . the best dietary advice for weight maintenance and for controlling hunger is to consume a low-fat, high-carbohydrate diet with a high fiber content." [Rolls (1995b)]

For example, use low-fat salad dressing. A salad dressing containing no fat at all will probably produce a pretty unpalatable salad. And it's important to make salads taste good, so that you will want to eat plenty of fresh raw garden vegetables. On the other hand a high fat salad dressing can negate the good effects of eating a salad in the first place. You might be surprised at the exorbitant number of Calories in many commercial salad dressings. Use a low-fat salad dressing such as one made with cold-pressed olive oil, perhaps mixed with a little lemon juice or apple cider vinegar. Or use avocado, very sparingly, as a salad dressing. A creamy low-fat dressing can be made from chickpeas (garbanzo beans) blitzed in a food processor with a little lemon juice and garlic.

Researchers at Ohio State University (USA) reported that eating fresh salad with some fat aids in the body's absorption of the antioxidants found in many vegetables. Without the presence of a little fat those antioxidants may not be as digestible.

Tips for including fat in the Satiety Diet.

- Eat "healthful" fats. The quality of the fat you eat is just as important as the amount.
- A low-fat diet is better for weight loss than a high fat diet or a no-fat diet. Choose foods that are not high fat, and not non-fat, but low-fat. A little fat helps nutrients absorb more readily. It also contributes to satiety. Non-fat foods can leave you feeling hungry. High fat foods contain a lot of Calories per unit of weight compared to other foods.
- If possible, avoid eating a combination of fat and sugar together in the same dish.
- For better satiety, include a little "healthful" fat with each meal.

Genetic resistance to fat.

Not everyone has the same physiology, so not everyone gains weight on a high fat diet. Some people are genetically "resistant" to the consequences of eating large amounts of fat. They stay lean, despite consuming a large proportion of fat with each meal. Scientists say they have "high-fat phenotypes", in contrast to people with "low-fat phenotypes" who gain weight on a high-fat diet. [Cooling & Blundell (2001)]

Macronutrients: Carbohydrates

Sugars, starches and dietary fibers are types of carbohydrate. Also known as "carbs", these molecules are made up of carbon, hydrogen and oxygen atoms in various configurations. They naturally exist in fruits, grains, vegetables and dairy products. Carb-rich foods are those that are sweet (like toffee and honey) or starchy (like bread and pasta) or both (like cake). Fiber can't be digested, but sugars and starches can, and these carbs are the body's main source of energy. They are vital for good health. Dietitians recommend that about 45-60% of our energy intake should come from carbohydrates.

The benefits of carbohydrates:
* They protect your muscles

When your body needs fuel, it uses the energy from carbohydrates first. If there's not enough carb-energy present in your system, it starts to use the energy in protein. Muscles are built from protein. When no carbs are available, your body breaks down your own muscles as an energy source. Carbs protect your muscles!

* They feed your microbiome.

Carbs also form part of many nutritious foods, and—*very* importantly—they can provide nutrients for the beneficial bacteria in your intestines that help you digest your food. This mass of gut bacteria is known as the microbiome, and its amazing role in combating obesity is only just being recognized.

* They boost satiety.

You need carbs for satiety. People who try eating nothing but meats, eggs and fish eventually find themselves craving for fruit, vegetables, bread and sweets. This is your Inner Guardian's way of telling you to go and find the sustenance you need for optimum health.

* They help you stick to a weight-loss diet.

A "zero carb diet" (also known as a ketogenic diet) is difficult to stick to. Low-carb diets are similarly hard to sustain. The body naturally desires carbohydrates, just as it desires protein and the other macronutrients. Cutting out an entire group of any macronutrient is detrimental not only to your health but also to your weight loss journey.

* They provide a wide range of nutrients.

For the sake of good nutrition, you need to eat foods that contain carbohydrates.

* The right kinds of carbs help regulate your blood sugar.

Complex carbs exist in whole, unrefined foods. As a general rule, these foods are high in dietary fiber and also richer in nutrients than processed foods.

Examples of processed foods include white rice and foods made with refined white flour, such as white bread, pizza, cakes, cookies and most pasta. Much of the natural fiber has been removed from these foods during processing.

Fiber-rich foods such as brown rice, nuts, seeds, legumes, whole grain bread and oatmeal are more slowly digested than low-fiber foods.

When food is digested slowly, glucose and other nutrients are released into the bloodstream gradually. Energy is supplied to the body continuously, keeping your blood sugar levels even.

Tip #1: When you eat carbs, eat complex ones. Whole grains can be included in side dishes, pilafs, salads, breads, crackers, snacks, and desserts.

Tip #2: Instead of regular pasta, choose pasta made from wholegrain wheat, buckwheat, brown rice, or pulses.

Refined, low-fiber carbs are digested rapidly. They release an intense burst of nutrients into your bloodstream. Your blood sugar soars rapidly to a spike, then plummets. Such spikes can trigger an insulin roller-coaster and leave you feeling hungry after they decline. Low blood sugar levels can activate your hunger hormones, causing cravings for more carbs. Keeping your blood sugar steady will help you lose weight. It may also improve your mood.

* Carbs can lift your mood.

Depression and weight problems are linked. Some people lose weight when they are seriously depressed, while others gain it. Those who gain weight may become even more depressed due to their changing body shape. In some cases it is unclear whether depression causes weight gain or vice versa, but being in low spirits can prompt people to eat as a way of comforting themselves, instead of eating to satisfy hunger. Using food to make you feel better, or to relieve stress or as a reward is called "emotional eating".

Dr. Judith J Wurtman, author of *The Carbohydrate Craver's Diet*, studied the relationship between emotional state, carbohydrate craving and brain serotonin. She found that overeating is frequently associated with a desire for stress relief. Eating carbohydrate-rich foods stimulates the production of the neurotransmitter serotonin in the brain. Serotonin is an important mood-regulator. Research suggests that your serotonin levels can affect not only your appetite, digestion, sleep, memory a nd sexual function, but also your emotions and mood. [Wurtman & Wurtman (1995), Fernstrom & Wurtman (1971), Wurtman & Wurtman (1989)]

About refined carbohydrates.

Refined carbs are found in highly processed or sugar-rich foods including:

- Many packaged breakfast cereals (such as puffed rice and corn flakes).
- Products made with refined white flour, such as pizza, white bread, bread snacks, dry biscuits/crackers, pasta, cookies and cake.
- French fries/crisps.
- White rice.
- Foods laden with refined sugar, such as regular sodas, sweets and candy.

The problem with eating lots of refined carbs is that you're consuming Calories with fewer nutrients, and you're missing out on the vital fiber that's so essential for the health of your gut microbes and so important for satiety.

Carbs boost satiety

In a 1988 study, Professor Wurtman found that when people ate modest portions of carbohydrate-rich foods at the beginning of a meal, they tended to eat less food overall. The carbs seemed to be boosting satiety. [Wurtman & Wurtman (1988)]

A study published in the International Journal of Food Science and Nutrition compared breakfasts of the same Calorie value but different macronutrient compositions. The breakfasts were:

* carbohydrate-rich, high-fiber
* carbohydrate-rich, low-fiber
* fat-rich, high-fiber
* fat-rich, low-fiber

Volunteers ate the breakfasts in random order on separate mornings. For the rest of the day they ate whatever they liked. The results?

The most filling meal, which made people eat fewer snacks throughout the morning and less food at lunch time, was the high-fiber, carbohydrate-rich breakfast. Satiety lasted longer after this breakfast than after any of the other meals.

The breakfast that came second in the satiety ratings was the carbohydrate-rich, low-fiber meal.

The fatty breakfasts came last. The researchers found that, "Both fat-rich breakfasts were . . . less satiating than the carbohydrate-rich meals and were followed by greater food intake during the morning."

The scientists watched the way the volunteers ate *after* breakfast, and noted that over the course of the day those who had eaten the fat-rich breakfasts consumed significantly more Calories than the eaters of the high-fiber, carb-rich meal. They had also eaten more fat, in total. [Holt et al., (1999)]

Another study, published in the European Journal of Clinical Nutrition, found that "...carbohydrate-rich foods are more satiating than fat-rich foods . . . The total amount of carbohydrate consumed at a meal . . . may partly determine the degree of hunger arising within the next 2 hours." [Holt et al., (1996)]

Why carbohydrates help you reach satiety.

When you eat carbs, the insulin released by your body propels glucose and amino acids into your muscle cells. The amino acids left behind in your bloodstream include tryptophan. Tryptophan can transfer itself from your blood into your brain, where it is converted to serotonin. So when you eat carbs, this relatively higher level of tryptophan in your blood leads to relatively higher levels of serotonin in your brain.

Remember what's so great about serotonin? It's a neurotransmitter that is associated with mood and appetite. Basically, it makes you happier, helps you sleep better and curbs your appetite.

What are the risks of low-carb diets?

The Inuit people of the Arctic and the Masai of Africa are two of the very few societies whose diet is traditionally very low-carb. The physiology of these populations has adapted, over thousands of years, to the consumption of mainly protein and fat. Even *they* need to eat carbs, however. Like the animals we call carnivores, they habitually consume the stomach and gut contents of their vegetarian prey.

In both populations, physical activity is a major way of life. Men, women and children operate at quite a marked Calorie deficit, which accounts for their leanness.

However even the health of the well-adapted Masai and Inuit people can suffer from the over-abundance of animal protein and fat, and under-consumption of carbs.

Researcher George V. Mann did an autopsy study of 50 Masai men and found that they had extensive atherosclerosis (hardened arteries). [Mann et al., (1971)]

Atherosclerosis puts people at risk of heart disease and stroke. A 2003 study of the Inuit concluded that, in general, heart disease was a significant cause of death among the population. [Bjerregaard et al., (2003)]

As we age, we tend to lose bone density. A 1974 study found that bone loss in older people began earlier and occurred with greater intensity for Inuit people. They surmised, "Nutrition factors of high protein, high nitrogen, high phosphorus, and low calcium intakes may be implicated." In other words, the diet of mainly meat played a part in bone loss. [Mazess et al., (1974)]

Unless you are a full-blooded Inuit or Masai person, you are unlikely to thrive on a low-carb diet, or even to be able to stick to it for more than a few months.

Very low-carb diets are not a solution to weight problems.

Significantly, very low-carbohydrate diets do not usually lead to long-term weight loss. The fashion of low-carb eating has been around for a long time now, yet people are still overweight.

146

Some scientists think that low-carb diets may actually cause people to put on weight. Researchers who set out to prove the benefits of the low-carb, high-fat "Paleo diet" have instead discovered it can cause significant and rapid weight gain. The study, by Melbourne University researchers, focused on two groups of overweight mice with pre-diabetes symptoms (impaired glucose intolerance). One group was put on the Paleo diet, and the other on their normal diet.

After only eight weeks, the mice on the Paleo diet gained 15 per cent of their body weight. Not only that, but their glucose intolerance became worse. [Lamont et al., (2016)]

One of the researchers, Associate Professor Andrikopoulos, said that he expected to see some weight loss in the Paleo-diet mice. Instead he was surprised by how much weight they gained. "The fat mice became even fatter and their glucose control became even worse," he said.

The test was conducted on mice, not human beings. However mice and men share genes and similar physiology.

Many people do lose weight on the Paleo diet—at least in the short term. This could be because they cut out refined, sugary foods such as soft drinks, alcohol, cakes, sweets and pastries. Anyone on any diet who stops eating the fatty, sugary, highly-processed foods they used to eat, is likely to lose weight.

In cutting out entire food groups, however, Paleo dieters are putting themselves at risk of cravings. When they stop dieting, they are likely to compensate for all the carbs they resisted, by eating more.

Gluten

Gluten is found in many carb-rich foods. For more about gluten, including a list of gluten-free, low GI foods, see *The Satiety Diet Weight Loss Toolkit* (book # 2 in the Satiety Diet series).

About whole grains.

Many people trying to lose weight avoid entire food groups in their efforts to be slim and healthy. Some have become convinced that eating grains causes inflammation, contrary to the overwhelming scientific evidence.

". . . whole grain intake is associated with a reduced risk of coronary heart disease, cardiovascular disease, and total cancer, and mortality from all causes, respiratory diseases, infectious diseases, diabetes, and all non-cardiovascular, non-cancer causes. These findings support dietary guidelines that recommend increased intake of whole grain to reduce the risk of chronic diseases and premature mortality." [Aune et al., (2016)]

It is thought, however, that consumption of *refined* grains may cause inflammation. [Masters, et al., (2010)]

But far from being inflammatory, consumption of whole grains appears to have the opposite effect. In fact, eating whole grains could reduce the risk of type 2 diabetes and cardiovascular disease, ". . . due to an effect on plasma inflammatory protein concentrations . . ." [Masters, et al., (2010)]

Nature delivers grains to us in whole form. An unprocessed grain is the entire seed of the plant, comprising the bran (the outer layer), the germ (the core), and the endosperm. Refining the grain removes the germ and the bran. This means that the valuable fiber, protein, and other essential nutrients are discarded.

The fiber in whole grains has an anti-inflammatory effect.

The beneficial microbes that live in your gut (and which are thought to help regulate appetite) rely on fiber for their survival. They use it as food. As a by-product of eating the fiber, they produce short-chain fatty acids (SCFAs). The body absorbs these SCFAs into the bloodstream. They are valuable to your health because they mitigate inflammation and help your immune system to function properly.

It's inflammation that puts us at risk of so many "Western diseases" such as diabetes and cardiovascular disease. When people fail to consume sufficient fiber in their daily diet, their gut microbes degenerate. As a result their immune systems may be ". . . existing in kind of a simmering pro-inflammatory state," says Professor Justin Sonnenburg, author of "The Good Gut". [Sonnenburg et al., (2015)]

Carbohydrates are part of the satiety solution.

When you eat food containing carbohydrates, your digestive system breaks down the digestible carbs into sugar, which enters your blood stream. As your blood sugar levels rise, your pancreas produces insulin, a hormone that prompts your cells to absorb blood sugar for energy or storage.

But this does not mean that insulin and sugar/carbohydrates are enemies of weight loss!

Insulin can actually *suppress* appetite [Pliquett et al., (2006)]. Furthermore, carbohydrates are better than dietary fat at helping you burn off the Calories in stored fat. [Acheson (1993)] This means you're probably storing more Calories when you eat fat than when you eat carbohydrates.

Protein can cause insulin spikes too, especially when processed. [Holt et al., (1997)]In fact, whey protein provides a higher insulin spike than white bread. [Salehi et al., (2012)]

Low protein, high carb diets can benefit your health.

It is well known in scientific circles that when people restrict their Calorie intake by around 40% they:

- Lose weight
- Live longer
- Improve their metabolic health
- Normalize their insulin levels and blood sugar levels
- Improve their levels of blood lipids (fats)
- Decrease their risk of cardiovascular disease
- Decrease their risk of diabetes

However, it is psychologically very difficult to sustain a diet in which Calories are restricted by 40% and hunger is ever-present. Besides, such severe energy restriction can adversely affect people's bone mass, libido, mood and fertility.

A 2015 study published in *Cell Reports* found that by adjusting the macronutrient balance of your diet to make it low in protein and high in carbohydrates, it might be possible to mimic the benefits of the 40% restricted Calorie diet.

The researcher found that when mice were allowed to eat as much as they wanted, Low Protein, High Carbohydrate diets ". . . delivered similar benefits to Calorie Restricted diets in terms of levels of insulin, glucose and blood lipids ... despite increased energy intake." [Solon-Biet (2015)]

When the mice were put on a combination of Calorie Restricted *and* Low Protein, High Carbohydrate diets, they received no extra health benefits compared with eating as much as they liked of the Low Protein, High Carbohydrate foods.

In other words, as long as they were eating Low Protein, High Carbohydrate foods, they didn't need to restrict their Calories in order to get fantastic health results!

Good news indeed!

But did the Low Protein High Carbohydrate diets also help with weight loss?

When the mice were freely eating as much as they wanted of the Low Protein, High Carbohydrate foods, they were naturally eating more Calories. But they also had much more energy to move around, play, socialize, explore etc. They *wanted* to exercise. By comparison, on the Calorie Restricted diet they ate fewer Calories and moved around a lot less.

By the end of the trials, the mice whose Calories were restricted weighed less than the mice who ate as much as they wanted. However the researchers found that the mice who ate freely of the Low Protein High Carbohydrate foods had a *lower percentage of body fat* than the Calorie Restricted mice and *did not gain any weight*! They had less "fat mass" relative to "lean mass".

Tip: Don't cut carbs out of your diet completely. Among many reasons, it could leave you low on energy and less likely to exercise, leading to muscle loss.

Carbs are better for satiety than fat.

Research suggests that foods high in carbs are more satiating than fatty foods.

People who eat more Calories in the form of carbohydrate than fat are less likely to be overweight or obese. [Astrup et al., (2000); Gaesser (2007)]

Furthermore, when people are presented with an assortment of high fat foods, they eat more Calories than when they are offered an array of high carb foods. [Blundell, et al., (1994)]

This may be because most of us are likely to think that a small serving of food will not be sufficient to fill us up, no matter how many Calories it contains, and fat contains more than twice as many Calories per gram as protein or carbs.

151

How to eat carbs and still lose weight.

You can eat carb-rich foods and still lose weight if you follow some simple rules.

* **Choose low GI foods containing complex, "slow" carbs.** This means whole foods, such as brown rice. When you eat low GI foods the sugars are broken down gradually and released more slowly into your bloodstream. You don't get a sudden flood of blood sugars that sends your insulin levels skyrocketing.

* **You can "slow down" carbs** by eating them in combination with other foods, especially foods rich in fiber. Nature helps us to do this—for example, sugar-rich fruits also contain fiber.

* **Eat your carbs last.** Save sweet and/or starchy foods for the end of your meal. A normal meal contains protein and fats, whose digestion requires a range of hormonal responses in the body. When these hormones are at work, they slow down the rate at which carbs are broken down and passed into your bloodstream. Thus, if you make sure you eat your carb-laden foods at least 15 minutes after you've eaten your proteins and fats, you'll help to even out your blood sugar levels and lower the risk of "spikes". Also, it takes around 20 minutes for the brain to receive satiety signals from eating carbs, and only about 5 minutes for signals from protein and fats, so with protein and fat in the first course of your meal, you'll feel full quicker and stop eating sooner.

Macronutrients: Protein.

You need to eat a certain amount of protein regularly to survive. Protein helps regulate your appetite, and is an essential building block for lean muscle, bones, cartilage, skin and other tissues. It is found in your hair, nails and blood. Protein is used in the manufacture of enzymes, hormones, and other chemicals vital for living.

Your body strives to meet a protein intake target. For every kilojoule of protein you need but don't eat, you are likely to overeat approximately 53 kJ of carbs and fat. [Brooks (2019)]

It is not necessary to eat meat in order to get protein. Populations around the world follow meatless diets while having plenty of protein to thrive on.

152

Amino Acids.

Protein is made up of chains of smaller chemicals called amino acids, which naturally occur in foods. Your body is capable of arranging amino acids in a number of different combinations. This is why it can manufacture thousands of different kinds of proteins from only 22 amino acids. It can also manufacture 13 of those amino acids all by itself, if you're eating a fairly well-balanced diet.

There are, however, 9 amino acids your body cannot manufacture. To remain healthy, you must eat these "essential" amino acids in certain proportions to each other. Your body uses amino acids in a particular ratio, so if you don't consume enough of one of them, the others cannot be used. All the amino acids work together. Your body will always balance them according to the scarcest amino acid. For example, if you consumed every essential amino acid except one, your body would be unable to use any of them as protein building blocks.

Nonetheless there's no need to be worried, because amino acids abound in a vast number of foods. Almost all foods contain the nine essential amino acids, though proportions do vary.

You don't need to eat eat animal-based foods or consume every essential amino acid at every meal, in order to get the complete protein your body requires. It's only necessary to eat some of each amino acid every day. Plant-based diets contain such a wide variety of amino acids that you can get all of your amino acids from them (and they give you added benefits, such as fiber).

For the best health outcome, vary your sources of protein. This helps you get a good balance of amino acids.

Protein promotes satiety.

Carbohydrates are more satiating than fat, but protein is more satiating than carbohydrates, and foods high in both protein and fiber are very satiating. That is why protein is important for weight loss. [Blundell (1986); Chambers et al. (2015); Yancy et al., (2004)]

Protein is digested relatively slowly, which is one of the reasons it staves off hunger and keeps you feeling satisfied for longer.

It is, of course, easier to lose weight if you eat foods that keep you feeling fuller for longer. Even just including 10% more protein in your breakfast can help you feel satisfied for longer, delay the onset of hunger and make you feel like having a smaller meal at lunchtime.

Eating at least 20 grams of protein for your first meal of the day may help with weight loss. You could, for example, eat baked beans on toast for breakfast, with a side of mushrooms (which are filling but low in Calories). Enjoy some protein-rich teff pancakes topped with berries and pepitas, or buckwheat porridge with crunchy walnuts.

When food passes through your digestive system it triggers the release of hormone called PYY into your bloodstream. When this enters your brain it suppresses hunger signals there and makes you feel fuller for longer. Protein triggers more PYY than any other foods.

Tip: To boost satiety (and help with weight loss), eat some protein at every meal. To boost satiety even more, eat protein that's combined with fiber. Examples include the plant proteins in such foods as teff, soy, chia, buckwheat, beans, nuts, seeds, lentils and quinoa. As an added bonus, plant-based protein is generally lower in saturated fat than animal-based protein.

Protein aids weight loss.

Research suggests that people who eat plenty of protein are more likely to lose weight and keep it off for at least a year. They are also more likely to keep eating healthful, lower-energy foods, if they are on a weight loss journey.

A 2004 study published in *The Journal of the American College of Nutrition* concluded that, "There is convincing evidence that a higher protein intake increases thermogenesis (heat production via Calorie-burning) and satiety compared to diets of lower protein content." The study's authors also reported that when people eat high protein meals they consume fewer Calories during the period after the meal. [Halton & Hu (2004)]

Other studies suggest that diets higher in protein result in an increased weight loss and fat loss as compared to diets lower in protein, but findings in this area have not been consistent.

There is also evidence that eating protein, especially with carbs, may help you to get a better night's sleep. Good sleep is also a valuable tool for weight loss. Feeling tired and sleepy can trigger "false hunger". [Zhou et al., (2016)]

Protein: Burn fat, not muscle.

When you're eating to become slimmer, the weight you want to lose is fat, not muscle. The scales might be telling you that you weigh less, but they cannot tell the difference between muscle and fat. How can you make sure you keep your muscles, instead of letting your body "burn" the protein in them for energy?

There are two things you can do in combination:

• Exercise regularly to keep your muscles intact and even increase your muscle mass.
• Eat plenty of protein.

A diet rich in protein, combined with regular exercise promotes loss of fat while protecting lean muscle mass. [Josse et al., (2011)]

Protein: Beware of decoys!

Healthy bodies instinctively crave protein. As already mentioned, amino acids are major building blocks of the body, and since our bodies cannot store them we need to eat protein regularly, to stay alive.

This is why your Inner Guardian uses all its wiles to lure you to eat foods that have the characteristics of protein. These characteristics generally include savoriness, umami flavor, saltiness, perhaps also the crunch of roasted crackling . . . Your Inner Guardian, however, is not really in tune with the 21st century. It does not know that modern foods with the characteristics of protein may not be protein at all.

All the sensory "protein characteristics" can be found in, say, industrially-processed potato crisps. Which is largely why we are drawn to them and "cannot stop at one"!

Based on the natural human desire for protein, industrial food companies produce cheap, low-protein processed foods that have the sensory characteristics of protein. These foods, which can encourage over-eating, are sometimes called "protein decoys".

Protein decoys were discussed on the ABC TV show "Catalyst" in 2015. To help explain what they are, here's part of the transcript, in which Professor Stephen Simpson, Executive Director of Obesity Australia, was interviewed.

Voiceover: "Your appetite control automatically gives priority to protein. If your diet runs short, you make up for it by getting energy from fats in carbohydrates that taste like protein."

Professor Stephen Simpson: "You know, the sort of lip-smacking, amino acid, umami [pleasant savory] flavors."

Voiceover: "Diluting protein makes food cheaper to make. Good for business, but bad for your appetite control."

Professor Stephen Simpson: "That's the savory snack food industry. Your potato chip is a protein decoy. It tastes like protein. Our bodies have evolved to associate those flavor cues with protein, but actually all you're getting is loaded up with more fat and carbs, leaving your protein appetite unfulfilled, and hence you're going to continue to snack and eat more." [Catalyst (2015)]

Tips for protein consumption:

- When on your weight loss journey, choose protein sources that are low in saturated fat and processed carbohydrates, and rich in diverse nutrients. Take into account the fats, carbohydrates, vitamins, minerals, and other nutrients that naturally occur in protein-rich foods. Bear in mind that while protein staves off hunger pangs, it's best if it's lean protein. For weight loss, keep counting Calories.
- Take note, also—if you eat more protein, you'll have to eat less of other foods to keep your daily Calorie intake at the same level.
- Beware of protein supplements. These are not whole foods. They are highly processed, and may not boost satiety. We recommend that you avoid protein supplements and obtain your protein from natural, whole, unprocessed foods that contain a balance of proteins and other nutrients, the way nature intended.

Protein is found in a wide range of foods.

When a food contains all nine of the essential amino acids in approximately equal amounts, it is said to provide a "complete" protein. Some people think that complete protein is only found in animal-based foods such as meat, fish, poultry, eggs and dairy products.

Far from it!

There is a huge variety of plant-based foods that provide complete protein. Many of the leanest and healthiest societies in the world thrive on vegan, vegetarian, or semi-vegetarian diets. These people obtain plenty of high quality protein from plant-based foods, without risking the cancers that may be caused by consumption of red meat such as beef, lamb and pork. And as already mentioned, the fiber that comes packaged naturally with plant proteins helps boost satiety.

Meatless meals are delicious. They have a number of other benefits, too. They are generally cheaper, the food tends to be lower in Calories, and eating plant-based foods may be better for the environment.

How much protein should you eat?

Research on the healthiest amount of protein to include in your diet is still continuing, and so far scientists have reached no agreement. The amount of protein people needs varies according to their age, their size, whether they are pregnant or not, and how much exercise they do each day.

As a general guideline, the Recommended Dietary Allowance (RDA)[16] for protein (for an average person) is 0.8 grams of protein per kilogram of body weight per day. The RDA is the amount of a nutrient you need to meet your basic nutritional requirements. Think of it as the minimum amount you need to keep your body functioning properly.

---

16   The RDA is the daily dietary intake level of a nutrient considered sufficient by the Food and Nutrition Board of the Institute of Medicine, a nonprofit, non-governmental organization in the USA.

Many nutritionists recommend estimating your minimum daily protein needs by multiplying your body weight in kilograms by 0.8, or weight in pounds by 0.37. The resulting figure is the minimum number of grams of protein you should eat each day.

Or, to make it even easier to visualize:

- A 150 pound (68 kg) person should eat about 55 grams of protein per day
- A 200-pound (90 kg) person should eat about 74 grams per day
- A 250-pound (113 kg) person should eat about 92 grams per day.

It's best for health and weight loss if your protein servings are split up into multiple meals, instead of being all eaten at one sitting.

Protein portion sizes.

Here are some ways to visualize how much protein the average person should consume in a single meal.

A protein portion is roughly the equivalent of:

- the size and thickness of the palm of your hand (not counting the fingers and thumb)
- the size of a bar of soap
- the size of a pack of cards
- Some people use plate size as a portion guide, allowing about a quarter of the space in the plate to be filled with a protein food— but this can lead to problems when dinner-plates are large!

As a general rule, women should have a single protein portion per meal, while men should have two portions. This book's section on portion sizes gives you helpful ways to visually gauge the amount of protein you should be eating at one sitting.

Is it possible to eat too much protein?

The body is only able to utilize a certain amount of protein. As with all foods, moderation is the key. Eating too much protein can result in unwanted side effects such as:

- Weight gain.
- Dehydration. Nitrogen is produced by your body during the metabolism of protein. Your kidneys use water to flush excess nitrogen out of your body, which can cause dehydration unless you make up for the water loss by drinking more.
- Digestive problems. If you eat a lot of animal proteins, the lack of fiber can cause constipation and/or diverticulitis.
- Eating too much protein can actually raise your insulin levels, which is not such a good thing.
- More serious side effects may include a greater risk of osteoporosis, kidney stones, and kidney disease.

Eating protein for satiety is all about balance.

While protein has been shown to promote satiety, eating lots of protein instead of carbs or fats does not necessarily make you lose weight. One of the secrets to using macronutrients for weight loss is to get the ratio right—in other words, to balance protein, carbs and fat.

Researchers still dispute whether or not high-protein diets work for weight loss. In fact, a high protein intake during childhood may actually have the reverse effect—it predisposes children to obesity in adulthood! A study published in the *International Journal of Obesity and Related Metabolic Disorders* reported that when kids ate a high percentage of protein during their first 2 years, they were more likely to get fat. By the age of eight years their body fat had significantly increased.

The researchers found a clear association between high protein consumption and obesity in children. They drew attention to the macronutrient composition of human milk, which is high in fat and low in protein. This is the diet nature intended for very young, growing children who use a lot of energy.

159

They wrote, "Our results suggest that high protein diet early in life could increase the risk of obesity and other pathologies later in life." [Rolland-Cachera et al., (1995)]

Your body can only use, and only requires, a certain amount of protein at any one time. Any more than that pretty much goes to waste. Protein can help you lose weight and adequate intake is vital for a healthy blood sugar level, but it is very important *not* to over-consume rich sources of protein such as animal-based foods or protein powders (which we recommend avoiding completely).

If you get most or all of your protein from vegetables, beans, nuts, seeds, legumes, and whole grains, your body's satiety signals will let you know when you've had enough. It's harder to over-consume plant-based protein.

Plant-based protein.

It's important to include the essential amino acids in your diet. If you prefer to avoid animal-based foods such as seafood, eggs, dairy products, poultry and meat, it's easy to find plant-based foods that provide "complete protein" (all the essential amino acids) either on their own, or when eaten with other plant-based foods.

Some foods, like soy and teff, naturally contain all the essential amino acids. Others only contain some of the essential amino acids, but meals with complete protein can conveniently be made by combining "complementary proteins."

Plant-based foods with complete protein.

Some plant foods that contain all 9 essential amino acids include:
- Amaranth grain: 9.3 grams of protein per 1 cup serving, cooked.
- Buckwheat: 6 grams of protein per 1 cup serving, cooked.
- Chia: 4 grams of protein per 2 tablespoon serving.
- Hemp-seed: 10 grams of protein per 2 tablespoon serving.
- Quinoa: 8 grams pf protein per 1 cup serving, cooked.
- Soy: 10 grams of protein per ½ cup serving (firm tofu), 15 grams per ½ cup serving (tempeh), 15 grams per ½ cup serving (natto).

160

- Teff: 9.8 grams of protein per 1 cup serving, cooked. This tiny, tasty grain is rich in protein, containing 15% high quality protein when cooked. It contains the essential amino acids required for the body's growth and maintenance. It also has abundant calcium, and contains manganese, phosphorous, iron, copper, aluminum, barium and thiamin. Teff also provides vitamin C, which is not normally found in grains. It's high in fiber, gluten-free, low in fat and low in sodium. Teff is the staple food of Ethiopia. In 2016 the CIA's "World Factbook" listed Ethiopia as the country with the leanest population of all the populations it surveyed in the world. [CIA (2016)]

Plant-based foods with complementary proteins.

"Complementary proteins" are two or more incomplete protein sources that can combine to provide of all the essential amino acids. Combining two or more foods with incomplete proteins can provide all the essential amino acids.

Complementary protein foods don't have to be eaten in the same meal in order for them to combine to make complete proteins. They can simply be eaten on the same day.

Protein groups in plant-based foods.

Dietary protein in plant-based foods can be grouped into the following categories:

- Grains. Examples include barley, buckwheat, bulgur, cracked wheat, corn, millet, oats, rice, wild rice, rye, triticale and wheat.
- Legumes. Examples include beans (black, broad, kidney, Lima, mung, navy, pea, and soy), black-eyed peas (cow-peas), chickpeas (garbanzos), lentils, peanuts, peas and tofu (made from soy beans).
- Seeds. Examples include amaranth, chia and salba seeds, cashews, flax seeds, pine nuts, pumpkin seeds/pepitas, seed sprouts (alfalfa seed, lentils, mung beans, peas, and soybeans), sesame seeds and sunflower seeds.

- Nuts. Examples include almonds, Brazil nuts, chestnuts, coconut (it's also called a fruit and a seed), filberts (hazelnuts), macadamias, pecans, pistachios and walnuts.

Examples of combining complementary proteins to make complete proteins include:

Grains together with legumes

Legumes together with seeds and nuts.

It is easy to mix complementary plant proteins. If, let's say, you eat legumes (such as beans, lentils, and peanuts), with grains (such as wheat, rice, and corn), you'd be getting the full range of essential amino acids.

People have been doing this for thousands of years—think Mexican corn and beans, or Indian dahl (made from lentils) with rice, or Lebanese hummus and pita. More recently, peanut butter sandwiches provide complete protein; peanuts being a legume, and bread usually being made from grains such as wheat or rye.

Some plant food combinations that provide complete protein:

- Ezekiel Bread: 8 grams of protein per 2 slice serving. This bread, whose recipe is mentioned in the Bible, is made from sprouted grains of wheat, barley, beans, lentils millet, and spelt.
- Oatmeal porridge with toppings of ground flaxseed, chia seeds, hemp seeds or a dollop of nut or seed butter: 10 grams of protein per cup of cooked steel-cut oats, in addition to the protein in your topping of choice. You can also cook your oatmeal in a high protein plant-based milk such as flax milk or almond milk.
- Rice and beans: 7 grams of protein per 1 cup serving.
- Spirulina with seeds, grains or nuts: 4 grams of protein per tablespoon.
- Seitan: 21 grams of protein per 1/3 cup serving. Seitan lacks the amino acid lysine, so cook it in a soy sauce-rich broth to make a complete protein. Seitan is made by mixing wheat

gluten[17] with herbs and spices and simmering it in broth. One of the bonuses of seitan is its chewy, meat-like texture.

Some examples of combining legumes and grains in diets around the world include:
- Refried beans and corn tortillas in Central America
- Chickpea falafels wrapped in whole wheat pita bread in the Middle East
- The Middle Eastern dip hummus, which is made from cooked chick peas and sesame seeds. It is often eaten with wheat bread, which adds an extra dimension of complementary protein.
- Lentil dahl with rice in India
- Rice and soybean products, such as tofu, in the Far East
- Daifuku, a Japanese dessert made from glutinous rice stuffed with sweet red bean paste made from adzuki beans
- Cornbread and pinto beans in the southern USA
- Rice with black-eyed peas
- Bean taco or tostada
- Split-pea soup with brown rice
- Bean soup with breadsticks
- Pasta salad with kidney beans
- Bean curd with sesame seeds
- Trail mix with toasted soybeans and pumpkin seeds
- Salad sprinkled with sunflower seeds and chickpeas
- Peanut butter on whole wheat bread

17 Wheat gluten has been receiving some bad press in recent times but unless you're non-celiac gluten sensitive (NCGS) or you have celiac disease, it's a food that is as good as any other. We list it in this book because we consider it a lightly-processed food; you can actually extract gluten from wheat in your own home kitchen. All you need is strong bread flour, salt and water. Mix it all together until it forms a dough, then start washing the dough by kneading it under running water. The water will wash away the starch, leaving behind the rubbery gluten. Yes, that's the same starch that can be used to stiffen your table linen or making wheat-starch paste! Seitan was originally created more than a thousand years ago as a meat substitute for Chinese Buddhist monks.

Benefits of plant-based protein vs. animal based protein
High protein foods from animal sources include:

- Seafood (fish, crustaceans, octopus etc.)
- Eggs
- Dairy products (butter, cheese, milk etc.)
- "Red meat" (Beef, pork, lamb etc.)
- "White meat" (Chicken, turkey and other fowls)

* Meat-based protein is associated with obesity.

In 2009 a study was published in the *International Journal of Obesity*. Titled "Meat consumption is associated with obesity and central [abdominal] obesity among US adults," the research found that obesity is associated with eating most of your protein in the form of meat. [Wang & Beydoun (2009)]

A 2016 study conducted in 170 countries found that the consumption of meat contributed to obesity just as much as fat and sugar. [You & Henneberg (2016)] This study, published in BMC *Nutrition*, was called, "Meat consumption providing a surplus energy in modern diet contributes to obesity prevalence."

Wenpeng You, the study's leading author, said, "Because meat protein is digested later than fats and carbohydrates, this makes the energy we receive from protein a surplus, which is then converted and stored as fat in the human body."

In the past, other studies have shown an association between meat consumption and obesity, but most people assumed it was the fat in meat that caused the problem. "On the contrary, we believe the protein in meat is directly contributing to obesity," You said.

Plant foods can provide good satiety. Plant protein is digested in a different fashion from meat protein, because of the fiber and other nutrients in plants.

Humans are animals. When we eat other animals, their proteins, which are the same as ours, are digested and absorbed more readily and rapidly than plant proteins. When food is digested more rapidly, it fails to keep us feeling full for longer.

Tip: Get most of your protein from plant sources!

* Animal-based foods may contain obesogens.

Animal based foods such as meat, poultry, eggs and dairy, may contain added growth hormones, antibiotics and other chemicals.

* Plant-based protein is rich in important dietary fibers.

Plant-based foods provide the valuable dietary fiber needed for satiety and a healthy microbiome. All kinds of fibers are abundant in these foods. The only dietary fiber to be got from animal sources is "chitin", which is the fiber found in the shells of shellfish. Few people are likely to much on unpalatable shellfish shells to obtain their daily dose of dietary fiber!

* Plant-based protein is lower in fat.

Plant based foods generally contain lower levels of fats and cholesterol than animal based foods. Animal sources of protein often contain saturated fat which is associated with raised low-density lipoprotein (LDL) cholesterol, a risk factor for heart disease.

* Plant-based foods are packed with nutrition.

If you obtain your protein from plant sources such as legumes, grains, nuts, seeds and pulses, then at the same time you are also consuming vitamins, minerals, carbohydrates, fat and fiber.

In other words you are getting a good balance of macronutrients.

Animal-based protein foods provide some minerals (mainly iron and zinc) and fat. They do not provide carbohydrates or any fiber, nor a wide range of vitamins. There is no Vitamin C in cooked meats.

Our human need for dietary fiber indicates that our bodies were built to cope with huge amounts of it. If people were built for low-carbohydrate diets, they would not become constipated while following them!

* Protein-packed plant-based foods are delicious and varied.

Countless plant-based food recipes are available in cookery books and on the Internet. Indian cuisine, for example, is famous for its spicy, tasty, protein-rich vegetable dishes.

* Plant-based protein saves money on groceries.
Beans, lentils and grains are usually much cheaper than meat.

* Production of food plants is more sustainable.
It is cheaper and more sustainable for farmers to produce plant-based protein instead of meat. The production of half a kilogram (about one pound) of beef on a typical US beef farm needs around 7 kilograms (approx. 16 lb) of corn, soy, as cattle feed. 7 kilograms of corn or soy would feed a lot more people than half a kilogram of meat!

In the USA, crops such as corn and soybeans grown just to feed cattle occupy at least half or more of the crop-growing acreage. Less land would be needed for farming if this were not the case.

* Eating plants is kinder to animals.
Large scale beef production, for example, is often cruel. In feedlots, cattle are allowed to eat grass in the way nature intended. Instead of their best-loved food, fresh green grass, they are given only high-protein soybeans and corn. The microorganisms in a cow's rumen work best when the cow eats grass, so when they are deprived of grass their health suffers. They are held in small pens to make sure they get fat because they cannot do any exercise, and often they are fed or injected with growth hormones to make them grow more quickly. Other chemicals with which they are treated include insecticides and antibiotics. Many drugs are required to treat or prevent or cure diseases caused by over-crowding in the pens.

Even dairy-farming is cruel. Millions of newborn male "bobby calves" are taken from their mothers every year and slaughtered, as "waste products" of the industry. For days or weeks on end, the distraught mothers call out for their lost babies, who they will never see again. The egg industry, too, is cruel. Male chicks are killed soon after hatching, and females are imprisoned in egg-laying factories, never to scratch in the green grass or feel the warmth of the sun.

* Eating too much animal-based protein can be a health risk.

It's true that eating protein helps you reach satiety, but it doesn't follow that eating loads more protein will have an even better effect. In fact, a 2014 study showed that eating more protein than your body needs can have seriously detrimental health effects, including a 75% increase in overall mortality, and a four-fold increase in the risk of dying from cancer. [Levine et al., (2014)]

* Eating more plant-based protein decreases health risks.

"These associations were either abolished or attenuated if the proteins were plant derived," the researchers concluded. In other words, the association between eating lots of protein and dying earlier or getting cancer was greatly reduced or simply didn't exist if the protein people were eating was plant-derived.

Referring to this study, Professor Mark Anthony of Austin Community College in Texas, USA wrote, "The startling results argue for the use of varied plant proteins, whole grains, legumes, nuts and seeds—all of which are associated with satiety **and healthy weight**." [Anthony (2014)]

* Red meat and processed meats can shorten life expectancy.

Researchers from the Harvard School of Medicine (USA) found that people who eat more than 1.5 ounces (42 grams) of red meat per day have a greatly increased risk of an early death from cancer or heart disease. This would be like eating one large steak per week.

Processed meats are even more risky. Processed meat differs from unprocessed meat in that it is cured by adding preservatives and/or other additives. Eating even small amounts of processed meats (e.g. sausages, salami, bacon, ham) can boost the risk of an early death by a fifth. This is a huge increase!

The daily amount of red meat, as recommended by the American Department of Health, is 2.5 ounces (70 grams), around twice the amount suggested by the Harvard study.

Dr. Frank Hu, co-author of the study, said: "Given the growing evidence that even modest amounts of red meat are associated with increased risk of chronic disease and premature death, 2.5 ounces (70 grams) per day seems (too) generous."

The leading author of the study, Dr. An Pan, wrote: "We found that greater consumption of unprocessed and processed red meats is associated with higher mortality risk. [An Pan et al., (2012)]

These results would suggest that for optimum health, you shouldn't eat red meat on a regular basis. Instead, only eat it rarely, if at all.

It is thought that the human body may identify red meat as a foreign invader, triggering an immune response that could lead to the formation of deadly tumors. [Samraja et al., (2015)]

The Cancer Council of Australia in its National Cancer Control Policy, says, "The consumption of red meat and processed meat is convincingly associated with a modest increased risk of bowel cancer. There is limited suggestive evidence that red meat may be associated with an increased risk of oesophageal, lung, pancreatic and endometrial cancer, and processed meat with oesophageal, lung, stomach and prostate cancer."

A study by the World Cancer Research Fund published in 2005 recommended that children should never be given any processed meat, such as salami, bacon or sausages.

More tips for protein consumption.

* Eat your protein as part of whole foods.

Protein curbs hunger pangs, but the protein should be eaten with the natural fats that exist within the protein-rich foods. Protein shakes, for example, are not whole foods. They have been highly processed.

* Eat tofu with miso or natto.

Tofu is made from soy beans that contain phytic acid, which can block the absorption of essential minerals. Vegetarians who rely on tofu as a meat substitute should follow the Japanese example and eat it with miso or natto, both of which contain bacteria that lower the phytic acid levels.

* Eat some protein for breakfast.

In particular, eating protein as part of your first meal of the day has been shown to help with weight loss.

Proportions of macronutrients.

In 2005 the National Academy of Sciences (a US, non-profit, non-government organization) published their latest Dietary Reference Intakes (DRIs). According to these recommendations the Acceptable Macronutrient Distribution Ranges for adults (AMDR), as a percentage of total Calories eaten in your diet, are as follows:

- Protein: 10-35%
- Fat: 20-35%
- Carbohydrate: 45-65%

For good health and weight control, this recommendation can be refined as follows:[18]

- Protein: 10-35%—mainly from plant sources.
- Fat: 20-35%—avoid or limit saturated and trans fats. Aim to eat equal proportions of Omega 6 and Omega 3 fats.
- Carbohydrate: 45-65%—choose whole, unprocessed carbohydrate foods
- Fiber: Women need to eat at least 25 grams of mixed dietary fibers per day and men need 38 grams per day.

Balancing your macronutrients.

You might ask, why is it important to balance the macronutrients in your diet?

If you're continuing to eat the same number of Calories each day but you change your diet to omit a group of macronutrients (such as carbs) then you will necessarily be eating more of one or both of the other two macronutrients—fats and protein. A high fat diet is generally pretty low in carbohydrate, for example, and a high protein diet is usually fairly low in carbohydrate and/or fat.

---

18   Recommendation of the National Academy of Medicine, an American nonprofit, non-government organization.

This could be dangerous to your health.

According to the Australian Government National Health and Medical Research Council, "There is a growing body of evidence that a major imbalance in the relative proportions of macronutrients can increase risk of chronic disease and may adversely affect micronutrient intake." [NHMRC (2016)]

For example, studies have shown that diets rich in fat can drastically alter the constituents of the gut microbiome. The international *Society for the Study of Ingestive Behavior* reports that high fat intake has been associated with increased insulin resistance and weaker satiety signals. [SCIB (2016)]

In another example, high protein diets have been associated with childhood obesity and—in adults—with the loss of calcium through urine, result in loss of bone, thus weakening the skeleton.

It's worth mentioning this again. "Five-year-old overweight children had a higher percentage intake of proteins at the age of 1 year than non overweight children, and lower intake of carbohydrates. Multiple logistic analysis confirmed that protein intake at 1 year of age was associated with overweight at 5 years. Conclusion— an early high protein intake may … influence the development of adiposity." [Scaglioni et al., (2000)]

Cutting out any macronutrient, whether it may be carbohydrates or fats or protein, will eventually throw your physiological and psychological systems out of balance, potentially raising the risk of risk nutritional deficiencies, weight gain and chronic disease.

"A diet that is balanced in its macronutrient distribution is recommended for lasting weight loss because unbalanced nutrient profiles may increase the risk of adverse health consequences." [Wilkinson & McCargar (2004)]

Choosing the right types of macronutrients.

While it is important, in a diverse diet, to include all macronutrients, its also important to choose the right types—those that can help weight loss and promote good health.

"... the form of fat (e.g. saturated, polyunsaturated or mono-unsaturated or specific fatty acids) or carbohydrate (e.g. starches or sugars; high or low glycemic) is also a major consideration in determining the optimal macronutrient balance in terms of chronic disease risk."[NHMRC (2016)]

- Carbs: Within the carbohydrate group, low glycemic foods (for example) are better for weight loss than high glycemic foods. High fiber foods are also more satisfying. Fructose consumption can increase appetite.
- Proteins: Every day, include in your diet sufficient essential amino acids to form complete protein. The protein found in plant-based foods can help with weight loss.
- Fats: Within the fat group, choose polyunsaturated, monounsaturated, and Omega-3s.

In summary:
- The macronutrient composition of a meal can influence your satiety.
- Unprocessed, complex carbohydrates, fiber, protein and small amounts of fat have an overall satiating effect.
- On the other hand, refined carbohydrates, fructose, and fat combined with sugar appear to increase appetite.
- For weight control, include in your meals real/whole foods containing fiber, protein, unprocessed carbohydrates and a small amount of "good" fat, balancing omega-6 fats with omega-3 fats.

Lay out your meal on the plate to judge proportions.

Here's a useful tip; a great way to keep track of the ratio of macro-nutrients you're eating at each meal is to arrange your food on the tableware before you begin a meal. This gives you a "map" of the quantities of protein-rich foods, vegetables, carbohydrate-rich foods and fats you're about to eat.

By organizing the elements of your food on your plate this way you'll be able to monitor the percentages of macronutrients in your diet. Thus, if you don't include enough vegetables in one meal, for example, you can make up for it by adding extra veggies in your next meal.

Sectioned "portion plates" can help

To help you get used to estimating your macronutrients, you could try using a sectioned plate. This type of plate is often used for picnics, or for serving food on airplanes, or in military canteens.

The plate is divided up into separate areas. Fill just under half the plate with NTS veggies while using a little over a quarter of the plate for starchy carbs and the remaining slightly-bigger-than-a-quarter for protein.

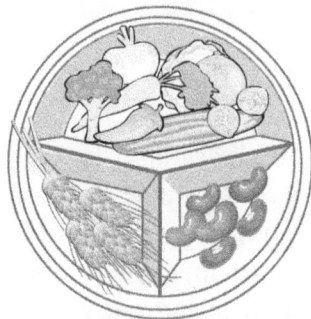

Dietary fiber.

What is dietary fiber and why do we need it?

Dietary fibers are indigestible carbohydrates. More specifically, "Though most carbohydrates are broken down into sugar molecules, fiber cannot be broken down into sugar molecules, and instead it passes through the body undigested." [Harvard (2017)]

Dietary fiber is also known as "roughage". It almost always obtained from plants (one exception is chitosan, which is found in the shells of shellfish). It is essential in any healthful diet for human beings and has many benefits, including:

- Improvement of bowel function.
- The boosting of fermentation in the intestines, which provides food for a healthy microbiome (the friendly microbes that live in the gut).
- Dietary fibers, especially soluble fiber, affect the body's absorption of ingested fatty acids. This is why eating foods that contain fiber can reduce blood cholesterol levels.

Fiber can boost satiety and help control weight.

Dietary fiber can help with weight loss for many reasons.[19] [Levine & Billington (1994)]

" . . . studies have shown that fiber intake is associated with a lower body weight," say the authors of an article in the *Journal of the American College of Nutrition.* [Clark & Slavin (2013)]

"Foods high in protein and fiber are satiating," report the authors of a 2015 review in *Trends in Food Science & Technology.* [Chambers et al. (2015)]

"A number of studies have shown that high-fiber foods consumed either at breakfast or lunch significantly reduce intake at the next meal when compared to low-fiber foods," says Barbara Rolls, the author of a 1995 article written for the US army. [Rolls (1995)]

In 2013 the result of a high-fiber diet study were published in the journal *Obesity.* Researchers noted that despite the fact that eating lots of fiber can reduce hunger and enhance satiety, most people on low-Calorie weight loss diets don't even consume the recommended daily allowance of fiber.

---

19 Note: In general, people who follow a low-FODMAP diet should avoid some types of fiber, including polyols, inulin, and oligofructose.

To test the effectiveness of low-Calorie, high fiber diets, they devised an experiment involving two such diets with different sources of fiber:

- Beans
- Fruits, vegetables, and whole grains

For four weeks one group of people followed the bean diet while the other derived their fiber from fruits, vegetables, and whole grains.

Both groups consumed significantly fewer Calories but experienced less hunger and better satiety, suggesting that fiber's properties play an important role in satiety, no matter whether it comes from beans or other plant sources. [Turner et al., (2013)]

Other researchers agree. According to the journal *Nutrition Reviews*, when people's diets all contain the same number of Calories, it's the people who eat more fiber who experience better satiety after meals.

The authors recommend, "In view of the fact that mean dietary fiber intake in the United States is currently only 15 grams per day … efforts to increase dietary fiber in individuals consuming less than 25 grams per day may help to decrease the currently high national prevalence of obesity." [Howarth et al., (2001)]

"Daily energy intake is lower on low-energy density, high-fiber diets than on high-fat, energy-dense diets." [Rolls (1995)]

Dietary fiber really can help increase satiety, thereby aiding weight loss. It works in a number of ways, depending on the type of fiber.

How does dietary fiber help with weight loss?
Fiber provides less energy.

All dietary fibers contribute less energy (dietary Calories) than sugars and starches, because they cannot be fully absorbed by the body. Insoluble fiber is almost completely indigestible and provides virtually no energy. Soluble fiber is partially fermented in the gut, and contributes some energy when broken down and absorbed by the body, but it's a relatively small amount.

"Regardless of the type of fiber, the body absorbs less than 17 kJ/g (4.1 kcal/g)." [Wikipedia (12th Aug. 2016)]

As a general rule, high-fiber foods, such as vegetables are low in Calories. When you eat the same volume of them as you would eat of low-fiber, high-Calorie foods, you can feel satiated on fewer Calories.

Fiber may obstruct absorption of some Calories.

Fiber can help to prevent weight gain by reducing the number of Calories the body *digests*, as distinct from the number of Calories *eaten*. Some fibers, such as insoluble fibers, may make it harder for the body to extract Calories from food. In other words, you may eat more fiber-rich foods than low-fiber foods, without absorbing as many Calories.

People on high fiber diets tend to have more abundant stools ("poop"), and some Calories may pass out of the body with these larger, more frequent stools. The fiber can carry Calories with it when it exits the body and is flushed away. [Wynne et al., (2005); Rolls et al., (2005)]

Fiber provides bulk.

Fiber makes your meal bigger, bulkier and more filling. It absorbs water and swells up, thus prompting your body to signal that your digestive tract is expanding. Fiber can form a gel in your stomach, which stretches your stomach and contributes towards the sensation of fullness. Thus it helps promote satiety.

"Like water, fiber is one of a dieter's greatest allies. Fiber swells up in the stomach, causing the stomach to distend and send signals to the brain telling it that you are full and you need to stop eating." [Harvard (2017)]

Both soluble and insoluble fibers add volume to your food without adding as many Calories as foods that contain digestible carbohydrates. They help provide satiety and can reduce appetite.

Fiber increases the viscosity of food.

Viscous foods have a thick, sticky, creamy, semi-fluid consistency; think of honey, custard, cream or glycerin. Viscous foods are more satiating (which is why food manufacturers spend billions of dollars creating alluring food products with viscous, creamy textures).

175

Fiber slows digestion.

Many fibers (such as guar gum and pectin) slow down the rate at which the rate at which your stomach empties food into your small intestine, thus making you feel fuller for longer.

Fiber evens out blood sugar levels.

By slowing down the digestion process, fiber may help to prevent blood glucose spikes. "Fiber helps regulate the body's use of sugars, helping to keep hunger and blood sugar in check." [Harvard (2017)]

Fiber boosts satiety signals.

Dietary fiber may influence some gastrointestinal hormones that moderate satiety and appetite, such as leptin. It possesses unique physical and chemical properties that help send early satiety signals to the brain and also produce increased or prolonged signals of satiety.

Fiber encourages chewing.

High-fiber foods take longer to chew than low-fiber foods that slip easily down the throat with little effort. Taking longer to eat meals can help you reach satiety before you have over-eaten, because it takes around 20 minutes for your body to generate satiety signals after you swallow food.

Fiber helps support the microbiome.

Significantly, fiber provides the right environment in which your microbiome can thrive. The microbes that live in your gut can have a powerful effect on your health and body weight.

Types of dietary fiber.

Scientists have discovered close to 100 different types of dietary fiber. Each type plays a different role in gut health. One study found that for every 10 g of cereal fiber people included in their daily diet, they had a 10% reduced risk of colorectal cancer. The same, however, did not apply to the fiber from fruits and vegetables, which indicates that each type of fiber possesses unique properties and serves a different purpose in the body.

Dietary fiber is classified into two main groups: soluble[20] and insoluble. A combination of "speedy" insoluble fiber and "slow" soluble fiber in the diet combines to perfectly regulate the movement of waste matter through the gut.

Soluble or "viscous" fiber.

The term "soluble fiber" is commonly used to describe types of dietary fibers that dissolve in water and form a gel in the digestive tract. These fibers are made up of polysaccharide compounds found in the walls of plant cells. Soluble fibers include inulin, oligofructose, mucilage, beta-glucans, pectin, gums, polydextrose, polyols, psyllium, resistant starch, and wheat dextrin.

Soluble fiber promotes good health.

Soluble fiber can be prebiotic. It can absorb water when it's mixed with water and cooked (like oat bran porridge) and it can also absorb water as it passes through your digestive system. After you eat it, the fiber passes through your digestive tract until it reaches your colon, where the microscopic creatures that make up your microbiome grab it and ferment it. They turn it into compounds that are essential for your good health.

But wait, there are more benefits! Soluble fiber also lowers total cholesterol and low-density lipoprotein (LDL) cholesterol, the "bad" cholesterol. This can reduce your risk of heart disease.

Soluble fiber's viscosity can boost satiety

Soluble fibers boost satiety more than fibers with less viscosity. Research has found that when people drink thick, viscous beverages instead of thin, watery beverages, they eat less food at the next meal, the drink passes through their stomach more slowly, and their satiety hormone levels are higher. [Vuksan et al., (2009); Juvonen et al., (2009)]

"Dietary fibers are believed to reduce subjective appetite, energy intake and body weight. However, different types of dietary fiber

---

20   Scientists at the National Academy of Medicine (USA) have recommended that the term "viscous" should be used instead of "soluble", because it's more accurate; however the term "soluble" is most widely used and accepted, so for now we will continue to use it.

may affect these outcomes differently. . . . fibers characterized as being more viscous (e.g. pectins, beta-glucans and guar gum) reduced appetite more often than those less viscous fibers." [Wanders et al., (2011)]

Scientists have yet to determine whether it's the sensory characteristics of such foods (their thick, creamy smooth texture) or something to do with the way foods with soluble fiber are digested that causes this appetite-reducing effect.

The same applies to foods as to drinks. Thick, creamy foods, such as porridge and thick soups, are more satiating.

Soluble fiber prolongs feelings of fullness.

Soluble fiber slows down the digestive process and delays the emptying of your stomach. In this way it promotes a prolonged feeling of fullness and satiety. After it has dissolved it looks like a mass of gelatinous, viscous, squishy stuff, sliding through your intestines. Despite the fact that it slows down the passage of food through the digestive system, it does not cause constipation—on the contrary, it regulates bowel motions. It does this by adding bulk to the feces moving through the gut; also by retaining water so that the bowel contents are moist and not hard and dry, so that stools are soft and easy to excrete.

Because it takes longer to digest, soluble fiber can make you feel full for longer, on fewer Calories.

Soluble fiber smooths out blood sugar levels.

Importantly, soluble fiber also delays your body's absorption of glucose, which decreases fluctuation (spikes and troughs) of blood sugar levels.

Food sources of soluble fiber.

Soluble fiber food sources include guar gum, oat bran, chia seeds and psyllium husks. It also exists in onions, beets, chicory roots, carrots, asparagus, Brussels sprouts, sweet potatoes, turnips and other vegetables, beans, peas, peanuts, lentils and other legumes, berries, unripened bananas, oranges, passionfruit, apples and other fruits, oats, barley, flaxseed, seeds, oatmeal, hazelnuts and other grains, nuts and seeds. There is no soluble fiber in animal-based foods.

Short chain fatty acids (SCFAs) may aid weight control.

Because soluble fiber can be digested it does (indirectly) deliver some Calories to the body. This is because your gut microbes use soluble fiber to manufacture short-chain fatty acids (SCFAs) which your body absorbs and uses to produce energy. Fortunately, the Calories obtained in this way from soluble fiber do not cause a spike in blood sugar levels.

SCFAs are not only hugely beneficial to your overall health, they may also contribute to weight control. One of these SCFAs is called butyrate. Experiments on obese mice and rats showed that after being treated with butyrate for five weeks, they lost 10% of their body fat.

The kind of soluble dietary fibers from which your gut microbes can produce abundant SCFAs include resistant starches, pectin, fructooligosaccharides (FOS), inulin, arabinoxylan[21] and guar gum[22].

In summary, soluble fiber:
- is found in a range of delicious foods.
- can prolong satiety and feelings of fullness, thus helping with weight loss.
- is fermented in the gut, into compounds that are essential for good health. This supports the microbiome, which may help with weight control.
- can reduce cholesterol and the risk of heart disease and diabetes.
- helps regulate blood sugar levels.
- may enhance immune function.
- helps regulate bowel movements and makes it easier to pass stools.

---

21 Arabinoxylan fiber is a major component of dietary fiber in cereal grains, and has been shown to help control blood sugar levels.

22 Guar gum is the ground-up endosperm of the guar bean, *Cyamopsis tetragonoloba*.

Insoluble fiber

Insoluble fiber gets its name because it does not dissolve in water. In contrast to soluble fiber, when insoluble fiber mixes with water it doesn't change much. This is because it is not very good at absorbing moisture. Like soluble fiber, however, it gives bulk to the contents of your gut, which helps regulate bowel movements.

Insoluble fiber can be prebiotic, which means that it is able to support your gut microbes. Eating plenty of insoluble fiber lowers the risk of bowel problems such as diverticulitis. The added bulk provided by insoluble fiber can also ease constipation.

Insoluble fibers include cellulose, some hemicellulose, chitosan and lignin.

Insoluble fiber for weight loss

Insoluble fiber cannot be digested, which means it passes right through your body and provides virtually no Calories.

"Eating insoluble fiber can reduce your appetite, lower your food intake, and even reduce your glycemic response to a meal you eat later. [Samra & Anderson (2007)]

In summary, insoluble fiber:
- can boost your satiety and feelings of fullness.
- provides virtually no Calories.
- supports your microbiome (which may also help with weight control and boost the immune system).
- is fermented into compounds that are essential for good health.
- is found in a range of delicious foods.
- can help dampen your appetite.
- can help lower your food intake.
- can help regulate your blood sugars (which also helps with weight control).
- helps ease constipation.

Food sources of insoluble fiber.

Most insoluble fiber comes from plants. It's found in leafy vegetables, fruit and vegetable skins, nuts, flax seeds, sesame seeds, and the bran layer of most whole grains—notably wheat, corn and rice. One particularly good source of insoluble fiber is crude corn bran. It contains fewer Calories than oat bran or wheat bran, and lots more dietary fiber.

Resistant starch.

Resistant starch is another carbohydrate. It's not really a fiber, although it's often considered as a third type of dietary fiber that can offer the same benefits as both soluble and insoluble fibers. It is sometimes compared to "fermentable insoluble fiber."

Scientists used to believe that any starch in the food we eat was fully broken down and absorbed in the small intestine. They thought that dietary fiber was the only food element that lasted long enough to pass into the large intestine.

Recently, it has been discovered that quite a large proportion of starch dodges or "resists" being digested in your small intestine and travels further in your gut, until it reaches your large intestine, where it produces effects similar to those generated by dietary fibers.

Research into resistant starch has revealed that it has some astonishing health benefits. Dr. David Topping, research scientist with CSIRO, said, "Resistant starch is turning out to be as important, and possibly more important, than fiber for the health of the human bowel."

Resistant starch can aid weight control.

There are several ways in which resistant starch can support weight loss.

Resistant starch supports the microbiome.

Resistant starch provides the health benefits of both insoluble and soluble fibers. It travels through your stomach and small intestine undigested. Just like soluble fiber, when it reaches your gut it feeds the "friendly" microbes that live there, increasing their health and number. These "good bugs" can then produce numerous compounds, including beneficial intestinal gases and short-chain fatty acids—notably butyric acid, which has enormous health benefits for the human body. A healthy microbiome can boost weight control.

Resistant starch provides fewer Calories.

When starch is cooked, then given time to cool down, its structure changes. It crystallizes into "resistant" forms that are harder for your digestive enzymes to break down. This means that you can eat pasta or pizza the day after it was cooked and absorb fewer Calories out of it than you would have absorbed if you'd eaten it when it was hot and freshly cooked.

Resistant starch doesn't make your blood sugar spike.

Resistant starch has an advantage over many other carbs—when you eat it, it doesn't raise your levels of blood sugar. And when you don't get blood sugar spikes, you don't get a strong insulin response that leads to a blood sugar crash accompanied by hunger and cravings.

Several studies show that resistant starch can improve insulin sensitivity. [Johnston et al., (2010)]

Resistant starch triggers glucagon release.

The hormone glucagon helps increase your body's fat-burning pace. Consumption of resistant starch stimulates the production of this hormone.

Resistant starch can help boost satiety.

Studies suggest that resistant starch may have a role in enhancing both short-term satiety . . . [Willis et al., (2009); Anderson et al., (2010)] and long-term satiety ... [Nilsson et al., (2008); Bodinham et al., (2009)]. It appears that the more resistant starch you consume, the more your satiety can improve.

How much resistant starch should you be eating?

Nutritionists recommend that you should aim to eat around 20 grams of resistant starch (RS) each day, to keep your gut healthy.

For more about resistant starch including food lists and how to treat RS for maximum benefit, see *The Satiety Diet Weight Loss Toolkit*, book #2 in the Satiety Diet series.

Resistant starch in summary.

To summarize, eating resistant starch can:

- increase your body's burning of Calories.
- boost your satiety hormones.
- decrease the number of Calories absorbed from the carbohydrates you eat.
- make you feel full.
- even out your blood sugar levels, reducing blood glucose "spikes" after eating.
- lower the glycemic index (GI) of foods.
- boost your immunity.
- help to keep your bowel motions regular.
- possibly reduce your cancer risk, by stimulating your gut bacteria to create short-chain fatty acids.

Note: If you eat a lot of resistant starch when you're not used to it you might end up with problems such as bloating, gas or bacterial overgrowth in the gut, so introduce it gradually into your diet.

Is resistant starch a "magic bullet"?

Is resistant starch the magic weight loss bullet we've all been hoping for?

No, but it's a useful helper. Losing weight and keeping yourself from putting it all back on requires the use of multiple tools in the Satiety Diet weight-loss toolkit.

Resistant starch is a wonderful substance that can help promote satiety and good health, but don't get too excited about it as a weight loss food. For a start, you have to be careful about the way you treat it. The way you process starchy foods can decrease their levels of resistant starch. Then, if you eat the non-resistant starch, your body will absorb it and use the Calories as energy or store them as fat.

Furthermore, resistant starch products such as Hi Maize® and potato starch are highly processed foods, not whole foods.

In the long run, however, incorporating more resistant starch into your eating plan may be beneficial to your health.

How you eat fiber is important.

Fiber in whole foods.

Fiber is more effective when eaten as part of whole foods than in processed foods. Nature intended for you to consume fiber as a natural component of fruits, nuts, seeds, vegetables, grains or legumes.

The best texture for fiber-rich foods.

If you want to reach satiety and keep feeling satisfied for longer, you can eat your fiber as part of some solid or viscous food. If you consume it in a thin, liquid form, as in a "shake", it will pass through your system more quickly than if you consume it in a solid or viscous form as, say, porridge or bran muffins. Slowing it down promotes satiety.

Processed fiber vs. naturally-occurring fiber.

Manufacturers sometimes add "isolated fiber" to foods to create "fiber-fortified foods". Isolated fibers may be chemically synthesized, or extracted from foods such as chicory root or coconut. Methods of extraction can include dry processing, wet processing, chemical, gravimetric, enzymatic, physical or microbial methods, or a combination of these methods.

Isolated fibers can be good for you, but adding fiber to low-fiber food may not be as beneficial as eating foods that are naturally fiber-abundant. Different dietary fibers have different roles in the digestive process. Many fiber-fortified foods contain only one kind of fiber, instead of the numerous kinds that exist in naturally fiber-abundant foods.

Isolated fiber may not possess all the properties of natural fiber, such as the stickiness of natural soluble fiber.

Furthermore, foods that are *naturally* high in dietary fiber come with nutritious vitamins, minerals and other plant compounds that may help your body utilize the fiber in the best possible way.

For best health outcomes and weight control, choose naturally high-fiber foods in preference to fiber-fortified foods.

Coarse fiber is more effective.

"The particle size of the fiber is all-important; coarse wheat bran being more effective [for satiety] than fine wheat bran." [Eastwood (2013)]

The removal of fiber from whole foods makes the resulting processed foods much less satisfying. But did you know that even when you leave the fiber in the food, if you mash it up and "disrupt" it before you eat it, you *decrease* fiber's satiety-inducing benefits? Puréeing fiber-rich foods reduces the satiety effect of the fiber. Consuming it may also cause spikes and troughs in your blood sugar levels, which can lead to sugar cravings.

Tip: don't smash up whole foods in those "magical" blenders! [Habera et al., (1977)] Yes, you will be drinking the fiber when you drink the blended liquid, but if your fiber is puréed:

- You'll consume the food more quickly than if it was whole (and slower eating is best for weight control).
- You won't reach satiety as easily as if you ate the whole food.
- You're likely to feel hungry sooner after you've consumed the liquid than if you'd eaten the whole food.

Eat different kinds of dietary fiber.

To get all the benefits of fiber it is essential to consume a wide variety of fiber-rich foods. When you eat fruits, vegetables, lentils, beans and whole grains you're obtaining not only dietary fiber, but also numerous other nutrients, and this is important for achieving satiety.

185

Soluble fibers, which include pectin, gum, mucilage and some hemicelluloses, are found across a range of different foods. The same goes for insoluble fibers such as cellulose, some hemicelluloses, and lignin. Variety is the key!

Focussing on eating, say, only soluble fiber with very little insoluble fiber, might slow down your digestion to the point of constipation. This is another good reason to eat a variety of fiber types.

If you find it difficult to eat the minimum amount of fiber you could take a fiber supplement, but make sure it's not your only daily source of fiber.

A tip from Chris Clark about fiber:

"I used to think that all I had to do was add a tablespoonful of wheat bran (insoluble fiber) and a tablespoonful of oat bran (soluble fiber) to my breakfast cereal every morning, and I'd have all the fiber I needed for the day.

"This did help my digestion, but it never seemed to curb my appetite or cravings. Eventually I realised that a) there are more than just two kinds of fiber out there in the world of food and b) eating fiber in its natural habitat, so to speak, increases its benefits. I had been eating fibers that had been separated from their mother-foods by processing methods. So I switched to eating a diverse range of whole-grain porridges garnished with seeds and nuts (and not necessarily just eating them for breakfast—they make a delicious dessert). Eating a variety of fibers as they naturally occurred in whole food significantly dampened my appetite and increased my sense of well-being."

How much fiber should we be eating?

The Hazda people of Tanzania still follow a "stone-age" diet, which is similar to the diet of prehistoric humans. Many people think that our bodies are still adapted to this ancient way of eating, and that the modern "Western" diet is not suited to human physiology.

Professor Stephen Simpson, the executive director of Obesity Australia, says, "An average person in the West, man or woman, is consuming less than 20g a day of dietary fiber. And to put that into an evolutionary perspective, six-month- to one-year-old Hadza kids are eating 50g to 200g of fiber a day, every day, and they do this throughout life." [ABC Catalyst (2016)]

Women need 25 grams of fiber per day, and men need 38 grams per day, according to the USA's National Academy of Medicine,[23]

Most people eat a lot less.

Want to start eating more fiber? If you are not accustomed to following a high fiber diet, you may have problems with gas at first. Introduce fiber gradually and make certain you drink plenty of liquids throughout the day.

* Fiber-rich "Satiety Porridge".

One way to ensure you get a good dose of fiber every day is to include a fiber-rich porridge with your breakfast—or with any meal for that matter! Porridge makes an excellent dessert too—just sweeten it with whole, fresh (or frozen) fruits and call it "pudding".

Some recipes for Satiety Porridge can be found in *Crispy, Creamy, Chewy: The Satiety Diet Cookbook.*

Gums, thickeners, jelling agents & other edible fibers.

When the dietary fibers listed below are mixed with water, they absorb the liquid and swell up. Eating these fibers can boost satiety by providing a feeling of fullness. They have close to zero Calories, and may regulate blood sugar and help lower cholesterol. These fibers should *never* be swallowed dry, as they can cause dangerous blockages of the digestive system. Always mix them with a liquid, such as water, and allow them to swell before you consume them. If you consume large amounts of these (or any) fibers when you're not accustomed to them, they can cause bloating and gas.

---

23 The National Academy of Medicine, formerly called the Institute of Medicine, is an American nonprofit, non-governmental organization.

Gums to enjoy.

- **Gum Arabic**—Of all the dietary fibers listed in this section, gum arabic appears to seems the least likely to cause digestive issues. Furthermore, it encourages the growth of beneficial microbes in the gut. Also known as acacia gum, is a natural gum composed of the solidified sap of various species of acacia trees.

- **Guar Gum**—Sometimes called gellan gum or guaran, this is a natural soluble fiber derived from guar beans.

- **Agar**—Also known as agar-agar, this is obtained by boiling certain species of seaweed. It has been used in Japanese cuisine since the 17th century, and is popular as a vegan gelling and sizing agent. In the 21st century a new weight loss fad called the "kanten diet" evolved. The scientific evidence supporting the efficacy of this diet is, however, sketchy.

- **Locust Bean (Carob Bean) Gum**—This substance is extracted from the seeds of the carob tree.

- **Konjac**—Konjac is a common name of the plant *Amorphophallus konjac*. The corms of this plant are known as "yams". In Japanese cuisine, noodles and "yam cake" are made from them. It is also used as a vegan substitute for gelatin.

Gums to avoid.

- **Tara Gum & Gellan Gum**—There is not a great deal of scientific research available concerning these two gums, which is why we recommend avoiding them. Gellan gum is produced by a bacterium.

- **Xanthan Gum**—This gum is produced by fermenting bacteria. It is not recommended for persons who suffer from histamine intolerance.

- **Carrageenan**—This is extracted from seaweed, so you'd think it was natural and safe. It has been used as a food additive. However carrageenan is an irritant, and can cause inflammation. In experimental laboratories it is used to induce inflammation in animals.

THE MICROBIOME

The human microbiome.

Microorganisms (microbes) inhabit just about every corner of the planet—every speck of soil and drop of water. They also live in and on animals, including humans.

Our bodies are home to trillions of "commensal microorganisms". These microscopic bacteria, fungi, viruses and archaea inhabit different body parts, such as the skin, the mouth, the nose, the vagina and the digestive tract.

There are thousands of species, and they cover every surface of our bodies, inside and out. They are living and dying within and upon your body right at this very moment. Collectively, they are called your "microbiota".

The term "microbiome" was coined by Joshua Lederberg to "...signify the ecological community of commensal, symbiotic, and pathogenic microorganisms that literally share our body space and have been all but ignored as determinants of health and disease." [Lederberg & McCray (2001)]

The word can also refer to the collective genomes of the microorganisms that reside in an environmental niche such as the human body. These symbiotic helpers are essential for our well-being.

Altogether, the body's microbes weigh about the same as the brain. Their activities affect our health, our body-weight and even—as many scientists think—our thoughts and behavior.

According to the University of Utah Health Sciences Genetic Science Learning Center, "Some scientists view our resident microbes as a newly discovered and largely unexplored organ, with many functions that are essential for life." [University of Utah (2016)]

How many microorganisms do we host?

Every body is different, and every community of microbiota is unique. The numbers of microorganisms hosted by each person's body can vary considerably. For example, some people might have twice as many or half as many microorganisms as other people.

Nobody is really sure exactly how many microbes make up the human microbiome, or even how many cells are in the human body, but we do have estimates. Scientists disagree on the proportions, however. "More than half your body is not human," is the headline of an article by James Gallagher, editor of BBC News Health. He writes, "Human cells make up only 43% of the body's total cell count, while the rest are microscopic colonists." [Gallagher (2018)]

Others say we're not outnumbered by our microbes, estimating the ratio as 1:1. [Sender et al., (2016)]

The second genome.

Our microbiota are so important they can be considered to be our second genome. Their genes vastly outnumber ours.

"...The human microbiome (all of our microbes' genes) can be considered a counterpart to the human genome (all of our genes). The genes in our microbiome outnumber the genes in our genome by about 100 to 1." [University of Utah (2016)]

Microbiologist Professor Sarkis Mazmanian, says, "...The genes of our microbiome present essentially a second genome which augment the activity of our own. What makes us human is, in my opinion, the combination of our own DNA, plus the DNA of our gut microbes." [Gallagher (2018); Grice & Segre (2012)]

How did we get our microbiota in the first place?

It started to happen when we were born. When babies are still in the womb, their bodies are sterile. As they pass down the birth canal on their journey into the outside world, their bodies pick up microbes from the mother. They may even acquire a few of Mom's gut bacteria from vestiges of her feces. This is good for newborns! As babies snuggle up to the breast and suckle on their mother's milk they receive not only any microbes that live on Mom's skin, but also many milk-sugars that they cannot digest, but which promote the growth of certain beneficial microorganisms in the gut.

Furthermore, "... there's increasing evidence that the milk itself is produced with bacteria in it." [ABC Catalyst (2016)]

190

The gut microbiome.

Most of your microbes inhabit your intestines. Each adult human has up to 2kg (4.4 pounds) of microorganisms living in their gut. Formerly called gut flora or gut bacteria, the crowd of microorganisms that inhabit the lower parts of our digestive systems are now known as "intestinal microbiota", "intestinal microbes", "gut microbiota" or "the gut microbiome".

The gut microbiome is the biggest, most diverse population of microbes in the human body. These microbes affect your life, and in turn their lives are affected by such factors as:

* The food you eat
* Where you live
* Where you work
* Where you socialize
* Where you exercise

Your gut microbes are essential for the breakdown and assimilation of nutrients from your food, enabling you to extract the vital dietary elements you need to survive. Without these tiny life forms, most of the food you eat would be indigestible. They are "symbiotic"—that is, they give you this service and in return you are their host, providing them with a welcoming environment in which to live. Not only are they an essential element of your digestive process, they also release beneficial substances in the normal course of their metabolic cycle.

The gut microbes help your body to produce vitamins and amino acids. Some of your intestinal microbes convert the undigested soluble fiber and resistant starch from your food into short-chain fatty acids. These travel out into your blood stream and slow down inflammation. They are a vital component in the functioning of your digestive and immune systems, your blood pressure and even your mental health! Imbalances in gut microbes have been linked to stress, anxiety and depression.

One of the short-chain fatty acids is called butyric acid, or butyrate. Amongst other health benefits it suppresses inflammation and contributes to the health of your gut lining. In mouse studies, it decreases the appetite for food.

Your gut bugs have a huge impact on your overall health. The food you eat feeds your gut bugs, so your diet could be contributing to your risk of obesity, heart disease, cancer, asthma, allergies, arthritis, autism, depression, multiple sclerosis, diabetes and more.

As if those tiny guys living in your intestines are not helpful enough already, scientists believe they may also play a role in making certain drugs work better. A small study conducted by researchers at the University of Texas (USA) reported found that cancer drugs worked better in patients who had a more diverse community of gut microbes.

The effect of the gut microbiome on health has become a field of intense research. For example, at the headquarters of the American Gut Project in Boulder, Colorado, Professor Rob Knight and his team are examining poop samples from a wide variety of people, with the aim of determining which microbiota are associated with which health problems.

Most amazingly of all, scientists have discovered that these microbes can actually talk to our brains, and even modify our genes!

The gut microbiome and obesity

Our intestinal microbes may play a part in dictating whether we are lean or overweight. Around the beginning of the 21st century scientists reported on the intriguing relationship between obesity and the microorganisms that inhabit our gut. The microbiota of obese people is quite different from the microbiota of lean people.

In a 2012 article entitled *Impact of the Gut Microbiota on the Development of Obesity*, the authors wrote, "The accumulating evidence strongly suggests that the gut microbiota play an important role in the regulation of energy balance and weight in animals and humans and may influence the development and progression of obesity and other metabolic disorders, including type 2 diabetes.

Although not a substitute for diet and exercise, manipulation of the gut microbiome represents a novel approach to treating obesity." [DiBaise et al., (2012)]

A 2014 study reported on, ". . . a case of a woman successfully treated with FMT who developed new-onset obesity after receiving stool from a healthy but overweight donor." [Alang & Kelly (2014)]

This patient had received fecal microbiota transplantation (FMT) as treatment for an infection in her digestive system. Also known as a "poop transplant", FMT involves cleaning out the intestines with large doses of broad-spectrum antibiotics to eradicate (as far as possible) the existing microbiome. Next, poop from a healthy donor is syringed into the almost sterile environment of t he patient's intestines. This new poop is teeming with microorganisms from the healthy donor, which are able to find a home and colonize the empty niches of the patient's gut. In this case, the patient had been of a normal weight, but after she received FMT from an overweight donor, she became obese. Scientists surmise that the new community of microbes may have been responsible for the patient's unexpected weight gain.

Experiments with mice found similar results.

In *Intestinal Microbiota and Obesity* researchers wrote, "The intestinal microbiota has recently been suggested to contribute to the development of obesity and the metabolic syndrome. Transplantation of gut microbiota from obese mice to non-obese, germ-free mice resulted in transfer of metabolic syndrome-associated features from the donor to the recipient." [Blaut & Klaus (2012)]

Researchers now know that an unbalanced microbiome can cause obesity in animals. A study published in the journal *Science* in September 2013 showed that slim, healthy mice turned into obese mice after gut microbes from obese humans were transferred into the gut of the mice. Similarly, when mice were transplanted with microbes from slim humans, they didn't put on excess weight. [Ridaura, et al., (2013)]

Certain gut microbiota are certainly associated with obesity. "The bacteria in fat people even seem better able to absorb Calories than those found in thin people," says Dr. Christoffer van Tulleken. [Van Tulleken (2013)]

Gut microbes can influence appetite and cravings via the "second brain".

There are many ways in which your gut microorganisms can influence your eating behavior. It's not only your brain that contains neurons (biological message transmitters). A closely packed, complex web of neurons also occupies your gut. This structure is called the enteric nervous system, and it regulates the biological operations of your gastrointestinal tract. Sometimes the enteric nervous system is called "the second brain".

The powerful signaling system that connects the bowel and the brain is called the "brain-bowel connection" or "the gut-brain axis". It's not an actual organ of the body, but rather a set of correlations between the brain and the gut.

These correlations fall into two categories:
- the circulatory system—that is, signals are sent back and forth via the lymphatic system and the blood stream.
- the vagus nerve (or the two paired vagus nerves, to be precise)— that is, signals travel up and down a long nerve pathway that stretches between the brain and the abdomen.

Appetite and food cravings may be governed by your gut microbes.

Gut microbes can produce neurotransmitters such as dopamine and serotonin, both of which involved in moderating your eating behavior. Many gut bacteria are also capable of releasing molecules that mimic your satiety and hunger hormones.

Many gut microbes can thrive on a wide variety of nutrients, but there are some species that prefer to consume their own particular food, such as dietary fiber, or carbohydrates, or a particular fat. For these "specialists", it's in their best interests to direct their human host to eat the food they want. Gut microbes can communicate with your brain, sending signals to manipulate your behavior. Sugar-loving microbes send "more sugar!" signals, while green leafy vegetable-loving microbes shout, "More kale!"

Researchers have found that when rats eat a lot of fatty foods, over a long period of time, they change the microbe population of their gut. This disrupts the "fullness" signals the gut sends to the brain, which in turn can lead to overeating and weight gain. If weight gain can be caused by a change in gut microbes, can the reverse be true? Could you make yourself lose weight by altering your microbiome?

It is thought that microbes could also affect "neuroplasticity", which is your brain's capacity to identify and form new neuronal routes and connections. It is the making of new pathways in the brain that gives you the ability to change your habits and break free of old, destructive habits such as "comfort eating".

These days, scientists are discovering more information about the associations between the gut microbiota and stress, depression, and anxiety—which are all emotional states that can have a huge impact on what you eat, how much you eat and when you eat, thus influencing your body weight.

Your gut microbes can indeed influence your appetite and your food cravings! Knowing this, perhaps we can manipulate our gut microbes, shaping them to help us lose weight.

Lean people tend to have a wider variety of gut microbes than obese people.

Scientists who study gut microbes in humans have found that lean people have a richly diverse microbiome, teeming with many species. In obese people, the microbiome is less varied. This raises the question, "Can you aid weight loss by making your own microbiome more diverse?"

Highly processed foods promote less gut microbe diversity, which is linked to obesity.

You can change (and improve) the ecosystem in your gut by changing your diet. Scientists have found that a narrower population of gut microbes is associated with a diet of highly processed foods. Habitually eating a wide range of unprocessed or lightly-processed foods can boost species diversity in your microbiome.

Antibiotics may contribute to obesity by altering the gut microbiome.

Modern use of antibiotics in humans, and in the animals that many humans eat, may be a factor in the rise of global obesity. Antibiotics are known to change the balance of gut microbiota, decimating some varieties while enabling others to proliferate.

Ever since the 1950s, antibiotics have been used in livestock production to promote weight gain. That is, farmer feed antibiotics to beef and dairy cattle, poultry, pigs, and other farm animals, *not* just to cure them of illnesses (these animals are perfectly healthy), but to increase their growth rate and make them put on weight.

Antibiotics change the composition of the animals' gut microbiomes, after which the animals gain weight. Could the same thing be happening in humans? When we consume antibiotics as medication, or when we eat the meat of animals that have been fed with antibiotics, are we altering our gut microbes in a way that makes it easier for us to gain excess weight?

Recent studies appear to confirm this idea, particularly in respect to children.

The authors of *Antibiotics in Early Life and Obesity* wrote, "Ultimately, antibiotics are important and potentially life-saving drugs that have considerably reduced the rates of human mortality and morbidity. Although these agents were thought to have minimal long-term metabolic side effects, we are now gaining clear insights to how these microbiota-modulating agents could contribute to obesity. [Cox & Blazer (2015)]

Researchers at the Johns Hopkins Bloomberg School of Public Health, USA, who examined the health records of 142,824 children between the ages of three and 18 years concluded that "… antibiotic use may influence weight gain throughout childhood and not just during the earliest years …" [Schwartz et al., (2015)]

In 2016, researchers at the University of Pennsylvania, USA, found that, "Administration of 3 or more courses of antibiotics before children reach an age of 2 years is associated with an increased risk of early childhood obesity." [Scott, et al., (2016)]

Not only can some antibiotics alter children's gut microbiome for up to two years, but antibiotic use is associated with both asthma and obesity. In 2016 researchers at the University of Helsinki in Finland wrote, "For the first time in human children, we demonstrate antibiotic-associated changes in the microbiome, which have previously been associated with metabolic diseases and obesity: [including] reduced diversity [of the microbiota] ..." [Korpela et al., (2016)]

Changing the microbiome.

If your gut microbiome can be changed to make you gain excess weight, can it also be changed to help make you become slimmer?

Let us review the facts:

- The non-obese woman who received a fecal transplant from an obese donor gained weight.
- Similarly, transplanting gut microbiota from obese mice to non-obese mice whose gut had previously contained no microbiota of their own, resulted in the non-obese mice getting fatter.
- An Israeli study has found that fatter people tend to have a less diverse range of microbiota in their gut than lean people.[24]
- A Finnish study found that antibiotics can reduce the diversity of the gut microbiota. Reduced diversity is linked with obesity. [Korpela et al., (2016)]
- Transferring "thin" microbes to mice that are genetically predisposed to obesity prevents them from gaining weight *even on a high Calorie diet!*

This evidence suggests that certain gut microorganisms tend to make us fat while others help make us lean.

---

24   The Personalized Nutrition Project is led by Prof. Eran Segal and Dr Eran Elinav of the Weizmann Institute of Science.

In fact, researchers have found that one particular gut microbe species, *Akkermansia muciniphila,* is associated with leanness and better glucose tolerance in mice. And in humans, higher levels of *Akkermansia* in the gut appear to have significant health benefits. [Everard, et al., (2013)]

Clearly it's a bad idea for you to take huge doses of antibiotics in order to wipe out your obesity-friendly gut microbes and make your intestines a sterile place, as researchers do to mice. This would be dangerous to your health. Besides, as soon as you went out into the world and started eating non-sterile food again, the microbes would start to re-colonize your gut.

So, if killing off our obesity-friendly microbes is not an option, is there any other way to change your microbiome?

Probiotic supplements may not help with weight loss.

Probiotic supplements contain live, beneficial bacteria that are good for your digestive system. They are available in yogurt, other dairy products, capsules and pills. Researchers have reported that certain strains of *Bifidobacterium* and *Lactobacillus* can not only act like antidepressants but also reduce anxiety levels. Depression and anxiety are known to influence people's eating behavior, so can boosting your levels of these specific microbes indirectly help with weight loss?

It is important to remember that just swallowing probiotic supplements may not help with weight loss, or indeed improve gut health, because:

- They are quite fragile little organisms and can be easily killed off by heat or stomach acid, before they even reach the gut.
- Furthermore, we cannot know which particular probiotic bacteria will best suit each individual person. Different bacterial strains may benefit some people but not others.
- If PRObiotics reach your gut they need plenty of PREbiotics to nourish them if they are going to survive. (A prebiotic is any substance in food which helps your gut microbes to thrive and thus benefits your health.)

198

People who take PRObiotic supplements without providing plenty of PREbiotics are gambling on the hope that:
- The microbes they are swallowing might not be destroyed before they reach the gut . . .
- And that if they do reach the gut, they will find the right prebiotics to keep them alive . . .
- And of those that stay alive, some might be particular strains that are helpful to their own, unique body.

The chance of all this happening is not good!

Prebiotics.

A prebiotic is a non-digestible food component, especially dietary fiber from plants (such as inulin), that promotes the growth of beneficial microbes in the gut. PREbiotics, unlike PRObiotics, cannot be exterminated by the body's stomach acids, or by heat or bacteria. They can:
- stimulate satiety hormones
- enable beneficial microbes to stick to the bowel wall
- provide food for beneficial microbes
- help to stimulate the growth of beneficial microbes
- selectively feed beneficial microbes instead of pathogens (harmful organisms).
- discourage the growth of pathogens.
- increase BDNF (Brain-Derived Neurotrophic Factor), a protein that affects brain function and parts of the nervous system.
- reduce the "awakening cortisol response" (a surge of cortisol that occurs about 30 minutes after people wake up in the morning, and which is more intense when people are under stress)
- help to reduce emotions of anxiety

[Schmidt et al., (2015); Parnell & Reimer (2012)]

PREbiotics act as a food, or fertilizer, to nourish the good bacteria. Probiotics are far more beneficial if they are combined with prebiotics. Without consuming plenty of PREbiotics you might be spending your money on PRObiotic supplements without getting the full benefit. If you don't have enough of the right prebiotics in your gut, the probiotic bacteria can simply die and be flushed away.

Even if some probiotic microbes swallowed in a drink managed to survive your stomach acids and reach your intestines, they would still have to compete against the huge numbers of microbes that are already living there.

It is, nonetheless, unlikely that PRObiotic supplements can give you the "thin" microbes. "Forget those trendy probiotic drinks—just eat more porridge!" writes Dr. Christoffer van Tulleken in The Daily Mail Australia, 22 October 2013. "The idea that there could be one simple drink with one simple bug in it that could make us all feel better is farcical."[25]

The gut microbiome has often been compared to a rainforest, brimming with thousands of species of living things, each with its own unique ecosystem. Simply throwing some more microbes into this complex mixture and thinking it will improve the whole system is a bit naive. Besides, the fat and sugar contained in some probiotic supplements can sabotage weight loss.

Okay, if drinking prebiotic products is fairly futile, what can you do instead? The answer is simple; *eat more fibers*. And one of the best ways to incorporate fibers into your diet is by eating whole grains, legumes and fresh vegetables. The beneficial microorganisms in your gut feed on the indigestible sugars in fiber, which play the role of prebiotics.

"To extend the rainforest analogy," writes Dr. van Tulleken, "if swigging a yoghurt drink is throwing a few seeds into the forest, significantly altering your diet is like changing the soil and the weather; get it right and the good stuff will flourish." [Van Tulleken (2013)]

---

25 He adds, however, that, "... There is evidence that taking probiotic supplements with particular species of bacteria in them will help in specific situations (such as infectious gastroenteritis, diarrhoea associated with taking antibiotics, or irritable bowel syndrome)."

You can make sure the microbes already living inside your gut are properly fed and supported, by providing them with prebiotics in the food you eat. The foods you choose to eat can either benefit your health or harm it, depending on how they alter your gut's bacteria populations and the biochemicals those bacteria release.

Foods high in prebiotic fibers include plantains, onions, garlic, sweet potatoes, dandelion greens, unprocessed wheat bran and rice bran. Prebiotics are also found in resistant starch.

Feeding all microbes indiscriminately is not helpful.

If the aim is to lose weight by feeding your gut microbiota with probiotics and prebiotics, the tactic of feeding all your existing gut microbes would work if you were starting off with a community of gut microbiota which promoted leanness. But in fact, if a person is already obese, their gut is more likely to be hosting the "obesity" microbes. Therefore nourishing them all may only serve to perpetuate the existing obesity.

Feeding all your existing gut microbiota indiscriminately may cause both the desirable and the undesirable microbe species to flourish. How can you just feed the microbes that can help you lose weight? How can you target them, while starving the "fatness" microbes?

Scientists have not yet finished making a list of which of the innumerable microbe species are the best for helping us lose weight, and even when they do, they will still have to work out what is the best way to make the "good guys" flourish in the intestines of any particular individual. Would it be by fecal transplant? By people taking "poop pills"? By wiping out every gut microbe and starting afresh?

Or can it be done through diet and supplements?

201

How to encourage "leanness" microbes.

Microbial diversity may help prevent food cravings.

Obese people generally have lower microbial diversity than people whose weight is normal and healthy. [Le Chatelier et al., (2013); Turnbaugh et al., (2009)]

Possibly this is because if you have lots of different species of microbes living in your gut, each individual species will find it harder to manipulate your behavior. The theory is that if your microbe diversity is low, a dominant microbe species gains enough power over the minor species to start sending signals demanding that you eat certain foods to satisfy its own needs. This shows up in your life as food cravings.

Having too few microbe species in your gut, may be one reason why it's difficult to lose weight.

Eat a wide range of nutritious foods.

You might be able to reduce food cravings by altering the composition of your microbiome. To increase the diversity of the microbes in your gut, you need to eat a greater variety of foods that contain a diversity of nutrients. This will encourage the growth of a wide range of microbes, decreasing the chances of a mere handful of species crowding out the rest and becoming dominant (and demanding!).

While changes in the microbiome can begin within a few hours of eating, it may take several months to really modify and boost your gut's microbiome diversity to the point at which your food cravings significantly diminish.

The importance of fiber to your gut microbiome.

Dietary fiber is prebiotic. The importance of fiber to your gut microbiota cannot be over-emphasized. When your gut microbes are nourished on fiber, they make major contributions to your good health.[26]

Whole foods, not fiber-fortified foods, give the best effect.

As mentioned earlier, some people try to increase their fiber intake by eating fiber-fortified processed foods. This, however, has been shown to be of relatively little benefit. Generally, food manufacturers add single fibers to their products. These don't nourish the gut like the more complex mixtures of different fiber types found in natural, whole or lightly-processed foods. It's plant-derived foods such as vegetables and whole grains that are not only packed with fiber, but also rich in various kids of fiber. These are the foods that encourage a diverse microbiome.

Fermented foods can promote beneficial gut bacteria.

Some people consume fermented foods like kimchi, kombucha, kefir and yoghurt, with the object of nourishing their gut microbiota.

In January 2017, BBC News reported on a four-week study conducted by Dr. Michael Mosley and the team from the TV show "Trust Me, I'm A Doctor". They wanted to find out which foods, if any, could populate the human gut with "good" microbes—the types of microbes that contribute to gut health.

They discovered that:
- Daily intake of prebiotic drinks from the supermarket had no significant effect on the gut microbe population of the volunteers.

---

26 Justin L. Sonnenburg, PhD, associate professor in the Department of Microbiology and Immunology at Stanford University USA), says, " … if you're not eating dietary fiber, your immune system may be existing in kind of a simmering pro-inflammatory state—the very state that predisposes us to different Western diseases. Our diet and deteriorated microbiota are really a major piece of the puzzle in trying to understand why Western diseases are rising like crazy."

- "Good" microbes multiplied significantly in the gut of people who consumed foods rich in prebiotic fiber.
- The numbers of "good" bacteria in the gut of people who drank kefir, a traditional fermented milk drink, rose quite dramatically.

(Note: Kefir and any other fermented foods and drinks are not considered suitable for people who suffer from histamine intolerance.[27])

Eat less "junk".

The mixture of your gut microbes changes depending on what you eat. Professor Stephen Simpson of the Charles Perkins Centre in Sydney, Australia says, "Diet changes what you're feeding to your bacteria. And because your bacterial species all have a slightly different requirement for nutrients, then you're going to support different communities." Different diets are associated with different gut microbiota. [De Filippo et al., (2010)]

"One day, we hope we might be able, through an altered diet or behavior, to shape the microbiota to improve health," says Professor Lawrence David, co-author of a study entitled *Diet Rapidly and Reproducibly Alters the Human Gut Microbiome*.

For every human gene, there are about 100 associated genes within your body's microbiome, your "second genome". The exciting thing is, you can alter this "second genome" by simple methods such as changing your diet. "What's interesting," says Professor David, "is that this second genome is potentially plastic and responsive to the way we choose to live our lives." [David et al., (2014)]

Eating a lot of highly processed foods supports inflammatory microbes in the gut, but when you swap "junk" food for "real" food, the inflammatory response declines.

---

27   See the book "Is Food Making You Sick? The Strictly Low-Histamine Diet".

Changing your diet rapidly changes your gut microbiome.

The colonies of microbes in your gut are extremely sensitive to the food you digest. Radical changes in your diet modify your gut microbiota composition, and the changes begin within hours!

Professor Katherine Samaras, an endocrinologist and clinical researcher at the Garvan Institute of Medical Research says, ". . . you can actually effect improvements in health within two or three days of changing your diet."

This is a relatively new field of research, but already it has been found that changes in gut microbiota due to changes in diet can affect satiety signals, insulin response and blood sugar levels, all of which are associated with obesity. After one month on a diverse, high fiber, whole food diet the improvements can be dramatic. [David et al., (2014)]

Changing your diet from "junk" foods to high-fiber "real" foods can be difficult at first. It's not easy to break a habit. Additionally, you'll be starving out the "bad" microbes in your gut, so they will be frantically sending signals to your brain demanding more of their specialty foods. However, once you've depleted your gut of those sugar-demanding, fat-demanding bugs, their place will be taken by microbes that love the fresh vegetables, legumes, whole grains, nuts and seeds etc. that you're now eating, and your cravings will diminish. These microbes include, for example, species such as oxalobacter, which thrive in your gut when you eat plenty of leafy green vegetables, such as spinach and kale.

It should be remembered, however, that if eating "good" food can rapidly change the populations of you gut, so can eating "bad" food.

Dr. Graham Phillips, host of ABC's "Catalyst" science show says, "If you want a good reason to start eating healthier food, consider this—just one meal of junk food could be enough for your body to have a bad reaction."

Exercise may change your gut microbiome for the better.
More research is needed, but a 2014 study showed that in mice, "Exercise induces a unique shift in the gut microbiota that is different from dietary effects." [Evans et al., (2014)]

Dysbiosis.

Populations of gut microbes can be seriously damaged by such factors as:

- An unhealthy diet
- Too much alcohol
- Antibiotics
- Food poisoning

If gut microbiota become unbalanced, this can lead to dysbiosis—a condition also known as "microbial imbalance", "bacterial imbalance", or "increased levels of harmful bacteria and reduced levels of beneficial bacteria".

When the balance of the microbial population in your gut is disturbed, the various clans of microbes lose the ability to stop each other from becoming too numerous. This can result in over-proliferation of one or more microbial groups. A vicious cycle can begin, wherein some smaller groups of beneficial microbes become overwhelmed by the larger ones. As more of the beneficial clans shrink or are wiped out, the imbalance snowballs. More of the larger groups expand, because the weakened groups are less able to hamper their growth. If this situation continues long enough, it leads to a chronic imbalance between groups. Your gut could end up lacking the health-giving diversity of many beneficial microbial clans.

Dysbiosis has been associated with a number of health problems including inflammatory bowel disease, chronic fatigue syndrome, obesity, cancer, and ulcerative colitis.

The microbiome and weight loss—a summary.

Dietary variety, whole foods and fiber promote a healthier and more diverse gut microbiome.

"All together, our low-fiber diets, antibiotics and Western ways have left us with very low diversity in our gut bacteria." [ABC Catalyst (2016)]

What scientists do know is that people whose gut hosts the highest diversity of microbiota species tend to be leaner than people with a narrow range of species.

And the highest diversity of microbiota species is achieved by:

- eating lots of naturally-occurring dietary fiber
- eating whole foods instead of processed foods
- eating a wide range of different foods
- not eating meat from animals (including poultry and fish) that have been treated with antibiotics
- keeping your own use of antibiotic medications to a minimum
- staying on the move; exercising, even moderately
- consuming naturally-fermented foods

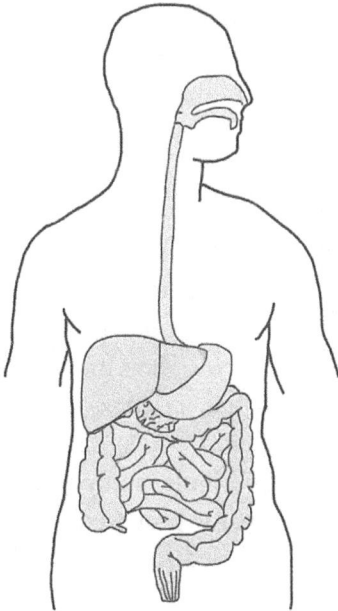

FOOD VARIETY

Have you ever tried to lose weight by following a monotonous diet? Diets that cut out certain foods or whole food groups fall into this category. Have you noticed that such diets aren't effective in the long term? Restricted diets can also create problems with your psychological relationship with food. In this section, we discuss issues associated with monotonous/restricted diets.

The Satiety Diet encourages food variety—the opposite of restriction and monotony. If your ultimate goal is to permanently lose weight and improve your health, the Satiety Diet is perfect for you.

Our definition of "real food".

What the authors of this book call "real food" is unprocessed or minimally processed food; food close to its natural state. Eating a wide range of this type of food is essential for weight loss. It also supports good health and helps ward off chronic disease.

Real food includes:

* *Food as nature formed it*—for example, food that has come straight out of the ground or off the plant or tree, or from the animal, bird or fish. This is food in its natural form, such as raw, organic fruit and vegetables, pastured eggs and free-range meats, with no artificial additives.

* *Minimally processed natural foods*—these are foods that you could produce in your home kitchen if you possessed the skills and equipment. They are foods that are still "real" because they have been modified very simply, in a way that our pre-industrial age forebears would have been able to achieve. They include fermented, cooked, strained, ground, cured, minced, dried, coagulated or frozen foods without artificial additives, and foods such as oils, which have been obtained by pressing. Maple syrup, yoghurt and porridge are some examples of minimally processed, natural foods that we call "real". Some canned or bottled foods also fall into this category.

Even corn that has been nixtamalized (processed with an alkaline solution such as limewater) can be called "minimally processed". Nixtamalization technology is not new. It dates from around 1200–1500 BCE. The people of South America have been preparing maize flour using this process for thousands of years.

Note that many of what we commonly call "foods" are really food combinations, or "dishes". Margherita pizza, for example, is basically a combination of grains, vegetables, and dairy products. The foods used to make a typical Margherita pizza would be wheat grains ground into flour, yeast, cheese, tomatoes, basil leaves, olives that have been cured in brine, garlic and salt. Of these ingredients, all would be classed as "real" except processed white flour, from which the bran has been removed. To make a real foods Margherita pizza you would swap the white flour for wholegrain flour.

Food variety and your Inner Guardian.

Your Inner Guardian receives body-speech signals from the outside world, to tell it how much food variety you are getting. How does this happen?

Sensory Input

In body-speech, food variety is indicated by external signals such as the following:
- Color (food can be any color, including black)
- Texture/consistency (e.g. creamy, crunchy, chewy, crispy), (see "Food textures")
- Flavor (e.g. sweet, sour, bitter, salty, tangy, sharp, umami) (see "Food flavors")
- Smell (piquant, fragrant, gamy, pungent, fruity, spicy, savory etc.)
- Shape and size.

Nutritional input

Your body has a complex range of internal physiological responses to the nutrients you consume. These responses affect your blood sugar levels, your hormone levels and a multitude of other biological processes. Your Inner Guardian interprets these signals to find out whether you're short of any nutrients you need for survival, and drives you to seek foods that contain any missing items.

Why sensory and nutritional food variety are important.

Most healthy people naturally enjoy eating a variety of foods.

- Sensory variety in food can lead to increased satiation and satiety, which are important for weight loss.
- Nutritional variety provides the widest range of nourishing substances, which your body utilizes for optimum health and which can help dampen food cravings. Healthy people tend to move more, which also helps with weight loss.

Sensory food variety.

As discussed, dietary diversity is one of the essential keys to satiety and thus one of the essential keys to weight loss. For best satiety, foods must not only *be* diverse, they must also also *appear diverse to your senses*. When you enjoy every sensory aspect of a meal, that meal becomes more satisfying and more memorable. Between meals, hunger can be staved off by recalling mental images of the last meal. When you eventually start to feel hungry again, it's pleasurable and calming to look forward to another meal that you know will provide a celebration of variety and tastiness. Eating like this can banish that sense of deprivation which frequently drives dieters to "break out", "fall off the wagon" and binge-eat.

Like strong flavors and interesting textures, deliciousness is important for mindful eating. You are more likely to take time to savor a pleasing flavor. It follows that you will be better able to recall it afterwards, when you visualize that meal. And if the food available to you is always delicious, you are less likely to want to gorge on it than if you only had access to delicious food every now and then.

Sensory enjoyment helps promote satiety.

For a meal that's exciting all the way through, the food needs to engage and delight you at every bite. This is why it's a good idea to mingle different sensory characteristics in the same dish. To food that's smooth and soft, for example, add elements that are rough and hard. Not only will your mouth register the change in texture and taste, your ears will hear the change from slurping to crunching.

With all this sensory novelty, your Inner Guardian re-awakens and takes a new interest. "What have we here?" it asks, stimulating your taste buds and trigeminal nerves to explore the novel substance. Not only do you become aware of the different food element, your awareness of all the other features of the dish also increases. The entire meal seems to become more delicious. You come to hope for a new sensory encounter with every mouthful.

Says Chris Clark: "To my amazement, I noticed that during the rare times I've been on an ocean cruise (once), or been staying in fancy hotels, or in any way living within easy reach of fabulous meals, I would always lose a little unwanted weight. I put this phenomenon down to the fact that as a person who's not interested in cooking, when I'm home I'd tend to grab some toast or cereal for dinner, or some canned or frozen food that you just heat and serve. Yes, I admit it.

"And then I'd feel hungry soon afterwards because the meal contained only a narrow range of nutrients, and wasn't truly satisfying. And I'd snack on some late-night chocolate. And I'd pile on the pounds.

"But when I was being offered, on a daily basis, a wide range of fresh, sumptuous, chef-prepared meals, I'd feel as if I didn't need to eat everything in sight because I knew all that food and more would be up for grabs again within a few hours or less. And it was satisfying food. So I guess that's why I lose weight more easily when I'm surrounded by an abundance of food diversity and deliciousness."

Use a variety of preparation methods.

In the ideal high-satiety meal, each dish is prepared in a way that makes every mouthful taste, feel and look slightly different. The food is plated in a way that displays variety, too, using garnishes and condiments to add an array of shapes, flavors, textures and colors.

Posh restaurateurs know that food's deliciousness and fascination is heightened by sensory variety, which is why their meals are often elaborate and artistically presented on the plate. Some chefs say that the most vital ingredient for diner satisfaction is variety.

Some examples of multi-textured, multi-flavored foods include creamy porridge with nuts and seeds stirred through, or creamy soups studded with crispy, crunchy, baked croutons.

In a single meal, try not to serve dishes prepared with the same cooking method more than once. For example, don't serve a savory pie as the main course, followed by a sweet pie for dessert. Different cooking methods create different sensory characteristics.

Different ways of preparing ingredients can add variety to the look of food, its textures and its flavor blends; for example:

- Soups, broth
- Stir fries
- Salads
- Steamed, roasted, baked, stewed or boiled foods
- Sauces, gravies, dressings
- Pies, quiches and tarts
- Casseroles and stews
- Roll-ups, wraps, burritos and rotolos

Food manufacturers know how profoundly sensory characteristics affect sales. There are massive, multi-billion dollar industries built on investigating and producing food textures, food colors and food flavors/smells.

Sensory-specific satiety.

There is a phenomenon called "sensory-specific satiety", which explains why people eat less food when their diet is monotonous. The more you eat of any particular food, the less you feel the desire to go on eating it, because your senses become sated with the characteristics of that food. The taste, texture, look and smell of the over-abundant food becomes uninteresting, and may even start to seem disgusting.

When you reach sensory-specific satiety, your appetite for other, different foods increases. You begin to yearn for the sensory qualities of the scarce food—for example, if you'd sipped nothing but soup for a few days you might long for crisp, crunchy foods to chew on, or if you'd lived on hard, dry rations for a long time you might develop a strong desire for moist, creamy foods.

Monotonous diets can induce cravings. People on low-carb diets often find themselves craving carbs. Sailors in days of yore, whose diet consisted mostly of ship's biscuit and salted beef, used to yearn for fresh fruit and vegetables, and gorge on them whenever they made landfall. Diners confronted with a buffet-style meal comprising an extensive selection of dishes they don't normally encounter, tend to consume a lot more food than they would eat at a standard meal with a narrower menu. [Raynor & Epstein (2001)]

When you're deprived of some sensory characteristics of food, you start to visualize the food you're craving as the ambrosia of the gods!

In fact, the sensory characteristics of the scarce food remain the same. It's your perception that alters.

This, of course, is an inbuilt survival mechanism. For optimum health your body requires a wide range of nutrients, so it's in the best interests of your Inner Guardian to decrease your appetite for foods of which you've eaten a great deal, and sharpen your appetite for foods you have not eaten recently.

Food preparation can change sensory characteristics.

Studies have shown that it's not simply the nutrient feedback from your gut to your brain that determines how bored you will be with eating a certain food; it is more likely to be the sensory qualities of the food. Sensory qualities can be changed by preparing the food in different ways. Wheat, for example, can be eaten as crunchy wheat toast or kibbled wheat porridge for breakfast, sandwiches or chewy wheat pasta for lunch, and tender wheat-flour-crusted pies for dinner, with crispy wheat-flour crackers for snacks between meals. The problem with eating the same ingredient presented in a variety of different ways is that it can lead to nutrition deficits. This can make it harder for you to reach satiety, so you're likely to want to go on eating.

Nutritional food variety.

Your body requires not only a certain quantity, but also a certain *variety* of nutrients in order to stay healthy. Quantity of food alone is not enough to provide satiety. No matter how much food you eat, if your diet is nutrient-poor your body will demand more, in an attempt to get the missing nutrition it needs. It will keep telling you that you need to eat more food, and this means you will find it hard to reach satiety. Unless you get a wide enough range of enough nutrients to give you satiety, you are likely to keep eating, and over-consume Calories.

A report from the British Nutrition Foundation states: "Apart from breastmilk as a food for babies, no single food contains all the essential nutrients the body needs to be healthy and function efficiently. The nutritional value of a person's diet depends on the overall balance of foods that is eaten over a period of time, as well as on the needs of the individual. A healthy diet is likely to include a variety of foods, from each of the main food groups, as this allows us to get all the nutrients that we need.

"Even within a single food group, different foods provide a different selection of nutrients, so variety is important to ensure we get the many nutrients we need to be healthy." [British Nutrition Foundation (2016)]

A varied diet is recommended for good health.

- Eating a wide variety of nutritious foods promotes good health and helps to protect against chronic disease.
- Eating a varied, well-balanced diet means eating a variety of foods from each of the five food groups daily, in the recommended amounts.
- It is also important to choose a variety of foods from within each food group because different foods provide different types and amounts of key nutrients.
- Choosing a variety of foods will help to make your meals interesting, so that you don't get bored with your diet.

[State Government, Victoria, Australia (2016)]

People who eat a wide variety of foods are more likely to get all the nutrition their bodies need. This means they are healthier, at a lower risk of disease and likely to live longer.

Healthy people are also better at losing weight and keeping it off, partly because they have more energy to move. They have the energy to plan and shop and cook and engage in exercise—all the things that lead to successful weight loss.

Nutritional deficiencies can boost appetite.

As already discussed, if your diet is deficient in just one nutrient, your appetite will drive you to eat until you satisfy the need for that nutrient.

Professor Stephen Simpson, Executive Director of Obesity Australia says, "Appetite isn't just a single thing. We have separate appetites for different major nutrient groups." And if you fail to satisfy those various appetites you are driven to go on eating until you have fulfilled your body's basic requirements.

Associate Professor Amanda Salis, weight loss researcher at Sydney's Garvan Institute is an advocate of eating a wide variety of foods to help weight loss. She agrees that if your diet is deficient in just one nutrient, your body will push you to eat until you meet that need.

For example, people tend to gorge on potato crisps, chips and instant noodles, because these foods taste like protein. Such foods have been called "protein decoys". They contain barely any protein, however, so the protein-craving Inner Guardian demands more food that tastes like protein... and so the overeating continues.

Yet it's not only protein that the body needs. There's a wide range of macronutrients and micronutrients, in certain proportions, that are required for your body's proper function and maintenance. Eating a wide variety of foods gives you a better chance of meeting all those needs without overeating.

Nutritional variety and balance.

Nutritional variety and balance both contribute to satiety. As your food passes from your stomach into your small intestine, body-speech signals flash through your body, from your gut to your brain. Hormones are released in response to the digestion and absorption of nutrients. Satiety signals are coordinated in areas of your brain responsible for the regulation of energy intake. These are the areas that give rise to your feeling of repleteness.

Your Inner Guardian learns exactly which nutrients have entered your gut, and in what quantities—right down to the tiniest micronutrients. This is important, because your Guardian then chooses to assimilate precisely the nutrients it needs to keep you healthy. If there are any "leftovers" (for example if you consumed too many vitamin or mineral supplements) the body tries to get rid of them by excreting them.

If you consume too much energy, on the other hand, your body stores it as fat. And no matter how many times you sit your body down in front of a mirror and give it a lecture on the fact that it is surrounded at all times by cheap, Calorie-dense foods within easy reach and that therefore it does not need to store fat, your Inner Guardian will not hear you. It only understands its ancient language, "body-speech"—the language you need to learn, if you wish to communicate with it.

Food variety at a single sitting.

Evolution has hard-wired our bodies to seek diversity in foods. When people sit down to a single meal containing what looks like a wider variety of foods than they are accustomed to, they are likely to consume around 30% more than usual. It is as if their Inner Guardian tells them, "It's a good harvest season. Seasons change, so stock up now! Eat all this variety while you can because, judging by past experience, it may not be available tomorrow!"

A 2012 study found that "...the greater the number of foods offered at a meal, the greater the spontaneous intake of those foods." The researchers offered people a pasta and vegetable stir fry dish, either:

- With the pasta and vegetables separate, served in small individual plates or bowls.
- With the pasta and vegetables mixed together as a "composite" meal.

Both meals consisted of the same ingredients, presented differently. Researchers noted that people ate less of the composite meals and more of the separated meals. The separate ingredients gave the illusion of more variety. [Levitsky et al., (2012)]

On the BBC TV show "10 Things You Need to Know About Losing Weight", a number of people were offered bowls of free candy. One bowl contained multi-colored candies and the other held only purple candy. People ate significantly more out of the bowl of multi-colored sweets. Again, it was as if their Inner Guardians were trying to ensure they consumed a wide range of nutrients. In the natural world, different food colors signal different nutrients.

The key phrase here is "what *appears* to be variety". As with the use of multi-colored candies, the appearance, division and arrangement of food can be used to trick your Inner Guardian into believing a meal's components are more diverse than they really are.

Use your desire for variety to help with weight loss.

The appearance of food variety at a single sitting tends to make you eat more—and you can use that trick to help you eat more of the foods that help with weight loss. By eating more Calorie-sparse, fiber-rich, nutrition-packed vegetables, you can more easily reach satiety without putting on pounds. You can take advantage of your natural, human inclination to eat more when there's more variety on offer, by serving light, fresh vegetable dishes in small individual plates or bowls, Japanese-style.

Human beings are natural omnivores.

In ancient times, human beings used to consume whatever edibles they could find or catch. Our cave-dwelling ancestors needed to eat a wide range of foods in order to survive. Their diet could include practically any kind of bird, beast, fish, egg, insect, larva, corm, stem, leaf, root, flower, seed, nut, rhizome, grain etc. They couldn't afford to be fussy. And if they ate an animal, they ate pretty much the whole thing—offal, stomach contents, stomach lining, brains, liver, feet, ears etc.

Healthy human beings are "programmed" to eat a variety of foods. Naturally, we are driven to seek a wide range of nutrients to keep us healthy.

A diverse diet signals "success" to your Inner Guardian.

When your diet includes a wide range of different foods, your body sends signals to your Inner Guardian saying, "My tribe is physically fit and healthy enough to be able to forage widely. The land over which my people ranges is fertile and productive enough to supply numerous and varied comestibles." Your Inner Guardian gets the message that you, the individual who is eating this food variety, are either healthy and fit enough to be able to go out and find it, or if not fit, you are such a valuable member of the tribe that they share good food with you.

Monotonous diets can have a rebound effect.

The first bite

The first bite of a meal is most important. No matter what you eat, it's always the first bite that most engages your attention and your senses. Your initial mouthful of food conveys multiple sensory signals to your brain. Your Inner Guardian wants to know, "What is this foreign substance that's entering my body? Is it poisonous? Should it be spat out? Is it delicious? What does it taste like? Is it full of energy?"

Habituation

After this inaugural surge of information, however, your brain becomes accustomed to the food you are eating and subsides into relative indifference. After the first bite your enjoyment of good food actually begins to decrease. This is called "habituation".

Adaptation

When your taste buds and other senses experience one particular flavor or sensation over a long period, they can become bored and jaded. That's why monotonous diets tend to make people eat less. This is called "adaptation".

Severely restricted and monotonous diets work in the short-term largely because "...the feeling of having had enough to eat, is specific to a particular food that has been consumed. If, for example, cheese is eaten until a subject has had all he or she wants, the rated pleasantness of the taste, smell, appearance, and texture of cheese will have declined." [Kissileff et al., (1984)]

When you eat a lot of one type of food day after day, that food becomes less appealing, although your appetite for very different foods won't have decreased (and, in fact, will probably *increase*). You simply become sick of eating the same type of food day in and day out, so you consume less of it. This is one reason why highly restrictive weight-loss diets that exclude entire food groups may work in the short-term.

219

Compensation—the rebound effect

In the long-term however, restrictive diets don't work. When you are deprived of particular foods or food groups, and limited to a narrow diet, you are highly likely to develop cravings. As soon as the diet ends, you'll probably compensate by eating large amounts of the previously unavailable foods. You seek out the foods that were "forbidden", and overindulge in them, thereby regaining all the weight that was lost, and more. "Deprivation causes craving and overeating, particularly in restrained eaters," is the conclusion of a 2005 study in the *International Journal of Eating Disorders*. [Polivy et al., (2005)]

This can occur for several reasons, including:

Nutritional compensation: To compensate for the vitamins, minerals, carbohydrates or proteins you've been missing out on.

Protection against future food shortages: Your Inner Guardian reasons that if there was a shortage of those foods once, it might happen again, so it drives you to cram as much into yourself as possible while the foods are still available.

Depletion of willpower: Eating a monotonous diet while being surrounded by and regularly exposed to the wide variety of foods available in developed countries has the psychological potential to increase cravings and cause rebound weight gain. The prolonged exertion of extreme willpower can deplete your resolve, eventually giving way to a bout of binge eating.

Sensory-specific satiety: Your appetite for the different sensory characteristics of foods motivates you to seek a variety of food textures, colors, shapes, smells etc. This drive to eat more food when there's a wide assortment of foods suddenly available can work to your detriment, especially if those foods are loaded with Calories. Not only do you eat more, but also, eating Calorie-dense foods actually dampens the triggering of sensory-specific satiety. [Rolls et al., (1983)] To avoid sensory-specific satiety, regularly eat a wide variety of foods prepared in diverse ways. Those foods should be as low in Calories as possible, as "real" as possible, as nutritious as possible, and rich in various sensory characteristics.

Chris Clark says, "I once went on the so-called Israeli Army Diet. It involved two days of eating nothing but apples, two days of cheese, two days of chicken and two days of salad. I lost weight all right, by but by the fifth day I was so fed up with those foods (literally) that I abandoned the diet and ate everything edible within reach, starting with bread. Needless to say I regained all the weight I had lost. To make matters worse, I was now burdened with a craving for carbs.

"The whole time I was on the Israeli Army Diet, or the Dukan® Diet, or the Beverley Hills Diet® or whichever fashionable restricted diet I happened to be enduring, all I could do was obsess about and yearn for the foods that were "off the list". When I finally surrendered to the insistent demands of my body and went off those narrow diets, I would gorge on the previously forbidden foods for weeks afterwards. My whole relationship with food went askew. It's my opinion that when it comes to monotonous diets willpower is a finite resource, and you can only use up a certain amount of it before you crack and undo most of your good work."

When you're on a diet of limited types of food you're constantly forced to fight against your Inner Guardian's directives to eat the un-available/forbidden foods. When you finally cease the diet your Inner Guardian is set free, and you "splurge" on the foods you previously denied yourself. This is one of the reasons why traditional dieting, in itself, promotes weight gain.

"It is now well established that the more people engage in dieting, the more they gain weight in the long-term." [Pietiläinen et al. (2011)]

A varied diet helps prevent overeating and cravings.

As we've explained, trying to lose weight by continually, chronically depriving yourself of foods that you love to eat can lead to cravings and eating binges. It's just a fact of human psychology. And of course, eating binges undermine your weight-loss efforts.

221

"... dieting causes bingeing." [Polivy & Herman (1985)]

Janet Polivy, a professor of psychology and psychiatry at the University of Toronto in Canada, writes, "A review of the literature and research on food restriction indicates that inhibiting food intake has consequences that may not have been anticipated by those attempting such restriction. Starvation and self-imposed dieting appear to result in eating binges once food is available and in psychological manifestations such as preoccupation with food and eating, increased emotional responsiveness and dysphoria [a profound state of unease or dissatisfaction], and distractibility. Caution is thus advisable in counseling clients to restrict their eating and diet to lose weight, as the negative sequelae may outweigh the benefits of restraining one's eating. Instead, healthful, balanced eating without specific food restrictions should be recommended as a long-term strategy to avoid the perils of restrictive dieting." [Polivy (1996)]

Monotonous diets are linked with obesity.

If food monotony leads to eating less, does food variety lead to eating more? The answer is "Yes—but only one meal at a time". People who are presented with a wide variety of foods at a single meal are likely to over-indulge. However, if your daily diet is already rich in variety, that one-meal binge is unlikely to happen. And if the wide variety includes foods that are energy-sparse, you're likely to consumer fewer Calories.

Studies have found links between a monotonous diet and obesity. "A 2010 study of young Iranian women found that those who consumed the least diverse diet were more likely to be obese." [Azadbakht & Esmaillzadeh (2010)]

Why people may eat a narrow range of foods:
1. Habit

Habits can lead to monotony. Sometimes people eat the same foods day in and day out, simply from force of habit. Some grocery stores and supermarkets reflect this. They tend to stock the most popular items, for example in the fresh foods section, where you're pretty much guaranteed to see piles of tomatoes, potatoes, green beans, pumpkins, apples, oranges and carrots. Not that there's anything wrong with these foods—far from it. It's just that the available food diversity is far greater than many of us realize. Where are the jicamas, the American ground nuts, the cardoons and the tigernuts, for example?

Fortunately it is possible to change your dietary habits. See our section on "Willpower and Creating Good Habits".

2. Fad diets that demonize food groups or nutrients.

In developed countries, with their abundance of food, people seem to be more confused about what to eat than ever before.

Some dieters avoid whole food groups in their efforts to become slim and healthy. This is not advisable. (See our section on "Carbohydrates—Whole Grains" for more information).

Food is about more than the macronutrients and micronutrients that it possesses. We eat food, not vitamins or minerals or protein or carbs or fat. Vilifying a single nutrient is counter-productive. Some weight loss "gurus" seem to be obsessed with one particular macronutrient or ingredient to the relative exclusion of most others. They have written books that condemn certain foods, even such nutritious foods as whole grains, despite the fact that their claims fly in the face of thousands of peer-reviewed studies showing evidence to the contrary, which have been published in scientific journals over many decades.

People can become so scared of certain food groups that they fearfully label raw carrots as "sugar on a stick", as if that nutrient-rich, fiber-rich, low-fat unprocessed vegetable is somehow the equivalent of a confection manufactured from refined sugar.

Nutritional scientists are now advocating a drastic review of our understanding of diet. They argue that instead of considering nutrients by themselves, we should be looking at the way blends of nutrients affect health.

Instead of blaming single nutrients or food groups as the cause of obesity, we should be looking at nutrient balance and diversity as the way to achieve weight loss.

Professor Stephen Simpson, academic director at the University of Sydney's Charles Perkins Centre says, ". . . when it comes to trying to understand the problems of over-nutrition, obesity and diabetes for example, focusing on single nutrients as the culprit or perhaps even the cure of these conditions, it doesn't work." [Oriti (2016)]

One example of demonizing single nutrients, Professor Simpson says, is the fad for singling out fat, carbohydrates or sugar by themselves and blaming them for the rise in obesity.

"Synergy" is defined as "the interaction of two or more agents to produce a combined effect greater than the sum of their separate effects." And, as highlighted in Dr. Michael Mosley's turmeric investigations[28], the nutrients in our food combine to have a synergistic effect on our health. They should not be considered as standing alone.

Diets that permit only a limited range of foods may work in the short term, because people become so jaded with that limited range that they prefer not to eat at all rather than to eat more of the food they are tired of. However, as discussed earlier, after the diet is over the weight is likely to be regained.

3. Eating disorders

In the 21st century an astonishing number of people in developed countries, where food is plentiful, suffer from forms of eating disorders. These range from "I don't like the taste of that particular food," to "I never eat any carbohydrates, or anything that's been cooked in any way, or anything that's not in season, or anything that's

---

28 Dr. Mosley found that turmeric's anti-inflammatory effects become far more powerful when the spice is mixed with food, especially with oils and pepper.

ever touched plastic, or anything that's not colored purple . . . " you get the idea.

"Restrained eating" is a disorder that can lead to bingeing. Deprivation of certain foods due to the practice of restrained eating can cause cravings and over-eating binges. This is another reason a varied diet is so helpful for weight loss. [Polivy et al., (2005)]

"Restrained eating" is not the same thing as fasting for cultural or religious reasons, nor should it be confused with avoiding certain foods because of a health problem such as celiac disease, histamine intolerance, FODMAP intolerance or diabetes.

"Chronic restrained eating" is an eating disorder. It is the practice of avoiding certain foods, entire food groups, or specific ingredients (e.g. fat or sugar), or eating in particular ways that cannot be altered to fit in with social situations. It involves thinking of foods as "good" or "bad", and may involve eating only at certain times of the day, or eating in certain rigorous patterns.

Note that "restrained eating" does not necessarily mean Calorie restriction for a weight loss diet. In fact, a person whose eating is very restrained, and who chooses to eat only a very narrow range of foods, may still eat too much of those foods and end up consuming more Calories than they expend.

People may, however, practice restrained eating because they are trying to lose weight. "In modern societies characterized by abundant and accessible foods, restrained eating may become an adaptive behavior to limit weight gain." [de Lauzon-Guillain et al., (2006)]

Ironically, restrained eating can have the opposite effect. It has been shown to heighten the risk of binge-eating. Cutting out foods or food groups, especially over a long period of time, leads to cravings so strong that people simply cannot help succumbing to them in the end. Restrained eating can also cause nutritional deficiencies.

"Research in normal weight individuals paradoxically suggests that measures of attempted eating restriction might represent robust predictors of weight gain." [Lowe, et al., (2013)]

One of the problems caused by restrained eating is the psychological effect. Certain foods are "forbidden' and restrained eaters force themselves to avoid them despite an intense longing to eat them. Ultimately if the restrained eater gives in and takes a single bite of the forbidden food, it's highly likely that their willpower will crash and they will end up gorging on that particular food, all in one sitting.

On the other hand, unrestrained eaters who are on a weight loss diet generally find themselves able to take a few bites of a palatable Calorie-dense food (such as chocolate) and be satisfied with that.

Research also shows that restrained eaters who have a long list of foods to avoid and a very short list of foods they allow themselves, are more likely to crash and binge. Once again, food variety with a focus on real, nutrient rich, lower Calorie foods is a key to weight loss!

Some people, in their efforts to pursue a healthy eating regime, may inadvertently descend into an eating disorder called "orthorexia nervosa."[29]

The term derives from the Greek "ortho," meaning correct or righteous. Sufferers strictly avoid specific foods that they believe to be harmful and eat only foods they believe are healthful.

Orthorexics become obsessed with the food they eat. They might fixate on the chemical composition of it, how "pure" it is, how much of it to consume, where it was sourced from, what time of year it was harvested, etc. Their diet dominates their thinking. Any deviation from their narrow path is considered catastrophic, and deserving of self-chastisement, such as strenuous exercise, or fasting. In the mind of an orthorexic, food seems to be more than just nourishment. It becomes symbolic of good and evil. Some orthorexics may view themselves as superior to people who don't follow their diet. Their philosophy of eating is a way of bolstering their image and self-esteem.

The dark side of orthorexia is that people can limit their "allowable" foods to such an extent that they fail to consume sufficient nutrients and energy for their bodies to function in optimum condition. Paradoxically, their commitment to good health can result in ill-health.

---

29 Orthorexia nervosa is not currently recognized as a clinical diagnosis in the DSM-5.

It takes a great deal of willpower to maintain such a rigorous regimen. Orthorexics' fixation with food can come to dominate their thinking, negatively affecting every aspect of life.

As mentioned, there are valid reasons why some of us need to avoid certain foods. These include people with histamine intolerance or celiac disease or fructose intolerance or food allergies. The 'Low FODMAP" diet is a good example of an eating regime that can be beneficial to many people with digestive symptoms, and the "Strictly Low Histamine Diet" has helped thousands of people with a wide range of health problems.

Most people, despite trends that come and go, are free from real food allergies and food intolerances. The majority of us can digest most foods without ill-effect.

4. The Western Dietary Pattern.

People who follow the 21st century Western dietary pattern eat a relatively limited range of foods, presented in many different ways that disguise the fact they are the same—for example, wheat flour is the main ingredient of pasta, pizza, brown bread, white bread, muffins, puffed wheat breakfast cereals, cakes, cookies and pancakes. And it's usually highly refined wheat flour, with the bran stripped away.

In bygone days—even as recently as the 1960s—the Western dietary pattern included a lot more offal than it does today. People's preferences have changed, and now, in general, muscle meats are more popular.

Insects and other bugs are a sustainable—and arguably more ethical—source of protein than mammals and fowls, but it's only a small proportion of the human population that relishes them. There are around 2,000 edible insect species in the world. Crickets, mealworms, grasshoppers, tarantulas, agave worms, scorpions, ant eggs and ticks are some of the high-protein delicacies prized in countries like Mexico, where insect eating—or entomophagy—has been practised for hundreds of years. Does the notion of eating bugs seem repugnant to you? Ideas can change. It was only around the end of the 20th century that Europeans began to embrace the concept of eating raw fish, and the popularity of sushi soared.

"Many foods in the Western diet have been engineered by the food industry to be 'hyperpalatable,' i.e., to contain an optimum balance of fat, sugar, and salt to promote consumption." [Johnson & Wardle (2014)]. Food manufacturers have increased the variety of sensory characteristics of these delicious, fattening foods; for example, sugary foods now come in a rainbow of colors, a wealth of flavors, and multiple textures. This "perceived variety" contributes to obesity.

In prehistoric times our lean ancestors consumed around 150 unique foods each week. Their microbiota must have been extremely diverse. In the 21st century, it's not uncommon for people to eat no more than about 20 different foods per week. And worse still—many of those foods are highly processed, low in microbe-nourishing fiber and riddled with excess fat and sugar.

The global obesity crisis has roots in a number of modern trends, including an increase in the variety and quantity of highly-processed, Calorie-dense foods available to consumers who follow the Western dietary pattern. These are sometimes called "obesogenic foods".

5. A decline in available "real" foods.

There has also been a decrease in the variety of unprocessed or lightly-processed foods available to consumers.

As the global human population rapidly increases, plant breeders are introducing new varieties of crops whose yield is much higher than the older, local plant varieties, and which may be genetically more resistant to pests and diseases. Farmers want to grow more food while reducing costs, so they replace their old, local crop varieties with the new global ones. This leads to a reduction in agrobiodiversity.

The UN Food and Agricultural Organization (FAO) estimates that:

- There are (or were) 250,000-300,000 known edible plant species.
- Humans now consume only 150-200 edible plant species.
- 75% of plant genetic diversity has been lost to crop-growers.
- 75% of the world's food is now generated from just 12 plants and five animal species.
- Only three species (rice, maize and wheat) provide 60% of Calories and proteins obtained by humans from plant crops.

Increases in obesity rates around the world have coincided with this decline in dietary diversity.

"Unique" foods.

Let's explain what we mean by "different", or "unique" foods. Unique means distinctive, individual; something that is the only one of its kind and unlike anything else.

Potatoes are botanically, genetically and nutritionally distinct from apples, for example, but a Pink Lady® apple is not sufficiently unlike a Red Delicious® apple to be considered "unique". By eating a Pink Lady® apple and a Red Delicious® apple, you are not eating two different/unique foods.

It's not always easy to differentiate between foods based on their common names alone. Look at their botanical, Latin names instead. As a general rule, foods sourced from different taxonomic ranks at or above the level of "genus" are likely to be unique. For example, wild rice (Zizania spp.) is not directly related to rice (Oryza sativa) and buckwheat (Fagopyrum esculentum) is not remotely associated with wheat (Triticum spp.) Buckwheat is not even a cereal grain.

Here are some examples of unique and non-unique foods:

- Foods that are all made from cows' milk, such as low-fat milk high and fat milk, or butter and cream, are considered to be the same food (not unique), just in a slightly different form.
- Cheeses are grouped together according to the animal from whose milk they were made: cows' milk cheese, goats' milk cheese, buffalo cheese etc.
- Rice includes the species Oryza sativa (Asian rice) and Oryza glaberrima (African rice). Asian and African rice are considered to be different, unique foods. Asian rice is the most widespread, with around 40,000 varieties. Worldwide there are four major categories of Asian rice: indica, japonica, aromatic and glutinous. Brown, red, black and white rice are one and the same grain, simply with or without the husk, so including both kinds in one's diet does not mean that the diet is more diverse. The same goes for basmati rice and jasmine rice, both of which are still Asian rice, and possessing close to identical nutritional profiles.
- Wild rice (also called Canada rice, Indian rice, and water oats) is a different, unique food in the genus Zizania.
- Whole wheat and refined wheat are still wheat, but of course whole foods are vastly better for you. Kamut (Triticum turanicum) and farro—which is a collective term for a group of three wheat species spelt (Triticum spelta), emmer (Triticum turgidum) and einkorn (Triticum monococcum)—are first cousins of wheat. While there are indeed nutritional differences between these four last-mentioned grains, those differences are relatively negligible and thus we can put them in the same "basket" as wheat.
- Different cultivars (varieties) of potatoes are all members of the same species, with little variation.
- Edible mushrooms, if they do not share the same genus, are sufficiently distinct from one another to have different nutritional profiles.

- Blue corn, red corn, white, purple, orange, yellow and black corn etc. are all members of the Zea mays species, They are not really diverse sources of nutrition. They do, however, contain different ratios of valuable anthocyanins, so when you eat corn, eat a range of colors.

How many unique "real" foods should you eat per week?

As we've mentioned, the Japanese are among the slimmest people in the world. The official Japanese Dietary Guidelines take the idea of variety seriously, recommending that people "eat a minimum of 30 or more different kinds of food daily and aim for 100 different foods a week".

Eating like this would certainly keep your microbiome diverse, and in a dynamic state of change. If you count three meals a day for a week, this works out at around five different real, unique foods per meal. Recipe books and online recipe websites can help you aim for this goal.

You don't have to reach this goal every week; simply aiming for it as best you can, is sufficient. It will challenge you to move out of your food "comfort zone". It will encourage you to re-try foods you've rejected in the past, and train yourself to appreciate them. It will motivate you to visit those niche sections in the supermarket with their "weird, foreign foods," or to peer into the corners of the fresh foods department looking for vegetables you cannot even give a name to!

Remember that to lose weight you would choose from foods that are Calorie-sparse.

A diverse diet helps weight loss.

A diverse diet of real, energy-sparse foods helps weight loss because:

- It dampens cravings. When you habitually eat a wide variety of flavorsome, nutritious, lower Calorie, lightly-processed foods you're less inclined to crave fattening, highly-processed foods laden with sugar, salt and fat. You do not feel as if your diet is restricted and boring.
- It decreases the likelihood of rebound weight gain when you "go off" the diet.
- It increases nutrition. This promotes better health, Healthy bodies are inclined to move more, which helps with fitness and weight loss.
- It keeps your microbiome in a healthy state of flux.
- It helps you feel full after eating fewer Calories.

Your body is always aiming to achieve the optimum balance for good health. When you provide the best nourishment, you give it the opportunity to regain its natural balance, with all its systems working properly. And when everything, including your appetite, is working as it should, there's a better chance of you returning to a healthy weight.

Eating delicious, varied foods can prevent compensatory gorging.

As discussed, people eat more when they are served with delicious rather than unpalatable foods, however, when you follow a diet that is unpalatable and/or monotonous you are more likely to overcompensate later. As soon as people have access to delicious, varied foods they tend to gorge on them. [Bobroff & Kissileff (1986); de Castro et al., (2000); Wansink & Park (2001)]

People also eat more when they are served with a variety of foods or flavors. [McCrory et al., (1999)] This works in your favor when you choose nutritious, Calorie-sparse foods.

Eating a wide variety of foods helps weight loss if you eat the right foods in the right way.

Choose foods that boost satiety and weight loss.

For satiety and weight loss, your diet should contain a wide range of foods, and clearly that means "real", nutrient-rich, relatively low-Calorie foods—not a wide range of highly processed, sugar-laden, fat-laden dishes. Diets that offer a wide variety of Calorie-dense foods tempt you to eat more, and make you put on weight. Even "real" foods can make you gain weight, if they are energy-dense. For example feasting on lavish amounts of coconut cream, avocados and honey would be a sure way to pack on the pounds.

While we advocate eating a wide variety of foods to give your body the best possible nutrition and sensory satisfaction—thus helping to dampen food cravings—we also suggest limiting the number of Calorie-dense foods at each meal. (Don't limit the vegetables!)

Researcher Eileen Kennedy in "Dietary Diversity, Diet Quality, and Body Weight Regulation" makes the comment that in general, the greater variety of food available in the Western diet can be considered beneficial, because it is indicative of good quality food from secure sources. "However," she writes, "variety in certain selected foods—energy-dense foods, for example—may contribute to over-weight and obesity." [Kennedy (2004)]

It's not only the narrowing of agrobiodiversity that limits your consumption of nutrients. It's also the fact that a relatively limited range of foods is processed into a dazzling array of delicious, enticing dishes that appear to be varied. (Again, think of the number of ways refined wheat flour is presented!)

People who are overweight or obese generally have fewer vitamins and minerals in their bloodstreams than leaner people. Their bodies could be producing more hunger-signals in an attempt to obtain the missing nutrients.

In a report titled "The Malnutrition of Obesity," New York-based endocrinologist Michael Via says, "Despite excessive dietary consumption, obese individuals have high rates of micronutrient deficiencies.

"...The medical care plan for obesity should include lifestyle changes [and] healthy food choices with high-nutrient content foods." [Via (2012)]

It is widely believed that there's no such thing as clinical malnutrition in developed countries, where food is cheap and varied. However, in the journal *Obesity Surgery* a team of researchers noted that in these countries, ". . . many people consume food that is either unhealthy or of poor nutritional value, that lacks proteins, vitamins, minerals, and fiber. ... The prevalence of vitamin deficiencies in the morbidly obese population ... is higher and more significant than previously believed." [Kaidar-Person et al., (2008)]

When you're eating a wider variety of nutritious, lower-Calorie, real foods, don't be tempted to continue eating as much Calorie-dense food as usual, in addition to the nutritious foods. Your new way of eating replaces your old way of eating.

Being offered a wide variety of delicious high-Calorie food is likely to encourage you to eat more. However if the wide variety includes abundant, delicious lower Calorie foods, you're likely to consume less energy. When you satisfy your appetite with lower-Calorie, real foods it will be easier to decreased your intake of energy-dense food.

"In the U.S. adults, variety in self-reported usual diet was associated with greater adiposity [fatness] across the majority of food groups examined, with the exception of fruits and vegetables, for which variety was associated with lower adiposity." [McCrory et al., (1999)]

Of course you can still eat Calorie-dense foods and lose weight, but eat them in small, mindfully-consumed portions.

Variety in your diet—but not all in one single meal!

When food variety is part of your daily life and you can expect diverse foods at every meal, you lose that sense of having to overeat in case of future deprivation. With multiple choices of food regularly on offer, there is no need to eat too much at one sitting. And if you consume a wide variety of nutrients, you can satisfy your body's nutritional needs and subdue food cravings.

When people have permanent, continual access to a wide variety of real foods, then after the first few splurges of eating around 30% more, they settle back into a normal eating pattern. Once your body's sensory, psychological and nutritional needs are satisfied, you don't need to eat as much food (and thereby consume extra Calories).

Chris Clark says: "When I travel, I lose weight. I guess it's because when I'm on the move I am exposed to a wider range of foods than I get at home (largely because I'm a lazy cook and tend to habitually shop for a narrow range of foods). When I travel, I eat out a lot, (though I am careful to order dishes with lots of veggies and no heavy sauces). At mealtimes I am presented with things I'd never normally see on a plate. My Inner Guardian stops saying, 'Look at all this food! You've got to take a mouthful of everything!' Instead it says, 'You don't have to eat all this now. There will be plenty of variety available whenever you want it.'"

Food diversity should be part of your eating plan all week, not simply at one or two meals. When various foods are eaten every day, but not set out simultaneously in one single meal, right in front of your eyes, the temptation to overindulge is not so great.

Plan, plan, plan!
Planning is an important tool for weight loss. For example, plan to have a different breakfast every day of the week. It's too easy to fall into the habit of eating the same breakfast, the same lunch, the same snacks day in and day out. Maybe that's why the pounds crept on in the first place!

Monotonous diets can affect your microbiome
One of the keys to weight loss lies in your microbiome. The more diverse your microbiota species are, the more likely you are to be slim.

Monotony of diet means little or no change in your microbiome. So if your microbiome composition is contributing to your being overweight, and it remains the same, you will always be faced with an uphill battle to lose weight.

To recap—your gut microbiota feed on undigested and partially digested foods you have consumed. Without food, they die. Certain microbes can only live on certain foods. Gut microbiota metabolize specific nutrients from your diet and produce specific substances that act as metabolic signals in your body. In return for the food you give them, your microbes protect you from harmful toxins and excrete important substances that are essential to your good health. One microbial species manufactures one set of substances, another produces different ones. The greater the variety of species your gut supports, the more health-giving molecules your body receives.

In other words, they are vital to your well-being as well as playing an important part in weight loss or weight gain.

When you eat a wide range of diverse foods from all food groups, you allow your microbiome to become diverse as well. Diversity is the most important factor in balancing any ecosystem, whether it's a rainforest or the population of beneficial microbes living in your gut. In general, healthier people have a wide variety of gut microbe species.

If for whatever reason (eg, illness, food shortages) several of your microbe species are wiped out, there will be others remaining to help the body thrive. This means that even if a few species die off for some reason, the microbiome as a whole can continue functioning properly. Indeed, there is an association between having a narrow range of gut microbe species and having type 2 diabetes, inflammatory bowel disease and/or obesity.

A general decline in food variety has led to a decrease in the number of microbe species inhabiting our digestive systems. Some scientists propose that this could be helping to fuel the rise in global obesity.

According to research published in *Molecular Metabolism* in 2016, "Changes in farming practices over the last 50 years have resulted in decreased agro-diversity which, in turn, has resulted in decreased dietary diversity.

". . . the reduction in dietary diversity has changed the richness of human gut microbiota, the community of microorganisms living in the gut." [Heiman & Greenway (2016)]

Restricted, fad diets can have a drastic effect on your microbiome. What do you think happens to the diversity of your gut microbiota when you stop eating a whole group of macronutrients— such as carbohydrates? Abolishing entire food groups from your diet supports certain microbial species and fails to sustain others. This can contribute to ill health or obesity, or both.

If you continue to follow restrictive diets that omit entire food groups, over time you will drastically alter the composition of your gut microbiome. This can happen in a relatively short time—a matter of just a few days. By eliminating one or more macronutrient groups, you'd be helping certain microbe species to thrive while starving others out of existence.

If you avoid a particular group of macronutrients (protein, carbs or fats) or foods (e.g. grains) for a short time, you'll decrease your gut's microbial diversity during that brief period, but it's highly unlikely you'll wipe out entire species.

If you exclude certain food groups over a longer period—months or years— then you risk permanently losing some valuable species. This can be detrimental to your health and put you at risk of problems with your bodyweight.

Your microbiome thrives on variety.

The authors of the study "A Healthy Gastrointestinal Microbiome is Dependent on Dietary Diversity," write, "The importance of microbiota diversity cannot be overstated." [Elsevier (2016); Heiman & Greenway (2016)]

Evidence overwhelmingly suggests that following weight-loss diets that exclude entire food groups decreases the diversity of your gut microbes. In the long run, this can put you at risk of regaining any lost weight and even making you fatter than before you started.

When your microbiome population is unbalanced, your digestive system does not function properly. This can lead to a drop in your energy levels, and a sense of fatigue. The stress of fatigue can trigger the release of the stress hormone cortisol, which in turn elevates your insulin and blood sugar levels, often resulting in weight gain.

All foods are permitted on the Satiety Diet.

No food is off-limits on the Satiety Diet. Having said that, it is important to remember that "real" food—food that loves you—is recommended for everyday consumption, while foods that are highly processed, nutrient-poor and Calorie-dense are to be eaten only sometimes, and mindfully, and in small portions. Completely banning the foods you love can make you feel deprived. And if you feel deprived you're more at risk of "falling off the wagon" and abandoning your weight loss journey.

Helpful tips for a varied, satisfying weight-loss diet:

1) Don't cease it, decrease it!

How can you avoid the vicious cycle of deprivation and bingeing? Quite simply, by not banning the foods you enjoy eating.

Of course, there's a proviso. (After all, it's eating large portions of the foods you love that contributed to weight gain in the first place.)

To dampen cravings, eat a small piece of the craved-for food. Eat it rarely and eat it mindfully!

To lose weight, you don't have to force yourself to eat large platefuls of low Calorie foods that you don't enjoy. Choose foods that have a few more Calories and taste better, but serve yourself with smaller portions. Or mix favorite foods into Calorie-sparse dishes.

If you experience a very strong craving, eat what you desire (chocolate is an example that keeps cropping up), but eat a small portion and consume it mindfully, extracting the utmost pleasure from every morsel. Four squares of a standard chocolate bar could be considered a "small portion". Choose the most intensely-flavored types, such as dark chocolate.

2) Don't ditch it, switch it!

Best of all, to stave off cravings—swap, swap, swap.

You don't have to make yourself miserable by forcing yourself to eat fat-free or low-Calorie foods that you don't enjoy. Instead of non-fat foods, choose low-fat foods. They are more likely to give satiety, and they certainly taste better, so you won't feel deprived.

238

Swap white, refined flour for wholegrain flour. Swap plain pasta for pasta made from wholegrain wheat, buckwheat, rice or pulses, and choose wholegrain bread in place of white bread. Exchange dried fruit for fresh fruit. Instead of drinking fruit juice, eat a piece of whole, fresh fruit (preferable low fructose) accompanied by a glass of cool water with a twist of lemon or a sprig of mint. You get the picture!

3) Use both tips together.

Some foods (and drinks) are hard to switch. For example, many people baulk at switching to water instead of alcohol, or carob instead of chocolate. On the Satiety Diet no food is off limits—all you have to do is downsize your portions of hard-to-switch foods. Enjoy those smaller portions and eat them mindfully. And, of course, only eat them sometimes, not every day.

Here's an alcoholic example; instead of drinking cocktails such as Piña Coladas, Mudslides or Grasshoppers, which are loaded with sugars and fats, choose a small glass of a light beer, or red or white wine.

If you prefer hard liquor, choose spirits such as vodka, tequila, whiskey, or gin. They are still high in Calories and devoid of nutrition, but a small amount is better for your waistline than a creamy, sugary cocktail. Accurately measure out a 30ml (1oz) shot of hard liquor. This can be mixed with plain water and ice, and garnished with a twist of fresh citrus.

Sip it slowly and make it last!

Keeping variation in your diet.

Eating a varied, well-balanced diet means eating a variety of foods from each of the food groups daily, in the recommended amounts. The food groups include:

- Vegetables and legumes
- Fruit
- Wholegrain cereals
- Protein-rich foods such as legumes, tofu, nuts, seeds, eggs, seafood, lean meats or poultry
- Reduced fat dairy products and/or alternatives made from soy, almonds etc.
- Unsaturated fats and oils

Choose a variety of foods from within each food group.

Some of these food groups contain only some of the macronutrients and micronutrients your body needs, while others may contain nearly all of them.

The Japanese, who (as we've often mentioned!) are among the leanest populations in the world, traditionally include an extensive range of tasty, mainly plant-based dishes in their satiating meals.

A typical homemade Japanese dinner would probably include:

- Rice
- Soup
- Pickled vegetables
- A salad of fresh, raw vegetables
- A dish of cooked vegetables
- Protein—usually seafood
- A dish of mixed protein and vegetables
- Seaweed (nori), furikake (a seasoning usually made from dried fish, sesame seeds, seaweed, sugar, salt and other ingredients), or tsukudani (a side dish made by simmering seaweeds in soy sauce and mirin.)
- Beverages such as green tea (matcha) or cold barley tea (mugicha)

For more about the Japanese way of eating, see *The Satiety Diet Weight Loss Toolkit*, book #2 in the Satiety Diet series.

Sources of diverse foods.

In developed nations, it is possible to purchase a greater variety of foods if we look beyond the supermarket shelves. Farmers' markets, health food stores, specialty shops online and our own backyard vegetable plot can provide some of the more unusual ingredients to keep us healthy and help us achieve satiety. Making the small effort to change old, narrow eating habits pays dividends in your quest for weight loss.

Buy fresh or grow your own.

Buying fresh produce from farmers' markets, growing your own edible plants, making sure you eat shop-bought food as soon as possible (instead if leaving it to languish in the refrigerator), and above all eating a diversity of whole, unprocessed foods—methods like these can help ensure that you are getting the best possible nutrition from real food. This also removes the need for swallowing vitamin and mineral pills or other dietary supplements.

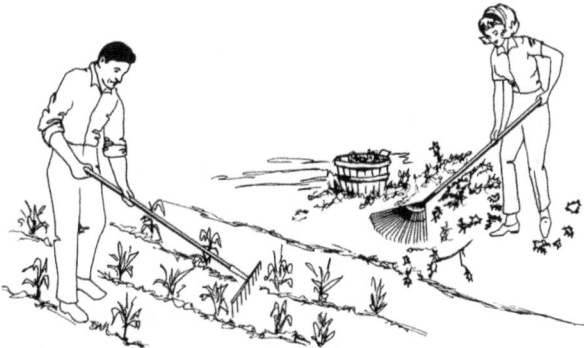

FULLNESS AND FOOD VOLUME
Food quantity and satiety.

One of the factors that contributes to satiety is the feeling of fullness. Your Inner Guardian wants you to eat enough food to provide the energy and nutrition for optimum health. Just one or two bites are not going to make you feel '"full". Unless you eat sufficient food to make you feel satiated, you are likely to keep eating and over-consume Calories.

When food enters your stomach, signals are sent to specific areas of your brain in response to the stomach's expansion. These signals help to inform your body about how much food is being eaten; i.e. the volume, or quantity of food. The expansion of your stomach is an important satiety signal.

Here are some tips for achieving that feeling of fullness without piling on excess weight:

Eat more fiber.

Fiber-rich foods can help you reach satiety without over-eating, by providing volume with fewer Calories.

Pay attention to your food.

Through years of eating without thinking about it, many people have lost the ability to measure their own fullness. Eating slowly and mindfully can help you become more aware of how full you are feeling.

Take notice of your meal's visual appeal and view all the courses laid out together. Your mind has significant power over your body. Certain mind-tricks can even, to a certain extent, fool your Inner Guardian. The amount of food you eat affects how full you feel, and whether you reach satiety. Amazingly, the amount of food you *think* you're eating can also influence satiety!

Here's where your eyes play a part. People who eat a meal in complete darkness, for example, tend to eat far more than they need. They also underestimate how much they have eaten. And even though they overeat, they don't feel particularly well-satiated afterwards.

Perceived portion size can affect how full you feel after a meal. Seeing your meal, "eating with your eyes", is extremely important for appetite control. That is why it's so helpful for you to view each meal in its entirety, with all the courses grouped together on the table in front of you. [Scheibehenne et al., (2010)]

Eat "big-looking" food that's low in Calories.

When food *looks* bigger, it's more likely to make you feel satiated. Even if it only looks bigger because it's full of air!

In a 2000 study, volunteers ate their breakfast, lunch, and dinner in a laboratory one day a week for four weeks. On three of those days they were given a milkshake 30 minutes before lunch (on one day they had no milkshake).

Researchers pumped air into two of the milkshakes so that they looked a lot bigger, up to double the size. When the study participants drank the bigger-looking milkshakes, they felt more satiated, and ate less food for lunch. This is despite the fact that all milkshakes were made from the same ingredients and there was no difference in their weight or Calorie content.

The researchers concluded that "...the volume of a [milkshake] independent of its energy density can influence satiety." [Rolls et al., 2000]

Use the power of suggestion.

Your expectations about food (whether right or wrong) have a powerful impact on your satiety. In a 2008 study, people were shown pictures of different foods and asked to rate how much satiety they thought each food would provide. It was found that there was " . . . a considerable mismatch . . . between satiety expectations and the energy content of foods." For example, people expected 200 kcal of pasta and 894 kcal of cashew nuts to provide equal satiety.

It was the *size* of the serving that influenced people's expectations of satiety, rather than the amount of energy contained within the foods.

The researchers also concluded that, " . . . expected-satiety judgments are learned," because people rated foods that were familiar to them as being more satiating than foods that were new to them.

"Humans have expectations about the satiety that is likely to develop after consuming particular foods," they wrote. "These expectations are potentially important, because they may influence decisions about meal size." [Brunstrom et al., 2008]

In a 2011 study, researchers gave each of the participants a smoothie to drink. All the smoothies were the same, but when the volunteers were told the drinks contained a lot more fruit, they not only expected to feel more satiated after drinking them, they actually *did* feel more satiated. [Brunstrom et al., 2011]

Eat out of heavier food containers.

Food's perceived weight can influence your satiety. People tend to think that if food weighs more, it will be more likely to provide satiety. Researchers gave food to people in two containers that looked identical—except that one container was heavier than the other. There was no difference in the food inside the containers, but the study's participants felt that the food in the heavier container was richer in Calories and more satiating than the food in the lighter container. [Piqueras-Fiszman & Spence, 2012]

Divide your food into more portions.

The number of food portions in a meal can greatly affect satiety levels. Do you remember the first time you ever bought something at a shop when you were a little child? You gave the storekeeper a single coin (of a high denomination) and in return, not only did she hand over the item you were buying, she also gave you a number of coins! The fact that these coins represented small change didn't mean much to a child. It probably seemed to you that the storekeeper was being extraordinarily generous and you were getting the best of the bargain. In return for one coin, you'd received a whole handful of coins, as well as something from the store, to boot.

As adults we know how money works, but deep down our minds operate in much the same way as they did when we were little kids. When we see many food items on the plate in front of us, we are tempted to see it as "more" food. Cutting up a large piece of food into smaller pieces can make you feel as if you are getting more to eat, thus contributing to satiety and making you feel satisfied with less food.

"... something as simple as segmenting the food into sub-portions can change perceptions of portion size and have beneficial effects on appetite control, presumably because people believed they were consuming more this way. [Chambers et al. (2015); Geier et al., (2012)]

Make food portions look different.

Food variety is important for satiety, but so is *perceived* food variety. Imagine taking a photograph of a normal-sized main course served on a large plate. The amount of food on the plate looks small by comparison to the vast expanses of the plate.

Now, divide up all the individual components of the meal and put each one into a small, individual dish, plate or bowl, all of different shapes and colors. Arrange these small dishes attractively on the table and take a second photograph.

The food is the same, but the second arrangement appears more filling and satiating.

Does an assortment of small, variously-shaped food dishes look familiar? This is how a traditional meal is served in Japan, a country with one of the lowest obesity rates in the world.

Eat until you feel satiated but not over-full.

Satiety is improved when you don't over-fill your stomach. *Hara hachi bu* or *hara hachi bun me* is a Japanese saying, based on a Confucian teaching that you should eat until your stomach is 80% full. It is practised widely in the Japanese island of Okinawa, where obesity is rare and the wider population is famously lean and long-lived.

Authors Wilcox, Wilcox and Suzuki surmise that *hara hachi bun me* assists in keeping the average Okinawan's Body Mass Index (BMI) low, because when the stomach is not regularly stretched to its utmost expansion, the stretch-receptors that send satiety signals to the brain remain sensitive. This means people can reach satiety more easily, without needing to eat as much food. [Willcox et al., (2002)]

It should be noted that "80% full" does not mean "80% satiated". By eating satiating foods slowly and mindfully, you can reach satiety without stuffing your stomach until it is over-full. For long term weight loss, it's important that you reach 100% satiety at mealtimes. Leaving yourself in a state of constant semi-hunger can make you open to nibbling and browsing and snacking.

CHEWING

We all need to chew. Malcolm Bourne[30] writes in his book "Food Texture and Viscosity, Concept and Measurement" that people have a "deeply ingrained need to chew".

Right from the time we, as babies, cut our first teeth until we grow so old that we may need dentures, chewing is an activity we find immensely satisfying. Babies grab objects within reach and bring them straight to their mouths, to gnaw on them with toothless gums. Mothers give rusks to infants to chomp on. In our later years, we visit the dentist to try to save our teeth—partly for cosmetic reasons, but also because we find it very satisfying to chomp on something chewy.

Human beings love to chew. The foods of every culture around the world include chewy foods. And by "chewy", we mean food that needs to be chewed hard, or for a relatively long time before being swallowed, usually because of its toughness or stickiness.

In theory, you could get all your nutrition from slurpy, puréed foods, but that's not enough for really good health, either psychologically or physiologically.

---

30   Malcolm Bourne is affiliated with Cornell University, Food Science and Technology, Geneva, New York, U.S.A.

Some benefits of thorough chewing include:

- Reaching satiety after eating less food. The action of chewing stimulates the release of certain hormones that are required to transmit satiety signals to the brain.
- Food that needs to be chewed takes longer to eat, thus increasing the likelihood of your satiety signals chipping in before you've over-eaten.
- Chewing also stimulates the flow of saliva—part of the first step in proper digestion.
- Better digestion. When your teeth and your saliva properly break down food in your mouth, it's easier for your body to extract and absorb the nutrients, thus helping to dampen cravings. Chewing also relaxes the pylorus, a muscle that regulates the movement of food from your stomach into your small intestine.
- Better weight control.
- Brain invigoration. The strong, rhythmic action of your jaws increases blood-flow to your brain, which stimulates the brain and may ward off dementia.
- Chewing is good for your teeth, and for the bones that hold your teeth in place. It keeps your teeth and jaw healthy.
- Feeling more relaxed and energized after meals When you digest your food properly your body receives better nutrition, which leads to better health and more energy. Life improves with chewing!
- Greater enjoyment of meals and satisfaction afterwards. Chewing means your food stays in your mouth for longer, giving you more time to enjoy the delicious flavors and textures.

Chewing promotes dental health.

A person who has the ability to chew vigorously and thoroughly probably has good teeth. In the Inner Guardian's ancient language of the body, having good teeth means that a) the chewer is probably young and/or b) the chewer is in good physical condition.

Your Inner Guardian reasons that if you have the ability to chew vigorously, without experiencing pain, you must possess at least *some* teeth that are firmly anchored in strong, healthy tissue and bone. Ergo, you are probably young and fit and strong—exactly the kind of person the tribe needs to help it survive. Good chewers, in the ancient language of the body, deserve to have their lives prolonged.

Tooth and gum diseases are also associated with other, major health problems. Inflammation of the gum tissue and periodontal disease can lead to cardiovascular disease, dementia, respiratory infections and diabetic complications.

Chewing and satiety.

For weight loss, it is vital to get the satiety message through to your brain, and one of the best ways to send this body-speech signal is by chewing—vigorous, hearty chewing!

Thorough chewing helps you eat more slowly, reach satiety more easily, and eat less.

When you take the time to properly chew your food, you're sending a stream of potent signals to your brain that tell it, "I am eating." Your jaw muscles are working. Your salivary glands are pumping and your tongue is performing a range of gymnastics as it moves the food around inside your mouth. Your teeth and gums are subject to pleasant pressures. The inner surfaces of your mouth are sensing textures. Your taste buds are experiencing flavors and your sense of smell is engaging with food aromas. Your eyes are witnessing the plate of as-yet-uneaten food that's still sitting in front of you while you chew. Your ears may be hearing the crunching sounds of food being broken down in your mouth. The reward centers of your brain are lighting up as you experience the satisfaction of eating.

When you chew your food thoroughly, all these intense events are happening for a longer period. On a physiological level, your brain is receiving a powerful message, "I am eating;" or even, "I have been eating for a long time, which means I must be getting plenty of food".

During the extended period of chewing, your digestive system has enough time to generate satiety signals in your gut and send them along their pathways to your brain. And when your Inner Guardian gets the message of that you've eaten plenty of food, it knows it can safely switch off your hunger drive and switch on your feelings of satiety.

By contrast, when you gulp down your food as quickly as possible, barely chewing it, or when you bypass chewing altogether by consuming your food in liquid form, you're not giving your brain the chance to really process the fact that you have eaten.

Your brain really needs all the input associated with chewing in order for it to determine that you've taken in sufficient food. Without that input, it can keep demanding food even after your stomach is full; long after you've consumed sufficient Calories and nutrients for your needs.

If you're in the habit of scarfing down your food, eating on the run, or swallowing each bite almost whole—don't despair. Habits can be broken. You can train yourself to "eat mindfully", focussing on each bite and chewing your food for longer. Eventually, chewing thoroughly becomes routine; something you always do without even thinking about it.

Chewy foods help you reach satiety.

Unfortunately for their waistlines, many people find it hard to change their habit of chomping down on their food with gusto, gulping as much as possible in one mouthful and swallowing it half-chewed.

How can you keep food in your mouth for longer?

Researchers have showed that when people choose harder foods, which require extra chewing, they keep food in their mouths for longer without even thinking about it. And this leads to eating less—without extra effort!

In a 2014 study, food science expert Professor Bolhuis and her colleagues conducted a study involving 50 volunteers. The researchers filmed the volunteers eating their lunch on two separate days.

On one of the days their lunch consisted of hard foods and on the other day, soft foods. On both days the diners were instructed to eat until they felt "comfortably full". The researchers analyzed the film footage, noting the size of the bites people took, and how long they chewed their food before swallowing it.

Five hours after their lunch was filmed, the volunteers were given dinner. This time the meal consisted of 60% noodles, 10% chicken, and 30% vegetables. The diners could eat as much of it as they liked, with no restrictions such as having to feel "comfortably full". The researchers calculated how many Calories each person consumed from their dinner.

The results showed that when people ate a lunch of harder foods they took smaller bites, chewed it for longer, and ended up eating significantly less food overall.

"Hard foods led to (an approximately)13% lower energy intake at lunch compared to soft foods," they wrote.

Interestingly, none of the volunteers compensated for this lower energy intake by eating extra food at dinner time. In other words, they ate a lot less during the day they had the hard foods for lunch, but they didn't feel as if they'd eaten less. All that chewing helped them consume fewer Calories without realizing it.

Imagine if you ate 13% fewer Calories every day for weeks or months, without really trying! Eventually you'd notice yourself losing weight. [Bolhuis et al., (2014)]

Thorough chewing slows down eating.

When your stomach becomes full during a meal, it takes around 20 minutes for the fullness signals to reach your brain. Chewing your food for longer is a good way to slowing down eating, so that you don't consume excess food even after your stomach is actually full. This can help with weight management.

Taking smaller bites of food and keeping it longer in your mouth before swallowing it tends to make you satisfied with eating less. The longer the food remains in your mouth, the better your brain registers that you are eating, and the more likely you are to reach satiety.

A 2013 study showed that people who chewed their food more thoroughly had lower body weights. [Fukuda et al., (2013)]

Chewing is one of the earliest satiety signal triggers.

Chewing your food sends a number of signals to your brain via your salivary glands, your jaw muscles, the roots of your teeth etc. In turn, your brain lets your stomach know that food will arrive soon. The action of chewing is a body-speech signal to your Inner Guardian that eating has begun. Already, as you chew, your body is preparing to increase production of satiety hormones and decrease hunger hormones.

A lot of chewing indicates that there is probably a lot of food. Your mouth is a remarkably sensitive area of your body. It needs to be, since it is the gateway and sentinel between the outside world and the internal world of the body.[31]

Chewy foods help with satiety. Potato crisps, for example, are less satisfying than dry crackers, because you have to chew the crackers for longer, which allows satiety signals more time to reach your brain. A study in which participants chewed almonds showed that those who chewed more times felt more sated than those who chewed less. [Cassady et al., (2009)]

Chewing helps you get better nutrition.

Thorough chewing breaks down your food. It also mixes it with saliva in your mouth, which is the first phase of digestion, and a very important one. Chewing crushes the food into smaller bits. This means there is more surface area for your salivary enzymes to come into contact with, so they can begin the process of digestion.

This process is already under way before the food slides down your throat. Enzymes in the saliva begin to decompose the food into its nutrient components even before you've swallowed it. For this, the rest of your digestive tract is grateful. The chewed food will be more easily assimilated later in the digestive process. Chewing makes it easier for your gut to absorb nutrients from food fragments as they

---

31 For example, the body relies on the mouth to tell it if something tastes nasty, because it might be poisonous, and should therefore be spat out. If something in the mouth feels too gritty to be chewed, it's unlikely to be digestible, and it also should be discarded.

travel through your body. If you swallow larger, insufficiently chewed food pieces, the rest of your digestive system may have a hard time dealing with them. They may not be completely broken down in your gut, possibly leading to indigestion and bacterial overgrowth.

When your body absorbs nutrients properly, it's less likely to send out hunger signals to drive you to to seek more food.

What's more, chewier foods tend to be less processed than soft foods, and they often contain more fiber. This means they are likely to be more healthful.

Chewing can improve the enjoyment of eating.

Another benefit of maximum chewing is that it seems to make food taste better. When you chew mindfully, really concentrating on the feeling and flavor of the food in your mouth, you begin to savor textures and flavor notes you may have missed before.

Choose real, solid food to promote chewing.

People in developed nations don't eat as many raw foods or whole foods as they did in the past. This means they do less chewing than their forebears. Highly processed food needs less chewing. Could this be one of the factors behind the obesity crisis? Simply by choosing to eat foods that are whole and unprocessed or lightly-processed, you will find yourself chewing more.

- Stop drinking shakes and smoothies, and start chewing. Study after study shows that when we chew our Calories we tend to eat less than if we swallow Calories in liquid form. "The energy delivered in drinks reportedly suppresses subsequent food intake less than the equivalent energy delivered in foods." [Rolls (1995)]
- Find recipes for chewy dishes. You can find recipes for a range of satisfying, jaw-working, chewy dishes in *Crispy, Creamy, Chewy: The Satiety Diet Cookbook*.

Avoid "nutritionally complete" drinks.

There is a huge industry churning out various brands of drinkable "nutritionally complete" foods, which are generally sold in the form of powders and liquids (although there are some solid ones). They are often called "meal replacement shakes". Some are made out of mixtures of various nutrients. Others are made out of foods that have been dried and pulverized. The assertion is that these foods free you from having to cook, while providing (theoretically) all your body's nutritional requirements.

When you drink your food there's no chewing involved, and no tasting of different flavors, and no texture other than the goopy texture of the drink, and nothing very attractive to look at or smell. Drinking is quicker than eating, so your meals don't last long.

Furthermore, drinkable "nutritionally complete" foods can never truly be nutritionally complete. Sharon R. Akabas, the director of the Master of Science program at the Institute of Human Nutrition at Columbia University, says it's impossible for any company to create the perfect food formula. "You would need hundreds of ingredients," she says, "and hundreds more that we don't even know about yet."

The bad news for people who want to lose weight is that no matter what the sales pitches claim, these foods are very unlikely to induce satiety. They may, in fact, lead to overeating and obesity.

How many times should you chew each bite?

If you want to keep stress out of your life, don't force yourself to count how many times you chew on a piece of food! And don't try and chew each piece 100 times, or even 50 times. The thing is, after you've chewed that mouthful a few times you'll probably get the urge to swallow. Then you'll have to fight the urge, so that you can keep chewing. And that's stressful! Instead of enjoying your food, you'll feel as if you're plowing through a chore. And you'll take ages to finish your meal, during which time you'll probably be worried about how much time you're wasting.

So simply chew your food until it reaches a pleasingly soft, gooey texture without any lumps and chunks. Then swallow it. That's probably more chewing than you usually do!

Chew more thoroughly, not much more slowly.

We recommend that when you practice mindful eating you don't try to chew much more slowly than usual. Chewing too slowly can make you feel as if you're holding yourself back from eating. In body-speech, this is akin to being deprived. It detracts from the enjoyment of eating.

Instead, simply chew each bite more thoroughly. This can have the effect of making you feel as if you're eating more food.

Thorough chewing can send calming signals to your Inner Guardian.

When you take the time to chew your food thoroughly, your brain is getting signals that you are not in a hurry. Your Inner Guardian deduces that there is no nearby danger for you to run away from. It reasons that you don't need you don't need a surge of cortisol or adrenaline, and you don't need to be prompted to seek extra energy/ Calories to help you run fast and survive that danger. Calmness promotes satiety.

THE EXPERIENCE OF EATING

The experience of eating plays as much of a role in weight loss as the actual food you consume. How you eat is just as important as what you eat.

How you eat refers to such factors as:
- how fast you eat
- the duration of meals
- how mindfully you eat (what you're thinking about while eating),
- the ambiance that surrounds you while you're eating (your dining environment).

Rate of eating.

For optimum satiety, it's important to eat relatively slowly. It takes about 20 minutes after you begin a meal for your digestive system to signal to your brain that you have eaten sufficient food. This is why eating at a leisurely pace can help your body register fullness before you eat too much. You'll be satisfied with smaller portions, which helps with weight loss.

Twenty minutes is just a rough guideline. In some people it can take up to 30 minutes for the digestive enzymes to release the hormones that signal "fullness" to the brain.

If you're shoveling in food rapidly, you may not give the "fullness" signals enough time to register, and you could still feel hungry despite having eaten a lot. Eating more slowly allows you to consume less food during the approximately twenty-minute window. Fast eaters consume a lot more food per minute than slow eaters. Eating slowly can help you reach satiety before you've over-eaten.

"... eating slowly may help to maximize satiation and reduce energy intake within meals," concluded the authors of a 2008 study published in *The Journal of the American Dietetic Association*. [Andrade et al., (2008)].

These results were supported the authors of a 2011 survey for The American Dietetic Association who said, " ...the results suggest that faster eating is associated with higher BMI in middle-aged women." [Sook Ling Leong et al., (2011)]

"Slow eating may be associated with reduced energy intake," wrote scientists who devised a 2011 study to examine the effectiveness of a bite-counting device. [Scisco et al., (2011)]

"...when foods can be ingested rapidly, food and energy intake is high. People may therefore be at risk of overconsumption, when consuming foods with a high eating rate," was the conclusion of a 2011 study in the journal *Appetite*. [Viskaal-van Dongen et al., (2011)]

Japanese researchers who conducted a 2006 study came up with results indicating that eating fast leads to obesity. [Otsuka et al., (2006)].

Psychologists studying people's eating behavior noted, "Eating slowly is associated with a lower Body Mass Index. . . eating slowly promotes self-reported satiation and satiety." [Ferriday et al., (2015)]

" ... eating slowly may help to maximize satiation and reduce energy intake within meals." [Andrade et al., (2008)]

"…when analysing satiation processes by the microstructure of meals in 4-year-old children, it was reported that mouthfuls of food per minute significantly predicted increased BMI and fat mass at 6 years of age." [Blundell & Bellisle (2013)]

"Slow spaced eating is associated with improved satiety and gut hormone responses in normal-weight participants. . . Slow spaced eating may be a useful prevention strategy, but might also help curb food intake in those already suffering from obesity and diabetes." [Angelopoulos et al., (2013)]

Duration of meals.

It follows that when people eat more slowly, their meals usually take longer to consume. "Increased meal length was associated with greater weight loss," wrote the authors of a 1991study published in the journal *Behavior Therapy*. [Spiegel, et al., (1991)]

Traditionally, the French allow a minimum of one hour per meal. No rushed ten-minute lunches or breakfast-on-the-run for them! Obesity rates in France are among the lowest in the OECD[32]. The habit of making every meal an occasion, instead of an after-thought, could be one of the reasons for longer meal duration. For better satiety and weight loss, slow down the rate at which you eat.

Here are some ways of prolonging meals:
- Chew your food as slowly as you can without becoming impatient.
- Put down your eating utensils between bites, and leave them lying on the table while you chew.
- Use chopsticks.
- Use your non-dominant hand.
- Take smaller forksful or spoonsful.
- Use smaller eating utensils.
- Include in your meal some foods that are chewy.
- Chew each mouthful thoroughly, until it has the consistency of puréed fruit.

---

32   The Organisation for Economic Co-operation and Development.

- Eat foods of lower Calorie-density. It could make you prolong your meal. "Eating time was significantly longer on the diet low in energy density by an average of 33% per day," say the authors of a 1983 study. [Duncan et al., (1983)]

Mindful eating.

A 2011 study published in the *Journal of Obesity* examined overweight women who were suffering from high levels of stress and emotional eating. The study found that when the women practised mindful eating they lost fat from around their abdomens without even dieting! [Daubenmier et al., (2011)]

Eating slowly and eating mindfully go hand in hand. Train yourself to eat mindfully, step by step. It's not easy to be completely mindful all at once, at every meal, when you've never tried it before. You could begin with one mindful bite per day for two or three days, then one mindful mouthful at every meal. Over the following days, increase the number to five or six mindful mouthfuls every time you eat. Eventually you will train yourself to eat mindfully at every meal, and even to eat snacks mindfully.

Chris Clark says: "When I first started the Satiety Diet, one of the things I found hardest to do was to eat mindfully. I found it surprisingly difficult to break my habit of eating while simultaneously watching TV or some other screen, or reading a book, or a newspaper, or the side of a breakfast cereal packet or the label on a peanut butter jar, or anything in print that was within eyeshot. This was a habit I hadn't even realised I had."

Mindless eating.

The opposite of mindful eating is mindless eating, which often leads to *over*eating. Mindless eating can include:

- Eating simply because you always eat at a certain time of day (e.g. you always eat lunch at 1 o'clock even if you're not hungry then).

257

- Eating simply because you always eat when you are in a certain place (e.g. you always buy a donut when you pass the donut store).
- Chewing your way through bags of popcorn or candy while watching movies at the cinema.
- Eating to relieve boredom.
- Eating as a form of comfort when you feel sad or lonely.
- Continuing to eat even after you feel full.

How to eat "mindfully":
1. Multitasking and distractions.
- Sit down at a table to eat (whenever possible).
- Eat in a place where there are no distractions such as sudden loud noises, or people making demands on you.
- Treat every meal as a special occasion. Some people view meals as a feeding process that interrupts their other daily activities. People who treat every meal as an enjoyable, relaxing occasion, worthy of mindful attention, are more likely to have a healthy body weight.
- Pay attention to your food. You eat more food if you are not concentrating on eating, so eliminate multitasking. Don't eat while driving, reading, watching television, walking around etc. Some people eat "on the run", usually as fast as possible, swallowing a shake as they tap away on their computer, or munching take-out food as they hurry down the street. When you are distracted, you are not tuning into your internal satiety signals. Distractions can also happen if you are eating in a social situation.
- Don't eat and walk at the same time. It's bad enough for mindfulness if you eat while watching TV, having a chat or reading, but if you eat while you're walking around, you could be even more likely to consume too much! A 2015 study published in the *Journal of Health Psychology* found that women who were dieting (restrained eaters), "... consumed more overall and more Calories (specifically five times more chocolate) if the cereal bar was eaten while walking."

They concluded that, "'Eating on the go' may disinhibit restrained eaters either as a form of distraction or by offering a justification to overeat." [Ogden et al., (2015)]

2. Your thoughts.

- Pay attention to every bite of your meal. Take time to enjoy your food and value the experience of eating.
- Focus your thoughts "in the moment" while you're eating, instead of pondering on what happened yesterday or making plans for tomorrow.
- Give yourself unconditional permission to eat as much of your nourishing, tasty, Calorie-sparse meal or snack as you need, in order to reach satiety without being over-full.
- Breathe deeply and feel calm. Calmness helps proper digestion.
- Think about the food nourishing you and filling you up.
- Feel free. Recognize that all food is available to you whenever you want (as long as you manage portion sizes). There is no "forbidden" food that could tempt you to binge.
- Let go of guilt. Many people are hypervigilant about what they eat. They feel bad if they eat something that they consider "wrong" or "bad". Give yourself permission to eat large portions of Calorie-sparse foods prepared in delicious ways, and small portions of the Calorie-dense foods you like. No food is off limits and all food should be savored and enjoyed.
- Recognize that you like some foods and you don't like others, and that this is just a matter of preference, not a vice or a virtue. Take the judgment out of eating and you'll feel more relaxed.
- Don't bargain Calories for exercise. If you develop the attitude of, "If I go to the gym I can eat this doughnut", you're likely to consume more Calories than you use up. Besides, when you think this way, eating can become a worry. It should be a joy!
- As you eat, remind yourself that you have chosen to enjoy your food, and that food is not your enemy, but the friend who gives you nourishment and pleasure.
- Don't worry about counting every single Calorie. Close approximation is fine.

259

3. Sensory enjoyment.

- Savor the flavor, texture/mouthfeel, smell, sound, temperature, sight and every other sensory quality of your food. When you really pay attention to your food, you'll get more pleasure from eating. It's important for satiety that you really relish your food. The texture, the taste, the smell. . . all these sensory inputs help to make you feel satisfied. Your Inner Guardian needs to register the sensory pleasure of food, so that it can be satisfied that your body has been fed.
- Do not eat in the dark!
- Select foods that are not only good for you, but also a pleasure to eat.
- Ideally, your dining table should be beautifully set, complete with condiments and small dishes of assorted sizes, shapes and colors, and perhaps a pretty table-cloth and a vase of fresh flowers (we are talking about a perfect situation here!) This sight will help you concentrate on the visual aspects of your meal.
- Enjoy the sight of all that colorful food on your plate. Look at it and remember it for later.
- Enjoy the smell, texture and taste of your delicious food by savoring each mouthful.

4. Mindfulness includes the rate at which you eat.

- Slow down your eating rate. Eat slowly and chew well.
- Allow yourself a minimum of half an hour for each meal. An hour is preferable.

5. Self-awareness.

- Eat when you're actually hungry. Not for any other reason.
- Be aware of your body's own internal hunger and satiety signals and be guided by them as to when to start and finish eating. In other words, it's best not to conform to some very strictly organized diet plan whereby you stop eating even when you have not reached satiety, or you start eating when you're not really hungry. Your Inner Guardian will soon misinterpret the signals you are sending it.

6. Mindful eating and sensory enjoyment.

It can be harder for obese people to enjoy their food. Bridget Benelam, of the British Nutrition Foundation says, "Studies looking at the sensory part of the brain being activated by food have found it is not as active in obese people—so theoretically they would have to consume more food to get the same pleasure as someone else." All the more reason for obese people to eat mindfully and derive as much pleasure as possible from their meals!

7. Eating mindfully works best in a quiet environment.

Concentrating on your food means listening to the sounds of food in your mouth and the soft sounds that accompany dining. It does not, however, mean listening to music or eating in a noisy environment. Quite the reverse!

A study published in the journal *Food Quality and Preference* found that people wearing headphones and listening to "white noise" to block out sound while eating crunchy foods ate more than people who could hear the crunchy sound of their food. It's as if the sounds of your eating help to give your Inner Guardian additional signals that you are, in fact, taking in nutrition. Yes your jaw is moving as you chew, yes you are feeling, tasting and smelling the food, yes you are swallowing it—but the sound confirms that all of this is happening. It is a vital piece of the satiety jigsaw. [Woods, et al., (2010)]

It is easier to eat mindfully when your dining environment is calm and peaceful. Ideally there should be no sudden loud noises (such as the clashing of metal cooking equipment from a nearby kitchen, or the shouting of orders from waiters).

Any dining companions who share your table should have a calm and relaxed attitude too. In a perfect world your dining companions would be mindful eaters, and not prone to too much conversation.

If you dine in the company of fast eaters, it is easy to start bolting your food too, without realizing it. And if you dine with constant talkers, your attention may be diverted from your food. In the perfect dining situation, all cell-phones, televisions and other devices would be switched off, and nobody (including small children!) would be making any demands on you.

Eating in a noisy environment can cause people to eat foods that are more Calorie-dense. In 2015, researchers conducted a study on sixty families. Thirty families in the experimental group experienced a continuous loud noise adjacent to the dining room during dinner, and the thirty in the control group experienced no additional noise.

"In general, more cookies were consumed in the noisy condition," say the researchers. [Fiese et al., (2015)] A quiet, calm environment is best for eating.

Other benefits of mindfulness.

Practicing mindfulness regularly has added bonuses.
- It has been shown to boost positive emotions while decreasing stress and negative emotions. [Weinstein et al., (2009)]
- Mindfulness can train you to ignore distractions. It can improve your focussing skills. [Kerr et al., (2011)]
- It can improve your " . . . levels of relationship happiness, relationship stress, stress coping efficacy, and overall stress." [Carson et al., (2002)]

Mindfulness can reduce stress as well as promoting satiety; thus it helps with weight loss in multiple ways.

TIPS FOR USING SATIETY FOR WEIGHT LOSS.

Make sure you reach satiation at every meal.

Repleteness is a message to the Inner Guardian, signaling that, "There is enough food in the immediate environment. You don't need to generate hunger signals to drive this human body to seek more food."

As mentioned earlier in this book, if you fail to reach satiation at each meal, it is highly unlikely that you will enjoy long-term satiety between meals. When you leave the dinner-table feeling slightly peckish, you're more likely to experience real hunger sooner after the meal. And then you'll be tempted to reach for the nearest snack.

Learn to recognize true satiation.

If it has been years since you last tuned into your body's satiation signals, it could take some time for you to begin to recognize them again.

It may be hard, at first, to read your body's signals and identify satiation when you've spent years sabotaging your own dieting efforts by grazing, and/or by leaving the dinner table while only half-full. When you start the Satiety Diet you will have to re-learn to listen to your body's silent cues, which have been ignored for so long.

Not-quite-satiated.

Some people try to lose weight by under-eating. They cease to eat when they are not quite satiated. They leave the dinner table feeling peckish or slightly hungry. There's a nagging feeling at the back of their minds that they really could have used a few extra bites, or something sweet for dessert, but they are trying to lose weight so, (they reason) they must resist; they must summon all their willpower and go without those few extra bites, or that sweet dessert...

Is this you?

For a time, after your unsatisfying meal, you might be able to stave off those nagging feelings. In the end, however, your Inner Guardian will probably win. By ceasing to eat before you feel replete, you are sending a message to your Inner Guardian that there is not quite enough food available in the environment to really fill your needs and satisfy you. Your Inner Guardian, therefore, thinks it should switch on your hunger hormones pretty soon after the meal, to drive you to seek more food.

Over-full.

On the other hand, satiation is *not* feeling over-stuffed or bloated with food.

True satiation.

Satiation is the feeling of "I have eaten exactly the right amount of food. I feel satisfied and pleasantly full, but not over-full." This is the best message to deliver to your Inner Guardian.

Don't "graze". Eat regular, satisfying meals instead.

Why is "grazing" unhelpful for weight loss? Because when you nibble on food lightly and often, you are unlikely to reach true satiation. Grazing doesn't send a "food is so plentiful in my environment that I can eat until I am pleasantly full" signal to your Inner Guardian. On the contrary—you are sending the message that, "I need to keep putting small amounts of food into my mouth as soon as it becomes available." Your Inner Guardian deduces that food must be scarce.

It is only when your Inner Guardian is perfectly certain that your environment offers a bounty of food that it will stop defending your fat stores by making you hungry and driving you to seek Calories.

In fact, if it is certain there's plenty of food available, your strong and protective Inner Guardian may even release biochemicals that *deter* you from seeking food.

For example, have you ever experienced that uncomfortable, over-stuffed feeling after you've indulged in a huge festive meal? Maybe you have thought to yourself, "Oh, if I even *look* at any more food I will feel sick. My belly feels boated and sore. I can't stand the thought of eating anything else!" That's due to your Inner Guardian firing off biochemicals such as the satiety hormone leptin, to protect you from overeating.

Eat only when your body really needs nourishment.

You can use this "protection from overeating" mechanism to your advantage. Refrain from eating between meals (you can drink as much water and milk-free tea as you like). Then when you eat a meal, eat mindfully until you reach satiation. These mini-fasts between meals help to shrink your stomach and accustom it to being less full. Your stomach's fullness-sensors become more sensitive. You become better tuned to your satiation signals and less likely to eat more than you need.

Be organised.

Plan, plan, plan! This is one of our mottoes! To really benefit from the Satiety Diet, you should plan ahead. Yes, we know it's boring to do that, but it's a small price to pay for freeing your body from the unwanted fat that's dragging it down!

- Always have your next meal planned—otherwise you risk being subject to real hunger and the temptation to reach for high Calorie snacks.
- Instead of shopping for food once a week (which can result in fresh food going stale), shop more often.
- Prepare meals at home more often.
- Freeze home-cooked meals for later, in sealed, labeled and date-marked containers. Having a range of satiety-friendly meals ready in the freezer can be very convenient.

Following the Satiety Diet at work.

- If you eat out at a cafe, choose one with a peaceful ambiance. Order a satisfying dish rich in vegetables and protein, and not drenched in oil or other fats.
- If you bring your own lunch to work, find somewhere to sit down and dine in peace. Spread out all your food in front of you, before you begin to eat. Take in the sight of all the colorful, nutrient-dense foods you are about to enjoy.
- Eat mindfully. Fill your mind with a sense of peace and calmness. Savoring the food's aroma, taste, texture, colors. Chew thoroughly. Eat slowly until you feel pleasantly full.
- Use the other tips and tricks from *The Satiety Diet Weight Loss Toolkit*, such as sipping some water before your meal.

Prolonging satiety between meals.

After a properly satiating meal, eaten mindfully, some people may not feel hungry for hours. Even up to 24 hours!

When you start to feel hungry between meals, use your imagination to visualize the last meal you ate. Remember how all the food looked, spread out in front of you. You consumed all that! It's inside you right now, nourishing you! Remembering your meal helps you to prolong satiety. Picturing the food you ate helps keep you feeling satisfied.

Use the tools in "The Satiety Diet Weight Loss Toolkit".

There was not enough space in this book to print the "Toolkit", so it's published as a separate volume, #2 in the Satiety Diet series. It offers lots more practical tools to help you get rid of the unwanted fat that's burdening your body. Read through the "Toolkit" and you'll find useful tips, such as:

- how to get a better night's sleep for easier weight loss
- meal preparation tools
- tools for keeping hunger at bay
- planning tools
- dining out tools
- tips on sweetness and sweeteners
- how to help prevent obesity in children
- stress reduction tools
- fasting tools
- more weight loss mind tricks
- tools for creating better habits
- thrifty weight loss

. . . and more.

PART THREE

HUNGER AND OVEREATING

Alert: Trigger words are used several times in the following section! It is preferable to read these words when you are feeling full and replete. Otherwise, when your brain decodes the words from print, it can spark off a physical reaction that increases your appetite. Stop reading now if you wish to avoid these words.

The trigger words are "hunger" and "hungry".

Hunger is the sensation you experience when you feel the physiological (and psychological) *need* to eat food. Appetite, on the other hand, is the *desire* to eat food. The sensation of hunger usually occurs after only a few hours without eating. Most people think of hunger as being an unpleasant feeling.

Hunger—a natural, beneficial feeling.

Believe it or not, hunger can be good. Feeling hungry can be a sign that your body is healthy and using up your fat stores.

Hunger naturally sharpens your appetite and actually makes food taste better. It can even make foods that you don't usually relish taste good. Besides, it's perfectly safe for normal, healthy people to go a few hours without eating. Hunger can even be lovable!

Hunger is also a sign that your body is working well, and your ever-loyal but perhaps sometimes misguided Inner Guardian is protecting you (as it supposes) by trying to compel you to stock up on energy and nutrition.

But it's also hunger that's the Great Enemy of weight loss. If we could switch it off whenever we wanted to, there would be no obesity crisis. Since it's hard to switch off, we can learn to love it instead.

TYPES OF HUNGER

Learn to differentiate between the different kinds of hunger you feel. Hunger can be classified into four levels:
- Level 1: False hunger (thoughts of food that are emotionally or cognitively induced)
- Level 2: Peckishness (low-level "real" hunger)
- Level 3: Mild hunger (mid-level "real" hunger)
- Level 4: Ravenous hunger (high-level "real" hunger)

Level 1: False hunger.

If you think you might be feeling hungry but you're not sure whether it's real hunger or whether your appetite has been aroused by some other factor, it's likely you're not experiencing real, physical hunger. "False" hunger is driven by habit, emotions, environmental cues etc.

Real hunger—physiological hunger—is a sensation in your body; for example, a sense of emptiness, a rumbling tummy, a feeling of low energy or fatigue, sometimes irritability or an inability to concentrate. Real hunger develops relatively slowly and gradually. It can be satisfied by any of many different foods.

Non-hungry eating, or "false" hunger, by contrast, is a thought. It can be a thought based on your emotions, or triggered by other factors, such as food images. It can happen quite quickly—suddenly, "I feel like chocolate", or "I feel like a bag of crisps". False hunger often manifests as a craving for a specific food, which is why it can be harder to satisfy with a lower-Calorie, more nutritious substitute.

False hunger has been called "not really hungry hunger". It's what happens when you think you desire food, but if someone offered you something low Calorie and relatively flavorless such as a lettuce leaf, you wouldn't want to eat it. False hunger can stem from situations such as these:

- Thirst, tiredness, stress, anxiety, anger or boredom.
- Exposure to a hunger trigger such as a picture of food on TV or in a magazine, hearing someone talking about food, reading words about food or seeing a movie about food. Even just imagining food can elicit chemical responses in the body. Picturing food, or hearing spoken words about food, or reading food-related words can all elicit similar physical reflexes. Browsing through cookbooks or online recipe websites can make you hungry.
- When you're procrastinating about doing something, you might turn to food to stall for time.
- Cultural/social time schedules such as morning or afternoon coffee breaks, when everyone else is eating and drinking.
- The habit of eating something at a certain time or in a certain place may have become so ingrained that it's almost an automatic reflex. For example, entering your kitchen might trigger the urge to eat, because eating often takes place there.
- False hunger can be a reaction to a sugar-overload; eating refined carbohydrates can result in an insulin surge. This can lead to a drop in blood-sugar which in turn makes you feel hungry, despite the fact you've recently eaten.
- Practising restrictive diets can also make people lose touch with their natural, inner hunger cues. Long periods of cutting out entire food groups, or living on very few Calories, or being

269

bulimic, can ruin your relationship with normal, healthy hunger. Denying hunger pangs becomes a deep-rooted habit. Often, people who have put themselves through these strict weight-loss regimes become terrified of submitting to their Inner Guardian's hungry command, "EAT!" They develop the idea that as soon as they surrender sufficiently to nibble a tiny morsel, they will lose all control and start binge-eating. And indeed, putting yourself through a self-induced "famine" does lead to a spike in your hunger hormone ghrelin and a dip in your satiety hormone leptin, which is why strict dieting often does go hand in hand with binge-eating.

Reconnecting with real hunger.

As the years pass, many adults learn to ignore their body's inner hunger cues and lose touch with "real hunger". For weight loss, it is vital to learn to reconnect with that feeling.

If you are unsure whether your hunger is real or false, ask yourself these questions:

- Did my hunger develop gradually or suddenly?
- Have I just experienced something that triggered an emotion such as anxiety or stress?
- Have I been looking at images of food, whether on TV or the Internet, in magazines or books, or on billboards etc.?
- Have I been seeing actual food on display, whether in food vending machines, or a shop window, in the supermarket, or on the counter at a gas station, or on a table etc?
- Have I just caught a whiff of baking bread or some other enticing food smell?
- Have I recently heard the sounds associated with eating, such as the clattering of cutlery and crockery, or the murmur of people dining?
- Have I been reading about food or talking about food?
- Am I thirsty?
- Am I bored?

- Am I procrastinating, trying to put off something I don't really feel like doing?
- Am I tired/sleepy?
- Right now, is it a time of day when I habitually eat something?
- Am I in a place where I habitually eat something?
- Have I recently eaten something sugary that might have spiked my blood sugar levels?

If the answer to any of these questions is "yes", then there's a good chance you're feeling false hunger instead of real hunger.

Dealing with false hunger.

What can be done to deal with false hunger (other than eating)?

- Recognise that it's not real hunger. It's not your body actually needing food.
- Recognise that false hunger is not a crisis but simply a passing thought.
- Recognise that you have control over false hunger (unlike real hunger which is controlled by your Inner Guardian).
- Distract yourself. Often, a bout of false hunger can fade from your consciousness if you find something else to distract your thoughts. Get busy and occupy your mind with interesting ideas that will push out those unwanted food thoughts. For example, watch TV, read a book, phone a friend, walk the dog, join Pinterest, visit Internet forums and contribute a post, go shopping (not for food!), clean out a closet, plan your next holiday, learn a new language, bath the dog, or do something nice for a family member or friend. Get passionately interested in whatever matters to you most.
- Exercise. You could go for a brisk walk, lie on the floor and do some sit-ups, pretend you're a boxer and punch an invisible opponent hard and fast, run up and down some stairs, or follow an exercise class on YouTube.
- Drink water, or some other low Calorie liquid *without* artificial sweeteners. Try a cup of warm water with a squeeze of lemon juice, or a glass of chilled water with a sprig of mint.

- Move away from whatever it was that triggered your false hunger—so far away that you cannot see/hear/smell/read/be reminded of those triggers.
- Don't go shopping for the weekly groceries when your stomach is empty.
- Meditate.
- Give yourself a massage, manicure or pedicure (or get someone to do it for you!).
- Have a long, luxurious bath, complete with bath oils and bubbles.
- If your blood sugar has crashed because you ate something sugary, eat a small amount of a high satiety food to bring your levels up to a stable, balanced state. If you really crave sweetness to the point of desperation, eat a piece of low fructose fruit such as an orange or a handful of berries, perhaps with a couple of teaspoonsful of rice malt syrup. Avoid sugary foods, and blood sugar crashes should not happen!

Importantly, remember that false hunger (and even real hunger) does not simply continue to grow until it reaches unbearably stratospheric levels. The way our bodies are wired, our hunger happens in waves. It comes and goes. This is an advantage, because if you can distract yourself for long enough, or remove yourself from hunger triggers for long enough, you can be sure that the wave of false hunger will pass. It *will* subside.

Levels 2 & 3: Peckishness and mild hunger.

Ravenous hunger is a highly unpleasant sensation. (More about that later.) Peckishness and mild hunger may not be exactly pleasant either, but sometimes you need to allow your body to experience them. It's natural to feel a little hungry from time to time—natural and desirable. As mentioned already, hunger means weight loss.

For many people trapped in the dieting cycle, the sensation of hunger can feel like a crisis. Over the years, for one reason or another, they have come to believe that the slightest twinge of hunger needs to be obliterated as soon as possible; that to exist while feeling hunger is a hardship to be avoided at all costs, and remedied by immediate eating. In contrast to those people with eating disorders who are terrified of eating, they become terrified of hunger.

The feeling of hunger, however, is not a medical emergency!

It is possible to teach yourself to tolerate or even to welcome feelings of peckishness or mild hunger. Your mind is a powerful thing, and you can use its power to your advantage.

Learn to love mild hunger.

If your body really is giving you genuine peckishness/mild hunger signals, you know it's a sign that you're probably losing weight. Your body is telling you it's run out of the food you consumed at your last meal, and it has now started drawing energy from your fat reserves.

Hallelujah! That's exactly what you want it to do!

But most people instinctively don't like this feeling of peckishness/mild hunger. It feels uncomfortable and annoying. Thoughts of food become intrusive.

While never allowing "hungry" to become "ravenous", it is important to accept and even to love peckishness and mild hunger. You know that as long as you're not yet ravenously hungry it's okay to feel peckish but how can you learn to love this feeling?

First of all, now is the time to check and make sure that you have on hand a supply of high satiety, low-Calorie food. This is the food you will sit down and eat mindfully just before you reach the "ravenously hungry" stage.

Okay, now that that's done, turn to our section on "Mind Tricks for Weight Loss" for helpful hints about make yourself love the mildly hungry feeling.

With **peckishness**, you can distract yourself. If you're thinking of food because you're bored, find something to occupy yourself. Aim to remove yourself from any hunger triggers, or remove them from your vicinity. This is a good level of hunger to have.

With **mild hunger**, simply acknowledge it and make sure your plans and preparations are in place for your next healthful meal, so that you don't end up grabbing the nearest Calorie-dense snack.

Tell yourself, "I acknowledge that I am feeling somewhat hungry, but I am quite okay with continuing to feel this way, because I know that a) it means my body is using up my fat stores and b) there is no need to panic, because I will soon be eating a delicious, satisfying meal."

Remind yourself that eventually, if this level of hunger doesn't subside naturally, then instead of reaching for the most convenient processed Calorie-dense "sometimes-food" that comes to hand, you can eat some delicious, nutritious lower-Calorie food that will boost your health and not your weight.

Over time, you can train yourself to experience mild hunger for quite a long while without being driven by strong urges to binge on Calorie-dense foods.

Level 4: Ravenous hunger.

It's fine to let yourself experience peckishness or mild hunger without eating anything to quell the sensation. But in order to lose weight on the Satiety Diet, you should never allow yourself to reach the "ravenously hungry" stage if you can possibly help it.

When you're ravenously hungry, your mind is dominated by thoughts of food. You feel obsessed with food. Ravenously hungry people often describe themselves as "starving". You might feel weak, dizzy, irritable, light-headed, tired; you could feel lethargic and low in energy, you might have trouble concentrating, and your empty stomach could be growling and/or aching with hunger pangs.

Feeling ravenously hungry sends alarm signals to your Inner Guardian, who responds by driving up your desire for Calorie-dense foods. If you try to ignore extreme hunger pangs, you'll probably end up looking for a "quick fix" to end the discomfort, and a quick fix is likely to be sugary, fatty food.

When you get ravenously hungry you're more likely to reach for the nearest candy bar. Your energy-conserving survival drive is usually, in the end, far stronger than your willpower.

The answer to dealing with ravenous hunger is to be prepared. Always have a Calorie-sparse, highly satiating snack within reach in case of emergencies. And eat meals that provide real satiety.

Ravenous hunger is extreme, all-consuming, and out of control. This kind of hunger may arise from situations such as:

- Not having eaten for several hours.
- Having eaten sugary foods (especially high-fructose foods) or high GI foods, leading to an insulin spike.
- Self-imposed dietary restrictions (e.g. avoiding whole food groups), leading to cravings for the nutrients that are lacking.

- Feeling hungry while being surrounded by hunger triggers (e.g. being on a low-carb diet while visiting a patisserie). Over-exertion of willpower can often lead to "giving in" and bingeing.
- Any combination of the above.

Ravenous hunger is a raging, obsessive hunger that won't leave you alone. It invades your thoughts, becoming the paramount imperative. It incessantly knocks on the door of your mind, driving you to seek of the highest-energy foodstuff you can find and eat it as quickly as possible in quantities as large as possible. In other words, it's the tyrannical hunger that causes binge-eating, and which often succeeds periods of self-imposed food deprivation (e.g. dieting).

It is important not to get to the stage of ravenous hunger in the first place. Aim to avoid reaching this stage by using all the tricks in the Satiety Diet's repertoire. However, if you do reach it and you don't have access to your nutritious satiating meal, then the first tools to try are:

- Distracting yourself with a pleasant alternative activity such as going for a walk, taking a bath or shower, or even going for a pedicure.
- Removing any nearby hunger triggers.
- Having "emergency" healthful foods on hand that you can access easily, or quickly prepare if you reach that Ravenous Hunger stage. Sit down and eat them slowly and mindfully. Let them be foods that are low in Calories, delicious and able

275

to satisfy your craving of the moment. This might be a craving for something sweet and creamy, or sweet and crunchy, or salty and crispy, or chewy and savory… in general, food cravings are as much about mouthfeel as flavor. Examples include tofu 'jerky' (salty and chewy), or silken tofu chocolate cream sweetened with stevia (sweet and creamy). If your healthful snack contains both protein and fiber that's an added satiating bonus! Use mental imagery to "photograph" your snack so that you can recall eating it.

DEALING WITH HUNGER

In summary—one of the keys to weight loss is to eat when you are really hungry.

Not when you're experiencing "false" hunger.

Not when you are merely peckish.

Eat when you are feeling mild hunger, before you get ravenously hungry.

- If you're feeling peckish or have false hunger, distract yourself.
- If you're feeling genuinely hungry, eat according to the Satiety Diet plan.
- Learn to reconnect with your natural feelings of satiation and satiety. Mindful eating and prolonged mealtimes can help achieve this.
- Don't let yourself get ravenously hungry. Keep Satiety Diet snacks on hand.

Don't eat when you are not hungry.

This seems an obvious statement, but another enemy of weight loss is eating when you are not hungry at all. Eating when you're not hungry sends confusing messages to your body. It also increases your chances of weight gain. Examples of non-hungry eating situations include:

- **Preventative eating**: Eating just in case you might become hungry later, when there's no food around. Preventative eating can happen when you're about to go to some place where they might not be any food at all, or any healthy food, or if you know you're about to go for several hours without food. Even if you're not hungry, you might eat something "just in case" you get hungry later. You might practise non-hungry preventative eating, as insurance against possibly having to feel hunger in the future, and also as insurance against being tempted to eat high-Calorie snack-foods. Preventative eating is helpful in some instances, but try to keep it to a minimum. Instead of eating "preventively" before you leave home, carry Satiety Diet snacks with you when you go out. Only eat them if you're really hungry, and then eat them mindfully.
- Social eating or drinking: Being obliged to eat or drink at certain social occasions, such as weddings or parties.
- Timed eating: Eating at pre-determined times of the day—for example, always dining at a certain hour, regardless of your actual hunger. Some people feel like eating at the time they usually eat, even if they are not really hungry.
- Eating for pleasure: Food cravings can be brought on by the desire for the pleasure of eating, rather than the need for nutrition or energy.

Tips for beating hunger when there's no "satiety food" available.

Have you ever found yourself feeling ravenous with only a food vending machine on hand—and it's filled with candy and crisps? What can you do if you feel hungry when you're in a place where there's either no food at all, or only unhealthful food?

- Adjust to the idea that hunger isn't a catastrophe, it's just a normal sensation; that it signifies that your body is using your fat stores; and that it doesn't just grow, it comes and goes.
- Dampen hunger by drinking some water, or by immersing yourself in a distracting activity, or by doing some exercise, such as walking.

277

Dealing with hunger: Snacks

Okay, so you've learned to listen to your body, and now you know whether what you're feeling is false hunger, or cravings, peckishness or real hunger, or ravenous hunger.

If you're at the stage of real (mild) hunger, then a snack is not going to be enough to give you satiety.

This is an important point.

Here's an example scenario: Many people tend to think: "It's mid-morning and I really feel hungry, but I've already eaten breakfast and it's not yet lunchtime, so I will have a snack to tide me over until I eat a high-satiety meal at lunchtime."

So they have a snack, but it's not enough to provide real satiety. Afterwards they still experience low level, annoying hunger; *unsatisfied hunger*, (which is not the same thing as a craving). Their Inner Guardian thinks, "There must be a food scarcity," and releases hunger hormones to prompt them to seek more food.

If you reach this point you can try to distract yourself by thinking of something other than food, or going for a walk, or using any of the Satiety Diet tools to deal with food cravings. Or you might eat a second snack, which may help assuage the worst of the hunger for a short time, but which does not provide satiety. This can lead to more low-level hunger, or a third snack... and so on. You could end up feeling so hungry that you keep picking at food and consuming extra Calories.

Too many snacks can promote weight gain, and prolonged low-level hunger can stimulate your hunger hormones.

Instead—break the vicious cycle!

The best thing to do in these circumstances is ignore the clock and listen to your body. If you're really hungry before it's officially "lunchtime", sit down and take the time to eat a nutritious, delicious meal mindfully, until you reach satiety.

Yes, according to the clock it's "too early for lunch", but your internal body-clock knows nothing about the measurement of time devised by humans. If you get mid-morning hunger pangs, you might find that thoroughly assuaging your hunger and reaching satiety mid-morning means you'll be hunger-free for most of the day.

It's vital to listen to your body so that you can tell whether it's a meal you need, or a snack, or simply a distraction.

"If you have an appetite that can be satisfied with just 100 Calories (400 kilojoules) it may be that you're not really hungry—you just want to snack," says Associate Professor Amanda Salis of the University of Sydney's Boden Institute of Obesity, Nutrition, Exercise and Eating Disorders. "If you're genuinely hungry you may be better off with a proper meal or a substantial snack like a small toasted sandwich or hummus with veggies that keep you satisfied and prevent grazing."

About skipping meals, especially breakfast.

Strictly speaking the word "breakfast" simply means "the first meal of the day after waking". You might eat your first meal of the day in the morning, or the afternoon. People have come to think of breakfast as a morning meal, but according to this definition, it need not be.

There is a popular myth that eating breakfast helps you avoid putting on weight. The theory is that if you don't eat breakfast you will get hungry later in the day and reach for high-Calorie foods.

There has been a lot written about the importance of eating breakfast, but if you don't feel hungry first thing in the morning, then don't eat. It's as simple as that. If you want to lose weight, don't eat when you're not hungry. You don't have to eat a morning meal unless you feel like it. Your Inner Guardian might be trying to tell you to eat breakfast later in the day.

Whether you eat a morning meal or not has no direct influence on weight loss, as more than one study has found. Scientists have discovered that contrary to what is widely believed, a recommendation to eat breakfast has "…no discernible effect on weight loss in adults." [Dhurandhar et al., (2014)]

A 2013 study reported that people who eat breakfast do not eat significantly less food for lunch. Consuming Calories early in the day did not necessarily mean the study's participants would consume fewer Calories later, so the breakfast Calories only added to their overall daily Calorie consumption. [Levitsky & Pacanowski (2013)]

Dr. Michael Mosley, on his TV show "10 Things You Need to Know About Losing Weight", skipped breakfast one day and then had a brain scan, while being shown images of different foods.

The scan showed that he had a significant desire for more Calorie-dense foods after he'd skipped breakfast, than when he looked at the same foods *after* eating breakfast. Areas of his brain "lit up" more intensely when he was hungry while looking at sugary, fatty foods.

The message would appear to be "don't skip meals"—however, the *real* message is:

- Eat when you're genuinely hungry, not just when the clock tells you it's time to eat.
- Don't allow yourself to become ravenous.
- If you are feeling hungry, avoid the sight/smell/mention of Calorie-dense foods and have satiating, lower Calorie foods ready on hand.

It is okay to skip meals if you're not hungry. Eating when you don't feel like eating can sabotage weight loss. If you're not hungry for breakfast, don't eat it. Just plan, plan, plan and make sure you have nutritious, satisfying, Calorie-sparse food on hand for later on in the day, when you start to experience real hunger.

CAUSES OF OVEREATING

HUNGER AND APPETITE TRIGGERS

Scientists used to think that hunger was the result of the body lacking energy, and that eating was the way our bodies regained that energy (the set-point theory). This has been superseded by the idea that we may not always desire food purely because we need energy, but because we know we'll enjoy the experience (the positive-incentive perspective).

". . . the evolutionary pressures of unexpected food shortages have shaped humans and all other warm blooded animals to take advantage of food when it is present. It is the presence of good food, or the mere anticipation of it that makes one hungry." [Wikipedia (29th May 2016)]

Even when you're not consciously thinking about food, your brain may be receiving food-related sensory inputs from your eyes and nose and even from your ears—sounds and images and smells from TV, billboards, radio, newspapers, magazines, cafes, restaurants, your home kitchen or other surroundings; food-related words spoken or read; and even other, more subtle cues such as the time of day. These factors can constantly remind you of food and thereby activate your appetite.

Hunger and appetite are regulated by -

- Physiological factors, such as your body's hormones, neuro-transmitters, organs and glands.
- Interactions between your body and the environment, including social and emotional circumstances.

The involuntary contractions of the stomach known as "hunger pangs" don't usually commence until 12 to 24 hours after you last ate. Emotional states such as sadness, anger or joy can suppress hunger contractions, while on the other hand low blood sugar levels can increase the intensity of hunger.

The rise and fall of leptin and ghrelin hormone levels in your body determine whether you feel hunger or satiety. To put it simply, when you eat, your body releases leptin, which reduces your desire to eat. After a few hours without food, your leptin levels drop significantly. Low levels of leptin trigger the release of the "hunger" hormone, ghrelin.

Nonetheless it's not just low leptin levels that can stimulate ghrelin release. Other factors, such as being in a stressful situation, can also make your ghrelin levels rise.

In an ideal world, the natural physiological mechanisms of your body would balance your appetite precisely. You would eat when you felt hungry and cease eating when you had consumed sufficient food for your energy and nutritional requirements.

Appetite, however, depends on more than biochemistry, and in the 21st century we are all vulnerable to numerous subtle eating prompts that, through body-speech, can actually override the natural programming of our bodies.

Eating when hungry and ceasing when satiety has been reached is an inborn trait. Yet, in many parts of the world where obesity has reached epidemic levels, this wise instinct has been "unlearned", and people only cease eating when they are unable to cram in another morsel.

Inputs that can trigger appetite may include:
- Thoughts of food
- Verbal or written descriptions of food
- Images of food still or moving
- The smell of food
- Actual sight of real food (don't leave food on display at home!)
- Sounds associated with food; e.g. sizzling, or clattering cutlery
- Colors and shapes
- Peripherals such as table settings and dishes
- Actions such as adding condiments, or sitting at a table, or shaking out a napkin/serviette
- Actions such as using a knife and fork to cut up food, or a spoon to scoop it, or hands to pick it up

Thoughts can affect appetite.

Simply thinking about food can stimulate your appetite. Food does not even have to be actually present, or even represented in pictures. For example, reading about food in recipe books or reading descriptions of food in novels can awaken a desire to eat, based on mental images created by your own imagination!

The well-known "imagine you are eating a lemon" visualization exercise demonstrates how powerfully your thoughts can act upon your body's parasympathetic and sympathetic nervous system. When you close your eyes and really concentrate on the look of a lemon, the feel of a lemon in your hand, the sharp, citric smell of a slice being cut and finally, when you imagine biting down into that slice, the astringent tang and explosion of juice in your mouth, it's likely you will experience a puckering of the mouth and a surge of saliva. Remarkably, such visualizations have been shown to significantly activate patterns in the human brain, and also to alter the pH levels of the tongue!

Simply imagining food can make you hungry. Your thoughts are powerful!

Environmental appetite triggers.

A range of signals from the world outside your body can trigger hunger and appetite. These environmental influences may drive you to eat when you're not really hungry. It's essential to identify your triggers, so that you can take steps to avoid or deal with them.

Some examples follow.

1a. Sensory triggers—sight.

"You first eat with your eyes", as all good chefs know. The very sight of food can make you want to eat more. One study found that people ate more from an uncovered bowl of chocolates than a covered bowl of chocolates. Human beings are drawn to food that is presented attractively, and in our minds certain colors (such as red) are associated with delicious flavors. The desire for food can be aroused by:

- Pictures or moving images of food.
- Watching movies about food (the movie *Chocolat* and the movie *Supersize Me* are renowned for triggering the desire for, respectively, chocolate and fast food).
- Watching food and cooking shows on TV, or commercials for foods and snacks.
- The sight of food, whether it be in shops or cafes or restaurants or the home kitchen.
- Watching other people eat.
- Being offered food.

1b. Sensory triggers—smell.

Your sense of smell, which is is closely linked to your memories and emotional associations, can also affect your appetite. Eating cues can include:

- The aroma of any food, especially freshly cooked food such as warm bread or barbecued meats.
- The aroma of a food you associate with a positive memory or emotion.

1c. Sensory triggers—sound.

- Hearing food spoken of can make you hungry—particularly if clever marketing vocabulary is used, such as the powerfully evocative words "crunchy, crispy, creamy, delicious".
- Hearing sounds suggestive of eating—such as the clatter of cutlery, the clinking of tableware, the murmur of voices in conversation over a dinner table—can trigger appetite.

1d. Sensory triggers—taste.

Highly palatable flavors such as those found in foods with high fat or sugar content can drive you to overeat.

Human beings prefer certain tastes and textures. In general, we are attracted to sweet, fatty, and "umami" (savory) foods. We are drawn to textures that are creamy or crunchy or chewy, and we also incline towards different tastes and textures mingled, such as crisp-creamy (think nachos and dips) or sweet-salty (think salted caramel).

2. Where and how food is displayed in your environment.

Food that looks and smells good incites appetite arousal. In an evolutionary sense, this used to be useful to our ancestors because it meant that they would eat good-looking and good-tasting foods even if they were not hungry. This helped insure against future food shortages.

Part of the modern lifestyle is the ready availability of food that looks and smells great, but our biology is out of whack with this environment.

Hunger and appetite can be regulated by:
- The size of dishes—we tend to eat more from larger plates.
- We tend to eat less from tableware of certain colors.
- Food availability: when food is in plain sight and easy to reach, people are strongly tempted to eat it.
- How close the food is to us. A Cornell University study found that people ate much more from a candy dish right in front of them than from a candy dish six feet away (2 meters). [Wansink et al., (2006)]

3. Social triggers.

Most of us want to "fit in" at social events. Your family, friends and colleagues influence your appetite and eating patterns. A celebration at the office, for example, can involve people bringing in Calorie-rich foods to share. It would seem unsociable not to eat with your work-mates.

Cultural signals prompt us to eat certain foods at certain times and in certain places. For example, it's not acceptable to eat during a job interview, lunch is generally eaten between 12 noon and 2pm in western societies, and throughout the year particular foods are traditionally consumed at festive times.

4. Emotional Triggers.

Emotional cues can trigger over eating. These can include
- Stress
- Unhappiness
- Anxiety
- Desire for comfort by means of "self-soothing"
- Feeling out of control of your life
- Remembered associations with a certain food, e.g. "eating pudding makes me feel better."

When your true needs are unmet, emotional triggers can retain their power and return repeatedly.

5. Routine and habit triggers.

Eating can be associated with certain situations. Your customary routines can prompt you to eat, whether or not you are actually hungry. These can include eating cake at birthday parties, over-indulging at Christmas festivities, having a beer with the boys on Friday afternoons, not leaving enough time to make breakfast in the morning before work (and instead buying fast food at a drive-through), and snacking while watching TV.

Habits, learned for some reason in the past that may not exist any more, or springing from no particular source, can cause you to over-eat. Such habits can include eating too fast and eating while distracted.

6. Cultural cues that can override appetite signals.

Overeating is discouraged in many cultures—for example in Japan and China, and in India's Ayurvedic tradition.

FACTORS THAT CAN DRIVE YOU TO OVEREAT

When you have lost touch with your body's natural satiety signals you may overeat or under-eat. Overeating or under-eating can lead to changes in your body's natural responses to food intake. People who eat too much may experience lethargy, brain fog, food cravings even when the stomach is full, heaviness in the gut, bloating, or excessive thirst. People who under-eat may experience anxiety or jitters, low energy, depression, irritability, or headaches.

There are many reasons why you may feel driven to consume too much food. Factors such as stress, loneliness, low serotonin and dopamine levels, depression, low blood sugar, and boredom can contribute to overeating. It may occur when you deliberately ignore your body's satiety signals, or when you are unaware of them, or when you become desensitized to them, or when external factors encourage you to ignore them, or when medications or a health problem interfere with those satiety signals. Some examples follow.

Overeating causes: Food.

Food: the ingredients and ingredient combinations in the western diet.

The combination of fat and sugar can be addictive. Foods that are "protein decoys" can make you want to eat more. Some food additives may stimulate hunger. Many characteristics of cheap, easily available, tasty but highly-processed foods can wreak havoc on your natural appetite.

Food: Availability.

Research shows that when food is readily available, people are more likely to eat it. This is why open plan living can be a cause of overeating—the kitchen, with all its edible bounty, is always on show. The refrigerator and pantry are within easy reach. In the kitchen, dishes of food such as fruit in bowls, or a loaf of bread, or packets of breakfast cereal, may be on constant display. Outside the home, food is never far away, either, at least in cities. Fast food outlets are to be seen on many street corners; cafes and restaurants and supermarkets are common.

Food: Portion size.

Large portions can also be a trigger for over-eating.

At any meal, people want to eat what they (consciously or sub-consciously) think is the "right amount" of food. The psychological definition of this desire is "unit bias". Often, without realizing it, we use tableware as a visual comparator to judge the "right amount" of food. For example, most of us have the idea that a satisfying food serving should fill up our bowl or our plate.

In 2005 behavioral scientist Brian Wansink and his team designed a study to illustrate the amazing influence of unit bias. They recruited 54 adults to sit down and eat a meal of soup. Unknown to the volunteers, half of them were eating from normal bowls while the other half were eating from bowls attached to a hidden apparatus that continuously refilled the bowls from below, at an imperceptible rate. The group eating from the self-filling bowls consumed a whopping 73% more food than the control group, but (and this is the interesting part), ". . . they did not believe they had consumed more, nor did they perceive themselves as more sated than those eating from normal bowls."

". . . people 'use their eyes to count Calories and not their stomachs," wrote the researchers. [Wansink et al., (2005)

Before you eat, take a good, hard look at the amount of food on the plate in front of you. Compare the portion sizes of each food with the serving sizes suggested in the dietary guidelines published by the U.S. Department of Health and Human Services (HHS). You might be astonished! The amount of food on your plate is likely to be far in excess of the recommended portions.

Food: Habitual overeating can lead to decreased sensitivity to satiety signals.

When you eat a large amount of food at one sitting, your stomach stretches to contain it all. A stomach that is frequently stretched to full capacity can gradually become accustomed to being over-full, and may lose sensitivity to satiety signals. This in turn means that you would have to eat more food to get the same sense of fullness.

See this book's section "Portion Size" for handy guides to estimating macronutrients.

Food: fad diets.

Fad diets are those which exclude certain foods or entire food groups, or which severely limit the amount of food you eat. Both of these extreme ways of eating can trigger over-eating.

Fad diets can stimulate strong cravings for the nutrients you are missing, leading to binge-eating. Avoid extreme diets if you want to achieve long-lasting weight loss.

Food: Eating modern foods may increase appetite.

It's not simply lack of willpower that makes people overweight. Many other factors play a role, including genes and hormones.

Food manufacturers have spent billions of dollars researching ways to create blends of fat, sugar and salt that are overwhelmingly attractive to the human palate because of our hormones and genes. Examples include salted caramel, deep fried candy bars, cheesecakes and bacon.

Overeating causes: The body.

The body: Your genes.
Your Inner Guardians hasn't yet adapted to the 21st century. It's still attuned to bygone times when food was scarce and humans had to work hard to get it. To survive, people had to eat as much as possible whenever food was available. It's hard-wired into our genes. This is why, in terms of evolutionary psychology, most of us tend to eat too much, and to prefer sugary, fatty, Calorie-dense foods.

In developed countries, those lean times are long-gone. Technology has given us machines and farming methods that allow the production of vast quantities of cheap food. We are now surrounded by an over-abundance of it.

Your environment has changed, but your Inner Guardian hasn't evolved in step with these changes. Genetic adaption takes a long time. Rapid evolution *can* occur over a few generations, but these changes tend to fade. It takes a million years to lay down evolutionary changes that really persist. [Uyeda, et al., (2011)]

Our instinctive drive to indulge in lots of sugary, fatty foods is now redundant. It would be wonderful to be able to simply tell our Inner Guardians to turn it off, but Mother Nature won't let that happen. The result is global obesity.

There are also some more specific genes that can cause obesity. One particular gene discovered in the early 21st century has been found to affect feelings of fullness after eating. Scientists discovered that people who possess certain variations of the "fat mass and obesity-associated (FTO) gene" have a bigger appetite and weigh more than people without those genes. The news is not all bad, however, because environmental factors can modify even your genetic heritage. People with the FTO over-eating gene can decrease its influence by eating fresh, whole foods and exercising regularly.

Prader-Willi syndrome is a genetic condition that causes people to develop an insatiable appetite, which leads to chronic overeating and obesity. Bardet–Biedl syndrome is another genetic condition that is characterized principally by obesity.

The body: Hormonal fluctuations.

Many women experience increased appetite every month, during the fortnight preceding menstruation. This is called the "luteal phase" of the menstrual cycle. During the luteal phase, there is a relative deficiency of the hormone estrogen. The "follicular phase" starts on the first day of menstruation and ends with ovulation. During this time women tend to eat less than during the luteal phase.

Testosterone, the most important male sex hormone, does not seem to have much effect on men's appetite, although some bodybuilders taking testosterone supplements do say their appetite increases.

The body: Dopamine.

We've discussed dopamine earlier in this book. Dopamine is a neurotransmitter that helps regulate the reward and pleasure centers in your brain. It also directs movement and emotional reactions, making it possible for you to not only perceive rewarding substances or activities, but to actually act to reach out and grasp them.

The levels of dopamine in your brain's reward pathways help to regulate your appetite. When food enters your digestive system the nutrients trigger the release of biochemicals from your gut, the pancreas and your stores of fat. These substances are involved in sending signals to your brain, telling it to release dopamine.

In healthy people this system is meant to balance their nutritional needs, keeping their appetite and body weight within normal parameters. Low levels of dopamine, however, can increase food intake.

In people who suffer from eating disorders such as uncontrollable bingeing, or anorexia nervosa, this system is not working properly. Dopamine may be released in response to starvation or gorging. It is such a strong motivator, its force is almost irresistible.

To demonstrate the impact of dopamine on appetite, scientists conducted experiments in which they caused mice to become dopamine deficient. Without any of this neurotransmitter circulating in their brains the animals simply give up eating and die, unless they are given a supplement of dopamine.

This does not mean that having low levels of dopamine will cause weight loss. Quite the contrary.

Some people's genes cause them to have lower levels of dopamine than normal. Researchers found that these people need to eat more food to reach satiety. They get a weaker lift in dopamine levels when they eat, which gives them a stronger urge to eat (to get more dopamine), which of course leads to them eating more food. This can result in obesity.

"Food reinforcement was greater in obese than in non-obese individuals, especially in obese individuals with [genetically low levels of dopamine]." [Epstein et al., (2007)]

Low dopamine levels, nonetheless, are not the whole picture. "Behavior and biology interact and influence each other," says leading researcher Epstein. "The genotype does not cause obesity; it is one of many factors that may contribute to it. I think the factors that make up eating behavior are in part genetic and in part learning history."

The body: Sleep deprivation.

Disrupted biological rhythms due to sleep deprivation or shift work have a powerfully arousing effect on the appetite.

Not getting enough sleep has been found to reduce levels of the "satiety hormone" leptin, which inhibits hunger, and increase levels of the "hunger hormone" ghrelin. Thus poor sleep can lead to weight gain. [Schmid et al., (2008); Copinschi (2005)]

The body: Mistaking thirst for hunger.

People often mistake thirst for hunger, because both of these needs send similar signals to your brain. If you sip water to stay hydrated throughout the day, you can ward off those seeming-hunger pangs.

The body: Spikes in blood sugar.

Spikes in blood sugar due to sugars and high GI starches can increase appetite. Eating foods that make your blood sugar levels soar quickly to reach a "spike" can make you feel much hungrier later, when those blood sugar levels drop. Those "high GI" foods, which usually contain a lot of refined sugar and carbohydrates, release a sudden surge of sugar into the bloodstream. In response, your body releases a load of insulin to cope with the sugar rush. This takes care of the blood sugar spike, bringing the blood sugar levels down. But because of the suddenness of the sugar overload, your body might have released more insulin than was precisely needed. The excess insulin pushed the blood sugar levels down much lower than they were before, and not long after you ate the high GI foods, you get a hunger attack.

High GI foods actually act as an appetite stimulant!

Avoid eating too many of them if you want to lose weight.

The body: Insulin resistance.

Insulin resistance can not only make it harder to lose weight, it may also lead to weight gain. This can become a vicious circle, because visceral obesity (an accumulation of fat in the abdomen, around the internal organs), can result in insulin resistance.

Insulin's job is to transport glucose from the bloodstream into the liver and muscle cells, where it can be used as energy. It regulates blood glucose levels, so that they neither drop too low nor soar too high. When people suffer from insulin resistance, their muscles and liver "resist" insulin's activity. They are unable to properly use the energy they consume, which leads to tiredness and cravings for sugary foods. In order to maintain normal levels of blood glucose, the body has to release extra amounts of insulin.

Insulin resistance has a number of other ill-effects. It can cause blood pressure to rise, it can make the body store fat more easily, and it can result in "fatty liver", a serious health problem.

The authors of a 2000 article published in the Journal of Clinical Investigation wrote, "There are also grounds for considering the ... possibility that insulin resistance ... in addition to being caused by obesity, can contribute to the development of obesity." [Kahn & Flier (2000)]

The opposite of insulin resistance is insulin sensitivity. The better your insulin sensitivity, the less your risk of getting diabetes. Therefore, anything that can improve your insulin sensitivity may also improve your chance of losing weight more easily.

The body: Overeating.

Overeating reduces satiety signals, leading to more eating.

When you regularly eat more food than you need, you can disrupt your body's normal satiety signals. Paradoxically, the disruption can lead to more overeating. This applies to both obese people and people who are of a normal weight. This is one of the reasons why it's so hard to lose excess weight and keep it off permanently.

One messenger that relays satiety signals from the gut to the brain is a hormone called uroguanylin. When your gut recognizes that it's received sufficient nutrition from your food, it sends this hormone to your brain where it generates a sensation of fullness. The authors of a 2016 study on mice found that uroguanylin production stops when the gut receives an overload of food energy. [Kim et al., (2016)]

One of the researchers was Dr. Scott Waldman, Chair of the Department of Pharmacology and Experimental Therapeutics at the Sidney Kimmel Medical College.

"What's interesting," said Dr. Waldman, "is that it didn't matter whether the mice [in the study] were lean and overfed, or obese and overfed—urogaunylin production stopped in both groups of animals when they got too many Calories. Here, it's not the obese state that's causing the problem but rather it's the Calories. Taken together, these experiments show that excess Calories—either from fat or carbohydrates—stress small intestinal cells so that they stop producing uroguanylin, which helps people feel full after eating."

How to break the vicious overeating cycle.

Stop eating when you satisfied. Satiety signals don't flash in front of your eyes like a neon sign. They are more subtle than that, and you have to be tuned in to your body in order to receive them. This is not as hard as you might think. You were tuned in to your body's signals as a child. If you have problems controlling your weight, it is likely that as you grew to adulthood you learned to habitually ignore your satiety signals.

How can you relearn to recognise them?

293

- Eat slowly to give your digestive system time to receive the food and generate satiety signals
- Eat mindfully to give your eyes a chance to see the food and your mouth a chance to really savor it, thus giving your brain a chance to really register that you are eating.

The body: Undereating.

Undereating, too, increases hunger signals—which may also lead to binge eating!

Trying to lose weight simply by significant, short-term food restriction (i.e. eating less food) doesn't seem to be working for most people. It doesn't appear to lead to healthy, sustained weight control.

If you do not eat when you are hungry, your body eventually tries to rectify the Calorie shortage by intensifying your appetite signals and stifling your satiety signals. The strongest trigger of binge eating? Dieting!

Dieting by way of severe cognitive (willpower-controlled) food restriction can actually lead to weight gain.

When you under-eat, your body doesn't get the energy and nutrients it needs. That's when your Inner Guardian steps in, enhancing your appetite for food to try to re-establish homeostasis (balance). This can result in bingeing. The cycle of bingeing and starving can be very destructive, both physically and mentally.

Restricting food—otherwise known as dieting—can intensify your preoccupation with food and weight, your feelings of guilt associated with eating and your cravings for food. It can lead to unhealthy weight fluctuations and a vicious cycle of restriction and bingeing. In the short term it may lead to weight loss, but once you tell yourself that you have lost enough weight and can now return to "normal" eating, you'll probably regain all the weight within two years. Why? Because "dieting" doesn't fix the reasons why weight was gained in the first place.

The solution? The Satiety Diet!

The body: The famine reaction/starvation mode.

People refer to something called the "Famine Reaction", otherwise known as "Starvation Mode". Professor Amanda Salis of the Boden Institute of Obesity, Nutrition, Exercise and Eating Disorders says, "...the body responds to energy restriction and weight loss with a series of adaptive responses that prevent ongoing weight loss and promote weight regain. This series of adaptive responses—referred to ... as the Famine Reaction—includes increased appetite, reduced energy expenditure, and alternations in circulating concentrations of hormones that tend to stimulate appetite and promote fat accumulation." [Cashin-Garbutt (2013)]

There's no need to worry about experiencing the "famine reaction" after you haven't eaten much food for a few hours, or even for a whole day or two, or three. It takes more than a few days of severe Calorie restriction for the body's metabolism to begin slowing down sufficiently for the famine reaction to set in.

Medical journalist Dr. Michael Mosley says that in the short term, there is no evidence that starvation mode is anything other than a myth. That is, in the *short* term! Most people on weight-loss diets do severely restrict their energy intake for more than three days, and their bodies often do succumb to the "famine reaction".

Researchers for the ABC's science show *Catalyst* say, "It sounds paradoxical, but your body actually defends itself from your efforts to lose weight by helping you to keep the kilos on. It's an in-built survival mechanism controlled by our brain, that we all share, and it's called 'the famine reaction'. One of the major effects of the famine reaction is that it makes you hungrier. It increases your drive to eat. Eight out of ten dieters who lose up to 10% of their bodyweight put it back on again within five years. Why is maintaining weight loss so difficult? And why do so many dieters hit a wall? . . . The longer you carry weight, the harder it is to lose it, because the hypothalamus in your brain resets the amount of fat your body defends. The famine reaction keeps you craving food. . . . It's a really difficult situation once you're obese to actually lose that weight again." [ABC Catalyst (2015)]

Why starving yourself to lose weight is a bad idea.

Starving yourself to lose weight does work, at first. Of course, if you're using up more energy than you're taking in, you will lose weight. In the long-term, however, it doesn't work. Your Inner Guardian gets the message that you're surrounded by famine. Convinced that there's limited energy available from the world around you, it tries to conserve the energy stores inside your body. It slows down your metabolism and acts to protect your fat stores. You become lethargic, and less inclined to move around. Your body uses Calories in your food more efficiently, to store fat.

Eventually, if you stop starving yourself and want to go back to eating in a normal, healthy way, you could find that your metabolism remains slow. You've re-set the rate at which your body burns energy. You need fewer Calories to just keep you at the same weight. In other words, if you return to eating the same way you did before you starved yourself, you're likely to gain weight more easily.

Starvation also has psychological effects. People who have suffered extreme starvation (such as concentration camp survivors or participants in some reality TV shows) become obsessed with food. This can last life-long. When they are restored to conditions of plenty, they may gravitate towards careers that involve food. A significant number take jobs as cooks or chefs. They frequently become overweight and they may feel compelled to hoard or hide food.

The body: Leptin resistance.
Homeostasis, the body's balancing mechanism.

Homeostasis is "the tendency of biological systems to maintain relatively constant conditions in the internal environment while continuously interacting with and adjusting to changes originating within or outside the system." [Free Dictionary (2018)]

In other words, homeostasis is the body's internal balance. Your body is usually expert at energy homeostasis too, juggling how much you eat and how much you shiver to keep your temperature constant in a cold environment, for example.

296

In theory, your body's homeostasis should work to increase your appetite when you are too thin, by releasing ghrelin, the "hunger hormone", and decrease appetite when you get too fat by releasing leptin, the "satiety hormone".

Yet the global obesity crisis is in full swing. So what's gone wrong?

Leptin resistance.

The fat storage cells of obese people are large, because they contain a great deal of body fat. It's those fat cells that produce leptin. The bigger the fat cell, the more leptin it produces. Therefore, obese people have very high levels of leptin in their bodies.

Leptin is the so-called satiety hormone, the one that's supposed to tell you to stop eating when you have consumed sufficient food for your needs. It is your body's way of signaling to your brain that sufficient energy is stored, which means you don't need to eat any more.

So why is it that obese people have high leptin levels? Surely with all that leptin circulating in their bodies, they should be eating a lot less. Surely they should not be obese at all!

There's a problem here. It's called "leptin resistance". All that leptin is present in the body, but for some reason the brain doesn't recognize it.

Robert H. Lustig, MD, professor of pediatrics at the University of California, San Francisco and a member of the Endocrine Society's Obesity Task Force, says, "In leptin resistance, your leptin is high, which means you're fat, but your brain can't see it. In other words, your brain is starved, while your body is obese. And that's what obesity is; it's brain starvation," he says.

What is preventing the leptin signals from working properly in obese people? Why is it that their energy homeostasis is not working as it should? What could be disrupting the satiety signals that leptin is generally so good at providing?

Let's take a closer look at leptin. This hormone is mostly produced by the body's fat cells. The more fat cells you have, the more leptin is released to inhibit hunger.

But leptin can work quite rapidly, taking action in your body long before there are any changes in your fat stores. You don't need to have lost or gained any weight for your leptin production to fall or rise. This is because it's the metabolic state of the fat cell that triggers changes in leptin levels. All the time, your body is constantly moving back and forth between a catabolic state (breaking down larger molecules into smaller molecules) and an anabolic state (building up and repairing tissue). Simply going without a meal can cause your fat cells to go catabolic. When this happens, leptin production drops and hunger sets in.

Possible causes of leptin resistance.

Recent studies are indicating that the chief components of the Western Dietary Pattern could be causing leptin resistance and boosting feelings of hunger. These components include dietary fat and sugar—more specifically, saturated fats, trans fats and fructose.

In addition to lots of leptin, obese people have high levels of inflammation, and raised levels of free fatty acids (FFA) in their bodies. Researchers believe that these are all potential causes of leptin resistance.

If that is the case, then adopting an anti-inflammatory lifestyle could be one way of controlling or even reversing) leptin resistance.

An anti-inflammatory lifestyle includes:

- Lowering your blood triglycerides. High levels of blood triglycerides can obstruct the delivery of leptin from the bloodstream to the brain. Eat small amounts of the "good" unsaturated fats and avoid the trans fats, cut down on fructose, eat more fiber, exercise and don't drink too much alcohol.
- Losing some weight. Yes, we know—that's why you're reading this book. But it's motivating to know that the more weight you lose, the easier it should get to lose even more weight, as your leptin resistance decreases. Losing weight also helps lower your blood triglycerides.

- Limiting your sugar intake. Sugar has been associated with inflammation.
- Avoiding highly-processed foods. Instead, eat whole, fresh food, preferably organic. It is thought that highly-processed foods may increase your appetite, as well as having an inflammatory effect. "Western dietary patterns warm up inflammation, while prudent dietary patterns cool it down," say the authors of a 2006 study. [Giugliano et al., (2006)]
- Eating soluble fiber.
- Eating foods that contain omega-3 fatty acids.
- Moving. Getting regular exercise may help to combat leptin resistance.
- Getting a good night's sleep.
- Eating whole foods that contain protein. Plant-based protein is recommended.

Overeating causes: The Mind.

The Mind: Being distracted while eating.

Being distracted or not paying attention to a meal tends to make you eat more at that meal.

Watching TV while eating can cause children to overeat. [Temple et al., (2007)] You are distracted if you eat while working, reading a book or newspaper, driving a vehicle, walking down the street, or having an argument with someone... Life is full of distractions.

Hurried eating is another pitfall. Eating more slowly and really enjoying your food can help you control how much you eat.

Eating mindfully is the opposite of distracted eating. Paying attention to a meal is linked to eating less later on. [Robinson et al., (2013)]

The mind: Thinking about food.

"Eating triggers", or "food cues" actually cause changes in the body's endocrine system. Merely thinking about delicious dishes can affect your body's inner workings in the same way as if you had really eaten the food, by raising your insulin levels, lowering your blood sugar levels and increasing ghrelin, the hunger hormone.

The mind: Emotions.

Many people succumb to emotion-driven eating, even if they have a conscious recognition that they are not particularly (physically) hungry. Both positive and negative emotions can motivate food intake. People may overeat when they feel lonely, sad, worried or bored, or even angry, frustrated or stressed. When you feel deprived of appreciation, comfort, or understanding, you might seek food as a form of solace.

Overeating can also be associated with positive feelings. People may feel happy when receiving playful items with food, or when eating in an environment that appears to be bright and joyful.

Marketing companies know how to use emotions to sell food using verbal, visual, or even olfactory triggers. Those that aim their products at children often package food in attractive little containers which, when opened, reveal plastic toys. Their advertising can be rich with emotive terms, for example; ". . . provides little moments of **delight** that **help** parents and children slow down to **enjoy** simple **play, sharing and togetherness**. . . . these moments of **excitement and surprise**. . ." [Ferrero (2017)] "Each McDonald's® **Happy** Meal® brings kids the **wonder and delight** of animals. . . " [McDonald's (2018)]

Through such toys, children can develop an emotional attachment to food which may continue into adulthood. When people associate positive feelings of happiness, delight, wonder etc. with certain foods, they are more likely to go on eating those foods throughout their lives. [Yale Rudd Center for Food Policy and Obesity (2013)]

The mind: Words can affect your appetite.

As discussed, it's not only images of food that can trigger a desire to eat. Words, whether spoken aloud or read silently, can conjure very real responses in your brain. Hearing or reading descriptions of food and food-related words can make you feel hungry. Even reading the word "hunger" can arouse appetite in some people!

Reading about food, about baking and cooking and eating food can stimulate a desire to eat. Reading this book might even make you start to feel hungry, because the topic involves food and hunger. (Read it anyway!)

Marketers for fast food companies *tell you what you're going to taste*. "If you market a hamburger as juicy, people eat it and think, 'Man, this is incredibly juicy,'" says Professor Brian Wansink, who is a leading expert on eating behavior and food marketing.

The actual taste and texture of the food has to be close to what has been promised to you by the advertisement, but the description of the food can really influence what you, the consumer, experiences when "chowing down". Advertisers know this, which is why food companies invent such slogans as "Finger lickin' good," (KFC®), or Subway's® "Eat fresh".

Without you even being aware of it, the words used by the marketers have trained you to believe in a taste that you have not yet experienced.

Marketing companies spend a lot of time and money on "neuromarketing", a method that uses neuropsychology to influence consumers' buying patterns. They study people's thoughts, their emotions and even their unconscious movements, in response to marketing strategies. They make lists of the most powerful and persuasive words and phrases, sometimes called "magic words," "smart copy," "emotional trigger words" or "words that sell".

These include words such as "new", "premium", "you", and "choose". Food ads may include emotive phrases that connect to hunger, nostalgia, or the desire for good health.

301

Those who write wine labels, restaurant menus, food articles in magazines, food labels etc. are well aware of the power of words to stimulate appetite—particularly words that describe food textures.

Celebrity chef Matt Preston says, "… when it comes to selling dishes on a menu 'creamy eggplant' always sells better than just eggplant, and 'crispy' anything sells better than just about anything!"

He goes on to explain, "What make this even more interesting is that many of these 'turn-on' food words refer to texture, rather than taste or flavor. " [Preston (2014)]

Chef Preston conjectures that the reason why people best respond to texture descriptions on menus is because it's easier to define and imagine textures than the vast range of flavors provided by food.

According to him, certain words exert a more powerful influence than others on our desire for food. These include:

- crispy (e.g. fried foods, chilled cucumber or fresh apples)
- crunchy (slightly harder than crispy, e.g. toasted nuts. Works well with creamy.)
- creamy (e.g. mashed potato, nut butters, blended silken tofu, porridge)
- silky (similar to creamy but with more fat added)
- nutty (includes nuts, cooked barley and brown rice, and other foods with roasty, toasty textures)

Fortunately, you can harness your brain's powerful suggestibility. You can use it to achieve weight loss rather than weight gain, if you know how. This idea is explored later in this book.

The mind: Procrastination.

A desire for distraction from a distasteful task or chore can drive you to eat. Eating becomes the substitute activity. You can tell yourself, "If I am eating then I have a valid excuse not to do that chore…"

The mind: Habits can even override your taste buds.

A study conducted by researchers at the University of Southern California found that one of the reasons we eat food is force of habit, and those habits can be stronger than our taste buds.

People were invited to a free movie screening, at which they were given a bucket of popcorn. Some received freshly-popped popcorn, while others were given stale popcorn that had been cooked more than a week earlier.

Stale popcorn doesn't taste nice, right? Eating it is something like eating cardboard. It's not completely disgusting, it's just disagreeable.

If people behaved rationally, then those who received the stale popcorn would probably have stopped eating it after the first bite (unless they were ravenously hungry!).

The movie-goers fell into two groups—

- Those who habitually bought popcorn every time they went to the movies
- Those who rarely or never bought popcorn when they went to the movies

The researchers found that people in the second group did indeed stop eating the stale popcorn after a bite or two.

However those for whom popcorn was part of the movie ritual automatically kept eating the stale popcorn, regardless of its flavor. Their behavior had been programmed by their past habits. In their minds, the idea of eating popcorn was less associated with feeling hungry or experiencing a pleasant taste, than with sitting in a seat in a cinema watching a movie.

To find out more about how habits can cause "automatic eating", the researchers then screened some movie clips in a boardroom. As before, they handed out buckets of fresh and stale popcorn. A boardroom is not a place that's usually associated with eating popcorn, so the force of habit no longer applied. As a result, people behaved rationally—everyone ate the fresh popcorn and nobody ate the stale stuff! [Neal et al., (2011)]

You can use the force of habit to your advantage. Indeed, you probably already do so, every day. For example brushing your teeth after meals is a good habit that benefits your health.

Take a look at the situations in which you find yourself eating purely from force of habit, rather than from real hunger. Do you always reach for food when you switch on the TV? Do you grab a snack every time you walk through the kitchen? Do you buy candy whenever you stop at a gas station to fill your car with fuel? Do you snack on crisps if you're in a bar? Or do you always eat dessert to finish a meal?

Such habits are strong, but you can overcome them. The first step is to identify the habit. The second step is to figure out a way to disrupt it. For example, you can disrupt habits by consciously changing your behavior—which requires some willpower. Instead of buying candy at the gas station, buy a newspaper or magazine. Instead of eating dessert, go for a walk. Alternatively you could simply avoid situations, environments and events that trigger automatic eating.

You are in control of your habits, after all.

Sensory inputs.

Sensory inputs: The smell of food.

There is a technique called "Aroma Marketing" that can make food products practically irresistible. Has the aroma of hot popcorn at the movies ever made you long to eat a bucketful? Has the savory smell of crispy French fries ever tempted you to buy some? Has the warm fragrance of freshly baked bread or cookies ever lured you into a supermarket, bakery or hot bread shop? If so, then you may have succumbed to a deliberate marketing stratagem.

The scent of food can trigger appetite arousal.

Even if you were not feeling hungry to begin with, when the smell of something delicious hits your nostrils, body-speech translates the signals to your Inner Guardian as, "desirable food is within reach". Your body reacts by boosting the production of ghrelin, the "hunger hormone", which stimulates your appetite. With your appetite aroused, you feel impelled to go and find that food, and consume it.

In May 2014 the *Wall Street Journal* reported that a chain of stores called Cinnabon™ deliberately installed its ovens near the front doors of its retail outlets so that the smell of baking cinnamon buns would lure in passers-by. They locate their bakeries in enclosed spaces such as railway stations and airports, so that the delicious smells were less likely to blow away and dissipate. So important was this aroma to maintaining a brisk trade, that some store managers warmed up cinnamon and brown sugar even when they were not baking buns. This kept the smell in the air and the customers walking in the door. Mentioned in the same report the Panera Bread Company™, at whose stores bread used to be baked overnight, chose to adopt day-time bread-baking so that the smell of freshly-baked loaves could entice customers. [Nassauer (2014)]

Why is your sense of smell such a powerful pathway for food marketers? In the first place you have to breathe to survive, so you are inhaling continuously. You take approximately 20,000 breaths each day. With each inhalation you experience the smell of your surroundings. You can shut off your other senses by closing your eyes and mouth or blocking your ears, but you have to go on smelling things whether you want to or not! You are always immersed in environmental smells, so food and fragrance marketers want to turn this to their advantage.

In the second place, your sense of smell is closely linked with your deepest emotions. This is because of the way your brain is made. The limbic system is a collection of structures inside the brain. It's the most ancient and primitive part of the brain, because it formed very early in human evolution. This system is responsible for your emotions, memories and moods.

Your olfactory receptors (the body parts that detect smells) are closely entwined with your limbic system. When you breathe in some air containing the molecules of a "smell", these receptors convert the experience into a message which travels first to your limbic system and then to the area of your brain whose job it is to identify the smell. None of your other senses travel such a pathway! None of your other senses are so closely associated with your emotions, memories and moods.

When people buy goods and services they tend to be strongly influenced by their emotions, memories and moods, whether they are aware of it or not. For this reason, there is a global, multi-million dollar industry based on creating smells that create a positive association between consumers and products. These products include food, fragrances, and even cars, computers and other merchandise. For example, a "new car smell air-freshener" is available for sale, and one company has even released a candle whose scent replicates the smell of newly-opened devices from Apple Inc®.

The smell of food can permeate the home kitchen, long after cooking is finished. This is another reason why open plan kitchens can contribute to over-eating.

Sensory inputs: The sight of food.
(See also "open plan living" and "habits".)

Visual cues can start you eating. Your desire to consume food can be triggered by environmental factors, on both the conscious and unconscious levels. Certain situations or events can encourage you to begin eating or to eat more, without you even releasing that you are being influenced. For example, when you see images of food your appetite can be aroused, and you may be unconsciously compelled to eat more.

As already mentioned, the sight of food includes images of food, as for example in in recipe books and magazines, on TV and on advertising billboards. Food may be depicted in photographs, drawings or moving images. The human brain makes little or no distinction between a colorful image of food, and actual food. Both can awaken cravings. When your eyes see these images, your Inner Guardian deems that you are in the presence of food and therefore it's time to eat. It unleashes the hunger hormones and starts the digestive process!

But why can images of food make you feel hungry? Because the ancient language of the body knows nothing of brightly-inked magazine pictures, or painted billboards, or printed plastic food wrappers, or TV screens. When the first humans lived on Planet

Earth, complete with their body-speech, food was scarce and hard-won. Body-speech takes no notice of 21st century food bounty and food excess. In the body's language, if your eyes are seeing images of food, that means food is within your reach. And if food is within reach that probably means your mouth is soon going to start tasting it and your stomach is soon going to receive it—which is why, at the very sight of food, your process of digestion is set in motion.

But what if that process is subsequently denied? What if your eyes see the food and your body-speech signals tell your hormones and juices to get ready for digestion, but no food enters your body? You cannot eat a brightly-inked magazine picture, or a painted billboards, or a printed plastic food wrapper, or a TV screen...

So your Inner Guardian having received the signals and been denied, begins to talk to you in a louder voice, like a kind but firm parent.

"Listen," it says to you in body-speech, "I am only saying this for your own good. There was food around and you didn't eat it. That was a bad move, survival-wise."

"Now," continues your Inner Guardian, "I am going to use hunger drive you. Whenever you see food I will send you strong urges to eat. If you don't eat food when your eyes see it, I am going to make you feel hungrier."

Your Inner Guardian is not going to put too fine a point on whether the chocolate cake your eyes are looking at is real, or whether it is a photo, or a screen full of pixels, or even a drawing. Your Inner Guardian, which is wired for a bygone age when the sight of food meant real food was nearby, says (in body-speech), "Right there within reach is some delicious high Calorie food. *We wants it*. Ghrelin, make my human hungry. Make the salivary glands start pumping. Drive my human towards this source of energy. I will remind you, my human, of how delicious that kind of energy is. I will make you, my human, want to reach out and take this energy source into his/her mouth and devour it."

This is why seeing images of food is often an appetite-trigger (and food advertisers know this).

307

Visual hunger is stimulated by beautiful food images.

A 2015 study titled "Eating with our eyes" found that the evolution of the brain and eyes is closely linked to our need to forage for food. The human body evolved in pre-technological times, when food was relatively scarce. Our ancestors' survival depended on being "wired" to respond to the sight of food, particularly energy-dense food. [Spence et al., (2016)]

When people are shown images of food, dramatic changes happen throughout the brain, body and nervous system. Viewing food images has a profound and measurable effect on us. The study's authors describe the concept of "visual hunger" as "the desire to view beautiful images of food, and consequent changes in organism."

There is a risk, warn the study's authors, of "… our growing exposure to beautifully presented images of food having detrimental consequences…" These colorful, high-definition images are often visually-enhanced, so that the food looks unrealistically inviting and delicious.

They wonder what effect "… our increasing exposure to images of desirable foods (what is often labeled 'food porn', or 'gastroporn') via digital interfaces [such as TV, Instagram and the Internet] might be having, and ask whether it might not inadvertently be exacerbating our desire for food (what we call 'visual hunger')." They call these images "Virtual food for hungry eyes."

And it's not just TV cookery shows and advertisements, Instagram and the Internet that bombard us with beautiful food images.

"…there are now so many more cookbooks out there than anyone could ever manage to cook from over a lifetime… From restaurants to supermarkets, from stories in the press through to the sides of product packaging, serving suggestions are often showcased with the foods themselves presented in the most favourable and desirable (albeit unrealistic) manner possible: Many such food images tend to be much more appetizing than the actual products that they portray. In some cases, dishes are created solely with the visual aesthetic in mind . . ." [Spence et al., (2016)]

Gorgeous images of colorful, high fat, sugar-rich foods increasingly bombard us both in reality and in the world of virtual food. These are the types of high-energy foods we are programmed to seek. It would seem that visual hunger, stimulated by an increasing abundance of beautiful food images, could be playing an important role in the obesity crisis.

We can combat over-eating triggers, cravings and food "addictions". Some suggestions follow.

How you can use visual hunger to your advantage.

The study's authors go on to say that you can use the power of visual images to boost your consumption of healthful foods or even to help you eat less. Examples include:

- Encouraging young children to like vegetables by showing them books containing attractive pictures of those vegetables.
- Teaching people to use the power of the imagination to visualize eating. The "simulation of consumption" can actually help reduce hunger! Researchers Morewedge et al. found that the simple process of visualizing themselves gorging on vast amounts of candy caused people to eat a lot less of the real candy later. [Morewedge et al., (2010)]
- Showing people picture of foods with a specific taste, for example a sweet, sugary taste, to decrease their enjoyment of that taste. Note that the study which achieved this result used 60 food images, because using 20 images didn't have the same effect. In fact, showing people only a few images can make them hungrier. The idea is to "mentally overindulge" in rich, sugar-laden confections to the point at which you start to feel you've eaten too many of them, and your taste for them declines. If you enjoy the taste less, you'll be likely to eat less of that food. [Larson et al., (2014)]

Hide the Calorie-dense foods. Or just don't buy them!

It's easy for your mind to overrule your body's satiety signals. A number of studies by behavioral eating researcher Brian Wansink have revealed that the more food you have within easy reach, and the more of it is on display in front of your eyes, the more of it you will eat. No matter whether you are hungry or not!

Researchers from Cornell Food and Brand Lab served volunteers with two identical meals. One of the meals was served from a counter that was far away from the dining table. The food for the other meal was placed directly on the table in serving dishes. When food was readily available on the table, people ate more. [Wansink et al., (2006)]

"Leaving serving bowls and dishes off the dinner table will decrease the amount consumed," say the editors of "Textbook of Obesity", published in 2012. [Akabas et al., (2012)]

Food displayed in front of you is very tempting. Bowls of fruit or candy arranged on a kitchen counter at home, racks of chocolate bars and snack foods in colorful wrappers on display at gas station pay windows; these are constant reminders of food. It is easy to reach out and grab these high-energy, good-tasting delights, and hard to keep dredging up enough willpower to resist the urge.

When you open a refrigerator door, you're probably inclined to grab the first foods you see, right in front of you. The solution—keep healthful foods at eye-level and within easy reach.

- If you don't want to eat it, don't keep it in the house.
- Don't leave leftover food on display.

Sensory inputs: Advertising.

Advertising bombards us on all sides. In the form of images (still and moving) words (spoken and written) sounds and even smells, it appears on TV, on billboards and other signs, on the radio, online, in magazines and newspaper, on Facebook, inside stores, in cinemas and gas stations etc. It seems that from the moment we wake up in the morning we are virtually swimming through an ocean of advertising.

And much of this advertising is about food.

TV Advertisements.

Television ads for food are highly effective at persuading children that they want sugary, fatty foods, particularly when they habitually watch a lot of TV. An article published in *Pediatrics*, confirms this. Researcher Emma Boyland of the University of Liverpool (UK) recruited 281 children aged 6 to 13. She and her team found that when the children watched a cartoon show punctuated by commercials featuring food, they then developed an appetite for fat-rich and carbohydrate-rich food items. The more TV the children usually watched, the more susceptible they were to the food advertising. [Boyland, et al., (2011)]

What holds true for children often holds true for adults, too.

A 2009 study by American psychologist Jennifer Harris showed that food advertising—in particular, ads displaying colorful images of food—can strongly influence your subconscious. Viewing such images can change your eating behavior without you being aware of it. [Harris et al., (2009)]

"Behavioral priming" describes the concept that when you are introduced to some kind of external thing or event, this conjures a mental image that can affect your behavior, usually without you noticing.

In a 2010 study entitled "Priming Effects of Television Food Advertising on Eating Behavior", researchers conducted television food advertising experiments on both children and adults. They found that, "Children consumed 45% more when exposed to food advertising. Adults consumed more of both healthy and unhealthy snack foods following exposure to snack food advertising compared to the other conditions. In both experiments, food advertising increased consumption of products not in the presented advertisements, and these effects were not related to reported hunger or other conscious influences."

The researchers concluded, "These experiments demonstrate the power of food advertising to prime automatic eating behaviors and thus influence far more than brand preference alone."

Eye-Catching Outdoor Advertisements.

Food companies spend hundreds of millions of dollars on advertising. Their preferred medium is television, followed closely by radio and outdoor advertising. Outdoor advertising includes billboards, posters and digital screens, which may be displayed on bus stops, hoardings, buildings, public transport vehicles etc.

The number of food ads displayed publicly in your neighborhood could be affecting your bodyweight and that of your community. A 2013 UCLA[33] study published in the journal *BMC Public Health* reported an association between outdoor food advertisements and a slightly higher risk of obesity. The researchers wrote, ". . . compared to an individual living in an area with no food ads, those living in areas in which 30% of ads were for food would have a 2.6% increase in the probability of being obese." [Lesser et al., (2013)]

Sensory inputs: Colors.

Color is an important element of brand identity. There's an interesting reason why fast food franchises such as McDonald's®, Hungry Jack's®, Burger King®, Pizza Hut® and Wendy's® all have the same red-and-yellow color palette. It's to do with the psychology of color. Those warm tones convey to the human brain a sense of deliciousness, and may stimulate the appetite.

The same magic works at home. One experiment offered party guests three rooms, all exactly alike in layout and size, but each painted a different color; red, yellow and blue. Each room contained the same type and quantity of food. The people at the party ate the most food in the yellow room, although they said that they found the food in both the red and yellow rooms to be equally tempting. They felt that the food in the blue room was much less appealing.

Of all the colors in the spectrum, blue, purples and blacks are the best appetite suppressants. Studies suggest that these cold colors may curb appetite because they remind people of spoiled or toxic foods.

---

33   **The University of California, Los Angeles**

Overeating causes: A cluttered environment.

Both obesity and "stuffocation" are bad for your health. Just as eating too much and being overweight is lousy for your physical well-being, so feeling overwhelmed by having too many material goods and feeling "stuffocated" can be damaging for your mental well-being.

Two psychologists who worked alongside the anthropologists at UCLA recorded how people feel about their homes and tested them for the stress hormone cortisol.

They found that women who have issues with clutter show the signature pattern of cortisol that is associated with people who have chronic fatigue, post-traumatic stress disorder, and a higher risk of mortality. High levels of stress hormones are also associated with obesity.

One solution to the problem of accumulating clutter is to recognise that happiness is more likely to be generated by experiences rather than "stuff".

Overeating causes: Culture.

Culture: Habitual over-eating.

The habit of eating at a certain time of day can cause you to overrule your body's natural appetite/satiety balance.

There may be a particular time of day, such as when you come home from school or work; or a particular activity, such as being in your car, or watching TV or studying, that is associated—in your mind—with eating. Such habits can be heard to break, though not impossible.

Other habits that can drive you to overeat include keeping high-Calorie low-nutrient foods like potato chips and candy in the home, eating while watching TV, reading or working on the computer (see 'being distracted while eating'), and ordering super-sized portions when dining out.

In a study by psychologist Paul Rozin, two men with such severe amnesia they could recall nothing that had happened longer ago than one minute, sat down and ate their lunch. The lunches were of a normal size, with standard portions of food.

Of course, one minute after they finished their meals and left the table, they had forgotten they had eaten lunch. Twenty minutes later the researchers offered them a second meal of the same size. They readily consumed an entire second lunch. Twenty minutes after the second lunch the researchers offered them a third lunch, and the same thing happened. This continued until the fourth meal was being eaten, when one of the men grumbled that his belly felt "a little tight".

This goes to show that the body's internal satiety signals can be overridden by eating cues such as "It's time for lunch," or "Someone in authority is giving me food".

Even people whose memory is intact can be influenced by eating cues.

It is important to consciously recall when and what you last ate, and to visualize that food as it looked on the plate in front of you. Doing so sends signals to your brain, saying, "This is the food you consumed recently. This food is inside your body now, nourishing you. Your body doesn't need any more food for a while."

Memory and visualization are useful tools to combat the effects of eating habits.

Culture: Social over-eating.

Social factors can cause you to ignore your body's natural appetite/satiety balance. These can include:

- the social pressure of eating when others eat
- the social pressure of eating when people of authority (such as parents) suggest it's time to eat.

Sharing food, or sharing a dining experience, is socially acceptable. It is a "social lubricant" that is present in every workplace, and at almost every social gathering. Holidays, parties or other social gatherings, eating out, doughnuts in the break room, birthday parties, barbecues—food is often consumed at social gatherings where it is plentiful and enticing. Watching other people eat can drive you to eat. Having easy, ready access to appealing food can have the same effect. Wanting to join in and be part of the crowd, in order to fit in—this is powerful social pressure. When others are eating, it's easy to feel awkward if you are not doing the same. When you eat in the company of other people, there's a temptation to eat the same food as everyone else, in the same quantities. This is not always a good idea—especially if you want to lose weight, and they don't.

Environmental factors such as our cultural heritage can also play a role in making us fat. In Polynesian culture, for example, large bodies have traditionally been viewed as more attractive.

" ... 'thrifty' genes are, at least in the human context, necessary but not sufficient factors in the causation of obesity. In actuality, the new discoveries in the genetics of obesity highlight our ignorance about the role of non-genetic or cultural factors . . . cultures have evolved behaviors and beliefs that appear to predispose individuals to develop obesity." [Brown (1991)]

Overeating causes: Obesogens.

What are obesogens?

To understand obesogens, you must first understand persistent organic pollutants (POPs).

Most natural organic compounds break down over time. They naturally rot and degrade by way of chemical, biological (being eaten by bacteria), and photolytic (being decomposed by light) processes. Think of such things as paper, apple cores, and wood. If you leave them for long enough, after a while they break down into simpler compounds—a kind of sludgy compost.

POPs, by contrast, are a class of organic compounds that are resistant to environmental degradation. Because of their persistence, POPs bioaccumulate, with potential harmful impacts on human/ animal health and the environment.

Everyone on the planet is continuously exposed to these toxic, man-made compounds, which may be from dietary, pharmaceutical, or industrial sources.

315

Dr. John Molot is a physician at the Environmental Health Clinic at Women's College Hospital in Toronto. He has focused his medical practice on environmental medicine.

"These chemicals don't break down," he says, speaking about POPs. "They get into the atmosphere and the water and travel around the world. They get into the food chain and climb up the food chain. They're found in newborn children, because their mothers have been exposed."

"The average person has maybe 300 different, synthetic chemicals in their body that weren't meant to be there," says Professor Gale Carey, Professor of Nutrition at the University of New Hampshire, USA.

POPs easily dissolve in fat. For this reason, they build up in adipose tissue (the body's fat stores).

Researchers have found evidence that some POPs possess the ability to disrupt the body's endocrine system, altering metabolic processes and predisposing many people to gain weight.

These chemicals are called "obesogens".

About obesogens.

Many health professionals still hold to the idea that a poor diet and lack of exercise are the only causes of obesity.

However, in the words of Robert H. Lustig, a professor of clinical pediatrics at the University of California, San Francisco, "Even those at the lower end of the BMI [Body Mass Index] curve are gaining weight. Whatever is happening is happening to everyone, suggesting an environmental trigger."

"There's no question that diet and exercise are the major players in the obesity epidemic. But the environment plays a significant role, too," Dr. Molot says. "There are many chemicals in the environment that make you gain weight and make it more difficult to lose weight." These are the chemicals that have come to be called obesogens.

The term "obesogens" was first coined in 2006 by Bruce Blumberg, a biology professor at the University of California, Irvine, USA. He was working with mice in a laboratory, when he noticed that mice exposed to tin-based compounds called "organotins" had a tendency to gain weight.

Following his discovery, many other compounds have been added to the list of obesogens. There are around twenty chemicals that have been shown to cause weight gain in animals who were exposed to those chemicals before birth or during their early, developmental years.

Not only humans, but also animals around the world "...have experienced increases in average body weight over the past several decades, trends not necessarily explained by diet and exercise," says science writer Wendee Holtcamp in "Obesogens: An Environmental Link to Obesity".

" . . . The role of environmental chemicals in obesity has garnered increased attention in academic and policy spheres, and was recently acknowledged by the Presidential Task Force on Childhood Obesity and the National Institutes of Health (NIH) Strategic Plan for Obesity Research." [Holtcamp (2012)]

Obesogens can affect future generations.

Obesogens can change the way your body works, so that even if you exercise and eat real, low-Calorie foods, you are pre-disposed to get fatter. It is thought that obesogens can even interfere with your DNA, predisposing future generations to obesity. These chemicals may affect not only your physiology, but the physiology of your children, and your children's descendants.

As Holtcamp wrote in the peer-reviewed journal *Environmental Health Perspectives*, "Some obesogenic effects may pass on to later generations through epigenetic changes, heritable modifications to DNA and histone proteins that affect when and how genes are expressed in cells, without altering the actual genetic code." [Holtcamp (2012)]

Adults are susceptible to problems caused by endocrine disruption, but obesogen exposure can be especially damaging in unborn children, young children and adolescents. The very early years are the ones during which the body is growing and developing, so changes in the number and size of fat calls, and the rate of metabolism, can affect children for the rest of their lives.

317

Baby mice in laboratories, who have been exposed to obesogens by consuming them or breathing them, or living in obesogenic environments, grow up to become obese adults. The alarming thing is, even if they then go on reduced Calorie diets and increase their amount of exercise, they remain obese.

Scientific research supports the idea of obesogens.

Is the concept of obesogens far-fetched? Not at all! A number of studies have linked levels of obesogenic chemicals in the blood of adult humans with obesity. Even the conservative American Medical Association supports the idea that obesogens play a significant role in the obesity crisis. [Grün (2006); Baillie-Hamilton (2002); Li et al., (2012); Grün et al., (2006)]

How do obesogenic chemicals make you fat?

When obesogens get inside your body, by being eaten, breathed in or absorbed through your skin, they disrupt the healthy chemical signals your hormones send to your cells. They can change these signals, or even block them. This is known as endocrine disruption.

Produced by your endocrine system, your hormones regulate a wide range of processes throughout your body. These include:
- your body's growth during your early years
- your body's development during your early years
- your metabolism
- the number and size of your fat storage cells

Endocrine disruption can cause adverse developmental, reproductive, neurological, and immune effects in both humans and wildlife.

Obesogenic chemicals can work in many different ways.

The role of fat cells in your body is not just to store fat, but also to produce hormones that regulate satiety and appetite, the rate at which you use up energy, and even your desire for certain foods. There are many different obesogens in the environment, and they can act on your body in a range of different ways that make you gain weight.

318

For example, they may:
- Increase the size of your fat cells
- Increase the number of your fat cells
- Interfere with the production of the hormones that help govern your bodyweight

A list of some obesogens.

Some particularly well-researched obesogens are listed in *The Satiety Diet Weight Loss Toolkit*, book #2 in the Satiety Diet series.

A growing list of potential obesogens.

Obesogenic chemicals are everywhere. They are impossible to avoid and they can be detected inside all of us. They can exist in many items we are exposed to every day. They may line the pipes of household water supplies, they are common in food packaging and they exist in high concentrations in the thermal papers of shop receipts. Obesogens can include:

- Chemicals in your food
- Pesticides in food and in the environment
- Growth hormones in your food
- Compounds used to manufacture the lining of microwave popcorn bags, the lining of containers for beverages such as baby formula and energy drinks, the lining of bottle tops, and the lining inside cans of such foods as soups, fish, beans and other vegetables
- Antibiotics in your food
- Antibiotics in medications
- Chemicals in cosmetics
- Chemicals in personal care products such as deodorants, lotions, shaving creams, and moisturizers
- Chemicals in detergents
- Chemicals in household items
- Compounds in plastic food and drink packaging

- Chemicals used to make plastics such as baby pacifiers, sports water bottles and plastic food wrap
- Chemicals in children's toys
- Chemicals in printed receipts from supermarkets and stores
- Chemicals such as flame retardants found in mattresses, pillows, computers, wall insulation and many other products may be obesogens. These chemicals can be inhaled when they adhere to tiny dust particles in the air that can't be seen.
- Chemicals in the atmosphere. Air pollution may be a risk factor for obesity, too.

Many known or suspected obesogens pervade our daily lives. A 2010 study discovered organotins—a class of POPS—in household products, such as wallpaper, floor tiles, vinyl window blinds, handbags and vacuum cleaner dust collected from 24 houses. [Kannan et al., (2010)]

Some obesogens that may contaminate our food supply.

Growth hormones, antibiotics, pesticides, preservative and other chemicals have found their way into food supplies all over the world. Many of these chemicals are obesogens.

* Growth hormones in our food.*

Livestock farmers, who raise animals to be slaughtered and used for meat, want the animals to grow quickly. The bigger they get while still very young, the faster they reach the size at which they can be profitably killed, and the more money the farmers make. This is why many meat producers across the world inject or feed the young animals with growth hormones.

In the USA, the meat and dairy industries use several different kinds of steroid hormones, including estradiol, progesterone, testosterone, recombinant bovine growth hormone, zeranol, trenbolone acetate, and melengestrol acetate. The first two on this list are female sex hormones, while testosterone is a male sex hormone. These three steroid hormones are produced naturally in the bodies of humans

320

and other animals, and they promote weight gain. When bodies receive larger than normal amounts of steroid hormones, the natural balance is disturbed and health problems can result.

The last three on the list are powerful, artificially-manufactured growth-promoting compounds. Synthetic hormones like these can accumulate in the body and may act as toxins. When you eat animal products such as meat (including chicken, turkey and other fowls), milk, cheese, and other dairy products, and even eggs, you may, yourself, ingest these hormones. You would then be subject to weight gain, just like the animals.

The fourth hormone on the list is recombinant bovine growth hormone (rBGH)—also known as recombinant bovine somatotropin (rBST).

Many dairy farmers inject this genetically engineered artificial hormone into cows to make them produce more milk. Research suggests that several health issues, such as cancer, may be associated with the consumption of dairy products from cows treated with rBGH. It is also thought that the use of rBGH encourages the proliferation of bacteria that are resistant to antibiotics. This is because rBGH appears to increase the rates of udder infections (mastitis) in cows, which means the cows have to be treated with antibiotics. The more animals that are treated with antibiotics, the more likely it is that drug-resistant bacteria can evolve. These bacteria can infect not only cows, but also humans. Some countries take these findings so seriously that their governments have banned the use of rBGH. Many countries, however—including some of the most developed countries—still use it.

Health authorities such as the FDA (the American Food and Drug Administration) hold the position that it's safe to give growth hormones to animals in the human food supply, but to date there have been no large, long-term studies performed in this area, so there is no real evidence to support this position.

* Obesogens in animal-based foods.

Most obesogens are fat-soluble, so they accumulate in fatty tissues. Fat is not always visible to the naked eye. Even cuts of meat that appear to be lean may have fat finely marbled through them. If you choose to eat meat, go for leaner cuts whenever possible and pick organic, free range, grass-fed beef that has been certified as hormone-free. Check the labels, as there are several grades of organic foods.

Note that whenever you eat animals, you also eat growth hormones. It's unavoidable. Growing animals produce growth hormones.

Growth hormones in meat, poultry, fish etc. don't have to be artificial ones added by food producers. Hormones exist naturally in all animals, as part of their physiology. Whenever you eat the flesh of a creature that was alive, you are eating the growth hormones nature bestowed on it so that it could grow and thrive. You are bringing another creature's growth hormones into your body.

Plant-based proteins, of course, do not come packaged with animal growth hormones.

* Antibiotics in our food.

Chickens, farmed fish, cattle, pigs, lambs and virtually any farmed animal are often fed or injected with antibiotics to promote growth and keep them healthy. And when animals (or humans) are kept crowded together in tight farm-pens, they are more susceptible to disease and infection, which means they need antibiotics. Antibiotics are obesogens. They can make animals (and humans) grow bigger more quickly. Even animals that are allowed to freely range on grassy farm pastures are often treated with antibiotics.

* Pesticides in our food.

Our daily food and drink is contaminated by numerous pesticides. Farmers use these lethal chemicals to protect their crops and animals. Pesticide residues can be found in virtually any food that is not certified organic. According to Stephen Perrine, author of "New American Diet," nine of the 10 most common pesticides we unintentionally consume every day are endocrine-disruptors, and are associated with overweight and obesity.

Polychlorinated biphenyls (PCBs) are organic chlorine compounds. They were once widely used in industrial manufacture, and they persist in the environment for a long time. In the 1960s it was discovered that they are toxic and cause major health problems, such as cancer, but they are still used by manufacturers to this day.

"Their production was banned by United States federal law in 1978, and by the Stockholm Convention on Persistent Organic Pollutants in 2001. Many rivers and buildings, including schools, parks, and other sites, are contaminated with PCBs and there has been contamination of food supplies with the substances." [Wikipedia, "Polychlorinated biphenyl" accessed June 2019]

Pesticides and PCBs may be found in non-organic fruit and vegetables. They tend to be more heavily concentrated in apples, pears, peaches, grapes and strawberries. Always wash any non-organically-certified fruits and vegetables thoroughly before eating them—although even washing may not completely get rid of all chemical residues. When you eat fruits that have to be peeled before being eaten (such as citrus fruits and melons) it's likely that much of the pesticide residue on the surface will be discarded along with the peel.

Pesticides and PCBs may also be found in:
• Beef or chicken that's been corn-fed or soy-fed
• Salmon that's been farmed instead of being wild-caught

* Other chemicals in our food.
Farmed animals may be fed or injected with other synthetic chemicals besides growth hormones and antibiotics. Consumers like to buy salmon whose flesh is deeply colored pink, so to ensure their fish are not pale, salmon-farmers may feed their fish with pink dye. The dye is mixed in with the pelleted fish-food. In the wild, salmon would gain a healthy pink hue because of the wide variety of fresh food available to them. Farmed salmon, on the other hand, get only pellets to eat, but they can be made to look healthier when their flesh is dyed.

* Preservatives, emulsifiers and other additives in our food.
If food manages to escape being affected by hormones, antibiotics, pesticides, dyes and so on, it may still be mixed with additives before it arrives on your plate. Food manufacturers use preservatives to prolong the shelf life of their products. Other chemicals, called emulsifiers, are used to make the texture of ice cream smoother, or to prevent mayonnaise from splitting into its separate components.

Unfortunately, some additives used in many highly-processed foods have been associated with obesity and digestive diseases.

A 2015 study published in *Nature* found that previously healthy mice who were fed with common dietary emulsifiers developed colitis and metabolic syndrome. [Chassaing et al., (2015)]

Metabolic syndrome is a cluster of at least three of the five following medical conditions:
- abdominal obesity
- high blood pressure
- high blood sugar
- high serum triglycerides
- low high-density lipoprotein (HDL) levels

How can you combat the effects of obesogens?

If we're all exposed to obesogens before we're even born, are we doomed to get fat or struggle with our weight all our lives? Not necessarily. Everyone can benefit from reducing exposure to obesogens as adults. It is in the best interests of your health to reduce your exposure to all kinds of endocrine-disrupting chemicals. For useful tips on avoiding obesogens, see *The Satiety Diet Weight Loss Toolkit*, book #2 in the Satiety Diet series.

Is soy an obesogen?

There is some public debate about whether soy contains substances that can promote obesity. This opinion may have arisen from the fact that soy contains isoflavones—plant compounds that act like the animal hormone estrogen. Some studies on rats suggest that consuming large amounts of soy's estrogen-like compounds might reduce fertility in females, trigger early puberty and disturb the development of baby rats in the womb, as well as juvenile rats.

It is not known whether the same applies to human beings, but in Japan, where consumption of soy is high, obesity rates are low. Still, if soy consumption bothers you, there are plenty of alternative vegan protein sources to choose from.

Other studies indicate that eating soy may actually be beneficial to weight loss. Phytoestrogens are plant-derived dietary compounds that are thought to be helpful in treating obesity and diabetes. They exist in a wide variety of foods, especially soy.

Soy is also a rich source of isoflavones, a class of phytoestrogens found predominantly in legumes and beans. "Soy protein is unique among the plant-based proteins because it is associated with isoflavones, a group of compounds with a variety of biological properties that may potentially benefit human health," say the authors of an article published in the *International Journal of Medical Sciences*. "An increasing body of literature suggests that soy protein and its isoflavones may have a beneficial role in obesity. Several nutritional intervention studies in animals and humans indicate that consumption of soy protein reduces body weight and fat mass in addition to lowering plasma cholesterol and triglycerides. . . . In obese humans, dietary soy protein also reduces body weight and body fat mass in addition to reducing plasma lipids." [Velasquez & Bhathena (2007)]

Evidence suggests that when people embark on a diet that includes plenty of soy protein (rich in isoflavones) and flaxseed (rich in lignans) their blood sugar levels even out and their insulin resistance improves.

Studies on animals have shown that a diet rich in soy protein can:

- restrict or even decrease the amount of fat accumulated in the body
- improve insulin resistance (which plays an important role in human obesity)
- reduce levels of insulin in the bloodstream

325

Studies on humans suggest that eating soy protein is good for people with obesity and/or diabetes because it appears to:
- improve high blood sugar
- reduce body weight
- decrease high levels of fat proteins in the blood (hyperlipidemia)
- reduce excess levels of insulin circulating in the blood (hyperinsulinemia)

[Velasquez & Bhathena (2007)]

In 2007, researchers found that eating soy while on a low Calorie diet boosted weight loss. "Soy-based low-Calorie diets significantly decreased serum total cholesterol and low-density lipoprotein cholesterol concentrations and had a greater effect on reducing body fat percentage than traditional low-Calorie diets. Thus, soy-based diets have health benefits in reducing weight and blood lipids."
[Liao et al., (2007)]

Overeating causes: Environmental factors.

Environmental eating triggers include such things as:
- The sight of Calorie-dense, highly palatable foods (especially if you've been deprived of such foods)
- Social occasions, with people expecting you and even urging you to eat and drink with them
- The sounds of dining such as clinking cutlery and the pouring of liquids
- The smells of food and drink
- The time of day (you can be habituated to eat at certain times of the day)
- Being a location where you normally would eat
- Stress

By being aware of your overeating triggers, you can take steps to deal with them. Just knowing that such triggers exist and knowing what they are is a good start, but it's not the final answer.

For example if you work in an office, and it's a colleague's birthday or farewell party or any other form of social gathering at which Calorie-dense foods are offered plentifully and at close range, what can you do? You know from past experience that it's a trigger situation. Look at those cakes. Look at those drinks. Your Inner Guardian is urging you to consume the pretty Calories!

Simply resisting the temptation is difficult, because the silent shouting of your Inner Guardian is compelling on a primal level. You know that if you sit there in front of that food for long enough, eventually you'll probably give in to the urge to eat those appealing sugar-laden, fat-rich foods.

What often happens is this: you resist the temptation at the time, but later on when you leave the office and go home or into another situation (such as a restaurant, the shops, a friend's place, the movies or a bar), the after-effects of that effort of resistance may take their toll on you.

Many people find that after they have exerted their willpower to abstain from appealing foods, it's as if they have exhausted their mental strength. Feeling "weakened", they are then tempted to binge on sugary or fatty foods, or whatever the tempting food was that they initially resisted—to make up for what they missed out on!

Clearly that's a bad outcome.

On the other hand, completely giving in to the trigger situation and over-indulging in the fatty, sugary deliciousness is also a bad outcome. You are likely to regret it later. What's the solution?

How to deal with environmental overeating triggers.

Beating over-eating triggers is all about being prepared. It's about:

- acknowledging that over-eating triggers exist
- acknowledging that those triggers are in general too strong for mere willpower to overcome
- having high satiety, low-Calorie emergency snack foods ready on hand
- eating small portions of the desired Calorie-dense foods so that you don't feel deprived
- ceasing to beat yourself up if you do give in those triggers

Tool #1: Be prepared.

When you are aware that a triggering social situation is about to take place—such as going out to dinner—eat a light, healthful, filling snack beforehand. This is one of the rare times when "preventative eating" is desirable.

Taking the edge off your appetite will help to stave off hunger and reduce the risk of eating everything within arm's length at the buffet. Snack on real, whole foods to decrease the likelihood that you will start to feel hungry when the party begins. That way you will already feel some degree of satiation by the time the appetite-triggering foods appear.

Tool #2: Move away.

Try to physically remove yourself from the sight, sound and smell of the trigger foods as far as is practically possible. If you cannot get right away from these sensory inputs, turn your back on the food You probably can't stop the smell reaching your nose or the sound of clinking plates reaching your ears, but at least you might have control over whether you have to look at the tempting morsels.

Tool #3: Don't cease it, decrease it.

We've mentioned this tool before. Select a small portion of the tempting food, put it on your plate and make it last as long as possible. Leave a long time between bites, chew the bites thoroughly, really admire the food, so that your eyes can tell your brain that yes, you are eating this food.

Savor the food. Eat it as mindfully as possible, even though you are in a social situation in which you are chatting to other people, and are therefore likely to be distracted. Enjoy that small portion and really make as much of it as you possibly can. Let it fill your senses. Enjoy the sight, smell, sound, taste, textures etc.

Tool #4: Drink water.

Arm yourself with a glass of water. Instead of eating, sip plain water, either still or sparkling (although recent research suggests that sparkling water may boost appetite, so be aware of this).

Tool #5: Eat before you shop.

Before you go to the supermarket or grocery store to buy food, have a light, filling, Calorie-sparse, high-satiety snack. At any food store you'll be exposed to the sight of food, and of colorful food images on packaging. This is another of the rare times when "preventative eating" is desirable.

Tool #6: Choose food substitutes.

Swap, swap, swap! Be aware that after the situation is over and you are no longer in a triggering environment, even if you have completely resisted all the Calorie-dense food or even if you have restrained yourself enough to only eat a small portion, the after-effects of having resisted strong temptation may linger with you.

You might be travelling on the train or in a car. You might be at the shops or at home. You're no longer at the party, yet you find yourself plagued with thoughts of the food you resisted. You might keep recalling that luscious cream-cake, or those salty, crunchy crisps and thinking, "I wish I'd eaten more of them while I had the chance!" Thoughts like this can lead to cravings.

To combat this, keep at hand substitutes for those foods you crave—lower Calorie, more healthful snacks that have a similar creaminess, or strong flavor, or crunchy texture, or whichever characteristic(s) your Inner Guardian is telling you it craves.

For example:
- Oven-baked vegetable crisps instead of high fat, oily, fried potato crisps
- A small tub of whipped silken tofu, low-fat ricotta or light coconut cream instead of creamy cheesecake
- Cocoa nibs instead of chocolate.

We cover this topic in more depth in *The Satiety Diet Weight Loss Toolkit*, book #2 in the Satiety Diet series.

Tool #7: Forgive yourself.

If you do find yourself unable to resist temptation and you binge on the foods that are likely to pile on the pounds, simply forgive yourself and move on. Don't blame yourself, don't agonize, and don't use it as an excuse to completely give up your dream of returning to the slim version of yourself. Just resume your healthful way of eating and keep going.

Overeating causes: Open plan living.

As discussed earlier, perhaps the most problematic drawback of open plan living—and kitchens in particular—is the fact that people in the main living areas are constantly exposed to reminders of food. Modern open-design homes often include kitchens and dining rooms that are part of the living area.

Foods on display in your kitchen can make you eat more. The refrigerator might be always within view. The kitchen counter might be strewn with foodstuffs such as packets of breakfast cereal or a bowl of fresh fruit. Savory or sweet smells drift from the oven or the toaster of the stovetop. Food odors permeate living-room furniture and remain noticeable for days or even weeks. Research suggests, again and again, that sensory cues like these really do contribute to over-eating.

Between mealtimes there is no escaping from the lingering smell of food, the sight of food-related objects such as the dinner table, kitchen appliances and the nearness of any foodstuffs left on the counter. With all these constant reminders of food, and the refrigerator situated so conveniently close at hand, the temptation is to graze at whim. Every extra bite of food adds to your Calorie intake.

Cornell University researchers found that they could actually predict the body weight of household members by looking at the foods displayed on their kitchen counters. Women whose kitchen counters were adorned with packets of breakfast cereal, or bottles of soda pop, tended to be much heavier than women whose counters displayed a bowl of fruit instead. [Wansink et al., (2015)]

A 2016 research article found that people ate more food when they were dining in an open plan environment. [Rollings & Wells (2016)] This is supported by numerous other studies showing that when you can see food, and when you have easy access to food, you're more likely to serve yourself more and eat more.

Open plan living has many benefits, but it also has some serious disadvantages. These include loss of privacy, loss of noise control and difficulties with heating and cooling. It costs more to heat or cool a larger space, and it's harder to cater for individual temperature preferences when everyone's occupying the same space. Furthermore, cooking is a messy business. Chopping, peeling, slicing, dicing—real cooking generates clutter and debris, not to mention stacks of dirty dishes. Clutter can contribute to stress and a rise in cortisol levels, which may prompt over-eating.

It can be difficult for home cooks to produce a good meal if they're trying to prepare it and chat to their guests at the same time. Besides, it can be awkward when visitors are milling about in the food preparation area while the cook is using sharp knives and hot utensils.

Experts advise people who have trouble sleeping to reserve the bedroom for sleep, and not to use it for waking-time activities such as studying, socializing or watching TV. Similarly, your living area should be for living in, not for eating. It should not provide contact cues to eat.

If you want to avoid eating triggers and you ever get the chance to design your own home, enclose the kitchen! Make sure that you can shut the door on it and keep your kitchen out of sight! Give your enclosed kitchen a large window or powerful exhaust fan, so that not only can you block food and food-related equipment from your field of vision, but you can also banish those tempting food aromas from your living space.

Even if your kitchen is not open-plan and merged with the main living areas of your home; even if it's a separate room tucked away in an isolated part of your house, it's important to keep any food stored or prepared there well hidden from view.

If you can't enclose your kitchen, do your best to store foodstuffs where you can't see them.

People who reply on willower to help them resist visible foods are fighting a losing battle. The conscious mind of a healthy person is no match for their Inner Guardian. Your Inner Guardian's purpose is to make you conserve energy stores in order to survive (as it views survival) in spite of your rational choice to be slim. If your eyes see food, your Inner Guardian is likely to demand that you eat it.

For more about open plan living and the rise of obesity, see *The Satiety Diet Weight Loss Toolkit* (book #2 in the Satiety Diet series).

Triggers of binge eating.

A study published in the journal *Psychological Medicine* focused on people with the eating disorder bulimia. With bulimia, episodes of gorging on food are usually followed by episodes of self-induced vomiting. Bulimia is linked to an obsession with body weight. People who have bulimia may also have anorexia nervosa. They may be of normal weight, or they may be obese people who have never been thin.

The authors of the study asked patients to describe what it was that triggered their episodes of ravenous overeating (binge-eating). They listed a variety of factors, twelve of which were commonly mentioned by most of the patients. [Abraham & Beaumont (1982)] Here they are in order of prevalence:

- tension
- eating something (anything at all)
- being alone
- craving specific foods
- thinking about food (which would involve visualizing food)
- going home (either after school or work, or after living away)
- feeling bored and lonely
- feeling hungry
- drinking alcohol
- going out on a romantic date
- eating out
- going to a party

To summarize, the binge eating triggers included:
- Emotions and moods (tension, feeling bored and lonely)
- The sense of sudden liberation from self-imposed restricted eating (drinking alcohol, which releases inhibitions; going out on a romantic date; eating out; going to a party; eating something; being alone—and therefore being able to eat unseen and unjudged by others; going home—where one may be able to relax self-imposed restrictions)
- Food visualization (thinking about food)
- Nutritional needs (craving specific foods, feeling hungry)

FOOD ADDICTION

IS FOOD ADDICTION REAL?

Can food and drink actually be addictive, in the same way as drugs of dependence? Is it possible that people may eat too much because they have become "addicted" to certain foods or beverages?

The problem for drug addicts is that consumption of certain substances, such as alcohol or heroin, stimulates reward pathways in the brain, and actually makes chemical alterations in the brain. This can lead to cravings and dependence. Can food really stimulate the brain's reward pathways in the same way as drugs?

Many people joke that they're "addicted to chocolate" or "can't resist eating bread". According to science however, there may be some truth in these statements.

The authors of a 2009 paper published in the *Journal of Nutrition* say, "The term ("food addiction") became especially popular in the second half of the twentieth century, driven by the 'obesity epidemic'.

"'Food addiction' is a concept that equates a person's behavioral and neurophysiological reactions to certain foods with the same reactions that exist in people with substance dependence. Whether or not food can be as addictive as drugs is a controversial subject. Expert opinions have been divided as to whether true food addiction exists, but recent studies appear to support the idea. [Corwin & Grigson (2009)]

Food "addictions" can manifest as increased appetite and cravings, so powerful that they override your body's natural mechanisms for regulating your energy needs.

" ...studies suggest that food addictions, similar to that of drug addictions, mainly exert their actions through the dopamine and opiate pathways," wrote the Yale University psychologists who authored a paper published in the journal *Appetite*. [Gearhardt et al., (2009)]

"Recent studies on food addiction have demonstrated that the neurobiological circuits involved in the development of drug addiction also play a role in food consumption," say the authors of a 2016 review published in the journal *Psychiatria Hungarica*. [Eördögh et al., (2016)]

"... a study conducted by the Scripps Research Institute found that rats fed a high-fat palatable diet for extended periods, overstimulated the brain's reward system, similar to brain activity in drug addiction." [Johnson & Kenny, (2014)]

A 2013 study published in *The American Journal of Clinical Nutrition* looked at the effect that food intake has on the pleasure centers of the brain. The research team, led by David Ludwig, director of the New Balance Foundation Obesity Prevention Center at Boston Children's Hospital in the USA, concluded that food addiction could, in fact, be a real issue. [Lennerz, et al., (2013)]

Professor Ludwig noted that, in addition to being involved with rewards and cravings, these pathways in the brain are "... also linked to substance abuse and dependence, which raises the question as to whether certain foods might be addictive".

Together, results like these appear to support the idea that dependency on certain foods can be as problematic as obsessive dependence on gambling, drugs or any other addiction.

Many scientists around the world now consider "food addiction" to be a disease, rather than just an overeating problem. America's National Institute on Drug Abuse holds an annual "Food Addiction Treatment Conference", an event in which the University of Massachusetts Department of Psychiatry and the Food Addiction Institute are also involved.

THE YALE FOOD ADDICTION SCALE

Given the possibility that in certain circumstances some foods can become addictive, in 2009 researchers at Yale University's Rudd Center for Food Policy and Obesity in the USA released a questionnaire called the "Yale Food Addiction Scale" (YFAS).

It contains 25 questions, based on classifications for substance dependence criteria, as listed in the *Diagnostic and Statistical Manual of Mental Disorders* (a manual published by the American Psychiatric Association). The purpose of the YFAS was to identify people who showed signs of dependency on certain foods.

The Yale researchers went further than a questionnaire—they also scanned people's brains using an MRI machine. The results clearly showed real differences in brain activity between people who scored high on the YFAS and those who scored low.

"Using functional magnetic resonance imaging (fMRI) subjects regardless of Body Mass Index(BMI), with high food addiction score compared to those with lower scores, showed significant differences in brain activity.

"Researchers found that the brain mechanisms in people with food addiction were similar to those in people with substance dependence, such as drug addicts."[Meule & Gearhardt (2014)]

"Foods most notably identified by YFAS to cause food addiction were those high in fat and high in sugar." [Wikipedia (5th Jan 2018)]

The YFAS survey seemed to show that particular foods more likely than others to stimulate the symptoms of dependence. These foods reflect the fat-rich, sugar-rich characteristics identified in previous food addiction studies.

The Yale Food Addiction Scale lists the following foods:
- Sugary sweets such as ice cream, chocolate, doughnuts, cookies, cake, candy
- Refined starches such as white bread, rolls, regular pasta, and white rice
- Salty snacks such as chips, pretzels, and crackers

335

- Fatty foods such as steak, bacon, hamburgers, cheeseburgers, pizza, and French fries
- Sugar-laden drinks such as soda pop

The results of the questionnaire showed that overweight and obese people scored higher for food addiction.

The results of a 2014 review of 196,211 people showed found that 19.9% of people fulfil the criteria for food addiction according to the Yale Food Addiction Scale. [Pursey et al., (2014)]

Five years after the development of the Yale Food Addiction Scale, psychologists Ashley Gearhardt and Adrian Meule concluded: "Although, the YFAS is not sufficient evidence that 'food addiction' exists, it does provide a standardized tool to identify individuals who are the most likely to be experiencing an addictive response to food."

THE ROLE OF DOPAMINE IN "FOOD ADDICTION"

Dopamine is a neurotransmitter released in the brain when the body is experiencing pleasurable sensations like the flavors and textures of food, a rise in blood sugar levels, satisfaction of appetite, the effects of various drugs, alcohol, sex etc. Dopamine makes it possible for you to see potential rewards in your life, and then to take action to move toward those rewards.

When scientists make laboratory animals dopamine-deficient, those animals die of starvation. Without any dopamine in their brains, they lose the motivation to seek food.

If a complete lack of dopamine makes animals stop eating, you would assume that having low levels of dopamine would make people lose weight, right?

Not at all!

People who are genetically predisposed to have lower dopamine levels (because they have fewer dopamine receptors in their brains) are, in fact, more motivated to eat than people with normal dopamine levels, and they also eat more. [Epstein et al., (2007)]

Scientists theorize that it is easier for people with more dopamine receptors to experience pleasure and satisfaction when they eat food, or drink alcohol, or interact with any sort of "rewarding substance". People with fewer receptors need to eat a lot more food, for example, to experience the same pleasure and satisfaction as people with the normal number of receptors.

Many obese people have a weak dopamine response to food consumption, so that they have to eat more to achieve satiety. When people have low levels of dopamine they are more likely to develop food cravings. However when they eat that food, they may derive less satisfaction from it. It's similar to drug addiction or alcoholism in that the more you consume, the more it takes to produce the same effect. Furthermore, binge eating activates the same dopamine reaction in the pleasure and reward centers of the brain' as do addictive drugs such as heroin and opioids.

This does not mean that everyone genetically predisposed to having fewer dopamine receptors will necessarily become obese. "Behavior and biology interact and influence each other," says Leonard H. Epstein, the leader of the aforementioned 2007 study. ". . . The genotype does not cause obesity; it is one of many factors that may contribute to it. I think the factors that make up eating behavior are in part genetic and in part learning history." [Reinholz et al., (2008)]

It is thought that increasing dopamine by methods other than eating, could help curb the appetite of dopamine-deficient people. Find tips on how to increase dopamine naturally, and more information about addictive foods and drinks, in *The Satiety Diet Weight Loss Toolkit*, book #2 in the Satiety Diet series.

OTHER POSSIBLE CAUSES OF "FOOD ADDICTION"

Food addiction: Eating disorders.

It's not only foods themselves that can cause "addiction". Restricted eating, extreme dieting, bulimia or other eating disorders can cause what is known as food addiction.

"Food is not ordinarily like a substance of abuse, but intermittent bingeing and deprivation changes that," wrote the authors of the sugar addiction review published in the journal *Neuroscience & Biobehavioral Reviews*. They were referring to a study in which rats were deprived of food for 12 hours every day, then were given access to a delicious Calorie-rich sugar solution and boring rat chow for 12 hours. "As a result, they learn to drink the sugar solution copiously, especially when it first becomes available each day."

The rats binged on sugar and became sugar-dependent. This, the researchers said, ". . . shares some aspects of the behavioral pattern of people diagnosed with binge-eating disorder or bulimia. Bulimics often restrict intake early in the day and then binge later in the evening, usually on palatable foods. . . These patients later purge the food, either by vomiting or laxative use, or in some cases by strenuous exercise." [Avena et al., (2008)]

Food addiction: Overeating.

A 2010 study investigated changes in the brain caused by excess food consumption. Over a period of time, overeating fat-rich foods can actually cause neurochemical changes in the brain, as demonstrated in studies of rats. This appears to make over-eaters crave food as if it were a drug of dependency. Alterations in the brain make it extremely difficult to quit, whether the substance in question is a drug such as cocaine, or a fat-rich food.

"Overconsumption of palatable (delicious) food triggers addiction-like neuroadaptive responses in brain reward circuitries and drives the development of compulsive eating," say the study's authors. [Johnson & Kenny (2010)]

Habitual overeating can become an addiction.

Studies show that dopamine signaling decreases after people experience a prolonged overstimulation of dopamine release. Such an overstimulation can be brought about by activities as chain smoking or overeating.

People who do not have a genetic predisposition to a weaker dopamine response can actually lower their dopamine response to food simply by persistent overeating or binge eating. Again, this means that they need to eat more food in order to feel satiated.

Several researchers have found evidence suggesting that chronic overeating or binge eating can turn into an addiction. [Gearhardt et al., (2011)]; Barry et al., (2009)]

Food addiction: Poor social connections.

Social connection and addiction.

How can social connection possibly affect addictive behaviors?

In the past, scientists generally believed that addiction stems from changes in body chemistry and a corresponding physiological need. New evidence, however, suggests that addictions (of any type, including food) can potentially be counteracted by replacing addictive substances with social connection.

You may have heard about the addictive qualities of cocaine or heroin as reported in experiments on rats. In the past, researchers put rodents in cages by themselves with two water bottles. One bottle contained pure water while the other was laced with cocaine or heroin. During the experimental period, the rats became so obsessed with the drugged drinks that they kept consuming the liquid until it killed them. The researchers concluded that cocaine and heroin were so addictive that nine out of ten lab rats would use them continually, until they overdosed.

The same was thought to be true of humans.

In the 1970s Bruce Alexander, a professor of psychology in Vancouver, Canada, noticed that the rats in the experiments were always kept alone. He wondered if their drug dependency had anything to do with their social status. To test his theory, the professor built what he called "Rat Park". This lush cage contained everything a rat could theoretically wish for, including not just lots of food and play-things, but also plenty of rodent friends.

Professor Alexander then repeated the drug-based experiment, with startling results. He found that the rats in Rat Park, with their full, social lives, didn't like the drugged water. In fact, not only did they not become addicted to the drink, they mostly shunned the laced concoction. They used less than a quarter of the drugs in comparison to the rats who were unhappy and alone. None of the rodents in Rat Park became heavy users at all, let alone died as a result of their consumption. By contrast, the rats who lived alone became dependent on drugs 100 percent of the time.

If you're wondering if this was a result limited to rodents, think again! Professor Alexander discovered that a human equivalent to this experiment actually took place, with similar results. This other "experiment" was the Vietnam War.

According to a 1975 study publishing in the *Archives of General Psychiatry*, around 20 percent of U.S. soldiers became addicted to heroin during active duty in the war. However, while it might be assumed that many veterans would have returned home as addicts when the war ended, in fact around 95% of the addicted soldiers simply stopped using drugs, and only small numbers of them had to go through rehabilitation to achieve this result. [Goodwin et al., (1975); Robins et al., (1974); Robins (1993)]

Professor Alexander believes that this was because they "shifted from a terrifying cage back to a pleasant one, so didn't want the drug any more". He argues that addiction, it seems, is more of an adaptation than it is a chemical response.

This is great news! If addiction is heavily influenced by our environment, instead of by our own physiology, then changing our circumstances can treat the addiction.

To test his theory further, Professor Alexander placed rats in isolation and let them use the drug-laced water for 57 days so that they would become well and truly hooked. Next, he took them out of their isolated cages and put them in Rat Park. Interestingly, he found that, even though these rodents had become addicted to drugs when alone, after a few noticeable twinges of withdrawal they gradually ceased their heavy usage of drugs and returned to a normal, drug-free life.

A Canadian doctor, Gabor Mate, also noticed the importance of social connection when it comes to drug usage. When doctors give hospital patients pain relief in the form of diamorphine (the medical name for heroin), the course of treatment often lasts for long periods—up to several months at a time. If the chemical-based theory of addiction were correct, in that it is purely drugs which cause an addiction and not psychological factors, then there should be high rates of people leaving hospital as addicts. However, Dr. Mate noted that this hardly ever happens, because most drug users simply stop when they leave hospital.

This reaffirms Professor Alexander's view that social interaction is the key. Patients leaving hospital typically return home to a life where they are comfortable and surrounded by loved ones. This is similar to the situation of those rats in Rat Park who weaned themselves off the drug-laced water with relative ease.

If pleasant, interesting surroundings and social interaction can cure men and rats of drug addiction, can these elements curb food addiction, too?

These studies provide a helpful insight into the issue of addiction, whether food or drug based. They demonstrate the fact that satisfied human beings who have deep and meaningful connections with others are not only more likely to steer clear of addictions in the first place, but also to escape from any previous addictions. On the other hand, people who struggle to form social bonds often try to find connection elsewhere—whether it be by injecting with syringes, popping pills, snorting powders, playing the slot machines, seeking solace in a bottle, or even by continually overeating.

[Davis et al., (2004); South & Huang, (2008); Palmiter (2007); Lerman et al., (2004)]

HOW TO OVERCOME "FOOD ADDICTION"

If you are affected by irresistible cravings and you feel unable to regulate your food intake despite your best efforts, then you might fulfil the Yale Food Addiction Scale criteria for what is controversially known as "food addiction".

Being a "food addict" make it almost impossible to lose weight on any diet regime, so it's important to fix this issue before you begin the Satiety Diet.

Keep in mind the fact that your eating behavior may be a result of your biochemistry, and you cannot always change it by simply using willpower. Therefore if you want to defeat cravings and lose weight, it's necessary to modify what's going on with your hormones and neurotransmitters. There are powerful ways to do this, including eating different foods, altering your mindset and making some lifestyle changes.

Here are some suggestions:

- Get professional help from a psychologist who specializes in the area of food addiction.
- If you're addicted to so-called "junk" foods, start eating a diverse range of nutrient-rich foods. When you're getting all the nutrition, flavors and textures your body needs and desires, cravings for junk food tend to subside. Your microbiome also changes for the better.
- Ditch foods and beverages that are likely to cause spikes in your blood sugar levels, such as sugar, honey, molasses, agave syrup, food products high in sugar, dried or candied fruits, soda and fruit juice, alcohol, artificial sugars and sugar substitutes.
- Include mainly low-GI foods in your diet. See our section on "Low-GI foods".

- Use something other than food to naturally boost dopamine levels and trigger feelings of satisfaction and reward in your brain.[34] See our section on "How to Boost Dopamine Levels Naturally".

- Break the vicious cycle of over-eating or binge eating. See our section on "Willpower and Creating Good Habits".

- Improve your social connections. Face to face social connection is the most rewarding, but you can also connect with like-minded others with a telephone call, or by joining online groups and forums.

- Reduce your exposure to food advertising. Food ads can appear on television, radio, social media, your phone etc. Not all food ads try to persuade you to buy "addictive" foods, but any reminder of food can trigger your appetite in any case.

- Quit smoking.

- Quit taking stimulants or sedatives, as long as your doctor is okay with this.

- Get regular exercise, even if it's just an hour of housework or 20 minutes of walking once a day.

- Drink plenty of water.

- Get better sleep.

- Learn relaxation techniques—and practice them.

- Keep a daily private journal recording your innermost feelings, for your eyes alone.

---

34 Note: It is important to use natural methods to boost dopamine, rather than drugs. Natural methods are unlikely to result in excessive dopamine levels. Having excessive dopamine in your system is linked to serious problems such as psychosis, increased impulsive behavior, nausea, vomiting and headache. Like most things, dopamine is good for you at the right levels—not too much and not too little.

FOOD CRAVINGS

Scientists are of the opinion that food cravings are the result of a number of social, cultural, psychological, and physiological elements. [Sharifi et al., (2013)]

The difference between hunger and food cravings.

It is important to distinguish between real hunger and food cravings. Hunger is your body's way of telling you it needs you to consume more nutrients and energy. One of the main differences between hunger and cravings is that eating any food will help quell your hunger and make the hunger signals subside. Cravings, on the other hand, are a fierce desire to eat a specific food, such as salty, crispy crisps or sweet, creamy chocolate. Food cravings are different from ordinary hunger and indeed, they may not even be associated with it.

In a 2014 article published in the journal *Frontiers in Psychiatry*, researchers described craving as "…a strong motivational state, which compels an individual to seek and ingest a particular substance. It usually refers to alcohol, tobacco, or drugs, but has become increasingly applied to food. Thus, food cravings refer to an intense desire or urge to eat a specific food."

They continued, "It is this specificity that distinguishes a craving from ordinary food choices and hunger. In Western societies, the most commonly craved foods are those high in fat, sugar, and salt, such as cake, chips, pizza, ice-cream, and in particular, chocolate. Most people experience cravings for such palatable foods on occasion without any problem. However, food cravings can pose significant health risks for some people. Most notably, they can contribute to the development of obesity and disordered eating, increasingly serious global health issues." [Kemps & Tiggemann (2014)]

Almost everyone has experienced food cravings at some time. Cravings are natural. They differ from so-called food addictions in that they tend to come and go. Cravings can be satisfied when the craved-for food is eaten, and after that the craving may not return for quite a while, or may never return at all. ("Addiction", however, remains.)

What causes food cravings?

There is no single explanation for what causes food cravings. They can spring from such triggers as:

- Your brain's chemical systems of pleasure and reward
- Your body seeking nutrients it lacks
- A sense of deprivation. A feasting-deprivation pattern of eating highly palatable foods for a few days or weeks, then forbidding yourself to eat any of those foods at all for the next few days or weeks, can intensify cravings. That's exactly what many dieters do, thus unintentionally setting themselves up for failure.
- Emotional states, such as boredom, or stress, or sadness
- Ravenous hunger
- The sight of food—images of food in a store or cafeteria, or on a billboard, TV etc.
- Insulin resistance
- Your microbiome
- Your body's circadian rhythms
- Non-diabetic hypoglycemia

If you experience a food craving, ask yourself why it happened. Only when you've identified the trigger can you address the problem.

Causes of food cravings: The brain's chemical systems.

Theories about food cravings involve the brain's chemical systems of pleasure and reward. It is argued that low serotonin levels affect the brain centers for appetite. Serotonin is one of the so-called happiness hormones. Consuming fats and carbohydrates may trigger the release of endorphins—another so-called happiness hormone. [Ronzio (2003)]

There is evidence that addiction and food craving activate some of the same brain areas. For example, when nicotine addicts view pictures of people smoking, the same "pleasure" areas of their brains are activated as in obese people when they look at pictures of food. [Brundige & Noll (2009)]. And not only obese people! Most humans derive pleasure, to some degree, from looking at pictures of food—or even from reading or hearing words describing food.

How to combat cravings triggered by the brain's chemistry of pleasure and reward.

Your brain's pleasure and reward systems are largely regulated by the so-called happiness hormones—endorphins, serotonin, dopamine, and oxytocin.

One way to help combat food cravings is to encourage the release of endorphins by natural methods, instead of by consumption of fattening foods such as chocolate and fries. Endorphins are natural chemicals released by your body. They are pain relievers, and they also stimulate pleasurable feelings, similar to the effect of morphine. Here are some suggestions:

- **Sleep:** Peaceful sound sleep every night encourages the release of endorphins in your body.

- **Addiction treatments:** Recent scientific findings suggest that in obese individuals, addiction treatments could be useful in learning to fight severe food cravings. That is, the same types of protocols that help overcome drug addiction can be used to help overcome food cravings.

- **Exercise:** Not only does exercise burn Calories and stimulate the release of endorphins, it can also help curb cravings—especially cravings for sweet foods. A study published in the journal *Appetite* showed that office-workers who went for a 15-minute brisk walk were half as likely to eat chocolate when they returned to their desks, compared with their colleagues, who rested for 15 minutes.[Ledochowski et al., (2015)]

- **Good food:** Your body's serotonin production may be enhanced by foods containing nutrients such as Vitamin C, B-complex vitamins (especially niacin) and zinc. See also our section in this book about how to enhance your dopamine and serotonin levels.

Causes of food cravings: Nutrient deficiencies.

Some cravings may be caused by the body seeking nutrients it lacks. Dr. Kevin Murphy, an endocrinologist from Imperial College, London, states: "Presumably we are evolutionarily programmed to recognise food sources and the brain remembers nutrient content so we can identify novel food stuffs. The most obvious evidence of this is when people stuck at sea start craving weird things like fish eyes because they provide the nutrients they're missing." [Topham (2011)]

The most craved-for foods include chocolate and sugar-rich confectioneries. The cravings for particular foods, however, may be associated with their ingredients. Chocolate for example, contains the amino acid phenylethylamine, which is important for the regulation of the body's release of endorphins.[Brundige & Noll (2009)] Endorphins trigger a positive feeling in the body, similar to the euphoric "high" of morphine.

Women may feel the most powerful yearning to eat chocolate just prior to and during menstruation. Chocolate also contains polyphenols, substances that are similar to estrogen. It is often suggested that consuming chocolate helps boost women's estrogen levels; however there is no evidence indicating a direct hormonal or physiological cause of chocolate cravings. Spinach can be another pre-menstrual craving. This green leafy vegetable is high in iron, a nutrient which is lost during the menstrual flow.

Cravings may focus on food's texture—for example, creamy or crunchy—or flavor—for example, sweet or salty.

One frequent craving is for salty foods. Craving salt may be partly due to a lack of electrolytes, perhaps lost during excessive sweating.

However there's more to salty food cravings than just mineral deficiencies.

Have you ever eaten just a single crunchy, salty potato crisp, only to feel compelled to eat the whole packet? You might actually be in need of protein!

Professor Stephen Simpson, the Executive Director of Obesity Australia says, "Your appetite control automatically gives priority to protein. If your diet runs short, you make up for it by getting energy from fats in carbohydrates that taste like protein, with that savory, piquant umami flavor. Your potato crisp is a 'protein decoy'. It tastes like protein. Our bodies have evolved to associate those flavor cues with protein, but actually all you're getting is loaded up with more fat and carbs, leaving your protein appetite unfulfilled, and hence you're gonna continue to snack and eat more." [Catalyst (2015)]

How to combat cravings triggered by nutrient deficiencies.
To ensure that you're getting as many macronutrients and micro-nutrients as possible, eat a wide variety of foods, preferably fresh, whole, organic and unprocessed!

Causes of food cravings: A sense of deprivation.
There is also more to cravings than just brain chemicals and nutrient deficiencies. Psychology is also part of the equation.

"Overall, the popularized account of cravings as elicited by specific nutritional need is having to give way to a more subtle and complex appreciation of human eating behavior." [Hill (2007)]

Researcher AJ Hill says, "Dieting or restrained eating generally increase the likelihood of food craving while fasting makes craving, like hunger, diminish. . . . Attempted restriction or deprivation of a particular food is associated with an increase in craving for the unavailable food."

How to combat food cravings triggered by a sense of deprivation.
If you ignore cravings, you do so at your peril! In the long run, your body's hunger systems are almost always stronger than your willpower. Denial of cravings often ends in bingeing. How can you defeat the deprivation-feasting pattern?

1. Pamper yourself a little! A small taste now could prevent binge-eating later. Resisting delicious, fattening food when you're at a party can be hard. Instead of depriving yourself until you buckle under the pressure, spoil yourself with a small serving of the food you fancy. It's quite possible that having a few mouthfuls will quell your longing. Simply serve yourself a small portion of the craved food and eat it mindfully. When you are experiencing a strong craving, the best way to deal with it is to eat a small amount of the craved-for food, rather than denying yourself completely.

2. **Seek the nutrients you might be lacking.** If you crave red meat, your Inner guardian might be prompting you to seek a source of iron. Other iron-rich foods include sunflower seeds, nuts, whole grains, dark leafy greens such as spinach, dark chocolate, and tofu. Teff is an ancient grain rich in protein and iron. A hearty veggie burger on a wholemeal bun could also satisfy this craving. If you do choose to eat meat, the best option is lean, home-cooked meat.

3. **Swap, swap, swap!** This is oe of our catch-cries. Substitution of a similar food that's lower in energy density may satisfy a craving for high-energy foods without piling on extra weight. If you can't get rid of the craving, substitute delicious foods that have the characteristics you're craving for but without so many Calories.

(See also our section on craving for sweet desserts after a meal.)

If you crave **ice cream**, your Inner Guardian might be on the hunt for a food that is cool, creamy and sweet. Try substituting pure low-fructose fruit sorbets, home-made silken tofu ice-cream (which is high in protein) or low-fat frozen yoghurt.

Your craving for **crisps/chips** might be deflected by choosing something else that's salty and crunchy but lower in energy. Swap crisps for tamari-seasoned rice crackers, or dip celery sticks or carrot sticks into hummus. You'll get a satisfying crunch with fewer Calories and more nutrients. Or make your own oven-baked, oil-free vegetable crisps. Use potato, sweet potato, carrot, kale, or zucchini.

Instead of eating an entire bar of **chocolate**, choose from these suggestions:

- A square of dark chocolate with a cacao content of around 70%. This contains less fat than standard milk chocolate, and studies report it might be beneficial for the heart.

- For a rich, satisfying liquid chocolate hit, place a couple of spoonsful of cocoa (or cacao) powder into a mug and mix to a paste with a little boiling water. When the powder is thoroughly moistened, pour in some warmed unsweetened almond milk or low-fat soy milk and stir. For sweetness you could add a tablespoon of rice malt syrup, or a couple of teaspoonsful of stevia and/or erythritol.
- Chocolate cravings may also be satisfied by eating a Chocolate Tofu Pot, which contains satisfying plant-protein, or a Vegan Chocolate Pudding, which is packed with nutrition. Both recipes can be found in *Crispy, Creamy, Chewy: The Satiety Diet Cookbook*.

Chris Clark says: "Oddly enough, some people have been known to quell chocolate cravings by eating a couple of slices of wholemeal bread topped with low-fat yoghurt, whipped silken tofu or fresh banana. This might indicate that their craving was less to do with a need for chocolate and more to do with a need for a creamy texture, or carbohydrates."

* Like potato crisps, **popcorn** can be the object of intense desire. Your memory plays a part in your food cravings, and like other cravings, the yen for popcorn is more likely to hit when you find yourself somewhere you've previously eaten (and enjoyed) that particular food. The cinema, for example, is a place where popcorn is often consumed. Plain, unsweetened, unsalted air-popped popcorn can be a reasonably healthful snack to enjoy in moderation, but the popcorn sold at cinemas is usually high in fat, sugar and salt. So bring your own home-made version, or buy the smallest portion-size of the commercial variety.

* Craving for **doughnuts**? (Or donuts!) Try substituting a wholemeal bagel spread a tiny smear of low-fat peanut butter, or a teaspoon of strawberry jam. Bagels and doughnuts share that chewy, cakey texture you're longing for.

* If **pizza** is your desire, it's easy to make one at home. Use a wholemeal base to add filling fiber, and instead of full-fat Mozzarella, choose a reduced-fat cheese or low Calorie vegan cheese. Toppings can include sliced fresh tomatoes, mushrooms, garlic, spinach, bell peppers (capsicums) sun-dried tomatoes, basil, grilled zucchini, red onions etc. Alternatively, just eat one of two slices of store-bought pizza instead of a larger portion.

* **Pasta** is good, filling food, as long as it's made with whole grain flour and not refined flour. Store-bought pasta sauces can have fats and sugars hidden in them, so read the label. Or make your own, easy pasta sauce with canned or fresh tomatoes as a base. Load it with scrumptious vegetables and you'll have a colorful, satisfying meal.

Of course, pasta doesn't have to be made out of wheat flour at all. It can, for example, be made from buckwheat, rice or pulses. For a lower Calorie, nutrition packed pasta dish:

- Buy or grow a "spaghetti squash" (Cucurbita pepo subsp. Pepo). This amazing vegetable, when cooked, yields beautiful golden strands of low Calorie, nutritious "spaghetti". Just add sauce and enjoy.

- Buy some shirataki noodles. These traditional Japanese noodles are made from the konjac yam, and they are very low in Calories but high in fiber.

- Make vegetable lasagna by substituting thin layers of parsnip or zucchini for sheets of grain lasagna.

- Make vegetable noodles (vegetti) using a spiralizer (often called a spiral vegetable slicer), a julienne peeler or a standard vegetable peeler. Vegetables suited to spiralizing include kholrabi (koloodles), zucchini (zoodles), carrot (coodles), parsnip (poodles), sweet potato (swoodles), turnip (toodles), broccoli stem (boodles—peel stem first), asparagus (aspoodles), kelp, radish and pumpkin.

* **French fries** are a commonly craved-for food. Soft on the inside, crispy on the outside, laden with salt and fat and offering that lip-smacking, savory umami taste, they can be close to irresistible. Standard French fries are astronomically high in Calories, so if

you're eating out try to limit yourself to less than half a dozen, while drinking plenty of water and filling up on salad. If you're at home when the craving hits, make your own low-oil oven-baked potato or sweet potato chips. If it's salt you're craving, you can add your own.

French fries can be a "protein decoy", and craving for them can mean your Inner Guardian is compelling you to look for protein, so eating some beans and whole-grains, or nuts and seeds, or fish or cheese or meat may help to dampen those cravings.

* Speaking of **nuts**, when you eat them opt for the ones that are still in their shells. These are as close to "natural" as possible and it takes longer to eat them because you have to break each one out of its shell. Nuts can be Calorie-dense, so only eat a few at a time, and try to completely abstain from "party food" nuts that have been roasted or fried in oil. (Check the label.)

* **Coffee** is not fattening in its "black" version, without cream, milk or sugar. So if you're craving coffee, drink it as close to black as you can. If you habitually drink it with sugar, gradually decrease the sugar load, over several weeks, until you get used to zero sugar coffee. If you're used to having coffee with cream, gradually switch to skim milk—and then to no milk at all, if you can handle it! Sweet syrups and coffee flavorings are, it goes without saying, just a way of sabotaging your weight loss!

Causes of food cravings: Emotional states.

Negative emotions such as nervousness, anxious or sadness can trigger cravings. This is called "emotional eating", and it is tied up with the brain's chemical systems of pleasure and reward. When you feel low in spirits, you might use eating as a way of making yourself feel better.

Combating food cravings triggered by emotional states.

If it's an emotion-based craving you're experiencing, deal with the emotion. Instead of reaching for a chocolate bar as comfort food, use stress management techniques such as meditation, yoga, a warm bath or shower, listening to calming music, phoning a friend or taking a brisk walk.

Causes of food cravings: Ravenous hunger.

It is natural, and indeed beneficial, to feel some peckishness or mild hunger between meals. However if you allow that hunger to escalate into ravenous hunger, your Inner Guardian is likely to start screaming, "You're starving! You need energy, fast! Grab the nearest high Calorie food and eat it!"

Ravenous hunger is such a powerful sensation that it can override your good intentions to eat only nutritious, Calorie-sparse foods. When you are in the grip of ravenous hunger, willpower is not enough. Your biochemicals are driving you to reach for the nearest Calorie-dense food and cram as much as possible of it into your mouth as fast as possible.

Ravenous hunger can lead to cravings for fatty, sugary, Calorie-dense foods.

Combating food cravings triggered by ravenous hunger.

If you're following the Satiety Diet and using the tips in *The Satiety Diet Weight Loss Toolkit* (book #2 in the Satiety Diet series), eventually you should get to the point at which you're rarely in danger of suffering from ravenous hunger. However, life can throw up unforeseen situations.

The answer, again is "be prepared". Planning your snacks and having them on hand at all times can help you stave off ravenous hunger and cravings. Eat these snacks only when your body tells you that your normal hunger (which is a sign you're burning fat and losing weight) is on the verge of turning into the ravenous kind.

Emergency satiety snacks should be small—preferably no more than 200 Calories.

Examples include:
- Carrot-sticks or celery-sticks with reduced-fat hummus dip.
- Chickpea snacks (see *Crispy, Creamy, Chewy: The Satiety Diet Cookbook*)
- Air-popped popcorn

It's also important not to snack all the time, and not to graze. You need to sit down to three satiating meals each day.

Causes of food cravings: Images of food.

Visions of food, whether it be the sight of real food, still photographs of food, moving images of food, drawings of food or even mental images of food conjured by words, can trigger appetite. Once triggered, appetite can turn into cravings.

Combating food cravings triggered by images of food.

If it's an image based craving, remove yourself from the images and use distraction techniques to refocus your thoughts.

Causes of food cravings: Insulin resistance.

If you often crave sugary foods, high insulin levels may be preventing you from losing weight. Ask your doctor to test you for insulin resistance.

Combating food cravings triggered by insulin resistance.

If your doctor has diagnosed you with insulin resistance, you may be placed on medication. Apart from drugs, there are things you can do yourself, to help control this issue, such as:
- Exercise regularly.
- Eat foods that are low in sugar and high in protein, fiber, and complex carbohydrates.
- Keep away from highly-processed, refined carbohydrates.
- Lose weight.
- Always get a good night's sleep.

Causes of food cravings: Your microbiome.

As discussed, each adult human has up to 2kg (4.4 pounds) of microbes living in their gut. They are essential for the healthy functioning of our bodies, and even play a vital role in the health of our minds. Collectively, the helpful microbes that live in and on our bodies are known as our "microbiome". The microbiome has been shown to affect disease, allergies and obesity.

It is thought that your body mass could be associated with the types of microbes living in your gut. Gut microbes may also affect food cravings.

The "second brain" of the gut microbiome is powerful!

As mentioned earlier, your body has a "second brain", and it's in your gut. The proper name for this "mini-brain" is "the enteric nervous system", and it's one of the main divisions of the nervous system; a network of neurons that regulates the operation of the gastrointestinal system.

The mini-brain in the gut and the brain in your skull are constantly sending signals back and forth to each other along what is called the "gut-brain axis". These signals are powerful. They can affect your health, your mood and even your behavior! They can prompt you to feel uplifted or depressed, they may persuade you to reach out to grab another bite of sugary, fatty food, and they may even govern your food cravings.

Fortunately, if you become aware of the power of your microbiome and how it works, you might be able to use that power to help you lose weight.

Different families of gut microbes can persuade you to eat different foods.

Down there in the gut, millions of tiny organisms are living and feeding and reproducing and dying. Different families (genera) of gut microbes thrive on different nutrients, so it's worth their while to try to persuade you to eat the foods that contain the nutrients they prefer! This sounds far-fetched at first glance, but remember that our microorganisms evolved in partnership with us. They evolved as we evolved. As with anything that evolves, the species that manage to obtain the best sustenance for themselves tend to be the most successful survivors. It's in the best interests of your microbes to tell you to eat the foods they like best!

Some microbe families can eat almost anything, but others require specialized nutrition—for example, dietary fiber, or certain fats, or carbohydrates.

But how can they tell you what to eat?

355

When microbes consume nutrients, they produce by-products called metabolites. These metabolites include several neuroactive agents—that is, substances that can affect or directly interact with your nervous system. These substances can be tiny enough to actually pass from your bloodstream into your brain. That's how your gut microbiome can "talk" to your brain, and in fact to your whole body.

The clever microbes can do more than that. They can, directly or indirectly, produce molecules that can mimic your body's own natural hunger or satiety hormones.

Your body, however, is also clever. If it detects fake hormones circulating about, it can manufacture antibodies against the fakes. This is because it's in your body's best interests to have total control over your hunger and satiety. The problem is, sometimes the antibodies get confused about which are the real hormones and which are the fakes. They may battle against the real ones.

So, not only can microbes influence your appetite, they can also affect your body's auto-immune response.

The gut microbiome can influence your moods.

The gut and its microbes produce approximately 30 neurotransmitters, including more than 50% of the dopamine in your body and around 90% of your serotonin. [Eisenhofer et al., (1997); Kim & Camilleri (2000)]

Both dopamine and serotonin play important roles in the management of the way you eat. [Koopman et al., (2016)]

Anxiety, stress, and depression have been shown to be associated with the gut microbiota. [De Palma et al (2015)] [Mahony et al., (2009)]

Feeling anxious, stressed or depressed is also linked with a greater risk of cravings for eating junk food or other food that is low in nutrition and often high in Calories. [Oliver et al., (2000)]

A healthy microbiome can help change bad habits.

Your microbiome is also thought to have an effect on your brain's capacity to adapt and develop and grow new pathways. [Olsen (2011)] And it is the brain's ability to alter that gives you the chance to change old habits and form new ones.

How to harness the power of your gut microbiome to combat food cravings.

The study of the microbes that live in the gut is still relatively new, but we know we can affect our microbiomes with lifestyle changes.

- Choose from a wide variety of foods
- Eat plenty of all types of fiber
- Eat some naturally fermented foods
- Avoid highly-processed, refined foods
- Exercise regularly

Causes of food cravings: Circadian rhythms.

Many people experience a strong desire for a sweet biscuit or a sugary beverage in the middle of the morning or the middle of the afternoon—or both. These are times in the circadian cycle when your energy is at its lowest.

Your blood sugar is regulated by daily fluctuations in hormones called glucocorticoids, which synchronize the biological clock.

"Glucose tolerance" refers to your body's ability to metabolize glucose. A glucose tolerance test measures how well your body's cells are able to absorb glucose, or sugar, after you ingest a given amount of sugar.

According to many studies, your 24-hour circadian clock plays a leading role in human glucose tolerance; for example, your glucose tolerance decreases during the evening hours[35]. This is probably because your Inner Guardian is expecting you to obey your melatonin signals and go to sleep when darkness falls. If you're asleep, you're

---

35   This puts shift workers at greater risk of diabetes.

not eating, so you don't need high glucose tolerance. Your glucose tolerance levels always drop during the evening, no matter whether you work throughout the night in well-lit surroundings, or go to sleep in a dark bedroom. [Morris et al., (2015)]

Combating food cravings triggered by circadian rhythms.

As mentioned, many people crave for Calorie-dense foods in the afternoon, around 3pm. There are many reasons this might be so.

* Eating Calorie-dense foods in the afternoon may have become a habit. If snacking on cookies during the afternoon has become part of your routine, it can be a habit that's hard to break. Be prepared by planning ahead and having delicious, satisfying whole-food snacks on hand. Gradually, over time, wean yourself off the junk and swap it for the whole, low-Calorie, low-GI foods. Also read our Satiety Diet tips on how to break bad habits and create good habits.

* Your blood sugar levels may be low. Foods containing carbohydrates, especially sugars, are a common target for cravings. Cravings can often occur because of a drop in blood sugar levels. The body needs to bring the level of blood sugar back to a higher level, so it sends out "craving signals", prompting you to seek Calorie-rich foods that will provide an instant fix.

However, if you eat those foods your blood sugar levels can rocket sky-high for a while before plummeting down again. They may drop even lower, leaving you even hungrier than before you ate.

The answer to this problem is the same as the answer above; turn to delicious, satisfying, Calorie-sparse whole-foods.

* You've skipped breakfast, or lunch, or both. If you've been busy all day without having eaten anything nutritious and satisfying, your body is not getting the nutritional support it needs, so by the time the afternoon comes around, your Inner Guardian sends out those craving signals. As a result, you are more likely to compensate by grabbing a quick, Calorie-dense nutrient-empty, processed snack.

We're not saying that eating a good meal of good food earlier in the day will guarantee you don't get the afternoon slump cravings—but it will make it less likely.

* **You haven't had enough sound, restful sleep.** Being sleep-deficient has a powerful effect on your appetite and cravings. Often, what you read as hunger-signals are actually tiredness-signals. Lack of sleep raises the body's levels of ghrelin (the hunger hormone) and decreases the levels of leptin (the satiety hormone).By the time the afternoon rolls around, you are starting to feel even more tired, and that's when you're tempted to grab the nearest junk food.

The solution—read our section on how to get better sleep. And act on it!

A tool for dealing with the circadian blood sugar slump.

Chris Clarke says: "Almost every day I experience a craving for sweet foods in the middle of the morning (at around 10:30) and again in the middle of the afternoon (around 3:30). My body seems quite clear about its own blood-sugar circadian rhythm.

It's no use my trying to deny the craving, because if I don't eat something sweet at those times I either end up desperately wanting to chew on anything even remotely edible, or I eat a lot of non-sweet foods that don't "hit the spot" to really satisfy the craving, and which probably have the same number of Calories as a small sweet treat in any case.

My solution is to answer the sweetness call, because I know I can't win anyway. But instead of ripping open a chocolate bar, I mindfully eat a low-sweetness, high protein snack, sweetened with a little low-fructose fruit or rice malt syrup. I take as long to eat it as possible, and really savor every mouthful so that my demanding Inner Guardian will really get the message that I've obeyed its command to consume something sweet. And then it can stop harassing me!

One of my favorite snacks is creamy white bean 'chocolate blancmange' sprinkled with a few walnuts for crunchiness."

Causes of food cravings: Hypoglycemia without diabetes.

If your blood sugar levels sometimes drop too low, you might have a condition called hypoglycemia. Hypoglycemia occurs in diabetics, but people without diabetes can get it, too.

As you know, your body produces insulin when you eat foods containing sugars. Insulin's purpose is to break down the sugar so that you can absorb it and use it for energy. Sometimes the insulin-sugar ratio in the body becomes unbalanced. If your body is not very good at stabilizing your blood sugar levels, or if it produces too much insulin after meals, too much of your blood sugar is broken down and you're left with levels that are too low.

Both adults and children can be hypoglycemic without being diabetic. Some people can have hypoglycemia without being aware of it. Others may suffer symptoms such as light-headedness, ravenous hunger, difficulty focusing on the task at hand, foggy thinking, irritability, weakness and headaches.

If you feel hungry within an hour or two of having eaten a filling meal, you might have "reactive hypoglycemia". It means your body is producing too much insulin. People with reactive hypoglycemia may be at risk for developing diabetes.

Non-reactive hypoglycemia occurs not in response to meals, but to other causes such as drinking too much alcohol, pregnancy, certain prescription medications, some eating disorders, pancreatic tumors (this is rare), hormone deficiencies and problems with the liver, heart, or kidneys.

People are most at risk of developing non-diabetic hypoglycemia if they are obese, have other health issues, or are related to diabetics. Stomach surgery to alleviate the symptoms of gastroesophageal reflux disease (GERD) can increase the risk of it, too.

If you think you might have non-diabetic hypoglycemia, consult your doctor right away. It is essential to control this problem in the long-term, because if left untreated it can cause health issues.

Combating food cravings triggered by hypoglycemia without diabetes.

You can guard against non-diabetic hypoglycemia. We recommend the following tips:

- Choose a variety of foods that are rich in protein, fiber, and complex carbohydrates.
- Avoid foods that are sugar-rich, high GI or made with refined, highly-processed ingredients.
- Plan meals and snacks ahead of time, to ensure you don't reach the stage of "ravenous hunger". This can help keep your blood sugar levels from plummeting.

Mental imagery and food cravings.

Mental imagery is at the heart of food cravings.

Dr. Robert Pretlow, a pediatrician and child obesity specialist, says that cravings are a vicious cycle of:

- stress, which induces the craving,
- more stress as a consequence of trying to resist the craving,
- more craving, as a result,
- until the person finally gives in, eats the food, then feels distressed, which provokes more stress ...

... and so the cycle repeats.

But this stressful cycle can be broken, by diverting the craver's attention.

How does this work?

One promising area of research focuses on the benefits of mental imagery as a tool to reduce food cravings.

Cravings are almost always accompanied by a mental image. Studies have shown that when people experience a craving for a certain food, they vividly picture the way the food looks, and how it tastes and smells. (They don't usually imagine the way it sounds!) [May et al., (2014); May et al., (2004); May et al., (2008); Tiggemann & Kemps (2005)]

In other studies, researchers have been able to actually induce food cravings by directing participants to imagine a visual image of themselves eating their favorite food. [Green et al., (2000)]

Mental pictures of a food's appearance, taste and smell are ". . . at the very heart of the craving experience".
[Kemps & Tiggemann (2014)]

How to use mental imagery to combat food cravings.

The intensity of food cravings can be reduced by distracting your thoughts in certain ways. Because your food cravings are strongly linked to vivid mental images of the food's look, taste and smell, you can dampen those cravings by disrupting the mental images. To combat cravings, you must occupy the same areas of the brain that were generating the food images, with images of other things. So for example, instead of picturing the craving-inducing appearance of food, you could imagine (or actually look at) a non-food image. When a person experiencing the craving substitutes a non-food related mental image, the food image is disrupted. Your mind can only really focus on one image at a time, so if you swap food imaginings for a different mental picture, the "craving image" disintegrates.

These non-food mental images are called "competing cognitive tasks".

". . . evidence from numerous laboratory studies has shown that engaging in a range of visual tasks can reduce food cravings. For example, imagining a series of non-food scenes (e.g., a rainbow) has been shown to reduce cravings for food in general, and for chocolate in particular." [Kemps & Tiggemann (2014); Kemps & Tiggemann (2017); [Steel et al, (2006)]

Visualizing a set of non-food images has been shown to reduce cravings for food in general, and especially for chocolate. [Harvey et al., (2005); Kemps & Tiggeman (2007)]

This seems obvious when you remember that simply thinking of food, and imagining it, can make you feel hungry. Combating cravings by thinking of non-food images is just doing the reverse. [Harvey et al., (2005)]

"… Other visual tasks, such as making hand or eye movements, watching a dynamic visual noise array, constructing shapes from modeling clay, and playing a game of 'Tetris', have also been shown to reduce food cravings." [Kemps & Tiggemann (2014); Littel et al., (2016); Knäuper et al., (2011)]

Dynamic visual noise can help curb food cravings.

"Dynamic visual noise" (DVN) is a flickering and meaningless display of pale dots or specks in motion against a dark background without any pattern or purpose. It is sometimes called "white noise".

Watching a display of DVN is another way of disrupting mental images of food and helping cravings to subside. [May et al., (2010)]

The random movement of the dancing dots distracts your attention from images of food, while the lack of any meaning or pattern does not provide anything to focus on. It provides an alternative target for your concentration. DVN also can help combat other cravings, such as the desire for nicotine.

DVN has a kind of hypnotizing quality. Watching the flickering, content-free movement can put you in a relaxed, almost trance-like state. Watching DVN can be calming and stress reducing. Relaxation reduces stress, which adds to the effect of breaking the craving cycle.

A number of studies have shown that your ability to retain an imaginary picture in your mind is disrupted when we look at DVN.

"…dynamic visual noise," say researchers, "may provide a useful tool for controlling problematic cravings in clinically overweight or obese individuals who are actively trying to lose weight." [Kemps et al., (2007); [Kemps and Tiggemen (2013)]

Where can we get some of this DVN?
- There are DVN apps available for your mobile device.
- Free online video sharing websites offer DVN clips of varying quality.

Other methods to combat food cravings.

You can significantly reduce your cravings—and your food intake —by doing one or several of the following things to deflect food cravings every time they hit:

- Instead of imagining the smell of your craved-for food, imagine a non-food smell. Imagine you're sniffing a non-food scent such as a flower's fragrance, furniture polish, eucalyptus oil or fresh paint.
- Alternatively, you can actually waft a bottle of non-food scents beneath your nose. Essential oils such as jasmine, camphor, cedarwood, cypress etc. can be enough to decrease food cravings. So if you want to use psychology to counteract cravings, use your imagination or break out a scent bottle. Make sure you don't use a delicious, food-related scent such as vanilla, cinnamon, orange etc!
- Start performing a task with your hands—one that requires your visual concentration. Handicrafts can be a good diversionary activity.
- Imagine you're occupied with your favorite activity (other than eating!)
- Watch dynamic visual noise on a device such as a computer tablet (there are videos on the Internet that can deliver this).
- Use a smartphone app that prompts you to imagine a non-food visual scene as a craving-disruption.
- You could even play a computer game called Tetris. It's been shown to focus and distract the mind enough to help reduce cravings. [Skorka-Brown et al., (2014)]

Note that the effect of using these craving-suppressant tools does not last for longer than the occasion on which you use them. The effect does not continue for the next few hours or days or weeks—it only works each time you use it for a particular craving.

This means you need to use the tool again, next time you have a craving, and each time after that.

The good news is that the effectiveness of these craving-curbing techniques does not decrease with repetition. Each time you use them they will be just as effective as the last time.

Craving-suppressant tools like those listed here should be used as an adjunct to other techniques. They may not completely overcome cravings, all by themselves. They might only help to dull the cravings, not completely eliminate them.

One of the great advantages of these techniques is that most of them require very little effort on your part. You can use your imagination in most circumstances, without needing any props. When these techniques do require props, they can be small objects, easily transported in your pocket or handbag, such as tiny bottles of scent or essential oils, or "food craving apps" or games of "Tetris" that can be stored on a smartphone.

If you're not near a source of DVN or a device on which you can play games, you can use your own powers of imagination to interrupt cravings, or build something out of modeling clay, another technique which has been shown to be effective.

Sweetness cravings after a meal.

Many people crave for dessert at the end of a meal. This holds true even if the meal was composed of healthful vegetables and high quality proteins.

Traditionally, dessert is a sweet dish and it's eaten last. There are good reasons for this. Some say the desire for sweet food after eating savory food is a culturally conditioned phenomenon—that is, it's a tradition in certain human societies.

But there is more to it.

When you eat food, your body breaks down any sugars to their simplest forms, such as glucose, galactose and fructose. These simple sugars pass into your bloodstream. Your body then releases insulin, which tells your muscles, liver and fatty tissues to extract glucose from your blood and store it in your body as glycogen.

Gradually the insulin rids your blood of its extra glucose (blood sugar), until your glucose levels return to normal. However, if your body has released more insulin than was required to deal with the amount of extra glucose in your blood, it can make your blood sugar levels drop *below* normal, and this is where the problem lies.

When your Inner Guardian senses that your blood sugar levels are lower than normal, it sends out a message: "You need to eat something sweet and sugary".

And you end up with a sugar craving.

Assuming you have not been diagnosed as hypoglycemic, insulin-resistant or diabetic, it's fine to eat a small amount of sweet food after a meal, if you are beset with sugar cravings. Research tells us that people feel more satisfied when a meal ends with a sweet course, and this decreases the probability that they might want to eat snacks later.

With these provisos:

- Delay eating dessert for 10 to 15 minutes. This gives your digestive system time to properly register the food you've eaten at the main meal, and generate satiety signals.
- Sweet dishes made from low fructose fruits, grains, nuts, seeds and vegetables are preferable because fructose can increase your appetite.
- Rice malt syrup is a sweetener that contains no fructose.
- Certain sweeteners such as stevia and erythritol may be used in small quantities, if you wish. See our section on "Sweeteners".
- If you choose to consume sugar, eat it in its natural, unprocessed, unrefined form.
- Train yourself to be accustomed to mild sweetness, instead of overly-sweet foods. Japanese confectionery (wagashi) and desserts are low in sugar. They have been eaten for hundreds of years by the people of Japan, a country which has one of the leanest populations.
- Eating sweet foods in conjuncion with fiber and protein is preferable.

366

Desserts to eat in moderation:

For a low-fructose, satisfying, natural, sweet and fruity dessert eaten in one sitting, choose from one of the following:

- a medium sized fresh banana or frozen, puréed banana ('banana ice cream').
- up to 60g blueberries.
- up to 160g cantaloupe (rock melon),
- carambola, clementine, kumquats, lemon, lime, mandarin, orange, dragonfruit, durian, guavas, passionfruit, pawpaw, prickly pear, pineapple, peeled plantain, raspberries, strawberries, rhubarb, starfruit,
- up to 1/4 cup fresh coconut
- up to 150g grapes.
- 2 small, peeled kiwi fruit.
- up to 10 longans.
- up to 90g honeydew melon.
- up to 10g tamarind.

You can mix and match desserts with small dollops of the following toppings/ingredients:

- Macadamia nuts, walnuts, brazil nuts, peanuts, pecans pine nuts, poppy seeds, sesame seeds, pumpkin seeds, and sunflower seeds. All raw and natural, not roasted.
- Low-fat vegan cream, whipped silken tofu, yoghurt, cottage cheese or ricotta.

Avoid artificial sweeteners, because they are thought to increase appetite. Use the following sweeteners in the recommended portions:

- 1 tbsp rice malt syrup
- 2 sachets (2g) pure stevia powder
- A stevia/erythritol blend such as Natvia®
- 1 tbsp brown sugar, palm sugar or raw sugar
- 1 tbsp CSR® Smart Sugar Blend (cane sugar blended with stevia)
- Up to 2 squares of dark chocolate

Examples of low-sweetness satiety desserts include Brown Rice Pudding or Japanese Pumpkin Pie.

Stress-induced sugar cravings.

Eating less sugar can be good for both your brain and your waistline.

But how can you deal with stress-induced sugar cravings?

Cravings for sweet foods can be triggered by such factors as circadian rhythms, blood sugar levels or a need for protein. They can also be triggered by stress, and that's what we're discussing here.

If stress is triggering your cravings for sweet, sugary foods, (or even for other "comfort" foods/beverages such as fatty or salty foods, or alcohol), learning how to deal with the stress in a new way can help.

Willpower alone is not sufficient to defeat the powerful ancient survival mechanisms of the brain that have worked for millennia to preserve the human race. Once you understand how these mechanisms operate, you will be empowered to work with them, instead of against them.

Eating sugary foods when you are stressed is actually a great way to survive—that is, if you're a human living in pre-modern times. It's not such a good idea when you're living in the 21st century, surrounded by easily-accessible Calorie-dense foods.

Stress causes your body to release cortisol and other hormones that, in the short term can help you, but over a long period of time can damage your health. To offset the harm wreaked by stress hormones, the Inner Guardian compels you to seek pleasure. When you experience pleasure, your body releases chemicals such as the mood-stabilizing hormone serotonin and endorphins (neurotrans-mitters that are natural stress and pain antidotes). By adhering to receptors in the brain, these compounds can decrease the harmful effect of chronic exposure to stress hormones.

The worse and more prolonged the stress is, the more powerful is the urge to offset it by finding pleasure.

Pleasure may be gained in various ways, some harmless and beneficial, others potentially not so good. The latter can include:
- consuming alcohol
- consuming sweet foods
- consuming other comfort foods
- gambling

Many pleasures can be addictive. Some can lead to weight gain. (And of course gambling can lead to financial problems which in turn can cause more stress).

Regular, long-term sugar consumption changes your brain—not in a good way! Research conducted by Professor Selena Bartlett from Queensland University of Technology's Institute of Health and Biomedical Innovation indicates that sugar could act in your body like a drug of addiction, and that regular, long-term sucrose consumption, like smoking and alcoholism, causes actual changes in the brain. So that when you eat sugary foods on a daily basis, over time, you need to eat more and more to experience the same level of pleasure. You develop a real "sugar tolerance."

"Excess sugar consumption has been shown to contribute directly to weight gain, thus contributing to the growing worldwide obesity epidemic. Interestingly, increased sugar consumption has been shown to repeatedly elevate dopamine levels in the . . . reward pathway of the brain, similar to many drugs of abuse." [Shariff et al., (2016)]

Not only can addictive substances change your brain and lead to tolerance, they can also cause disorders of the nervous system and the mind, affecting your mood and motivation. Sugar triggers the release of dopamine, which binds to receptors in your brain in the same way as alcohol and nicotine. Regular consumption of sugar, alcohol and nicotine alters the brain, leading to the need to consume more and more to feel the same level of pleasure.

"Just like alcohol and nicotine," says Professor Bartlett, "a sudden decrease in sugar consumption will lead to withdrawal symptoms and cravings."

Yes, you can really get "sugar withdrawal symptoms".

Combating sugar cravings.

So how can you break free of the cycle of bingeing, withdrawal, craving and bingeing again?

Think of the stress-sugar cycle like this: Trigger-Behavior-Reward.

- Trigger; a stressful event occurs and you feel bad.
- Behavior; you reach for the chocolate/candy/ice cream etc.
- Reward; you feel pleasure, and the bad feelings temporarily fade.

The problem is, the sugary reward in this case is only a short-term reward. In the long term it leads to weight gain, which is not a reward but a "punishment". And that punishment can lead to more stress…

You can't remove all triggers. Stressful events are always going to happen at times in your life.

But you can change the way you respond to triggers. You can break the cycle by changing the behavior that rewards you.

Step 1: Recognise the moment in which a stressful situation is triggering your urge to eat sugary foods, (or smoke, or drink, or whatever your pleasure source may be). Acknowledge and identify that this is a feeling produced by chemicals in your brain. It's not a feeling you get because you are a weak, bad person with no willpower! It is a powerful, compelling drive springing from an ancient area of your brain; an imperative that was originally designed to protect you.

Step 2: Replace your usual (unwanted) response with a better one. But what can possibly make you feel as good as that chocolate bar or that drink? Believe it or not, your body and your brain will get a surge of pleasure if you move your body and make your heart beat faster. You can indulge in high intensity exercise such as running or skipping or a series of rapid push-ups, or dancing. Even brisk walking can help. If for any reason it's impossible to do any of those things, try stretching, or deep breathing. Moving feels good! When you were a child you used to love running and playing. Your body remembers that, deep down. Moving not only feels good—it floods your body with the natural chemicals of pleasure (endorphins, serotonin etc) which reward and heal your brain.

If you repeat Steps 1 and 2 consistently, it becomes a habit. Your brain changes back to its normal, healthy mode. Sugar tolerance fades.

BAD HABITS CAN REWIRE YOUR BRAIN
BUT
GOOD HABITS CAN HEAL YOUR BRAIN

... and when your brain gets back to normal, good habits become much easier!

For more information on breaking a food addiction see our section on "Willpower and Creating Good Habits" and our section on "Food Addiction".

Helping to curb chocolate cravings.

Many people are prone to intense cravings for chocolate. Here are some suggestions for dealing with those insistent demands from your body!

- Stay away from images of chocolate, reminders of chocolate, the word chocolate being spoken within your hearing, or even the word chocolate written down. In fact, after you've read this section in this book, just remember it and try not to look at it again! As Chris Clark says: "One of my biggest chocolate-eating triggers is that wonderful movie I love so much—*Chocolat* starring Juliette Binoche. Whenever I watch it, I have to have a chocolate stash on hand. I just go crazy for chocolate, because of seeing so much of it on screen!"
- Don't just deny the cravings and hope they will go away by themselves. They *might* go away, but more likely they will plague you until you give in and eat chocolate... and then more chocolate... and more... and you might end up bingeing on chocolate. Recognize the cravings and do something about them. Preferably go for a run!

- Mindfully eat a chocolatey food that's not as Calorie-dense as an actual chocolate bar, and which has many of the same characteristics. An example is Satiety Diet Chocolate Pudding, which can be made with cocoa/cacao for flavor, puréed white beans for protein and fiber, oat bran for extra viscosity, fiber and protein, and either rice malt syrup or erythritol/stevia, with some coarsely chopped almonds thrown in to offset the velvety creaminess with crunchiness.

- If you really must eat chocolate, then instead of reaching for a whole block of milk chocolate, eat 2 small pieces of dark chocolate that contains a minimum of 70% cocoa. This will satisfy those cravings better, according to 2011 research published in *Nutrition and Diabetes*. Dark chocolate's bitterness helps trigger the release of satiety hormones, and its stearic acid content acts to slow down the process of digestion and keep you feeling fuller for longer. [Sørensen & Astrup (2011)]

RESET YOUR NATURAL APPETITE

How do you know if you are really hungry?

And how can you tell if you are really experiencing satiety?

To reset your natural appetite, you have to re-learn to listen to your body.

CHILDREN ARE ATTUNED TO THEIR BODIES' SIGNALS

Many nutritionists say that healthy children are born with an ability to listen to their body and choose the foods they need. They appear to have an inborn nutrition-seeking mechanism that can guide them to make the right food choices.

In a well-known experiment conducted in the early 20th century, researcher Clara M. Davis observed infants from six months to 11 months who had never been given any food other than their mothers' breast-milk.

372

When the infants were provided with a wide range of healthful foods and allowed to freely eat of whatever foods they liked in whatever quantities they liked, they chose the foods containing the nutrients their bodies required. They intuitively selected a balanced diet, with precisely the nutrition and energy to supply their individual needs on a daily basis. Even the influential pediatrician Dr. Spock supported this principle. [Davis (1928)]

Modern day researchers aren't convinced by Davis's theory, but it makes sense to imagine that most of us were born with an innate ability to recognize our own hunger and satiety signals. Infants and toddlers generally push away food when they've had enough to eat. As they grow older, other experiences can override and erode that inner wisdom.[36] As adults we can, however, re-learn it.

When you deliberately become aware of your physical, mental and emotional state, you are more likely to be able to tune in to your body's real needs.

Everyone is different, so it's a matter of re-learning to listen to your own body.

FACTORS THAT MAY OVERRIDE YOUR NATURAL APPETITE.

Many of us have lost touch with the signals our bodies send to us. We may eat at the times we are accustomed to eating—not necessarily when we are actually hungry. You may eat certain foods purely from habit—not because your body is telling you you need that food.

---

36 Note that some people retain, at least partially, the ability to hear what their Inner Guardian is telling them about nutrition. Women may crave chocolate and spinach in the week leading up to their menstrual period. Green leafy vegetables can provide the iron their bodies need to replace the iron-rich blood they are about to lose. Almost half the American women studied in dozens of articles on cravings, reported that they experienced intense chocolate cravings during the few days before and the first couple of days of menstruation. It is sometimes claimed that premenstrual chocolate cravings are a culturally-induced craving, but perhaps they are the body's signal that it needs the psychoactive substances found in chocolate such as theobromine, caffeine, phenylethyl-amine (PEA), and anandamide. These compounds have a huge impact on the brain and may help counteract premenstrual dysphoric disorder. Chocolate also contains substances that are similar to the female hormone estrogen.

It's likely that during the years since you left childhood, you've been learning to ignore your Inner Guardian's signals. Certain events and situations override your natural appetite rhythms. Instead of ceasing to eat because you'd receive sufficient nutrition and energy, you learned to stop eating because:

- you'd cleaned your plate
- you'd had your usual number of courses
- you'd consumed your diet portion
- someone told you to
- you thought you ought to
- cultural pressures made you feel obligated to fast
- you didn't like the food
- there wasn't enough food
- according to the clock, it was time to stop

Or a myriad other reasons. But hardly ever (except when a child) because you were *satisfied*.

Similarly, instead of eating because you felt hungry, you learned to eat because:

- your plate still had food on it
- you felt obliged to eat at least part of every course in a meal
- someone commanded you to
- you thought you ought to
- cultural pressures made you feel obligated to feast
- easily available food was fatty, sugary and tempting
- food was available—visible and within easy reach
- food was plentiful
- according to the clock, it was time to eat
- you smelled food
- you saw food, or images of food

If people are indeed born with an innate ability to seek a diet of balanced nutrients, why do they tend to lose touch with it as they grow from babies to toddlers and through adolescence into adulthood? Being exposed to processed food, junk food, obesogens and food advertising probably has something to do with it.

Some examples: You find it hard to stop eating salty chips/crisps because you are really craving protein. With their savory, umami flavor, salty chips are a "protein decoy".

Or you eat excessive amounts of sugar because you ate something sugary earlier in the day, and it produced a spike in your blood sugar levels, followed by a sharp fall and the resulting hunger surge.

LISTENING TO YOUR BODY

Listening to your Inner Guardian and understanding its body-speech can help you lose weight. Fortunately it is possible to reset your body's natural appetite by gradually switching to eating only "real foods". It may take a few weeks to really restore that healthy balance, but it's worth the journey—because when your appetite is back to normal and you are listening to your body's silent but powerful demands for various nutrients, you will be free to follow a satisfying diet and shed excess pounds.

Start listening to your body's signals again. Be patient and persistent. It will take you some time to get used to acknowledging them, interpreting them and responding to them.

1. Tune in to your appetite.

Tune in to your appetite, as you did when you were a little child. If you feel like ordering a vegetarian dish when everyone else is having meat, go right ahead. If you feel like eating oatmeal for lunch instead of breakfast, go with your inclinations. You don't have to eat what everyone else is eating, or eat certain foods at certain times.

2. Don't cut out entire food groups.

If you feel a strong urge to eat a certain food and you have to use a lot of willpower to resist the urge, you could be sending your Inner Guardian into a panic! Diets that cut out entire food groups can set you up for failure.

3. Don't deprive yourself.

Free yourself from food restrictions by tuning in to your body's needs. Give yourself permission to eat whatever you want whenever you genuinely feel hungry—as long as you choose suitably small portions of any foods that are Calorie-dense, and eat them mindfully.

4. Accept that every day is nutritionally different.

For your body's nutritional needs, every day is different. The food that satisfied you yesterday at 3 o'clock will not necessarily do the same today at 3 o'clock. For your body, every day is slightly different. Your energy and nutrient needs vary daily, depending on the complex interplay of nuanced variables in your environment, such as:

— the things you did that day

— the emotions you felt

— your time of the month (men too)

— the amount of nutrition in the food you ate yesterday or last week. Food nutrition is never static; even a potato's nutrition varies imperceptibly depending on where it was grown, what the season was like, when it was harvested how far it has travelled to your plate etc. We can't always tell the difference, but the body can. The body's Inner Guardian knows what nutrients you lack, and it tries to tell you. You may not be listening, or you might be led astray. For example, when your Inner Guardian tries to tell you you need protein, you might eat a protein decoy—a food that tastes like protein but isn't. Your senses are saying, "This must be protein, because it tastes like protein," but your body is saying, "It may taste like protein, but down here in the digestive system we are not receiving any protein. Eat more protein!" And that is why you end up eating a whole bag of potato chips/crisps.

5. Don't eat unless you are hungry.

This seems logical, especially if you want to lose weight, but due to our busy daily schedules it's not always easy or possible to obey your body's signals. If possible, in the mornings, don't eat an early meal unless you are hungry. If you really are hungry when you get up in the morning, then do have breakfast, but make sure you eat a Satiety Breakfast in a mindful way, including only foods that will help you achieve satiety.

Plan, plan, plan! Be organised to ensure you have all your satiety meals ready to assemble or cook, and all your satiety snacks ready to eat.

6. Embrace hunger, instead of being frightened of it.

You could be undermining your weight loss efforts because you're scared of your natural hunger signals.

Unfortunately many people panic and seek food, as soon as they start to feel hungry. The moment you feel the first niggling sign of hunger there's no need to grab a packet of cookies right away. Your body is built to tolerate hunger. Besides, when you allow yourself to fast between meals you can lose weight, as well as improving your blood pressure, cholesterol and insulin sensitivity.

7. Identify your own feelings of real hunger.

Earlier in this book, we divided hunger into four levels.
- Level 1: False hunger (thoughts of food that are emotionally or cognitively induced)
- Level 2: Peckishness (low-level "real" hunger)
- Level 3: Mild hunger (mid-level "real" hunger)
- Level 4: Ravenous hunger (high-level "real" hunger)

You can learn to differentiate between the different kinds of hunger you feel.

Some signs associated with peckishness:
- Feeling bored
- Having a desire to experience a flavor or texture
- Experiencing thirst
- Eating at a certain time of day due to habit
- Feeling upset or stressed and wanting to "comfort eat"

377

Signs of real hunger include:

- A rumbling stomach
- Intrusive, compelling thoughts of food
- A feeling of light-headedness

Signs of satiety include:

- Stomach feeling full
- Feeling satisfied
- Not feeling a strong desire to eat any more

Become aware of your body's hunger and satiety signs. Next time you sit down to eat a meal[37], really focus on your physical feelings.

Let's say you are about to eat a High Satiety Meal, with the appropriate combinations of macronutrients, textures, colors, tableware design, a calm environment etc.

First, make a mental note of your hunger levels before eating.

Then take note of the way your body responds while you mindfully eat the meal, taking at least 20 minutes to do so. Remember that meals lasting for an hour are preferable, as they are more likely to provide optimum satiety.

Notice your body's feedback after you've finished the meal. Ideally, you should feel replete, content, relaxed and satisfied, but not overfull, gorged or bloated. You should have no desire to eat any more food.

> Chris Clark says: "I have a self-test to find out if what I am feeling is real hunger or just peckishness. Celery is a vegetable I don't like very much. So I say to myself 'Am I hungry enough to eat a stalk of celery?' and if the answer is 'Yes,' then I know my hunger is real!"

---

37   . . . and all meals should be eaten while sitting down—not while standing up, or walking, or driving, or lying down etc.

Under normal circumstances, around two hours after you've finished your meal you might start feeling a little peckish. If you reached satiety at that last meal, you should not be feeling really hungry yet.

Three to four hours after finishing the meal you will probably be feeling the signs of increasing hunger. Of course this can vary from person to person. It also depends on your environment, your level of physical activity and a number of other variables such as whether you are bored, stressed, excited and so on.

After 4 hours have elapsed it's likely that you really are hungry. You're probably experiencing all those hunger signals again. This is a good time to sit down and mindfully eat satiating foods.

If you deny the demands of your appetite and put off eating, your hunger levels are likely to increase. By denying yourself food when you are hungry, you are telling your Inner Guardian that there's a food shortage. In response, your Inner Guardian ramps up the urgent hunger signals, predisposing you to reach for high-energy (Calorie-dense) foods, to make up for what it perceives as a scarcity of energy sources. The risk of you making bad food choices escalates. This is when good planning pays off; if you have delicious, nutritious, low-Calorie foods close at hand, you can reach for them instead.

In conclusion: Being aware of your body's hunger and satiety signals can help you lose weight.

- Eating when you are not hungry is a recipe for weight gain.
- Feeling peckish or mildly hungry between meals is fine.
- Eating a lot of food in response to merely feeling peckish or mildly hungry is not a good idea.
- It's advantageous to wait until you are truly hungry before you eat.
- However it's disadvantageous to put off eating until you feel ravenous, because then you are more likely to overeat.

8. Use mindfulness meditation.

Researchers have found that "mindfulness meditation", focussing on your body, can lead you to tune in to your body's appetite signals. This form of mediation can help you recognise whether you are hungry or full. [van de Veer et al., (2015)]

They wrote, ". . . after a mindful body meditation, consumers are more aware of physiological cues that develop after [eating a meal] rather than of the amount they have previously eaten.

"Furthermore ... only mindful attention with a focus on the body [instead of the environment] stimulates compensation for previous consumption and awareness of satiety cues."

Broadly speaking, in order to meditate mindfully focussing on the body, you would:

- Go to a calm place that is free from distractions.
- Sit or lie in a comfortable position
- Close your eyes or unfocus your gaze.
- Relax your muscles
- Breathe slowly and deeply
- Simply let any thoughts or images that appear in your mind's eye come and go, without focusing on them.
- Pay attention to your experience of breathing.
- Simply notice how your body feels at this moment. Pay attention to its physical feelings, rhythms and pulses. Be calmly aware of your thoughts and emotions. Observe them without reacting, without judgment or expectation.
- If your mind wanders, don't worry—that's normal. Simply return your attention to your breathing, your body and your feelings.
- There's no time limit. When you feel ready, take another deep breath and gently return your attention to the outside world.

IN CONCLUSION: YOU CAN RE-SET YOUR APPETITE

Change your eating habits. Eventually you will get used to having a better relationship with food, and it will become second nature.

- Recognise real hunger.
- Satisfy hunger before it becomes ravenous.
- Trick yourself into feeling full by using visual mechanisms and controlling your environment.
- Visibility effects appetite. Put food where you can't see it unless you're ready for a proper meal.
- Teach yourself to eat smaller portions.
- Train yourself not to snack too frequently—and when you do snack, eat wisely.

MEDS THAT CAN MAKE YOU GAIN WEIGHT

Certain prescription drugs and over-the-counter medications can make you pile on the pounds. Many people are unaware of this, and wonder why they find it hard to lose weight.

Check out this list, to see whether your meds might be sabotaging your efforts. If they are, ask your doctor if you can switch to another medication that doesn't have the same side-effects. If that's not possible, simply being aware that the problem may be due to the drugs, not your "lack of willpower", can make you feel better.

The lists given here are not exhaustive. We have only mentioned some of the most common drugs. Note that we list their generic names, rather than the brand names. For example, the drug triamcinolone is sold under at least three different brand names. Check the information on the packet or ask your doctor or pharmacist if you are unsure.

Whatever you do, don't stop taking your prescribed meds without first consulting a medical practitioner!

ANTIHISTAMINES

These medicines are used relieve the symptoms of allergies, including hay fever, hives and some food intolerances.

One group of antihistamines, called H1 antagonists, are appetite stimulants, and have been linked with obesity. This applies when they are swallowed orally, as distinct from being smeared onto the skin. H1 antagonists include (but are not limited to):

- Acrivastine
- Astemizole
- Bepotastine
- Bilastine
- Cetirizine
- Desloratadine
- Ebastine
- Fexofenadine
- Ketotifen
- Levocetirizine
- Loratadine
- Mizolastine
- Quifenadine
- Rupatadine
- Terfenadine

ANTIDEPRESSANTS, SEIZURE PREVENTATIVES ETC.

- Amytriptyline
- Chlorpromazine
- Citalopram
- Fluoxetine
- Fluvoxamine
- Mirtazapine
- Nortriptyline (used to treat both pain and depression)
- Olanzapine
- Paroxetine
- Pregabalin (used to treat both seizures and pain)
- Sertraline
- Valproic Acid

CORTICOSTEROIDS

These are valuable and powerful drugs with a wide range of uses.

- Cortisone
- Dexamethasone
- Ethamethasoneb
- Fludrocortisone
- Hydrocortisone
- Methylprednisolone
- Prednisolone
- Prednisone
- Triamcinolone

DIABETES MEDICATIONS

- Chlorpropamide
- Insulin

BETA-BLOCKERS

These medications are used to treat such issues as high blood pressure, anxiety and heart problems.

- Acebutolol
- Atenolol
- Atenolol
- Metoprolol
- Propranolol

ANTIBIOTICS

Taking antibiotics causes changes in the gut microbiome. This can make laboratory mice gain weight. It is thought that the same process could happen in human beings.

PAIN RELIEVERS

- Nortriptyline (used to treat both pain and depression)
- Pregabalin (used to treat both seizures and pain)
- Opioids (may cause weight gain or weight loss)

PART FOUR

FOOD AND DRINK

UNDERSTANDING CALORIES

"Count your Calories," they say.

Oh please! Will the nagging of the weight-loss pundits ever cease?

Can't we simply shed unwanted pounds by controlling our hunger with satiety?

The simple answer: no.

It is true that while controlling your hunger is more useful for weight loss than counting Calories, it is still essential to choose mainly Calorie-sparse foods.

CALORIE ABSORPTION

The number of Calories you actually absorb from food varies a lot. In theory it doesn't matter what proportions of carbohydrate, protein and fat you include in your diet, as long as you eat fewer Calories than you use up by staying alive and moving around. Reducing your Calorie consumption is vital to weight loss.

No matter which diet you choose to follow, you will lose weight as long as the Calories you consume are fewer than the Calories your body burns.

Having said that, we must also say that the food-form in which Calories are delivered to your body can make a huge difference to weight loss.

Same number of Calories, different satiety value.

Food's satiety value can affect how much you eat.

After you eat candy, for example, you are likely to feel hungrier, sooner, than after you eat the same number of Calories in wholegrain porridge garnished with nuts and seeds.

Digesting food uses up Calories.

Your body uses different amounts of energy to digest different foods. For example a Calorie that you eat may not be equal to a Calorie available to your body. For example:

- of every 100 Calories of fat you eat, your body will have access to 98 Calories.
- of every 100 Calories of carbs you eat, your body will be able to use 90 to 95 Calories.
- of every 100 Calories of protein you eat, your body will receive only 75 Calories.

But that's only if you were eating pure fat, carbs or protein.

Food's "potential energy" varies.

You generally eat a mixture of macronutrients in your food. All foods contain energy, but the amount of potential energy stored in each food varies significantly, depending on the type of food, and not all of the Calories are available to your body. For example when you eat whole, unprocessed almonds with their skins on, about one-third of their Calories are not absorbed into the body. Instead they pass right through, undigested.

Food processing changes how many Calories you absorb.

Depending on the way you prepare you food, you can make more or fewer Calories available to your body. The more your food is processed, the more Calories it gives up to your body.

If you want to GAIN weight, some ways to INCREASE the available Calories in food is to -

- grind or pound the food to increase its surface area
- cook it (by frying, boiling, baking, grilling etc.)
- ferment it

. . . which indicates that by eating most of your food raw or only lightly-processed, you can eat the same number of Calories but absorb fewer.

(Note that many foods do need to be cooked in order to make them digestible.)

Whole foods.

Your body must use more energy to process whole foods than processed foods. Not only do processed foods give you more Calories, they use fewer Calories to be digested. Once again, whole foods win in the weight-loss stakes.

The microbiome.

The composition of your microbiome affects the number of Calories your body extracts from food. Every body is unique. Everybody's gut bacteria population is unique too. Some populations are better than others at extracting more energy from food.

The Calorie count of the foods you eat.

It's important to remember that not all Calories have the same effect on weight loss. The Calories in the different types of foods you eat can have different effects on your body. Some Calories are in foods that aid weight loss, while others are to be found in foods that promote weight GAIN.

The Calories in foods that promote weight gain: Sugars

Sugary foods are among the foods that can make you fat. You rapidly digest the Calories in sugars, whether they are refined sugars or naturally-occurring sugars such as agave syrup, honey, maple syrup or palm sugar. Desserts, cakes, candies and sugary drinks can all cause a spike in blood glucose levels, followed by a sharp drop in blood glucose, which triggers hunger again.

The Calories in foods that can help weight loss: Fiber

High-fiber foods are among those that can help you lose weight.
- Your body digests fiber-rich foods more slowly than fiber-poor foods. The food stays in your digestive tract for longer, thus prolonging satiety. This can help prevent over-eating.
- Soluble fiber can absorb water and swell, making your stomach feel fuller.

- In contrast to the rapid assimilation of sugary foods, your body gradually assimilates the Calories in fiber-rich foods.
- Only around half the Calories in dietary fiber get absorbed into your body. The other Calories are not digested. They pass through your gut and get flushed away.

COUNTING CALORIES

To lose weight you don't have to count Calories obsessively. Everyone knows that you gain weight when you consume more Calories than you burn. This does not mean, however, that when you want to lose weight you have to calculate the quantities of Calories in every food, and weigh and measure and add and subtract and multiply. Such a time-consuming and difficult task would take the fun out of eating—and out of life in general!

A better way is to teach yourself to be "Calorie informed"; in other words, learn to know:

- the approximate number of Calories you need to eat each day
- the approximate Calorie-count of the foods you eat

1. The number of Calories you need each day.

Your Calorie needs vary according to your age, sex, health, body size and level of physical activity. According to the 2015-2020 Dietary Guidelines for Americans[38], most women need 1,600 to 2,400 Calories a day, while men need 2,000 to 3,000. To find out your own individual Calorie needs, ask your doctor or search on the Internet for online Calorie calculators.

2, The approximate Calorie count of your food.

You can also find food Calorie counters in bookshops and libraries, and on apps for your devices. Once you start learning the calorific value of foods, you might be surprised. Standard mayonnaise, for

---

38 Published by the U.S. Department of Health and Human Services (HHS) and the U.S. Department of Agriculture (USDA).

example, is frighteningly high in Calories. As for soda drinks, they are crammed with them! You'd have to run fast, non-stop for around 20 minutes to use up the Calories in one can of soda. It is easy to inadvertently eat more Calories than you need.

3. How many Calories do you need, to lose weight?

The way to *gain* weight is to eat few extra unneeded Calories each day. This is the way most people accumulate excess weight—bit by bit. It only takes one superfluous 49-Calorie cookie a day, over the course of a year, to add 17,885 Calories worth of fat to your body.

Conversely when you want to *lose* weight, you need to eat a few Calories *less* than you burn, every day.

Pure fat contains about 9 Calories per gram—252 Calories per ounce—so you'd think that if you ate 252 fewer Calories per day than you burned, you'd lose an ounce of body fat per day, right?

No. It's more complicated than that.

Body fat is not pure fat. It's mixed with some fluids and proteins. This means that there are slightly fewer Calories in an ounce of body fat than in an ounce of pure fat. It has been estimated that a pound of body fat (approx. 0.45 kg) may contain anywhere between 3,436 and 3,752 Calories. Per ounce, that's between 214 Calories and 234 Calories.

That's good news!

The UK's National Health Service recommends that when you're following a weight-loss regime, you should aim to lose around 0.5-1kg (1lb-2lb) per week until you reach your goal weight. If you lose more than this, you could be endangering your health and also putting yourself at risk of rebound weight gain later on. If you lose less than this, it can be discouraging.

Losing this amount of fat requires you to eat around 500-600 Calories less than you expend, each day. There is, however, a proviso…

How to stop weight loss from slowing down over time.

When you begin a new weight loss regime, the pounds/kilos can drop away relatively easily, over the first week or two. Then your Inner Guardian awakens from its peaceful slumber, notices that you're losing precious energy stores and swings into action.

It releases more hunger hormones, prompts you to exercise less to conserve energy, and boosts your digestive efficiency to extract every morsel of energy from your food. If you move around less, you may also lose muscle mass. Muscle mass increases the rate at which you burn Calories, so losing it is also going to slow down your weight loss.

Your Inner Guardian thinks it is protecting you from a famine.

The trick to weight loss is to give your Inner Guardian the message that there is NO famine, so that it will stop guarding your fat stores and instead allow them to be used up.

Thus, if you want to keep losing body-fat at the recommended rate (around 0.5kg-1kg or 1lb-2lb per week), take note of the following:

- Consume fewer Calories.
- Choose unprocessed foods rather than highly-processed foods.
- Choose low GI foods rather than high GI foods.
- Eat plenty of NTS vegetables.
- When craving sweetness, go for low-fructose foods.
- Eat smaller portions of Calorie-rich foods, if you crave them.
- Lull your Inner Guardian into a sense of "food abundance" by reaching satiety at each meal
- Allow yourself to become mildly hungry between meals, but never ravenously hungry. Hunger = weight loss. Ravenous hunger = a "famine" signal to your Inner Guardian.
- Boost your exercise levels. It is said that successful weight loss is due to "20% exercise and 80% what foods you eat," but that 20% it very important—not only to aid weight loss, but to keep you healthy!
- Weight lifting and resistance training can help prevent loss of muscle mass and help to increase the number of Calories you burn.
- Employ as many tools from *The Satiety Diet Weight Loss Toolkit* as you find useful.

4. Tips about Calories.

You really can eat more food and still lose weight with these Calorie tips.

Take into account all the Calories you eat, even those in healthful foods.

Some people blame their metabolism for their inability to lose weight, but it might be a case of simply forgetting about some of the Calories they consume, or not realizing that they consumed them. Studies show that even people who record daily food diaries can unintentionally under-report as much as 50% of the foods they've eaten. Why?

- You might forget that all the extras, such as snacks, drinks, condiments and sauces, also contain Calories and add to your daily total.
- Even whole, fresh fruit, which really is healthful, can tempt you to over-consume Calories because you underestimate how many Calories they contain.
- You think the Calories in "healthy" foods don't count. Beware of "healthy" foods that are really candy in disguise! Food manufacturers often tout foods such as breakfast cereals, granola, smoothies, fruit juices, dried fruits and snack bars as "healthy", but they can be loaded with Calories. Healthful-looking snack bars can be packed with sugary fruit juice, flavors and concentrates. They are labeled with words such as "natural", which give them a "health halo". Many "low-fat" foods marketed as being healthful can contain up to five times more sugar than their "full fat" counterparts. Manufactured foods labeled as "low-fat" or "low Calorie" may be worse for your health than the more natural versions of those foods, because of the chemicals that are added to make them taste good despite their lack of fat or sugar. Sugar added to low-fat products and artificial sweeteners added to low Calorie products are thought to contribute not only to rising levels of obesity but also to serious health problems such as diabetes, heart disease and cancer.

Hidden Calories.

Do some research into how many Calories really are in your food, and what form those Calories take. Read the labels on processed foods. They may contain hidden sugars. Even savory foods such as baked beans, pasta sauce and bread can contain added sugar. Smoothies can be particularly loaded with sugars.

5. Swapping Calorie-dense for Calorie-sparse foods can help you lose weight more easily.

There is no doubt that lower Calorie, higher-fiber foods can promote satiety and weight loss.

According to the Committee on Military Nutrition Research (USA), "Energy density of foods can affect daily energy intake and body weight. In one study, obese and normal-weight subjects had access to one of two different diets, for 5 days each. One diet had twice the energy density of the other; the low-energy-density diet was low in fats and sugars and high in fiber. The subjects consumed three meals a day and were allowed to eat as much of the available foods as they liked at each meal.

"Subjects on the high-energy-density diet consumed nearly twice as many Calories as those on the low-energy-density diet. Subjects on the low-energy-density diet were slightly hungrier at mealtimes but found the meals to be satiating.

"The diets in this study differed not only in energy density, but also in the fat content and in the amount of fiber, both of which could affect the amount of food consumed." [Marriott 1995)]

Swap, swap, swap!

Swap high Calorie foods for low Calorie foods, sugary foods for naturally sweet, whole, low-fructose foods, and low-fiber foods for high fiber foods.

A series of small changes in your diet can add up to a huge difference in your Calorie consumption. By switching to low Calorie, low sugar, high fiber versions of your favorite foods you could halve your daily Calorie intake.

For example:

- Drink black coffee instead of cappuccino.
- Choose wholegrain toast instead of a pastry.
- Enjoy a plain garden salad instead of a salad with cheesy croutons and a creamy dressing.
- Eat a piece of low-fructose fruit such as oranges, plums and berries instead of chocolate.
- Have a thin crust pizza instead of deep pan.
- If you're drinking cocktails, a Bloody Mary has fewer Calories than a Piña Colada.
- Instead of buying sugar-laden, high-fat granola or muesli, make your own breakfast mix or Satiety Porridge
- Replace fruit juices, smoothies, shakes, sodas and diet sodas with still water, sparkling water, coffee, tea, or herbal infusions.

6. How much exercise burns off how many Calories?

To what extent does exercise help with weight loss? You can find free "Calories Burned Calculators" online. They are useful for estimating how many Calories you would use up during an exercise session.

For example, for a female 172 cm (5 feet 8 inches) tall, weighing 70 kg (154 pouds) and aged 35, doing 20 minutes of Pilates would use up approximately 72 Calories.

For a male 172 cm tall, weighing 85 kg (187 pounds) and aged 35, doing 20 minutes of Pilates would use up approximately 90 Calories.

That same male would burn 232 Calories by running cross country for 20 minutes, while that same female would burn 185 Calories.

PROCESSED VS UNPROCESSED FOODS

Many popular weight-loss diets are effective in the short-term, though they may lead to rebound weight gain afterwards. The one element that almost all *long-term effective* diets have in common is that they recommend eating whole plant foods and they all limit processed foods. Processed foods can be defined as foods that have been interfered with by humans. People have been processing food for thousands of years—drying fish and fruit, for example, or pickling vegetables. Those simple, traditional forms of light processing that can be performed in your home kitchen are not the problem. The problem lies with foods that have been processed by food manufacturing companies whose aim is usually to profit by persuading consumers to eat as much of their product as possible. They use many techniques to achieve this aim, including:
- wrapping their foods in eye-catching, attractive packaging
- refining the food's carbohydrates, and adding "bad" fats and extra sugars.

FOOD: DEGREES OF PROCESSING

We can classify foods into three categories: unprocessed, lightly-processed and processed/ultra-processed.

Unprocessed foods.

Just about all natural, unprocessed, whole foods that are prepared properly and without chemical additives, are healthful foods.

Lightly-processed foods.

Most lightly-processed natural foods are in the "healthful" category. For example, the pressing of olives is a process and olive oil, consumed in moderation, is a valuable addition to a healthful diet. Canning is considered to be light processing, as long as the food that's canned has not been combined with additives. Freezing is also

395

viewed as light processing—again, only if the frozen food contains no additives. Drying, cooking, fermenting and even pasteurizing are forms of light processing. All these light processing methods can be undertaken in the home kitchen.

Some natural foods require light processing to make them safe to eat—for example quinoa, legumes and cassava.

Light processing is not always a good thing for weight loss, however. The pressing of oranges yields orange juice, which is oranges separated from their fiber and from their chewy, textural characteristics. Calories drunk as a liquid are less likely to give rise to satiety than Calories consumed as a solid. This is why slowly and mindfully eating a whole, peeled orange is better for weight loss than drinking the juice of that same orange.

Highly-processed/ultra-processed foods.

What we usually think of as "processed foods" are foods that have undergone extensive changes in an industrial food manufacturing plant.

These foods are not necessarily unhealthful, (depending on the way they've been processed) but any food that's been altered this way may contain added salt, sugar, fat, preservatives, colors, stabilizers, flavors and other additives.

Satiety is best achieved by consuming unprocessed foods. Ironically, commercial food manufacturing companies are aware of this, and are busy producing processed foods that are touted as "promoting satiety".

The more highly-processed a food is, the less likely it is to have health benefits. It's pretty easy to spot these foods in supermarkets.

- They are the ones that you wouldn't find growing in a rural landscape.
- They are the ones your pre-20th century ancestors wouldn't recognise.
- They are the ones whose ingredients list contain words that may be hard to pronounce—such as "hydrogenated" or butylated hydroxyanisole"!

Scientists have now coined the term "ultra-processed foods". A 2019 trial titled "Ultra-Processed Diets Cause Excess Calorie Intake and Weight Gain", suggests that consuming these foods actually makes you eat more and gain weight—possibly by influencing your hunger hormones. [Hall et al., (2019).]

Examples of common processed foods include:
- breakfast cereals
- cheese
- tinned vegetables
- bread
- savory snacks, such as crisps
- meat products, such as bacon
- "convenience foods", such as microwave meals or ready meals
- drinks, such as milk, soda and soft drinks

HOME-PREPARED MEALS

You can't really know what goes into food that you buy from fast food outlets or restaurants or cafes. The aim of food-sellers is generally to make food taste nice, not necessarily to feed you what's good for you.

That said, there are plenty of excellent eateries that do sell fresh wholesome food—but are you prepared to fork out extra money for this? It's usually cheaper to prepare meals at home, and that way you know exactly what ingredients have been used and how fresh they are.

There can be good reasons for eating out—one advantage of dining in a restaurant of cafe is that you're likely to get more variety. Eateries may offer foods you wouldn't have usually thought of buying for yourself.

But don't make eating out a habit, and especially avoid high fat, sugary fast food.

One habit that can really help you lose weight is eating home prepared meals—meals assembled or cooked from scratch as opposed to processed meals out of packets and cans. (Canned fish is fine, particularly if canned in water, because it's a principal, unique food.)

If you're keen to lose weight, be prepared to either:
- Spend time in your home kitchen preparing food, or
- Find a friend or loved one to spend time in the kitchen preparing food, or
- Pay someone else to spend time in the kitchen preparing food.

Some people join weight-loss programs run by companies who deliver their food to your door.

Chris Clark says, "I've tried those meal-delivery weight-loss programs, and they didn't work for me. To be honest, I felt terribly hungry most of the time. Almost every meal included a lot of white bread slices or dinner-rolls, which didn't seem healthy to me. And the program was expensive!"

Think of buying (or growing your own) ingredients and preparing your own food as a kind of homage to your body; a meditative ritual leading to healthy weight loss. It doesn't have to be a chore. Preparing food can be relaxing and rewarding. Plenty of people do it as a hobby. Creating your own dishes can be satisfying—not only to your taste buds but to your sense of self-worth and your sense of nurturing yourself.

Preparation of healthful food can be incredibly simply and quick. It can be as easy as tearing up some fresh salad leaves and putting them on a plate with some tuna canned in spring-water, topped with low-fat hummus and a sprinkling of cracked pepper.

One of your best friends in the home is a freezer. Fresh-frozen foods (within their use-by date!) are the next best thing to fresh foods. When you cook, make double the quantity and freeze half for later. This saves time.

REAL, WHOLE FOODS HELP PROMOTE WEIGHT LOSS

All foods contain some level of nutrition, and strictly speaking we should not call foods "good" or "bad"; but those that contribute to over-nutrition really are bad news for people who are trying to lose weight and become healthier.

Eating nutrient-dense foods in their most natural form provides the best chance of satiety and weight loss. When you eat raw, unprocessed food you are more likely to control your weight. If you eat the same food refined or otherwise processed, you are more likely to get more Calories out of it and gain weight.

Same number of Calories, different result.

The labels on processed foods tell you how many Calories a food contains, but it's not as simple as that. The point is, the number of Calories you actually absorb from your food can depend on how highly processed it is.

1. Finely-ground foods are less satiating than whole foods.

A 1994 study published in the *European Journal of Clinical Nutrition* found that "The smaller the particle size of the food, the higher the glycemic-insulin response and the lower the satiety rating." [Holt & Miller (1994)]

In other words, when whole food is ground down into finer particles, it makes it easier for your body to rapidly digest all the Calories. This leads to a spike in blood sugars, followed by a fall, which stimulates hunger. It also means that your food passes more rapidly through your digestive tract and then your stomach feels empty—again stimulating hunger.

Food processing can involve grinding, blending or mashing, all of which renders the food particles smaller and frequently softer. Soft foods are easier to digest, so your body burns up less energy during the process of digestion. Your body also digests processed foods more completely, extracting more Calories out of it.

2. Processed foods usually contain less fiber.

Processing often involves reducing the fiber content of foods. Fiber promotes satiety, and many of the Calories in fiber-rich foods can pass through your body undigested.

3. Processed foods tend to have more "empty Calories".

When you eat a lot of highly-refined, nutrient-depleted food products such as sugar and flour, or processed foods containing preservatives and artificial ingredients, you are missing out on the complex nutrients found in whole foods. It's not primarily Calories that give you satiety—it's nutrients: vitamins, minerals, fiber, protein, and "good" fats. The more nutrition you feed your body and the fewer "empty Calories" you consume, the less you will crave for the nutrients you're missing, and the less you will be driven to find them by eating more food. It will be easier for you to reach satiety as your hunger signals subside.

4. Processed foods are often very energy-dense.

"Energy-dense" foods are those that deliver more Calories per gram/ounce. By contrast to processed/manufactured foods, whole foods such as raw vegetables, seeds, nuts and fruits need a lot of chewing, and their fiber content makes you feel full for longer, so they provide more satiety per bite.

5. It's easier to gain weight when eating "ready meals".

"Ready meals", "TV dinners" and other packaged meals that you buy already prepared and cooked, so that you only have to heat or thaw them before eating them, are convenient and easy to use. The picture on the front of the packet makes you think they are healthful. So what's bad about them?

a) Read the label. They may be high in sugars and fats, not to mention salt!

b) Keep reading the label. Are you seeing ingredients you don't recognize, or would not be able to buy at your local grocery store, or whose names are unfamiliar and hard to pronounce? Are there ingredients your grandmother wouldn't have been able to identify? These are chemical additives, generally used to make the meal look better or last longer. They may be good for the manufacturer's profit margins, but they may not be all that good for your health.

c) What is *not* written on the label is just as important, but harder to discover. Many processing methods cause vitamins and minerals to be leached out of food or destroyed. Nutrients such as antioxidants, Vitamin C, B vitamins, glucosinolates may be missing from ready meals, depending on how the manufacture cooks them. If vitamins and minerals are mentioned on the label, the manufacturer may be referring to the raw ingredients, not the processed versions. The nutritional value of ready meals is important for your health and important for satiety.

d) Ready meal manufacturers may substitute cheaper ingredients for traditional ones. Sometimes, for example, extra virgin olive oil is swapped for inferior vegetable oils that have not been shown to possess the same health-giving characteristics.

6. Choose whole fruit rather than processed fruit.

Processed fruit is more fattening than whole, fresh fruit. Choose whole fruit rather than fruit juice. Whole fruit contains more fiber than the juiced version. Whole fruit needs chewing. It takes a lot longer to eat two oranges than it does to drink two oranges' worth of juice—and a lot more chewing! Fruit juices and smoothies bring you plenty of Calories, rapidly consumed, high in sugars and low in fiber. Juicing is *not* a good weight loss tool. Fruit juices do contain nutrients and sometimes the fiber is left in, but fruit in liquid form is "pre-chewed" by a juicing machine. It is more likely to make you put on weight than fruit in its natural, unprocessed form. Even if you chew slowly and mindfully, it's unlikely your teeth will pulverize your food as efficiently as the whizzing steel blades of a powerful, motorized machine.

7. Processed foods can trigger cravings.

The more you eat highly processed foods such as sugars, salt, fat and refined carbohydrates, the more you want them. Such foods may be "addictive". Making a habit of eating whole, "real" foods can be a powerful way of suppressing cravings and binge eating.

VEGETABLES

1. NOURISHING, TASTY, SLIMMING VEGETABLES

Veggies, especially NTS veggies, are Calorie-sparse. Eat as many of them as you like, but as with any food, eat only until you are satisfied, not over-full.

What are NTS vegetables?

Those vegetables that contain fewer Calories (chiefly in the form of starches and/or sugars) than other vegetables, we call Nourishing, Tasty, Slimming (NTS) vegetables. They are generally rich in water and fiber—and, of course, nutrients.

For a given number of Calories, you can eat larger quantities of these nutritious, Calorie-sparse NTS vegetables than you could eat of starchy/sugary vegetables.

On the Satiety Diet all plant-based foods are considered desirable. All vegetables are good for you, but to lose weight, eat smaller portions of vegetables that are not on the NTS list. We single out the NTS veggies because they are the ones you can eat freely, without counting their Calories or assigning them a portion size. As a rule of thumb, NTS vegetables do not include grains and seeds, or very starchy/sugary vegetables such as sweet potatoes, yams, and potatoes.

Here's the exception to the rule:

Some NTS vegetables are a little more starchy and energy-dense than others—for example corn, winter squashes, parsnips, peas, Jerusalem artichokes, legumes and salsify—but research shows that people are unlikely to overdose on them! They are nutritious and delicious, so do eat them. They add to your food variety.

NTS vegetables include (but are not limited to):

- Amaranth leaves (Chinese spinach)
- Artichoke (globe and Jerusalem)
- Arugula (rocket)
- Asparagus
- Aubergine (egg plant)
- Bamboo shoots
- Bean sprouts
- Beet greens
- Belgian endive
- Bell pepper (capsicum)
- Bok choy/bok choi/pak choy
- Broccoli
- Brussels sprouts
- Cabbages of all kinds
- Calabash (gourd)
- Capers
- Carrot
- Cauliflower
- Celery
- Celery root/celeriac
- Chayote (pear squash, vegetable pear, choko)
- Chicory
- Courgette (zucchini)
- Chinese broccoli/kai-lan
- Corn
- Collard greens
- Cucumber/ gherkin/ pickling cucumbers
- Daikon radish
- Edamame/ soy beans
- Endive and escarole
- Fennel
- Galangal
- Garlic

- Ginger
- Grape leaves
- Green beans of all kinds[39]
- Greens and green leafy vegetables such as:
  Beet greens
  Collard greens
  Dandelion greens
  Fiddlehead greens
  Kale
  Kohlrabi greens
  Mustard greens
  Rapini
  Spinach
  Swiss chard / silver beet
  Turnip greens
- Hearts of Palm
- Herbs (parsley, cilantro, basil, rosemary, thyme, etc.)
- Horseradish
- Leeks
- Legumes (beans, peas and lentils)
- Lemongrass
- Lettuce of all kinds
- Marrows (squashes)
- Mushrooms of all kinds
- Napa cabbage
- Nopales
- Okra
- Onions of all kinds including green onions/ scallions
- Parsnip
- Peas
- Pumpkin

---

39 For example string beans, snap beans, French beans, string beans, runner beans, mangetout.

- Purslane
- Radicchio
- Radish
- Rutabaga (swede)
- Salsify
- Sea vegetables, e.g. seaweeds
- Shallots
- Sorrel
- Snow peas or pea pods
- Squashes of all kinds
- Tomatillo
- Tomato
- Turnip
- Water Chestnut
- Water Spinach
- Watercress

2. EAT MORE FOOD, LOSE MORE WEIGHT!

Along with eating some protein at each meal, consuming more NTS vegetables is one of the keys to weight loss. When you eat loads of veggies you can fill up your plate with a rainbow variety of colors and textures, and feel as if you're not on a restricted diet. As well as being packed with vitamins, minerals and antioxidants, veggies are loaded with filling fiber and water. Vegetables add color, flavor, and texture to a meal whether raw, steamed, or roasted.

3. HOW TO EAT MORE VEGETABLES

We all know that eating more energy-sparse vegetables will help us lose weight. Furthermore, nutritionists and dietitians are always telling us that we should eat plenty of vegetables for good health, but not many people eat "between five and 13 servings of vegetables and fruits each day" (according to the 2005 Dietary Guidelines for Americans).

How can you make yourself eat more vegetables?

4. HOW TO MAKE VEGETABLES TASTE BETTER

Vegetables are packed with delicious flavors, but some people say they don't like them. Here are some tips to make vegetables taste even better.

- **Tip #1: Choose baby vegetables.** The flavor of young vegetables is less intense, and often they are sweeter.

- **Tip #2: Add zest with a well-chosen garnish or condiment**. To bring out the flavor in vegetables add mint or lemon juice, or sprinkle with herb salt or chopped, fresh parsley, or coriander, or garnish with finely chopped fresh or dried chili, or top with some grated Parmesan cheese. Drizzle a little extra-virgin olive oil on your veggies (not too much!) or sprinkle them with herbs.

- **Tip #3: Blanch your vegetables to prevent over-strong flavors from developing.** Blanching reduces the bitterness of cruciferous vegetables better than steaming or microwaving. Take a small batch of vegetables freshly-cut into uniform pieces. Pour enough water into a saucepan to just cover the vegetables, and bring it to the boil. Use as little water as possible, to help retain nutrients. A pinch of salt is optional. Add the vegetables to the boiling water and allow to boil for 30 seconds to 3 minutes, depending on the vegetable. When tender but still firm, remove vegetables with a slotted spoon and plunge them into a bowl of cold, iced water. When cool, remove and drain.

- **Tip #4: Get fresh.** Stale vegetables not only lose flavor, they also lose nutrients. Buy fresh vegetables from farmers' markets—or grow your own.

- **Tip #5: Use your freezer.** Frozen veg can contain as many nutrients as fresh ones— and sometimes more. They add instant variety to your diet and help avoid wastage.

406

- **Tip #6: Go undercover.** Sneak vegetables into your diet "by stealth". For example:
  * Disguise veggies in frittatas, quiches, and pasta sauces.
  * Add chopped green beans and diced carrots to a Shepherd's Pie/ Cottage Pie.
  * Toss in some extra vegetables to bulk up pasta sauces.
  * Enjoy a fresh side-salad with your meals.
  * Pile extra vegetables on top of pizzas.
  * If you're having a stew or curry, pour in a load of vegetables. They will take on the flavor of the stew or curry.

- **Tip #7: Use the power of your mind.** Think about veggies doing you good. It becomes easier for you to tolerate foods that are good for you but whose flavor you don't like, when you understand *why* the foods are good for you. For best results, this should be combined with repeated, regular exposure to those foods. [Stein (nd)]

- **Tip #8: Wield the wok.** Stir-fry loads of vegetables to preserve their fresh flavors and crispy textures. Include some tofu or other protein, slathered in some low-Calorie stir-fry sauce.

- **Tip #9: Eat vegetables you don't usually eat.** Many people get stuck in a rut when it comes to food. At some time in the past they have decided "I eat this, and I never eat that". They walk straight past the "unusual vegetables" section of the supermarket or greengrocer's store. It's time to break out of that rut and be adventurous, because you're missing out on lots of amazing flavors and textures. Artichokes, cardoon, okra, celeriac, pea shoots etc.—find a good recipe and give them a try!

- **Tip #10: Bring out the natural sweetness.** Natural sugars exist in most vegetables—the kind of sugars that nature has blended with fiber and nutrients in the perfect ratio to give good health to those who eat them. If you're going to really appreciate the delicious taste of these sugars, you may have to eat your vegetables cooked. Certain types of cooking can unlock the sweetness of vegetables. It can also concentrate their flavors by removing moisture, caramelize the natural sugars to add an almost toffee-like sweetness, and mask any bitterness that might be present. Roasting and frying, which are called "dry cooking" techniques, are recommended. (Examples of "wet cooking" include steaming and boiling.) Generally, a light coating of oil is needed to obtain the best caramelization. Oil is Calorie-dense, so use a light spritz of spray oil, rather than pouring oil from a bottle. When oil-sprayed veggies are roasted or fried, the "Maillard reaction" occurs, giving you caramelized veggies which can be crisp and intensely-flavored on the outside and tender on the inside. You can cook most vegetables this way to bring out their sweetness, although it works best with harder vegetables such as carrots, potatoes, pumpkin/squash, parsnips, garlic, turnips, swede, onions, beetroots—even courgettes (zucchini). Line the roasting tray with baking paper (parchment) and use a minimum of oil. You can sprinkle roasted veggies with a variety of seasonings such as rosemary, cayenne pepper, or garlic.

- **Tip #11: Enjoy it hot!** Buy some sugar-free curry paste or make it from scratch using fresh ingredients. You can choose to have it as mild or as hot as you wish. Mix the curry paste with pure tomato passata and cook your vegetables in this vibrant mixture. The delicious, spicy flavors will dominate.

- **Tip #12: Dip and crunch.** Eat raw carrot, celery or cucumber sticks with tasty dips such as low-fat dressings, salsa, or low-fat hummus.

- **Tip #13: Spiralize your veggies.** For some reason, vegetables cut into "noodles" tend to taste better. As mention elsewhere in this book, you can make vegetable noodles (vegetti) using a spiralizer (often called a spiral vegetable slicer), a julienne peeler or a standard vegetable peeler.

- **Tip #14 Make vegetable lasagna.** Simply substitute thin layers of parsnip, eggplant or zucchini for sheets of grain lasagna.

- **Tip #15: Get the perfect texture.** For crunchiness, eat vegetables raw. If you want crunchiness in cooked vegetables, steam them instead of boiling them. Note, however, that steaming green leafy vegetables (such as spinach and kale) can make their color fade somewhat. If you want silky-smooth mashed potatoes or pumpkin/squash, boil the vegetables before mashing them. Boiling tenderizes them more rapidly than steaming. Most vegetables need to be cooked at a high temperature before they become tender. If the cooking temperature is too low, you could end up with vegetables that are too hard.

- **Tip #16 Keep the color in cooked green vegetables.** We "eat with our eyes" and when food has beautiful vivid colors, it seems to taste better too. Some people add baking soda when they cook leafy vegetables, to make them keep their color. This is not advisable, since baking soda can destroy some of the valuable nutrients, such as vitamin C, vitamin D, riboflavin and thiamine. Steaming makes them lose color more than boiling does. To help preserve that gorgeous green, you can blanch the vegetables— see Tip #3.

5. CHRIS CLARK'S VEGETABLE PHILOSOPHY

Chris Clark says, "Here's a mind-trick to help you plan meals. Say to yourself, 'All foods that are *not* NTS vegetables exist purely to make NTS vegetables taste good.' If you approach meal-planning with this attitude, you'll base pretty much every course around nutritious, filling, fiber-rich vegetables— even desserts and sweets! Your protein, fats and other carbs will be added to the veg in ways that make them taste truly delicious.

"Examples include:
* Stir-fried vegetables
* Vegetable soups
* Raw vegetable salads
* Crustless vegetable quiches
* Sweet pumpkin pie
* Rice pudding made with 'cauliflower rice' instead of rice."

6. RENAME YOUR VEGGIE DISHES

Giving vegetables attractive names makes them more appealing.

Another way to make vegetables taste better is by using the power of the mind. It sounds far-fetched but researchers at Stanford University in the USA have come up with some interesting results. [Turnwald (2017)] They found that when vegetables were given enticing descriptions that made them sound luxuriously scrumptious, people piled more of those vegetables on their plates.

To conduct the experiment, the same vegetable dishes were served at different times, rotated to ensure variety, and given different titles. The titles fell into four categories:
- "Basic"—a straightforward description such as "green beans"
- "Healthy restrictive"—e.g. "Light 'n' low-carb green beans and shallots"
- "Health positive"—e.g. "Healthy energy-boosting green beans and shallots"
- "Indulgent"—e.g. "Sweet sizzlin' green beans and crispy shallots"

Indulgent descriptors had the biggest impact on people's food choices. Flavorful, exciting, and indulgent names such as "Sweet sizzlin' green beans and crispy shallots", "Dynamite chili and tangy lime-seasoned beets" and "Slow-roasted caramelized zucchini bites" tempted diners to relish their vegetables.

Interestingly, the foods with "healthy restrictive" labeling proved to be the least popular. The researchers suggest that this is because our food choices are generally guided by taste and flavor—and we tend to think of "healthier options" as less flavorful!

Perhaps also it's because we subconsciously like to think we're getting "more" rather than "less" when we eat.

"Labels really can influence our sensory experience, affecting how tasty and filling we think food will be," says researcher Brad Turnwald, "so we wanted to reframe how people view vegetables, using indulgent labels."

Though the researchers were not able to measure how much food each diner actually consumed, other research has shown that people usually "eat 92% of self-served food, regardless of portion size and food type."

So, how can you help yourself or your family and friends get healthier and lose weight by eating more vegetables? One low-cost way is to simply follow low-Calorie vegetable recipes with names that make them sound lush, gourmet, interesting and delicious. Or even invent your own names!

7. TRAIN YOURSELF TO LIKE VEGETABLES MORE

Great news! It's actually possible to train yourself to like vegetables more than you do right now. Researchers at Coventry University in the UK found that when children ate a green vegetable they didn't really like (kale) as part of their diet every day for fifteen days, at the end of that time most of the children liked it more than they had to begin with! And they certainly liked it more than a second group of children who had eaten raisins instead of kale for fifteen days. Familiarity can breed appreciation. [Fogel and Blisset (2017)]

Some of us might take longer than fifteen days to start appreciating the taste of strongly-flavored foods and bitter foods. That is because about 25% of the population is highly sensitive to taste. The message is, "persevere with eating vegetables, because the more you eat them, the better you'll like them."

FOODS AND DRINKS THAT HELP WEIGHT LOSS

Good food choices for weight loss are low-fat, protein-rich foods, fiber-rich foods like beans and lentils, whole grain products, low Calorie foods and foods that contain a relatively large amount of water. Of course, vegetables are particularly helpful for weight loss. As well as being filling and delicious (when prepared the right way), they contain loads of nutrients and very few Calories.

In this section we give you some examples of foods (and drinks) that can help with weight loss by improving satiety.

1. DRINKS THAT CAN HELP WEIGHT LOSS: WATER

Water. All life requires it, to survive. It's cheap and free from side-affects. An adequate intake of water is an effective weight loss tool—but only if used properly!

Dampen "thirsty" hunger by drinking water.

Thirst can mimic hunger. A study published in the journal *Physiology & Behavior* found that in 60% of cases, people who were thirsty responded to their thirst not by drinking, but by eating. [Mattes (2010)]

Inside the human brain, hormones produced by the hypothalmus govern physiologic functions including hunger and thirst. At times, these signals can become confused; you can have the idea that you're hungry when in fact your brain is trying to tell you that you need to drink some water.

If your body is constantly under-hydrated it can adjust to obtaining more water from food. It learns to send hunger signals for food in order to get the liquid it requires.

412

Studies have shown that in a majority of cases, people are more likely to respond to thirst by eating instead of drinking. And if they do drink, they will often choose a Calorie-dense liquid, such as sugary coffee, or a milkshake or a soft drink/soda. Both eating when you're thirsty, and consuming Calories in liquid form are almost guaranteed to make you gain weight.

Plain water is the best thirst-quencher. It can be flavored with natural herbs or teas, or a squeeze of citrus juice, or a slice of raw ginger root—but make sure you do not sip on water that contains added Calories. If you buy a bottle of commercial water—read the label!

So, when you feel like something to eat between meals, drink a cup of plain water instead—with a squeeze of lemon, or a sprig of mint, or a few ice cubes. Wait 20 minutes to see what happens to your appetite. If you're still hungry, then eat something (preferably a Satiety Diet snack). If drinking water dampens your desire for food then, in the long term, it will help you lose weight.

Sip water throughout the day.

Carry water with you, and if you think you're starting to feel hungry, take a few sips. You might not be hungry—you might actually be a little dehydrated.

Reach satiety more easily by pre-loading with water.

Timing is the key.

You can drink water to help with weight loss, but is there an optimal time to do it and if so, when is it? You know it's a good idea to sip water throughout the day, but should you also swallow a glassful during meals? After meals?

One way to take full advantage of the weight loss benefits of water, is to sip some before you eat a meal. Drinking water before meals helps you eat less.

Imbibing around 2 cups of water before you eat a meal makes you feel fuller more quickly, so that you don't eat as much food at that meal. This can reduce your daily Calorie intake significantly.

413

Instead of just carelessly sipping on your water during the course of the meal, relax and swallow the entire amount before you even pick up your knife and fork.

A 2010 study published in the journal *Obesity* concluded that drinking two cups of water about half an hour before meals helped people consume 75 to 90 fewer Calories over the course of the meal. The researchers concluded that " . . . when combined with a hypocaloric diet (a diet in which you eat fewer Calories than you burn), consuming 500 ml water (2 cups) prior to each main meal leads to greater weight loss than a hypocaloric diet alone in middle-aged and older adults." People who drank the water before meals lost 44% more weight than those who didn't. [Dennis, et al., (2010)]

A 2015 study published in the same journal, *Obesity*, supported this conclusion. It was found that volunteers on a weight-loss diet who drank 500 ml of water (two cups) 30 min before their main meals lost more weight over 12 weeks than volunteers who simply practiced visualizing that their stomach was full before meals.

"There is preliminary evidence that water preloading before main meals leads to a moderate weight loss at follow up," wrote the study's authors. [Parretti at al., (2015)]

Why do people eat less food after a drink of water? Probably because the water expands the stomach before the food arrives. Then when the food enters the stomach the water combines with it, filling and swelling the stomach even more. Sensing that there's no space left for any more food, the distended stomach sends satiety signals to the brain, suppressing the appetite, and the person stops eating.

Does sparkling/fizzy water work?

Until quite recently, it was thought that both still/flat water and fizzy/sparkling water (with no additives) had the same effect on the body. It was supposed that you could sip on plain water either with or without bubbles, to help dampen your appetite.

A 2016 study suggests that this may not be so. The study's title says it all: "Carbon dioxide in carbonated beverages induces ghrelin release and increased food consumption in male rats: Implications on the onset of obesity." [Eweis et al., (2016)]

414

Another study, conducted on humans instead of rats, came up with conflicting evidence. [Wakisaka et al., (2012)] These results suggested that carbonated water curbs people's appetite even more efficiently than still water. The researchers wrote, "Our data suggest that carbonated water may induce a short-term, but significant, satiating effect . . ." What if those tiny bubbles whizzing around in your stomach could stimulate your satiety signals? If this is so, then fizzing up your pre-meal water would magnify the benefits, and drinking two cups of fizzy water before meals might aid weight loss.

While the jury is still out, listen to your body and be aware of how drinking the fizzy stuff, (such as plain soda water or plain mineral water) affects your appetite.

Does it have to be water?

Other liquids can stretch your stomach to trick it into sending satiety signals to your brain, but water is the liquid with no Calories whatsoever, so water is best for weight loss (and proper rehydration!).

That said, there are other liquids which also have very few Calories—such as weak green tea, herbal tea or black tea. These are good substitutes. If you prefer not to drink hot tea, sip cold tea with lemon, mint, lemon verbena or cinnamon. Ice cubes can add freshness and a satisfying tinkling sound.

Before meals, avoid drinking fruit juices, smoothies, shakes, soda or any other drink laden with Calories. In fact don't drink them at all, ever! (Unless for a one-off "treat" you can't resist.)

One of the worst things you can drink, either before meals or at any time of day, is diet soda. Manufacturers may market them as containing no Calories, but their sweetness and flavor may distort and flaw the satiety signals sent from your digestive system to your brain.

Instead of drinking diet soda, choose a glass of plain water, still or sparkling, perhaps flavored with a twist of lemon, a slice of cucumber or a sprig of fresh mint. Float some frozen raspberries in it.

We don't recommend drinking vegetable juice because it's quite highly processed. Even drinking juice made from NTS vegetables, and even if the fiber is retained in the juice, it is not as good for weight loss as eating those same vegetables in their solid, natural form.

Water can speed up your metabolic rate.

Drinking water can boost metabolism by 24-30% over a period of 1-1.5 hours, helping you burn off a few more Calories, according to two studies in *The Journal of Clinical Endocrinology & Metabolism*. [Boschmann et al., (2003); Boschmann et al., (2007)]

Yes, it is possible to drink too much water.

Don't drink lots of water if you're not thirsty. In general, healthy people should let their thirst be their guide.

There's a popular idea that we should all drink eight glasses of water per day, in addition to what we usually eat and drink.

In an October 2013 article for BBC News Magazine, Dr. Chris van Tulleken explained that there is no scientific basis for this idea. In fact, it could be bad for you!

As Dr. van Tulleken wrote, "Saying that you should drink more water than your body asks for is like saying that you should consciously breathe more often than you feel like because if a little oxygen is good for you then more must be better." [Valtin (2002)]

Following a 2016 study, researchers advised people to "drink to thirst", because over-hydration can actually be more harmful than under-hydration. [Saker et al., (2016)]

One of the study's authors, Associate Professor Farrell, added the proviso that elderly people frequently do not drink enough, and should consciously try to keep up their fluid intake.

How much water should you drink each day?

Experts recommend that:
- Men should drink about 13 cups (3 liters) of fluid per day
- Women should drink about 9 cups (2.2 liters) of fluid per day.
- For every hour of vigorous exercise you should drink an extra 500ml to 800ml of water. The exact amount depends on your individual needs and the local climate—i.e. if you sweat a lot and it's hot, you'll need more.

That said, a few people—particularly the elderly—seem to have a low awareness of their own thirst levels and their body's need for water. If you're one of these people, look for one or more of these signs of dangerous under-hydration, and fix it by drinking water more often!

- Constant hunger
- Headache
- Dry mouth, eyes, and skin
- Dark-colored urine
- A feeling of disorientation
- Low energy levels
- Frequent muscular spasms or cramps
- Failure to sweat during exercise

Can coffee help with weight loss?

Good quality coffee (preferably black) is loaded with antioxidants, and may have numerous health benefits.

Studies show that the caffeine in coffee can boost your metabolism by 3-11%, and increase fat burning by up to 10-29%. Just don't drink caffeine-rich beverages before bedtime, or you might not sleep well! [Koot & Deurenberg (1995); Dulloo et al., (1989); Bracco et al., (1995)]

Also, make sure *not* to add a bunch of sugar, cream or other high-Calorie ingredients to it. That will negate any benefit you get from the coffee.

2. FOODS THAT CAN HELP WEIGHT LOSS: LEGUMES/PULSES

Legumes.

The word "legume" refers to a family of plants known as the Fabaceae (or Leguminosae). It also refers to the fruits or seeds of those plants.

"Well-known legumes include alfalfa, clover, peas, beans, chickpeas, lentils, sweet lupin bean, mesquite, carob, soybeans, peanuts and tamarind." [Wikipedia (10th Feb 2018]

Pulses.

The dried seeds of legumes are called "pulses". The word pulse comes from the Latin "puls", meaning a seed or grain that can be cooked into a thick, viscous stew, potage, soup or porridge. In other words, dishes with a highly satiating texture!

Pulses are very good at promoting satiety, because they contain protein, fiber and—when properly cooked—water. Like the other edible legumes, they are also low in fat and high in nutrients. Pulses have a low glycemic index—which means they are digested slowly, without causing rapid, sharp spikes in blood sugar levels.

The most common pulses include:
- Edible beans, such as butter beans, haricot beans (also known as navy beans), red kidney beans, adzuki beans, black-eyed beans and soybeans. The "white bean" family includes cannellini, great northern and white garden beans. These are the most common beans—there are lots more.
- Dried peas (which can be green or yellow and are available either whole or split)
- Chickpeas (also known as Bengal gram, or garbanzo bean)
- Lentils, which come in several colors such as brown, green and red.

... and back to legumes.

Legumes are rich in protein and fiber, and generally low in fat. They are among the cheapest forms of dietary protein. When you eat them with high protein whole grains such as buckwheat, brown rice or teff, you are getting the full range of essential amino acids required by humans.

The seeds of legumes can be eaten in their fresh, raw form. Legumes that can be eaten fresh include:

- green garden peas, snow peas
- peanuts
- carob
- green beans, string beans, runner beans

Versatile pulses.

Pulses can be used in many dishes, both savory and sweet.

You can prepare beans and lentils in numerous savory ways—for example in dips, in soups and casseroles or on toast. Ground legume flours such as chickpea (garbanzo bean), lentil and broad bean (fava bean) can be used in baking, although baking is "dry cooking" and we recommend sampling small quantities to begin with (see our section on "Lectins"). Preferably use legume flours in "wet cooking", such as a replacement for cornflour, a thickener for soups or stews, or as a base for porridge. Note that you'll probably absorb more energy from legume flours than from whole, unprocessed legumes.

There are also delicious ways to enjoy pulses as sweet desserts. Cooked black beans can be used to make luscious Satiety Diet Black Bean Brownies. Add puréed beans and lentils to sweet slices and cupcakes (see the Satiety Diet Cookbook for cupcakes made with kidney beans).

The Japanese, Vietnamese, Chinese, Koreans and others from Asian cultures have been eating bean-based sweets for centuries. For example, sweet adzuki bean paste (sometimes called red bean jam) is a staple in Japanese cuisine and confectionery.

419

The science of pulses and weight loss.

Scientists have been studying the relationship between edible legumes and weight loss. The results are interesting!

Eating pulses can help with weight loss—and improve health.

A study in the journal *Advances in Nutrition*, found that people who were on a low Calorie diet lost significantly more weight when they ate 2 cups (for women) or 3 cups (for men) of pulses every day as part of that diet. In fact they lost up to four times as much weight as the people who ate very few pulses. [McCrory et al., (2010)]

In another study, published in the *European Journal of Nutrition*, obese adults lost significantly more weight on a diet rich in lentils, chickpeas, peas, or beans. Their blood pressure and cholesterol levels also improved.

The authors of a 2014 scientific review stated that, "Replacing energy-dense foods with legumes has been shown to have beneficial effects on the prevention and management of obesity and related disorders . . ." [Rebello et al., (2014)]

It is thought that eating pea flour and chick peas may help to reduce the fat that accumulates around the abdomen. Eating pea flour can also lower insulin resistance. [Marinangeli & Jones (2010)]

Eating pulses may help burn Calories.

Faba beans (*Vicia faba*), have many names including, broad beans, English beans, horse beans, and pigeon beans. Along with peas and lentils, faba beans are rich in arginine, an amino acid that has been shown to stimulate the burning of both carbohydrate and fat. Animal studies show that the addition of pea flour to the diet can raise the metabolic rate.

Faba beans and lentils also contain glutamine, another amino acid. Studies on humans show that glutamine is associated with a 50% increase in the number of Calories burned after a meal.

420

Eating chick peas can promote satiety.

A study published in the *Journal of the American College of Nutrition* showed that when as little as 100g (3 1/2 ounces) of chick peas (garbanzo beans) was added to people's normal diet they tended to eat less food overall. They said that they felt more satisfied when they were having the chick pea supplement. [Pittaway et al., (2006)]

You become healthier with pulses.

You can lose as much weight by eating pulses as by cutting out carbs—but you get healthier.

The results of a study published in the *Journal of Human Nutrition and Dietetics* showed that there was no significant difference in weight loss between overweight people who ate a high-fiber, pulse-rich diet and those who followed a low-carb diet. There was, however, a significant difference in their health after the trial finished. The people on the pulse diet had a lower risk of heart disease—and that lower risk lasted for at least a year!

The researchers concluded: "A high-fiber bean-rich diet was as effective as a low-carbohydrate diet for weight loss, although only the bean-rich diet lowered atherogenic lipid (the formation of fatty deposits in the arteries)." [Tonstad et al., (2013)]

Arguably, the healthier you feel, the more likely you are to enjoy movement and exercise—and this can help with weight loss.

Eating pulses quickly curbs hunger.

A review published in the journal *Obesity* reported that eating pulses may increase "acute satiety". Acute satiety means satiety that is quickly achieved. The review's authors concluded that these results might "… explain some of the long-term weight loss benefits associated with dietary pulse consumption by supporting adherence to weight loss diets." In other words, when people quickly achieve satiety by eating pulses, there may be more chance that they will stick to meal plans that can help them lose weight. [Li et al., (2014)]

Pulses may keep you slim.

After you've successfully shed some pounds, eating pulses may help maintain your new, lower weight. A 2016 review in *The American Journal of Clinical Nutrition* indicated that eating pulses can not only help you lose weight, but also help you to keep it off.

The reviewers examined 21 clinical trials in which 940 adult men and women took part. The participants lost an average of 0.75 pounds (340 grams) over the course of six weeks, simply by adding a single serve of pulses to their usual diet. Even better, the weight loss occurred without the volunteers making a conscious attempt to cut down on other foods. A single 130 gram serving of pulses per day (less than a cupful) provided people with extra satiety, and helped them to lose weight.

Review leader Dr. de Souza said: "Though the weight loss was small, our findings suggest that simply including pulses in your diet may help you lose weight, and we think more importantly, prevent you from gaining it back after you lose it. [Kim et al, (2016)]

Beans and blood sugar.

Some kinds of beans can help stabilize blood sugar levels. There is evidence that beans eaten with grains (such as rice) can lower blood sugar, thus decreasing the risk of blood-sugar related health problems such as obesity, diabetes and heart disease. A study published in *Nutrition Journal* reported that "Pinto, dark red kidney and black beans with rice attenuate the glycemic response compared to rice alone." [Thompson et al., (2012); Hutchins et al., (2012); Olmedilla-Alonso et al., (2012)]

Peanuts.

Protein-rich, nutrient-rich peanuts are legumes that are quite energy dense. They are, however, very satiating, and may curb your appetite for longer than many other foods. So satisfying are peanuts that they may help you eat fewer Calories overall.

"Despite being energy dense, peanuts have a high satiety value and chronic ingestion (eating a lot) evokes strong dietary compensation and little change in energy balance," concluded the authors of a study published in the *International Journal of Obesity and Related Metabolic Disorders*. [Alper & Mattes (2002)]

Peanuts can be included in a weight-loss diet, but be aware of how many Calories you should be eating per day and include peanuts as part of that allowance. Eat them raw, not roasted in extra oil. Preferably buy them still in their shells and crack them open just before you eat them. This not only uses more energy than simply scooping pre-shelled peanuts into your mouth, it also slows down your eating. You might choose to eat peanuts as a substitute for highly-processed snacks.

What about lectins?

Some people follow a way of eating called the "lectin avoidance diet". It excludes grains, beans, nuts, seeds, most potatoes and all dairy products. This restricted eating regimen is based on the idea that lectins, which are proteins, are "bad for your health".

While it's true that some types of lectins can cause health issues and all lectins can be problematic if eaten the wrong way, people have been consuming lectins in a wide range of foods for thousands of years—long enough to figure out how to treat those foods so that the lectins are rendered harmless, and in fact nutritious. Soaking, fermenting, sprouting and cooking are all processes that reduce lectin levels in foods and release nutrients for you to digest.

Lectins are not alone in their need for pre-processing. There are numerous other foods that have to be treated before they become digestible, such as eggs, which should not be consumed raw in large amounts.

Medical researcher Dr. Art Ayers says, "Some people think that humans and other mammals must be protected from lectins, and that this protection is shown in human and cow's milk in the form of antibodies against lectins. This seems to be a misunderstanding. It is possible for people to be allergic to lectins, but this is unlikely. For example, peanut allergies involve proteins other than the peanut lectins."

Dr Ayers continues, ". . . lectins add to the nutrition of cooked beans and grains that have been the foundations for several thriving civilizations. The longest living [human] members of the bean and grain cultures are typically older and more fit than comparable individuals with a modern, inflammatory diet. . . " [Ayers (2008)]

Lectins are resistant to dry heat, so if you bake with raw legume flours, such as lupin or chick pea flour, start by eating only small amounts of the finished product to see if you have any adverse reaction.

Foods rich in mucilaginous fiber can bind lectins and virtually neutralize them. Such foods include flaxseeds, chia seeds, psyllium, aloe vera, okra, figs, and the seaweeds kelp and agar agar.

Phytic acid or phytate.

Phytate is a compound that exists in all edible plant seeds, including grains, nuts and legumes. It can reduce the bioavailability of iron, zinc and calcium, but the phytate content of foods is easily reduced by soaking, sprouting or fermenting.

How to reduce flatulence from eating beans.

We're always hearing the advice that we should be eating more legumes/pulses (such as beans) because they are packed with protein, fiber and other important nutrients. Eating beans with grains gives us complete protein. However some of us are put off by the possible side effects of eating beans—namely, gas!

Fortunately there is an answer to this problem. After all, beans are a staple and traditional food of many Asian communities. Years ago they worked out how to overcome the uncomfortable and anti-social flatulence, or "wind" problem!

Step by step, here's how to do it.

- If you're switching from a low-fiber diet to a high-fiber diet including legumes, do it gradually. Allow your gut microbes to get used to the new source of nutrition. Give them time to build up populations of the species that deal with legumes, thriving on them, and processing them efficiently. Over, say, a week, introduce small amounts of beans into your diet, slowly increasing the amount. Your body, and your microbiome, adapt quite rapidly if you persevere. After three weeks on a high-legume diet there should be very few side effects and after 8 weeks, practically none at all.

- Begin by eating legumes that contain fewer of the complex sugars that are harder for your digestive enzymes to break down. These more easily-digested legumes include mung beans, adzuki beans and lentils.

- Lentils, tofu, split peas, and canned beans tend to produce less gas.

- Soaking dried beans overnight and throwing out the soaking water before cooking helps reduce the gassiness of beans. Repeated soaking can also help.

- When boiling beans, skim off and discard any foam that rises to the surface.

- Cook dry beans by boiling them at least three times. Each time you boil them, throw out the used water and cover the beans with fresh water before replacing the pot on the heat.

- Properly chew beans before you swallow them. Digestion begins in the mouth. Take time to chew them into small fragments, while enjoying their flavors and textures. Using your teeth to start the break-down process means that your gut microbes will have less work to do later.

- The sulfurous odor of flatulence gasses is caused mainly by the digestion of foods rich in sulfur, so avoid eating meat or eggs in combination with beans. You might also want to avoid cauliflower and garlic.

- Sugars mingling with legumes in the gut may contribute to gassiness. To minimise this, eat any sugary foods or fruits 2 to 3 hours *before* or 2 to 3 hours *after* a meal containing beans. Having said that, note that sugar-sweetened bean pastes are popular in Asian cuisine. Anko is sweet red bean paste made with adzuki beans, while Shiro-an is sweet white bean paste. Neither of these preparations appears to cause flatulence problems, probably because of the way they are prepared, with repeated cooking. (They are also delicious and rich in protein.)

- Eating seaweed with beans may make them more digestible. In traditional Japanese cuisine, a piece of seaweed such as kombu, kelp or wakame is often eaten with beans. Sea vegetables are also loaded with nutrients.

- Intensifying the flavors of your meal of beans by cooking them with particular spices may also help to reduce gassiness. Indian cooks may add ginger, turmeric, fennel, cumin and sometimes asafetida to bean dishes. These are sometimes called "digestive spices".

- When you eat beans, eat them in combination with plenty of vegetables. Aim for a ratio of approximately one part beans to three parts vegetables.

- Some people avoid eating potatoes in combination with beans, to reduce flatulence.

- If all else fails, dietary supplements such as "Beano®", containing the alpha-galactosidase enzyme can break up bean sugars and decrease flatulence.

How to cook dried beans.

Many people prefer to use dried beans because they are cheaper than canned beans, and come with no additives. Here's how to cook them.

- Before you cook them, soak them in fresh cold water for at least eight hours. You could soak them overnight if you wish.

- Pour the beans into a colander/strainer. Drain and rinse them thoroughly. Throw out the soaking and rinsing water (you could water your garden with it!). Some people like to repeat this soaking and process twice, or even several times, to get a better result.

- Place the beans into a cooking pot with plenty of fresh, clean water (read the packet for directions on the ratio of water to beans).

- To the pot, you could add some seaweed and/or some spices to help with digestion, if you like.

- Place the pot on the heat and bring to the boil. Cook for the period of time recommended on the packet. Skim off and discard any foam that forms on the surface. Discard the cooking water after the beans have become tender and ready to eat.

3. FOODS THAT CAN HELP WEIGHT LOSS: SPICES & HERBS

Spices and herbs are your weight loss friends.

Your taste-buds will be glad of this news! Not only can you make your meals taste better, but you may also be able to improve your health and satiety just by adding spices and herbs.

When you eat foods that are rich in strong flavors, your Inner Guardian gets the message that you really have dined well, and so there is no need to trigger the release of any more "hunger hormones". Imagine eating nothing but bland, insipid foods, day after day… surely you would start to have cravings!

Some people think of "spicy" as meaning "hot"—that is, with hot chillies added. The Merriam-Webster dictionary, however, defines spices as "any of various aromatic vegetable products (as pepper or nutmeg) used to season or flavor foods". Spice has another meaning: "Something that gives zest or relish". And indeed, that's exactly what spices do to food.

For clarification, we classify spices as "sweet" (cinnamon, nutmeg, cardamom, ginger, cloves, turmeric etc.) or "hot" (Spices derived from chillies or peppers containing capsaicin and/or related compounds called capsaicinoids.)

"Herbs" include garlic, sage, thyme, rosemary, parsley and so on.

Blood sugar and blood fats.

Both spices and herbs may help curb blood sugar spikes. Researchers from Penn State University (USA) showed that adding some spice to a meal can actually make digestion easier. They added herbs and spices including rosemary, oregano, cinnamon, turmeric, black pepper, cloves, garlic powder and paprika to the meals of overweight volunteers. The addition of spices lowered the volunteers' blood insulin spike by around 20%. The researchers concluded, "The incorporation of spices into the diet may help normalize postprandial [after-eating] insulin and triglycerides [blood fats] and enhance antioxidant defenses." [Skulas-Ray et al., (2011)]

The hot spices.

Burning more energy and curbing appetite, the hot spices include mustard, cayenne pepper, horseradish, wasabi, and chili peppers.

Red hot chili peppers

Chilies, or chili peppers, are plants in the botanical genus Capsicum. Like cayenne pepper, they contain a compound called capsaicin, which can help with weight loss.

"Addition of capsaicin . . . to the diet has been shown to increase energy expenditure; therefore capsaicin is an interesting target for anti-obesity therapy," say researchers. [Janssens et al., (2013)]

Study after study contributes supporting evidence that eating hot spicy foods can help you lose weight. [Inoue et al., (2007); Yoshioka et al., (1999); Reinbach et al., (2009)]

It has even been suggested that hot chili peppers could be used as a drug to fight obesity. [Leung (2014)]

A study published in the journal *Physiology & Behavior* found that when people ate food spiced with hot red peppers, it not only increased their energy expenditure and core temperature (thus burning more Calories!) but it also reduced their appetite, so that they ate less food. The hot red peppers had to be eaten as part of a meal, and not consumed in capsule form as a dietary supplement. The spicy meals given to volunteers were "hedonically acceptable"— which means they were not too hot for the diners' preferences and didn't cause them discomfort!

Interestingly, the hot spicy food only had a Calorie-burning/ appetite-reducing effect on people who were not accustomed to eating it. The researchers concluded that "Desensitization to red pepper's effects may occur with long-term spicy food intake."

So if you're going to use hot spices to help you lose weight, don't eat them every day. [Ludy & Mattes (2011)]

In summary, adding hot chili peppers to some meals may:
- Curb your appetite so that you want to eat less food
- Speed up your metabolism so that you burn more Calories
- Decrease your desire to eat fat
- Make you eat more slowly, so that you reach satiety earlier in your meal

Chili peppers can be used fresh, dried, or dried and ground to a powder. Add them to your meals in different ways.

- As a hot, spicy sauce such as sriracha, or Tabasco®, poured over your food
- In hot curry paste
- In the form of dried, powdered or chopped chilies sprinkled on meals or cooked into dishes
- In the form of cayenne pepper

The sweet spices.
Cinnamon.

Eating cinnamon (*Cinnamomum verum*) can lower blood sugar levels. A 2007 study published in *The American Journal of Clinical Nutrition* [Hlebowicz et al., (2007)] reported that the addition of cinnamon to a rice pudding dessert:

- Significantly delayed gastric emptying—that is, it made the pudding-eaters feel fuller for longer.
- Lowered the "postprandial glucose response"—that is, it decreased the blood sugar spike usually associated with eating sweet desserts like rice pudding.

Turmeric.

Turmeric (*Curcuma longa*) is rich in curcumin, which may help curb weight gain. In 2009, researchers at the Jean Mayer USDA Human Nutrition Research Center on Aging at Tufts University published the results of a test on mice who were fed high-fat diets. When the researchers included curcumin in the food of the mice, the growth of the mice's fat cells appeared to be suppressed and their weight gain was reduced. [Ejaz et al., (2009)]

Fenugreek

The fiber in fenugreek (*Trigonella foenum-graecum*) can boost satiety. It is a plant that is used as an herb (dried or fresh leaves), spice (seeds), and vegetable (fresh leaves, sprouts, and microgreens). The seeds are frequently included in the cuisines of the Indian subcontinent, incorporated into pickles, vegetable dishes, daals, and spice mixes. In their raw state the seeds have a touch of bitterness, but roasting decreases this as well as improving the flavor. After roasting they can be ground into a powder or used whole.

A 2009 study published in *Phytotherapy Research* found that when overweight people included 8 grams of fenugreek fiber in their meals, it "significantly increased satiety and reduced energy intake at lunch, suggesting it may have short-term beneficial effects in obese subjects." [Mathern et al., (2009)]

Other benefits of spices.
Healthier genes?

It is thought that turmeric may be able to decrease your risk of disease. As mentioned, turmeric contains a compound called curcumin, which gives it that rich, golden color. In our section "Can we replace food with dietary supplements?" we discussed Dr. Michael Mosley's experiments with turmeric.

To refresh your memory: Professor Widschwendter of University College, London, said, "… the group [of test volunteers] who mixed turmeric powder into their food [showed] quite substantial changes. It was really exciting, to be honest. We found one particular gene which showed the biggest difference. And what's interesting is that we know this particular gene is involved in three specific diseases: depression, asthma and eczema, and cancer. This is a really striking finding."

Longer life?

A 2017 research article published in the journal *PLOS One* found that eating a lot of red hot chillies was associated with longer life! [Chopan & Littenberg (2017)]

4. FOODS THAT CAN HELP WEIGHT LOSS: SOUP

Soup is good for satiety.

As a general rule, a meal that is drunk in the form of a liquid beverage tends to gives less satiety than the same meal in the form of solids that have to be bitten and chewed. Solid foods are usually more filling than liquid foods.

Soup, however, is the exception to this rule!
[Mourao et al., (2007)]

"Energy-yielding fluids generally have lower satiety value than solid foods. However, despite high water content, soups reportedly are satiating," say the authors of a 2004 study published in Physiology & Behavior. " … these data support the high satiety value of soups." [Mattes (2004)]

"Soup is an example of a food that is highly satiating," say the authors of a 1995 report. "A clinical survey in which intakes were analyzed from food diaries found that meals that included soup were associated both with lower caloric intakes within the meals and with lower daily caloric intakes than those meals without soup. Several studies have confirmed that soup is a highly satiating food. At least part of the explanation is the low energy density of soup." [Marriott (1995)]

The right kinds of soups can help you lose weight. They can make you feel replete and full on fewer Calories, even when you're eating a larger volume of food. The best high-satiety soups for weight loss are:

- satisfying and filling
- low in Calories
- rich in fiber
- nutritious
- full of flavor
- abounding in water
- low in fat

How does soup help with weight loss?

Soup is mainly liquid, but it's nutritious liquid, teeming with food particles. A 2013 study published in the *European Journal of Clinical Nutrition* aimed to find out why so many previous studies had established the satiety-power of soups compared with solid foods. The researchers wanted to discover the mechanisms controlling soup-induced satiety. They wrote, "This study aimed to understand the physiological mechanisms causing soup to be more satiating."

They gave three different meals to volunteers; a solid meal, a chunky soup and a smooth soup. After each meal they measured:

- How fast the food passed out of the stomach into the intestines (the rate of gastric emptying)
- Fluctuations in the volunteers' blood sugar levels
- How satiated the volunteers said they felt

The volunteers gave the smooth, viscous soup the best rating for satiety. The smooth soup also stayed on their stomachs for longer (which helps to explain the feeling of prolonged fullness). Perhaps surprisingly, the smooth soup also had the greatest impact on blood sugar levels. This seems to contradict what we've been told about the Glycemic Index, but there is an explanation. Because the tiny particles of food in soup are easier for the body to absorb than big chunks, it's not long after you start eating soup that your bloodstream receives a dose of carbohydrates. This triggers the sending of certain signals to the brain. Very early in your soup-eating experience, your Inner Guardian gets the message that "food is incoming". The hunger hormone ghrelin is then turned down, while the satiety hormone leptin is turned up. Your appetite diminishes.

The researchers concluded: "The smooth soup induced greater fullness compared with the solid meal because of a combination of delayed gastric emptying, leading to feelings of gastric distension and rapid accessibility of nutrients causing a greater glycemic response." [Clegg et al., (2013)]

Different forms of ingredients.

Eating the same ingredients in different forms changes their satiety power. Visualize a typical evening (western-style) meal; for example, meat and three vegetables washed down with a glass of water. After you've eaten and drunk, you probably won't feel hungry again for at least an hour or two. Yet, if you put that same meal into a blender and pulverize it until it becomes a creamy soup, eating that soup will keep you feeling fuller for longer.

Water content.

Soup's water content keeps the soup in your stomach for longer. When you eat the solid meat and vegetables, and drink the very runny water, you might imagine that the chewed foods would blend with the water to form a smooth soup inside your stomach in any case. Yet this is not so.

After you eat a meal, your pyloric sphincter valve (a band of smooth muscle at the junction between your stomach and your small intestine) closes off. It needs to hold the food in your stomach, so that the stomach has enough time to properly churn the food and mix it with digestive juices. Anything that's as runny as water is still able to easily escape through the pyloric sphincter valve. When you drink water, it goes pretty much straight from your mouth to your intestines. It doesn't stay in your stomach for very long at all, and thus it cannot make you feel full.

However, when you drink water that's been mixed with fine food particles—i.e. soup—those food particles slow down the water. They keep it in the stomach for longer. The stomach remains stretched for longer, and while it is stretched it is sending out "fullness" signals to your brain. Yet it's partly full of water—and there are no Calories in water!

How to use soup as a weight loss tool.

Researchers recommend eating soup as a first course, or "preload", to help you lose weight. One study found that soup was just as satiating whether it was thin like consommé, bouillon and broth, thick like mulligatawny or somewhere in between, like minestrone.

" . . . consuming soup as a preload can significantly reduce subsequent entrée [main course] intake, as well as total energy intake at the meal. . . . varying the form and viscosity of soup, by changing the way in which identical ingredients were blended, [does] not significantly affect energy intake or satiety. Therefore, consuming a preload of low-energy-dense soup, in a variety of forms, is one strategy that can be used to moderate energy intake in adults." [Flood & Rolls (2007)]

When meal ingredients are puréed into the form of a thick and viscous soup, they provide more satiety than those same ingredients eaten in solid form.

Soup's viscosity and temperature.

However, given that other food studies indicate that viscous textures tend to be the most highly satiating, we would recommend that thicker soups would be most helpful for weight loss. We have as yet found no data on cold soups versus hot soups, but anecdotal evidence suggests that hot soup would be most satisfying.

Satiety Diet soups

Canned, ready-made or other processed soups may be satiating, but they may not be suitable for the Satiety Diet. Many contain added sugars, oils, fats and starches. Read the label! Real Satiety Diet soups are more like a home-cooked meal blended with a glass of water—very thick and more like a purée than soup. Dry-baked croutons and other crunchy bits can be added for an extra-satisfying texture. "Crispy, Creamy, Chewy: The Satiety Diet Cookbook" (book #3 in the series) provides recipes for satisfying soups.

5. FOODS THAT CAN HELP WEIGHT LOSS: COLORFUL FOODS

As the saying goes, "Eat the rainbow".

Colorful foods are rich in valuable nutrients. When you "eat the rainbow" you are benefiting from all these different nutrients, and warding off the nutritional deficiencies that can lead to over-eating.

Colorful foods also provide important sensory enjoyment, in that a plate full of colorful foods is more pleasant to look at than a plate of foods that are all drab colors. Imagine a salad plate of purple cabbage, red tomatoes, orange carrots, yellow bell peppers and green basil leaves compared with a plate of white cabbage, white potato salad, and blanched cauliflower florets. Most people would prefer the plate of many colors!

As mentioned elsewhere in this book, putting three food items of three different colors on your plate is more likely to satisfy you on a subconscious level, if you're an adult, while children seem to prefer seven different items and six colors. [Zampollo et al., (2012)]

Orange and yellow foods.

Many fruits and vegetables come in shades of orange and yellow. Apricots, for example, and cantaloupe (rock melon), mangoes, peaches, papayas, citrus fruits, pineapple, carrots, sweet potatoes, butternut squash, sweetcorn, pumpkin, and capsicums (peppers).

Fruit of these colors contain zeaxanthin, flavonoids, lycopene, potassium, vitamin C and beta-carotene (vitamin A).

The yellow and orange hues in these fruits and vegetables is largely produced by their beta-carotene content. This strongly colored red-orange pigment is a powerful antioxidant that benefits the health of your eyes and has been shown to slow down the decline of cognitive function in older people.

Green foods.

Green is the color of freshness. It's the color of springtime and new leaves. Green is one of the appetizing colors. What makes plants green is a pigment called chlorophyll. The plants with the darkest green color contain the most chlorophyll.

436

Chlorophyll is a valuable phytonutrient that promotes good health in a number of ways, including helping with the repair of damaged DNA and promoting the healing of wounds.

Green foods include:
- leafy greens such as silver beet (chard), spinach, kale, watercress, rocket (aragula).
- fresh herbs such as cilantro (coriander), mint, basil.
- green vegetables such as asparagus, peas, celery and broccoli.
- green fruits such as kiwifruit and grapes.
- sea vegetables (seaweed)

Red foods.

Our brains are wired to prefer red foods over foods of other colors. It is thought that this is because in nature, red foods generally have more Calories or protein (e.g. meat) than foods of other colors. [Foroni et al., (2016)] Red, of course, is also the color of ripeness.

Knowing that red is a color associated with appetizing food, marketing experts favor red shades for food packaging and advertising.

The red color of many plant foods comes from anthocyanins, those bright, attractive pigments with a wide range of health benefits. Red anthocyanins can be found in such foods as strawberries, cranberries, raspberries. tomatoes, rhubarb and red cabbage.

Anthocyanins in colorful foods.

We discuss anthocyanins further in our section on Colorful Foods: Purple Foods. Just a reminder—anthocyanins are pigments that occur in the tissues of certain plants, including leaves, stems, roots, flowers, and fruits. They can appear in shades of red, purple, or blue. They belong to a parent class of molecules called flavonoids.

Anthocyanins act as antioxidants in plants and also in laboratory test tubes, but after you eat anthocyanin-rich foods these colorful compounds lose this antioxidant effect. Nonetheless, studies show that after you eat them, the antioxidant capacity of your blood increases. Experts surmise that this beneficial effect "…may not be caused directly by the anthocyanins, but instead may result from increased uric acid levels derived from metabolism of flavonoids." [Stauth (2007)]

Purple and blue anthocyanins can be found in purple carrots, blackcurrants, purple cabbage, black rice, purple plums, blueberries and mulberries.

Blue foods.

The color blue, in foods, is said to be an appetite suppressant. Blue is a beautiful color, so why is it considered to be unappetizing?

Perhaps because in nature, blue—the color of a clear summer sky—is a color rarely found in anything that's edible. Most foods we call "blue" are really purple or purplish-black—think of blueberries, blue corn etc. The few edible exceptions include flower petals such as those of the butterfly blue pea (*Clitoria ternatea*) and cornflower (*Centaurea cyanus*).

Naturally sky-blue food is uncommon. Meat doesn't come in shades of blue and neither do leafy vegetables. (That said, the Japanese are famous for their artistic use of food colorings, including blue!)

As we've mentioned elsewhere, research from around the world shows that it is hard to persuade people to taste blue-colored foods. In one study, people sat down to a delicious meal on a plate, comprising colorful foods in yellows, reds, and greens etc. Before they started eating, the lighting in the room was changed to blue. The meal and the surroundings all took on a blue tinge. Under these conditions, the study's participants consumed the meal that they knew— cognitively—was really composed of multi colored ingredients. However their eyes told them a different story, and they struggled to finish the meal. Some of them even felt sick afterwards.

Weight loss and food colors.

Why should you choose food colors that increase appetite, if you're aiming for weight loss?

Based on the premise that the color blue suppresses appetite, some weight loss gurus suggest strategies such as eating off blue tableware, installing a blue light in the dining room or kitchen, dyeing your food blue and wearing blue-tinted sunglasses. We don't recommend these practices, however. When you're aiming for weight loss, choose food colors that promote satiety, not colors that put you off your meal.

Satiety is inextricably associated with satisfaction. If you're presented with a meal that's all one bland color, for example, or if you're offered a meal in which everything is dyed with unappetizing shades of blue, you're not going to get as much satisfaction from that meal.

After the unsatisfying meal is over, as you go about your daily activities you're likely to glimpse images of better-colored, more appetizing-looking foods, or to conjure mental images of them. That kind of thinking leads to cravings, because your Inner Guardian is more likely to be on the lookout for foods of the colors it missed.

Purple foods.

Like purple, blue is a "cold" color, but purple has some red in it, which makes it "warmer". Most of us enjoy eating purple foods such as blueberries, grapes, aubergines, plums and purple carrots.

While psychologists and researchers tell us that we find warm-colored foods most attractive, it's vibrantly-colored foods—in particular purple foods—that can bring us a host of health benefits, including weight loss!

Purple foods may boost weight loss.

If you become obese your swollen fat cells can burst, allowing fat to leak into your bloodstream and causing low-grade inflammation. Over time, this inflammation can cause damage to any and every one of your internal organs, leading to diseases such as heart problems, fatty liver, diabetes and insulin resistance. [ABC Catalyst (2015)]

If you lose weight, you can stop the inflammation.

Professor Lindsay Brown of the University of Southern Queensland (Australia) has been conducting research into whether purple fruits and vegetables can actually help obese people to lose weight, so that their levels of inflammation will subside and their overall health will be improved.

The purple coloring in plant-based foods is bestowed anthocyanins. Anthocyanins may appear red, purple, or blue depending on their pH. The more acidic the pH, the redder the hue of the anthocyanin. The more alkaline (basic) the pH, the more the color shifts to purple and then to blue. This would indicate that purple foods have a fairly neutral pH.

Plants use anthocyanins to keep themselves in good health. These compounds can do the same for us.

Professor Brown and his team fed rats a high-carbohydrate, high-fat diet. They became obese, and developed high blood pressure, a fatty liver, poor heart function and arthritis. Then, without changing anything else, the researchers added purple plum juice or carrot juice to the unhealthful diet of the obese, unwell rats.

The rats lost weight. Not only that but their blood pressure, fat levels, liver function and heart function all returned to normal.

Professor Brown was surprised by the spectacular results.

"When purple carrots or Queen Garnet® plums were ingested, even in the presence of eating a high fat, high sugar diet, weight loss occurred. Not only that, but heart health improved, liver function and architecture were normalized, blood pressure returned to normal, and glucose was taken up normally by the body once more," he said. "… the anthocyanins in purple carrots, in Queen Garnet® plums … completely reverse all of those [obesity-related ill-health] changes, so we haven't changed the diet—they're still getting this high-carbo-hydrate, high-fat diet—and yet with that intervention, all of those parameters that characterize obesity are back to normal."

Can eating purple carrots help with weight loss?

The next step is human trials, but until they are completed, it might be worthwhile to incorporate purple carrots into your diet (assuming you can't get hold of any Queen Garnet plums® yet). Queen Garnet® plums may have the highest anthocyanin content of any fruit, but purple carrots have the highest anthocyanin content of any vegetable.

Purple foods can help curb weight gain.

Blueberries and mulberries, rich in purple-blue anthocyanins, have been shown to help curb weight gain.

A 2013 study published in the journal *PLOS One* aimed to establish "...whether blueberry (*Vaccinium ashei*) and mulberry (*Morus australis Poir*) juice, anthocyanin rich fruit juice, may help counteract obesity."

In this trial, the researchers fed mice a high fat diet. One group received only high fat food, while the other group ate the same high fat food in addition to blueberry juice and mulberry juice. The mice that ate only fatty foods got fatter and heavier. Their insulin resistance increased, and so did their blood fats and the fats in their livers. By contrast, the mice that received the dark purple fruit juices did not gain weight. They enjoyed other health benefits, too!

"These results indicate that blueberry and mulberry juice may help counteract obesity," wrote the study's authors. [Tao Wu et al., (2013)]

441

Brown and beige foods.

Brown and beige foods may not sound very exciting at first glance, but they belong on the rainbow too. They include cinnamon, nuts, cocoa and cacao, chocolate, mushrooms, brown rice, fresh ginger, chickpeas and hummus,

Black foods.

Black is another color that is said to make food look repellent, but this is debatable. In Vietnamese cuisine for example the plant ramie (*Boehmeria nivea*) is prized for its black food dye.

The trendy Western palate delights in black rice, black pasta, black beans, black sesame, black corn chips, strong coffee, dark chocolate, foods colored with squid ink, black beans and other black foods.

The color in many "black" foods is caused by dark purple anthocyanins, natural compounds that are beneficial for your health.

White foods.

White foods sometimes get a "bad rap", because highly-processed, nutrition-sparse foods are often pale. Take, for example, white bread, white pasta and products made from refined flour and table sugar.

White foods are not "on the rainbow", but they can be delicious and nutritious, and naturally occurring white foods should be included in a diverse diet. The very first food that ever passed your lips was white in color—milk. Other naturally white foods (or close to white) include cauliflower, tofu, chick peas, parsnips, and potatoes.

6. FOODS THAT CAN HELP WEIGHT LOSS: OLIVE OIL

Olive oil contains oleic acid which may help weight loss by helping create a sense of satiety. That said, olive oil is rich in Calories so consume it sparingly! Choose cold pressed extra virgin olive oil. [Schwartz et al., (2008)]

7. FOODS THAT CAN HELP WEIGHT LOSS: GRAPEFRUIT

In the 1980s a craze for eating grapefruit to lose weight swept the western world. Eating grapefruit is harmless unless you are taking certain medications, whose bioavailability may be compromised (read the instructions on your medications). Grapefruit is nutritious, relatively low in Calories, high in vitamin C and considered to be a "low-fructose" fruit.

A 2006 study published in *The Journal of Medicinal Food* shows that grapefruit may indeed help with weight loss. Over 12 weeks the volunteers lost between 3.3 and 10 pounds (1.5 - 4.5 kilograms).

The researchers wrote, "Half of a fresh grapefruit eaten before meals was associated with significant weight loss. ...Insulin resistance was improved with fresh grapefruit. Although the mechanism of this weight loss is unknown it would appear reasonable to include grapefruit in a weight reduction diet."

The study was conducted with obese human volunteers.

[Fujioka et al., (2006)]

8. FOODS THAT CAN HELP WEIGHT LOSS: NUTS

You'd think that nuts would be "forbidden" to people who want to lose weight, because they are relatively Calorie-dense. You can eat them now and then in small quantities, however, and still lose weight. Studies indicate that people who eat peanuts and tree nuts (e.g. almonds, walnuts, pecans) on a regular basis are more likely to be slimmer than people who don't. Furthermore, a 2008 study found that people on low Calorie weight-loss diets are more likely to stick to the diet if they allow themselves to eat nuts from time to time, and thus they tend to lose more weight!

The researchers wrote: "The few trials contrasting weight loss through regimens that include or exclude nuts indicate improved compliance and greater weight loss when nuts are permitted. This consistent literature suggests nuts may be included in the diet, in moderation, to enhance palatability and nutrient quality without posing a threat for weight gain." [Mattes et al., (2008)]

9. FOODS THAT CAN HELP WEIGHT LOSS: KUDZU

Kudzu can help curb alcohol consumption, which in turn helps with weight loss. Also known as Japanese arrowroot, kudzu (*Pueraria lobata*, also called *Radix puerariae*) is an ancient vine that has been a popular food in Japan, Korea and China for thousands of years. The young leaves can be eaten, as well as the flowers and the roots. The tuberous roots that dried and pounded into a starchy, nutritious powder that has multiple uses in Asian cuisine. It's often used to thicken soups and sauces, or to make batter to coat foods for deep-frying.

In addition to being high in fiber, protein and vitamins A and D, kudzu root contains certain isoflavonones. Consumption of these compounds as a herbal extract has been proven to reduce alcohol intake. Kudzu doesn't curb cravings for alcohol, but it has been shown to make people drink less without really noticing it, and without any nasty side effects.

10. FOODS THAT CAN HELP WEIGHT LOSS: BREAKFAST FOODS

Here's what *not* to eat for breakfast when you want to lose weight:
- Those conveniently pre-packaged, heavily processed and heavily sugared foods manufacturers call 'breakfast cereal'. It's really candy in disguise.
- Those "grab and go' convenience breakfasts
- Liquid breakfasts, such as shakes or smoothies or protein drinks
- Bakery foods made with refined flour

Here's what to eat:
- Protein, unrefined carbs, fiber, a small amount of healthful fats
- Food of many textures and colors
- Foods that take a lot of chewing
- Porridge that needs a lot of cooking, e.g. steel cut oats or whole oat groats, rather than instant oats.
- Finish your breakfast meal with something sweet, if you feel like it. Choose low fructose fruits or a low fructose dessert. Your body processes sugars best early in the day.

444

11. FOODS THAT CAN HELP WEIGHT LOSS: FIBER-RICH FOODS

Foods that are high in dietary fiber tend to be more satiating than low-fiber foods. A fiber-rich diet can help with weight control.

A 2012 study found that people who ate whole grains (such as brown rice instead of white rice) had a lower risk of weight gain. [Ye et al., (2012)]

In 2003, researchers reported that women who consumed high fiber foods weighed less than women who followed a low-fiber diet. [Liu et al., (2003)]

Another study found that when white rice was replaced with a mixture of brown and black rice in meals, overweight women lost weight and body fat. [Kim et al., (2008)]

Eating brown rice instead of white rice can also help normalize blood sugar responses. [Mohan et al., (2014)]

In 2008, researchers conducted a study to determine whether including whole-grain foods in a low-Calorie diet could help with weight loss. They reported "There were significantly greater decreases in ... percentage body fat in the abdominal region in participants consuming whole grains than in those consuming refined grains." [Katcher, et al., (2008)]

Brown rice contains fewer Calories per gram (or ounce) than white rice because it contains fiber, which is not digested, and water, which is Calorie-free. This means it can make you feel full on fewer Calories, which in turn makes losing weight less difficult.

Other excellent sources of dietary fiber include legumes/pulses such as beans, peas and lentils.

12. FOODS THAT CAN HELP WEIGHT LOSS: HIGH PROTEIN, LOW-FAT FOODS WITH FIBER

Protein boosts satiety. It is considered to be a powerful appetite suppressant. "We found that an additional 20-30 grams of protein or a 3-4 ounce portion of lean protein was enough to influence appetite," says Purdue University nutrition professor Wayne Campbell, PhD, who has helped conduct several studies into the relationship pf protein to appetite. "We have also shown that when diets are inadequate in the amount of protein and don't meet national recommendations, the desire to eat increases." [Leidy et al., (2007); Leidy et al., (2010); Leidy et al., (2011)]

You can eat lean protein at any meal, but studies indicate that eating it at breakfast time could be especially beneficial.

Enjoy lean protein at every meal and as part of any snack. At mealtimes, it helps boost satiety when you eat protein as part of your first course ("appetizer" in US terminology; "starter" or "entrée" in UK terminology).

For weight loss, choose lean protein over high-fat protein. Except in soy, the fat in beans is negligible. Unprocessed, whole grains are low in fats. Peanuts and some seeds are high in fats, but they tend to be beneficial fats.

High protein plant-based foods.

Protein is a proven satiety-giving food, and so is fiber. You can get both of these packaged together as nature intended, with extra nutrients thrown in (as well as plenty of flavor), if you choose plant-based protein. Make sure you choose whole foods, which come complete with their natural fiber. For example, choose brown rice instead of white rice, and whole-wheat flour instead of white flour.

"Complete protein" contains all essential amino acids. Our bodies cannot manufacture essential amino acids, which is why we must get them from food. The nine essential amino acids are: histidine, isoleucine, leucine, lysine, methionine, phenylalanine, threonine, tryptophan, and valine.

Different plant-based foods contain amino acids in various concentrations and proportions. By mixing together a number of varied plant-based foods, you can obtain all the essential acids needed to make complete protein. The following are some examples of high protein plant-based foods. Many more exist!

Seeds.
Hemp seed
Hemp seeds contain all the essential amino acids. However, the protein in hemp is not considered to be a complete protein source, because it is low in lysine. Its leucine content is also relatively low, but it contains satisfactory amounts of both L-tyrosine and arginine.
Chia seed
Chia seeds contain 18 of the 22 amino acids, including all nine essential amino acids: isoleucine, leucine, lysine, methionine, phenylalanine, threonine, tryptophan, valine, and histadine.

Grains.
Teff
Teff is a tiny, ancient grain that's rich in almost-complete protein, gluten-free, very low in saturated fat and packed with vitamins, minerals and fiber. Traditionally it is the staple foodstuff or people in Eritrea and Ethiopia. It is also delicious and versatile. Teff is a satiating food that is valuable ingredient for body-weight management.

Legumes.
Soy
Whole, unprocessed soy beans are good sources of protein, as are oy products such as tempeh, miso, edamame and tofu. Soy contains all eight essential amino acids. It is also a rich source of iron and calcium and many valuable dietary minerals.
Peanuts
A celery stick dipped in a little peanut butter provides a satisfying blend of fat and protein for a snack.
Chickpeas (garbanzo beans)
High in protein but low in fat, chick peas are also cheap and nutritious. They contain 23% protein, and when eaten with grains or seeds (such as rice or sesame seeds) they hep provide complete protein.

Pseudocereals.

Quinoa

A serving of quinoa contains the following amino acids: isoleucine, leucine, lysine, phenylalanine, tyrosine, cysteine, methionine, threonine, histidine, tryptophan and valine.

Animal sources of protein.

You can also get low-fat protein from Greek yogurt, cottage cheese, eggs, and lean meats. Animal based protein, however, contains no fiber.

13. FOODS THAT CAN HELP WEIGHT LOSS: CALORIE-SPARSE FOODS

Foods that are Calorie-sparse (i.e. with low energy-density) are foods that contain few Calories per unit of weight. Imagine two foods of the same weight. If Food "A" has a low number of Calories and Food "B" has a high number of Calories, then Food "A" has a lower energy density—it is more "Calorie-sparse".

Dr. Adam Drewnowski, Director of the Nutritional Sciences Program at the University of Washington in the USA, writes that when people are free to eat whatever they like, they "… tend to consume a constant weight of food rather than a constant quantity of energy."

He goes on to say that "Foods with lower energy density (i.e. fewer Calories per unit weight) deliver fewer Calories per eating occasion than do energy-rich foods. In contrast, higher energy density is associated with higher energy intake per meal. According to current theories, high energy density, rather than the fat content of foods, is the main reason for overeating and for the growing prevalence of overweight." [Drewnowski (1998)]

The satiety benefits of Calorie-sparse foods.

When you eat foods that are Calorie-sparse, you can feel full and reach satiety after eating fewer Calories. Conversely, if you eat a lot of Calorie-dense foods, you will probably end up eating more Calories to make you feel full.

Including foods low in Calorie-density as part of your regular diet enables you to lose weight without feeling as if you're deprived or restricted.

By eating this way you can reduce Calories while still filling your plate with plenty of food. Your eyes will see a plate loaded with food, which is a visual cue to your Inner Guardian, conveying the message that you're having a lot to eat. The Guardian then thinks it can safely start releasing leptin, the satiety hormone, and curbing ghrelin, the hunger hormone. And because Calorie-sparse foods stay in the stomach for longer, you're unlikely to be tormented by continual hunger.

"We have found in numerous studies that when you allow people to eat as much as they want of foods that are high in volume yet low in density (Calories), they eat less at the meal or during the day," says Researcher Barbara Rolls, PhD, of Pennsylvania State University in the USA.

By choosing the right foods, you can actually eat more and still lose weight!

The composition of Calorie-sparse foods.

Foods containing the same ingredients can have different Calorie densities depending on how they are composed. Here's a simple example:

Cup #1 holds water mixed with half a teaspoon of sugar. The liquid weighs 225 grams (8 ounces). Cup #2 holds water mixed with 3 tablespoonsful of sugar. The liquid also weighs 225 grams (8 ounces).

Both containers hold sugar syrup, but the syrup in #1 has more water in it than the syrup in #2. Therefore it is less Calorie dense.

Water and sugar are not satiety-promoting foods. The sugar syrup example is given just to show how Calorie density works. It takes more than just low energy density to make a food worthy of the Satiety Diet!

449

What makes foods Calorie-sparse?

Water is one of the ingredients that can make foods less Calorie dense, because water has zero Calories. **Fiber** can also reduce the Calorie-density of foods because it is bulky but largely indigestible. **Air** is another ingredient which, when it forms part of a food, acts to distend the stomach and give a feeling of fullness while providing zero Calories.

The water, fiber or air must be part of the food.

As we discussed in our section on "Soup", simply drinking water with meals does not enhance satiety. Eating Calorie-rich food and drinking water at the same time is not sufficient to change the fattening food into a low Calorie-density snack.

The water has to be IN THE FOOD.

This is because:

- When water is thoroughly pre-blended with the food, the food stays in the stomach for longer and keeps you feeling full for longer.

- It takes you longer to eat bulkier, water-rich foods than it does to eat solid foods and drink some water. This gives your body time to release satiety hormones before you've eaten too much.

- When you take longer to eat a meal, your senses are being stimulated for longer. You see, hear, and taste the food for longer, so that your Inner Guardian really gets the message that you've eaten and sends out body-messages to stop eating.

The same goes for air. If you manage to swallow some air while you're eating, it's unlikely to have any satiety-power. However when you eat a low-Calorie whipped pudding, full of tiny air bubbles, you can get that sensation of fullness on fewer Calories.

Foods that may curb appetite and help with weight loss include soups and salads, because they contain more water and fiber.

There's no doubt that eating more fiber-rich, water-rich, Calorie-sparse whole foods helps people lose weight. [Sartorelli et al., (2008)]

Some Calorie-sparse foods.

For better weight loss, make vegetables the main bulk of your meals. (You can even make desserts from veggies!)

All foods contain at least a few Calories (except things like salt). Theoretically if you gorged on several pounds of blueberries in one sitting, for example, you could gain weight. But you're unlikely to do so—factors such as sensory monotony and stomach distension would probably make you stop eating.

Here's a list of some foods that are recommended for weight loss due to their relative Calorie-sparseness, high fiber content or other characteristics. These are foods that can be eaten freely, because you're unlikely to "overdose" on them!

Acorn squash	Agar agar (also called kanten)
Aragula (rocket)	Artichoke hearts
Asparagus	Bamboo shoots
Beans and lentils (protein)	Bean sprouts
Beets	Bell peppers (capsicums)
Blackberries	Blueberries
Bok Choy	Broccoli & broccolini
Broccoli rabe	Brussels sprouts
Butternut squash	Cabbage
Carrots	Cauliflower
Celery	Clementines
Cranberries (fresh)	Cucumber
Eggplant (aubergine)	Endive
Escarole	Fennel
Gelatin (sugar-free)	Grape leaves
Grapefruit	Hearts of palm
Horseradish	Hot chili peppers
Jalapeno peppers	Jicama

Kimchi	Kohlrabi
Leeks	Lemons
Lettuce (all kinds)	Limes
Mixed greens	Mushrooms
Mustard	Okra
Oranges	Pumpkin
Radishes	Raspberries
Rhubarb	Rutabaga
Salsa	Sauerkraut
Scallions	Garden salad (no dressing)
Seaweed	Snow peas
Spaghetti squash	Squash (all types of winter and summer)
Strawberries	String Beans
Spinach & Silverbeet	Sugar snap peas
Tangerines	Tomatoes
Turnips	Water chestnuts
Watercress	Zucchini

Examples of low-Calorie foods for the Satiety Diet:

- Soups made with low Calorie ingredients such as vegetables. Beans and lentils are great additions to soups because they provide satiating protein. Avoid adding cream to soups.
- Stews and casseroles made from vegetables, beans, lentils or lean meats.
- Leafy greens, such as kale, lettuce, spinach, aragula (rocket), microgreens, and radicchio. If you make them into a salad, use a low-Calorie dressing.
- NTS vegetables (non-starchy vegetables) such as asparagus, broccoli, carrots, cauliflower, celery, cucumbers, tomatoes and winter squash.
- High-fiber foods such as pulses, brassicas (e.g. broccoli, cabbages, Asian greens, Brussels sprouts) berries and bran.
- Low-fructose fruits such as berries and citrus fruits.
- Popcorn with no added fats

Swapping Calorie-rich for Calorie-sparse.

Why don't people who want to lose weight simply switch to foods with low Calorie density?

As a rule, foods with a high Calorie density are more delicious than low Calorie density foods because their Calorie density is high. People prefer sugary, fatty, starchy foods because they usually taste better!

This is due to an inbuilt survival mechanism. Sugar and fat are concentrated and readily available energy sources, which is what we humans needed back in the days when we were hunter-gatherers. When young children are given a choice between foods with more Calories per weight—such as candy—and foods with low Calorie-density—such as lettuce—they tend to select the candy!

Tips to help you eat more Calorie-sparse foods.

To fully utilize the satiety-power of low Calorie-density foods:

- Begin meals with a low-Calorie soup or salad before your main course. Make your soup or salad a high protein dish by including lentils, beans, nuts, tofu, fish, eggs, lean meats or poultry. This will help you feel fuller on fewer Calories.
- Eat foods containing as much water, air, or fiber as possible, as long as you don't sacrifice flavor. (For example, a bowl of water-soaked bran contains lots of water and fiber but may not be very palatable.)
- Choose low-fat foods, but don't avoid all fat. We all need a little fat in our diet for optimum health. Many dishes require a small amount of fat to boost flavor, and of course experiencing strong flavors helps your Inner Guardian recognize that you've eaten a good meal and you don't need any more hunger hormones surging through your system.
- Make Calorie-sparse foods taste good. Cooking with herbs and spices and strong-flavored vegetables, for example.
- Mimic the desirable sensory qualities of Calorie-dense foods: the creamy mouth-feel of fat can be mimicked in many ways, using foods of lower energy density.
- Eat smaller amounts of Calorie-dense foods—e.g. a couple of squares of chocolate instead of the whole block.
- Eat Calorie-dense foods mindfully, so that we can prolong and fully enjoy the sensory experience.
- Get as many veggies into your meals as possible. Add shredded or chopped vegetables to pasta sauces and curries. Thickly slather pizzas with extra vegetables.
- Eat whole fresh or frozen fruits, instead of dried fruits, canned fruits with additives, fruit juices or smoothies. Always eat fruit in conjunction with other foods, for example as part of a dessert.
- Use a blender to whip air into sauces and frothy puddings. Or air-pop some popcorn.
- Eat brown rice, and whole-grain cereals, breads and pastas.
- Dip raw vegetables into a black bean and corn salsa for a high protein, low Calorie snack.

Mix calorie-sparse foods with low-fat protein

Including both high protein, low-fat foods and low Calorie-density foods in your meals can help you lose weight more easily.

Dawn Jackson Blatner, registered dietitian and spokeswoman for the American Dietetic Association says, "If you have at least one or more foods that are high in water or fiber and lean protein at all meals, you will feel full on fewer Calories."

> Chris Clark says "I don't mean to harp on endlessly about legumes, but cooked beans and lentils, when eaten with whole grains, really do provide the perfect package of lean protein, water and satiating soluble fiber. They are also rich in complex carbohydrates that help slow digestion and keep you feeling fuller for longer!"

14. FOODS THAT CAN HELP WEIGHT LOSS: TEXTURED FOODS

Foods with solid or viscous textures provide best satiety.

Liquids: The least satiating.

The food textures that have the least satiety-power are thin, runny liquids; beverages, sodas, smoothies, shakes etc. These are foods that are so liquid that you drink them rather than eat them. It's true that drinking water or tea can curb appetite, but it's a weak effect and generally only works:

- if thirst has been mistaken for hunger
- if you find that keeping your mouth busy sipping water or tea can help stop you from putting Calorie-dense food in your mouth.

Solid foods: More filling than liquids.

Solid foods generally make you feel fuller than liquid foods. (One exception is soup.)

"Beverages high in water do not last as long in the stomach as solid foods," says Purdue University professor of nutrition Wayne Campbell, PhD. "Hunger will not be reduced as much with a liquid as with a solid, so if you are choosing between a meal replacement drink or a meal replacement bar, go for the bar for greater satiety."

Chewy foods: Satiety boosters.

If you're going to eat solid foods, choose chewy ones. When you have to really chew your food, not only are you using up a few extra Calories by working your jaw, but you're also experiencing the sensory characteristics of the food in your mouth for longer, giving your Inner Guardian more time to register that you're full. The very act of chewing sends signals to your digestive system that can help satiety. Nuts, whole fruits and vegetables, chewy udon noodles, brown rice, French breads, buckwheat and freekeh groats—these are some of the chewy foods that can help you feel satisfied. Choose whole foods in their most natural form—raw carrots instead of juiced carrots, for example. High fiber foods are often chewy, and they have the added advantage of keeping you feeling fuller for longer.

Highly viscous foods: Better satiety-power.

Viscous of "semi-solid" foods such as thick soups, porridges, dips, sauces and certain puddings, have been shown to promote satiety. These foods take longer to consume than foods in the form of thin liquids, and they stay in the stomach for longer.

"A slower eating rate and a delayed gastric emptying rate can partly explain the stronger satiating properties of high viscous semi-solid foods," say the authors of a study published in *Nutrition Bulletin*. [Slavin & Green (2007)]

A study in the journal *Physiology & Behavior* provides more evidence, with the statement, ". . . the semi-solid [food] product is apparently considered more satisfying than the liquid [food]." [Zijlstra et al., (2009)]

Very viscous foods often have quite a high water content, too, which lowers their Calorie-density.

15. FOODS THAT CAN HELP WEIGHT LOSS: "EMERGENCY" FOODS

Imagine it's mid-afternoon and you're feeling famished. You don't have a beautifully-prepared high-satiety meal on hand. You're tempted to find the nearest fast-food outlet and grab some highly-process, low-fiber, Calorie-dense food to quell your food cravings.

What's a better appetite-curbing solution for weight loss? Use this step by step snack solution.

- #1 Drink some water.
- #2 Have some hot, low-Calorie, high-protein soup, such as bean soup.
- #3 Snack on raw Nourishing, Tasty, Slimming (NTS) Vegetables, with no dressing or with a low Calorie dressing. Thrown in a handful of canned beans for extra protein, or purée some canned garbanzo beans (chickpeas) with garlic and lemon juice to make a tasty, fiber-and-protein rich, low-fat, satisfying dip.
- #4 Snack on an NTS Vegetable stir-fry. Flavor it with plenty of herbs and spices, and some canned lentils for extra fiber and satiety.
- #5 Eat some natural pickles that don't contain any added sugar, or artificial colors or flavors. Pickles are so strongly-flavored that they can help curb appetite.
- #6 If you're hankering for sweetness, whip up a Satiety Chocolate Pudding.
- #7 Still craving sweets? Make Emergency Vanilla Pudding. Place 2 cups of low-fat soy milk or unsweetened almond milk in a blender with a scoop of unsweetened soy protein powder. Add vanilla and a pinch of cardamom or cinnamon, some sweetener of your choice.[40] Turn on the blender and mix ingredients thoroughly. While the machine is running, add 1 teaspoon of guar gum powder or xanthan gum powder to thicken the mixture. When it's all well-blended, pour it into a bowl, sprinkle it with chopped non-blanched almonds to give crunchiness, and enjoy.

---

40   For example stevia powder, or erythritol, or a mixture of stevia and erythritol, or a spoonful of rice malt syrup.

16. FOODS THAT CAN HELP WEIGHT LOSS: LOW GI FOODS

As mentioned, the relative ability of a food to increase the level of glucose in the blood is called the Glycemic Index, or GI. For weight loss, choose foods with a low GI. They are digested more slowly and their glucose is released into the bloodstream more evenly, without sharp rises and falls that can trigger a roller-coaster of insulin levels.

Sudden floods of insulin, caused by high glycemic foods such as white bread and sugary, refined foods, are associated with diabetes and weight gain.

Refined, low-fiber carbs are digested rapidly. These high GI foods release a burst of nutrients into the bloodstream. Your blood sugar soars rapidly to a spike, then plummets. Low blood sugar levels may then trigger your hunger hormones, causing cravings for more carbs. Eating high GI foods can actually make you feel hungrier later. Keeping your blood sugar steady will help you lose weight.

Low GI foods can boost satiety.

When people eat foods containing low-GI carbohydrates instead of higher-GI carbs, they tend to stay satiated for longer and eat fewer Calories at the following meal, according to a 2003 study published in *Nutrition in Clinical Care*. The researchers who undertook the study suggested that there is "...a potential role for low-GI carbohydrates in weight-reducing regimens." [Roberts (2003)]

The GI is a rough but useful guide.

The Glycemic Index is a hierarchy of foods ranked according to their capacity to raise blood glucose levels. It should be used only as a rough guide, however, because a food's effect on blood glucose levels also varies due to many additional factors, such as:
- fiber, protein or fat content of foods eaten at the same meal—more fat, protein or fiber lowers the GI
- ripeness—the riper the food, the higher the GI
- cooking time—lengthy cooking raises the GI
- the time of day at which the food is consumed

458

- the blood insulin levels of the consumer
- how processed foods are—the more highly processed, the higher the GI
- the wholeness of foods—the closer foods are to their natural form, the lower their GI

Some low GI foods.

The lower a food's glycemic index is, the better that food is at keeping your blood sugar levels smooth and spike-free.

High GI Foods: GI 70 +
Medium GI Foods: GI 55-69
Low GI Foods: GI > 55

Foods with a low glycemic index include whole grains and most vegetables. Exceptions include some of the "starchy" vegetables such as corn and sweet potatoes, which can still be eaten when you want to lose weight, but in smaller amounts and accompanied by low GI foods.

There are many lists of low GI foods freely available online.

Suggestions for low GI meals include pulses and steamed greens, tofu and vegetable curries, ratatouille or thick vegetable soups. For dessert, enjoy almonds, citrus fruits such as mandarins, oranges and tangelos, or berries such as blueberries, raspberries, blackberries and strawberries, or baked desserts incorporating wholemeal flour or whole black beans/adzuki beans.

Low-carb vs low-fat vs low GI

A 2012 study published in the Journal of the American Medical Association evaluated the benefits of three popular diets compared side by side:

- Low-carbohydrate Diet
- Low-fat Diet
- Low GI Diet

They concluded that out of all three, a low GI diet of foods with high quality nutrients is the best regime for healthy long-term weight loss and weight management.

" . . . from a metabolic perspective, all Calories are not alike," said Dr. David Ludwig, one of the researchers. "The quality of the Calories going in affects the number of Calories going out."

Dr. Ludwig adds, "For weight loss . . . avoid diets that severely restrict any major nutrient, either fat or carbohydrate. Instead, focus on reducing the highly processed carbohydrates that cause surges and crashes in blood sugar. " [Ebbeling et al., (2012)]

PORTION SIZE

1. IT'S TEMPTING TO EAT EVERYTHING ON YOUR PLATE

Many people feel compelled to eat all the food they are served— that is, to "clean the plate". In an article for Cornell University's Food and Brand Lab, researchers wrote, "Individuals who ate soup out of self-refilling bowls ate more than those who ate out of normal bowls, but did not feel any more satiated."

They were discussing an experiment we've already mentioned in this book. Called " Bottomless Bowls: Why Visual Cues of Portion Size May Influence Intake," it found that participants eating from "bottomless" bowls consumed an astonishing 73% more than those eating from normal bowls.

"Bottomless soup bowls show. . . we eat with our eyes," said the researchers. "Environmental cues have an impact on how much we eat, and we don't even know it. So, next time you sit down for a meal, keep in mind that relying on visual cues like an empty bowl might actually lead you to overeat!" [Wansink et al., (2005)]

People tend to eat all the food on their plate, no matter whether there is a lot or a little. Thus portion size—the amount of food served in a meal—affects the total amount of food you eat. Over time, meals containing large portions add up to an intake of many excess Calories and can lead to obesity.

460

According to a 1979 study published in the journal *Behavior Research and Therapy*, basic alterations in the way food is presented at mealtimes can have a significant effect on how much food is eaten. Most of us are inclined to finish the food that is served to us. It follows that if food portion sizes are reduced, people will eat less. [Krassner et al., (1979)]

2. SMALLER PORTIONS HELP WITH WEIGHT LOSS

For weight loss, portion sizes should be small.

"The way that foods are presented, such as the portion size, can affect the amount consumed." So say the authors of a 1995 report, in which nutritionists looked into why many soldiers lose weight because they "often do not eat their Military Operational Rations in amounts adequate to meet energy expenditures." They found that when the soldiers were offered small portion sizes, they ate less. [Marriott (1995)]

One powerful way to boost weight loss is to decrease portion sizes. Study after study reinforces the conclusion that portion size really does influence energy intake. [Ello-Martin et al., (2005)]

3. THE DIFFERENCE BETWEEN A PORTION AND A SERVE

The terms "serve" and "portion" often are used interchangeably, but in fact they have different meanings. A portion is the amount of a particular food that you choose to eat for a meal, in one sitting. The size of a portion is up to you: it can be large or small. For example a 113g (4oz) plain bagel can be a portion. It could contain 2 serves of starchy carbs.

A serve, or serving is a measured amount of food or drink, such as one slice of bread or one cup of milk. It's the amount of food recommended by government health departments and some weight loss protocols. Serve-sizes are used to provide consumers with dietary recommendations.

A single portion of food may contain several serves/servings, or it may be less than one serve.

461

4. SMALLER PORTIONS CAN HELP INCREASE SATIETY

One factor affecting the obesity crisis is increasing portion sizes. Both inside and outside our homes, the amount of food that gets piled on our plates has grown bigger. Most of us are eating much larger portions of food than we need.

Eating large portions can make you less sensitive to your satiety signals. By eating smaller portions you can help your body reach satiety more easily.

The stomach can be thought of as a bag made of strong, stretchy muscles. Its job begins after you have tasted, chewed and swallowed your food. The muscular stomach walls contract and expand with a wavelike motion, churning up the food and disintegrating it into tiny fragments. Meanwhile, glands in the stomach walls release digestive juices to mix with the food. These extremely acidic fluids are a mixture of mucus, enzymes, and hydrochloric acid (HCl), and they begin to break down proteins and fats into their component parts of amino acids and fatty acids.

Your stomach turns your food into a mushy soup called 'chyme', then pushes the chyme into your small intestine. It's here that the nutrients from the food begin to pass into your body, and satiety signals are generated.

Loading your stomach with too much food actually resets the sense of feeling full, and can lead to increased appetite. There's a tension-sensitive nerve in your stomach. When your stomach is stretched by food, the nerve activity increases the signals to your brain, to tell the brain that your stomach is full, so you can stop eating.

"This is central to regulating appetite, because without it, the brain wouldn't know when to stop eating. And here's the key: When . . . the stomachs of lean mice [are compared with] with obese ones, the response to stretch is dramatically reduced in the obese mice and doesn't return to normal. The same thing happens in humans."[ABC Catalyst (2015)]

Associate Professor Amanda Page, a neurologist investigating the ways the appetite-controlling nerves allow the stomach to communicate with the brain, comments, "People will say, 'Why won't an obese person just stop eating? It's easy to stop eating.' But, actually, they're not getting those signals of fullness, so they can't."

"Eating less food won't shrink your stomach," says Mark Moyad, MD, director of preventive and alternative medicine at the University of Michigan Medical Center in Ann Arbor (USA), "but it can help to reset your 'appetite thermostat' so you won't feel as hungry."

It's important to remember that if you eat a lot of food in one sitting (that is, at one meal) your stomach will stretch a lot. This over-stretching actually serves to decrease your body's natural sensitivity to knowing how full of food you are. In other words it means it's harder for you to achieve satiety when your stomach is often over-filled and over-stretched.

This is why you have to make sure you get your food portion sizes right.

Portions should be sufficient to:
- Enable you to reach satiety. Your stomach should be stretched sufficiently to trigger satiety signals, sending them to your brain to tell you you're full.
- Not over-stretch your stomach. Over-stretching can decrease your satiety signals and make it more likely you will overeat.

Being aware of the size of your portions at every meal and reaching satiety while not over filling your stomach is a very useful tool discussed in *The Satiety Diet Weight Loss Toolkit* (book #2 in the Satiety Diet series).

As mentioned earlier, "*Hara hachi bun me*" is the philosophy of eating until you feel 80% full. It is practised by Okinawans in Japan, and it is worth noting that Okinawans are the world's longest-lived people. Researchers believe that *hara hachi bun me* may act as a form of Calorie restriction, thus extending practitioners' life expectancy by helping to keep the average Okinawan slim. This effect is thought to be due to sensitivity in the stomach stretch receptors that help signal satiety. The result of habitual over-eating is continual stretching of the stomach, which in turn means people need to eat more food to feel full. [Willcox et al., (2002)]

"Stop eating when you are 80% full" does not necessarily mean "stop eating when you are 80% satiated". That feeling of satiation is the key to weight loss. It's the body-speech signal telling your body that there is so much nutritious food surrounding you that there is no need to store food as fat, and therefore there is no need to send out extra hunger signals.

If you do not reach satiety at mealtimes, your appetite is likely to be aroused sooner after the meal. You might find yourself grazing on snacks throughout the hours until the next mealtime, and in total, the Calories in these snacks can add up to far more than the Calories you would have eaten, had you consumed enough to reach satiety at that last meal.

Of course satiety isn't only driven by how full your stomach is. That's only one element contributing to your sense of repleteness. There are numerous other factors, including your blood sugar levels, insulin levels, mental images, attitudes (such as your perception of how energy dense a food is), and sensory inputs such as what your eyes see, what your nose smells etc.

Stomach fullness is a very important element, however and it is one of many, which is why the Satiety Diet gives you multiple tools to tackle obesity.

5. SMALLER PORTIONS CAN REALLY SATISFY

There's no need to worry that eating less food will make you feel deprived. A 2012 study published in the *Journal of Food Quality and Preference* found that people can eat only 25% of their usual snack portion and feel just as satisfied 15 minutes after eating, as if they had eaten the full 100%. [van Kleef et al., (2013)]

6. HOW MUCH FOOD CAN YOUR STOMACH HOLD?

Portion size is associated with stomach size. After you reach adulthood your stomach doesn't grow any more. The fact is, the size of an obese person's stomach is not much different from the stomach size of a slim person.

- **Empty:** When empty, the capacity of the average human stomach is around two hundred milliliters (1 U.S. cup). Your stomach is normally the size of your fist and it stretches to accommodate the amount of food you consume.
- **Comfortably full:** Most adults feel full after consuming about one liter of food (4 1/2 U.S. cups), but the stomach can stretch to hold a lot more than that.
- **Uncomfortably full:** 1.5 - 2 liters (6 - 8 U.S. cups)
- **Uncomfortably overfull:** The greatest volume of food a normal human stomach can hold is about three to four liters (12 - 18 U.S. cups).

After your food has passed from your stomach into your small intestine, your stomach returns to its original size.

It's important to see your whole meal set out in front of you before you take the first bite. Imagine that food inside your fist-sized stomach. How much will your stomach have to stretch?

In summary—when estimating how much food to serve yourself at a single meal, aim for a total intake of between 2 and 4 fist sizes (not fistfuls but fist equivalents).

7. PERCENTAGE OF MACRONUTRIENTS IN YOUR DIET

It's all very well to make portion sizes smaller, but what kinds of foods should those portions contain? Clearly it would be unhelpful to eat a small portion of say, mashed potatoes only, for dinner. We all need variety. What are the ideal proportions of nutrients to provide both good health and weight loss?

Imagine a meal set out in front of you. There might be a bowl of soup, a plate containing your main meal, a dish of dessert, and a glass or cup filled with some beverage.

All the food on all your plates and cups in that single meal is 100% of that meal.

The AMDR recommendations.

The Food and Nutrition Board of the Institute of Medicine calls the range of relative intakes of macronutrients we need for good health in our overall diet, the "Acceptable Macronutrient Distribution Range" (AMDR). These are the recommendations for avoiding the risk of chronic disease, not necessarily the recommendations for weight loss.

AMDR recommendations:

Protein: 10-35% of your meal

Fat: 20-35% of your meal

Carbohydrate: 45-65% of your meal

The Satiety Diet recommendations.

As a rough rule of thumb for weight loss, these are the approximate macronutrient proportions to aim for—either at each meal, or in your overall diet:

- **Protein** (e.g. beans, tofu, seafood, teff, nuts): 25-30%
- **Starchy carbohydrates** (e.g. whole grains and legumes): 10-25%
- **Low-Calorie carbohydrates** (e.g. salad leaves, zucchinis, tomatoes, broccoli, kale, sweet peppers, herbs)" 30-50%
- **Low-fructose fruits:** up to 2 serves per day
- **Fat** (e.g. avocado, olive oil, butter, coconut cream): the AMDR for fat is that it should comprise 20-35% of your diet. For weight loss, aim for 20%.

More about fat; Aiming for a fat intake of 20% does not mean dividing your dinner plate into 5 sections and covering one of those sections with butter! Since fat is a natural component of so many foods, it is not always easy to estimate just how much fat you're actually eating. There might be oils and fats in your salad dressing, or marbled through your steak, or in your cheesy pasta sauce, or in the peanuts from which your satay sauce is made. Fat from various food sources can quickly add up to a high percentage, so to make portion-estimation easier, just choose low-fat foods or smaller portions of fatty foods.

For example:

- 1 tbsp avocado instead of a whole one.
- Use oil sprays for baking or frying, to spread a thin layer, instead of pouring oil from the bottle.
- Lean, low-fat fish such as tuna, cod, flounder or sole.
- Unsweetened almond milk instead of dairy milk

Note that the type of fat you eat is also important. "Desirable" fat is unsaturated fat, while, in general, "undesirable" fat is saturated fat and trans fat.

You'll have noticed that the above percentages do not add up to 100. That's because they are expressed in the form of a range, to give you freedom to choose within those guidelines. For example you might choose to eat in one meal:

25% protein
10% starchy carbs
30% non-starchy carbs
15% low fructose fruit
20% "good" fats

8. ESTIMATING PORTIONS AND MACRONUTRIENTS

As discussed, making your food portion sizes smaller is yet another excellent tool in the weight loss toolkit.

But how can it be done?

There are many ways to measure food portion sizes. You could use a set of kitchen scales, or cup measures, for example; or you could calculate the Calories per gram/ounce of every food you are about to eat. This can be time-consuming and annoying. The most convenient methods are:

- Using your hands as a rough guide
- Comparing food portions to familiar, everyday objects
- Using your plate size as a rough guide

Your hands.

Make a fist. Look at it. That's about the size of your empty stomach.

Your hands are very useful tools for measuring portion sizes. At Arizona State University (USA), nutritionists recommend using your hands as guides to portion size. "Unlike . . . measuring cups or other visual images, hands are always at the table with you," says Simin Levinson, lecturer at ASU's School of Nutrition and Health Promotion. "They are practical and accurate."

* Protein

At each meal, your portion of protein (e.g. beans, teff, tofu, beef, fish, poultry or other protein) should be equivalent to the size and thickness of the palm of your hand; that is, the palm only, not including the fingers and thumb. Hold out your hand and imagine your protein portion sitting on the palm. That's the amount of protein that should be on your plate at each meal. It would probably occupy around one quarter of your plate (depending on your plate size).

* Starchy carbohydrates

At each meal, your portion of starchy carbohydrates (e.g. brown rice, potatoes, corn, bread, pasta)should be no bigger than the size of your fist. Note that your pasta should be equal in volume to the pasta sauce.

* Calorie-sparse, fiber- and water-rich foods

NTS vegetables such as lettuce, asparagus, broccoli, cauliflower, cucumber, spinach, mushrooms, onions, peppers and tomatoes, are different. Without over-stretching your stomach to the point at which it loses satiety-sensitivity, aim to eat as many different colors of NTS vegetables as possible with each meal. They are nutritious and filling, low in Calories and high in fiber. If you can do so while still reaching satiety, try swapping your fistful of carbs for an added fistful of NTS vegetables.

* Fruit

One portion of fruit is equivalent to how much fruit would fit in the palm of one hand.

* Fat

A one-portion serving of fat, such as coconut cream, dairy butter, peanut butter or olive oil, should be about half the size of your thumb.

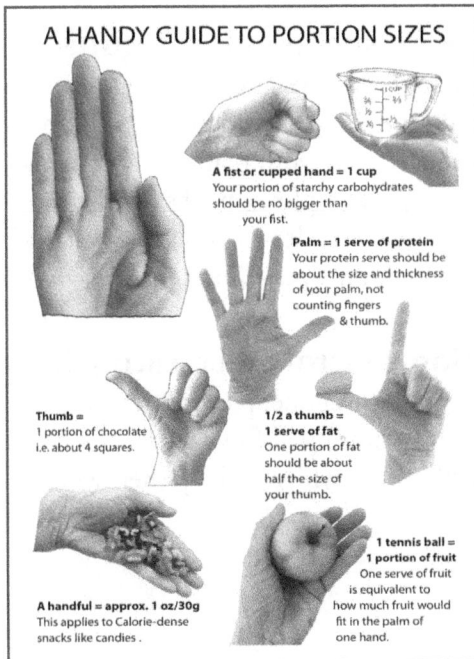

A HANDY GUIDE TO PORTION SIZES

A fist or cupped hand = 1 cup
Your portion of starchy carbohydrates should be no bigger than your fist.

Palm = 1 serve of protein
Your protein serve should be about the size and thickness of your palm, not counting fingers & thumb.

Thumb =
1 portion of chocolate i.e. about 4 squares.

1/2 a thumb =
1 serve of fat
One portion of fat should be about half the size of your thumb.

1 tennis ball =
1 portion of fruit
One serve of fruit is equivalent to how much fruit would fit in the palm of one hand.

A handful = approx. 1 oz/30g
This applies to Calorie-dense snacks like candies .

Comparing food portions to familiar objects.

Another way to estimate your portion sizes is to compare your food to visualizations of everyday objects you know well. Here are some examples of a portion size in one meal:

- **Protein**—about the size of a bar of soap or a pack of cards.

- **Starchy carbohydrates**—about the size of a coffee mug.

- **Fruit**—about the size of a tennis ball.

- **Fat**—A one-portion serving of fat is approximately:
  * The contents of one teaspoon.
  * The size of a stock cube.
  * The size of a soda-bottle cap.
  * The size of a poker chip.
  * One portion of chocolate=a lipstick tube, i.e. about 4 squares.

Using your plate size as a rough guide.

Imagine that your entire meal fits on a single dinner plate. Visualize that plate divided into sections. Use percentages to mentally arrange the different food groups on your plate—e.g. roughly 1/4 of the plate might be filled with protein plus some fat, 1/4 with starchy carbs and half with low-Calorie carbs. It's in your best weight-loss interests to choose a small or medium-sized dinner plate!

Tip for portion control when eating in groups.

If you're dining with other people who are weight-conscious, don't provide them with a communal food source, such as a casserole dish on the dinner table, from which to help themselves.

9. BE KIND TO YOURSELF—ESTIMATES ARE FINE

If you start measuring your macronutrient percentages down to the last ounce, or gram, or Calorie, eating can become stressful. Eating should be a pleasure, not a chore. Estimating your portion sizes and nutrient percentages doesn't have to be an exact science. Approximations are permitted. There is no need to worry about being utterly precise. Your body's needs aren't mathematically calibrated from day to day, but change according to many variables.

Portion sizes and macronutrient percentages are all general rules. You don't have to stick to them religiously. Use them as guidelines.

Relax!

Listen to your body.

Your body's nutrient needs can change from hour to hour, depending on how well you absorb nutrients, how active you are, whether you're exposed to pollutants, and a range of other variables. Learn to listen to what your Inner Guardian is telling you about what macronutrients your body requires. *Really* listen—don't just let your appetite be triggered by external hunger cues such as pictures of food.

For example, at some point in your day you may experience an overwhelming feeling that you need protein; the sense that protein is the only thing that will satisfy you. If that happens, increase the percentage of protein in your meal!

It is not necessary for you to slavishly follow the recommended protein/carbs/fat ratio at every meal, but that ratio is a good basic framework to aim for, especially when you feel as if your body isn't giving you any specific messages about what type of nutrition it requires.

10. USEFUL TOOLS TO HELP YOU WITH PORTION CONTROL
The size of your plate.

If you've just served yourself a palm-sized portion of this, and a fist-sized portion of that, and a thumb sized portion of something else, and you're sitting at the table with a deprived feeling, staring at what appears to be a vast expanse of emptiness on your plate, here's a fantastic tip:

Downsize your tableware.

Use a smaller plate. Research has proved that this is a great way to get people to reach satiety while eating less food. On a smaller plate, it looks as if you are getting more food, so your eyes and brain begin to feel satisfied even before you take the first bite. See our section on "Tableware" for more information.

Increasing portion sizes, but not your waistline.

Do you still feel as if your plate is not full enough? Fill the empty nooks with delicious foods that help with weight loss. Add as many different lightly cooked NTS vegetables or raw, NTS salad vegetables as you like—or at least as many as you can eat without overstretching your stomach!

SWEETNESS AND SWEETENERS

Human beings of all ages, races, and cultures love sweet tastes. Most sweet tastes come from sugar, in one form or another. Sugars are not "good" or "evil"—they are just a source of energy.

The Satiety Diet "Sweetness" section is so extensive that there's not enough room for it here, and we've had to divide it in two. Part 1 can be found in this book. The second part has been published in *The Satiety Diet Weight Loss Toolkit* (book #2 in the Satiety Diet series).

While not "evil", sweet foods and beverages are thought to be major contributors to the global obesity epidemic. The added sugar consumed by modern humans comes hidden in foods such as sodas, flavored milks, sweetened grains (such as breakfast cereals), table sugar, candy, snacks, syrups and ice creams.

1. TYPES OF SWEETENERS

We can roughly put sweeteners into these classes, some of which intersect:

- Non-free sugars—These are sugars found naturally in completely unrefined foods, such as lactose (found naturally in milks/ milk products) and fructose (found naturally in whole fruits).

- Free sugars—These are those sugars that have been, to some extent, refined, either by humans or by bees. They are sugars added to foods by the manufacturer or consumer. They are also sugars that are naturally present in honey, natural syrups (such as agave and maple) and fruit juices.

- Natural "sugar substitutes"—Some people try to lose weight or improve their health by using sugars that don't look like white refined table sugar. The idea is that because they are natural and not white and granular, they are better for you. Indeed, they usually contain more nutrition than white refined sugar, but the Calorie count is still high, and their fructose levels may be exorbitant. Examples include honey, dates, coconut sugar, maple syrup, agave syrup, blackstrap molasses, yacon syrup, treacle.

- Natural low Calorie or zero Calorie sweeteners that are not sugars—Some naturally occurring plant compounds, such as stevia, miraculin and glycyrrhizin can "trick" your taste-buds into sensing sugary-sweetness.

- Sugar alcohols—These are not considered to be artificial sweeteners, because they're derived from natural sources. Arguably the most popular sugar alcohols for sweetening are erythritol and xylitol.

- Artificial sweeteners—these are man-made substances such as saccharin and cyclamate.

473

2. FREE SUGARS

Free sugars are defined by the World Health Organization and the UN Food and Agriculture Organization in multiple reports as "all monosaccharides (such as glucose and fructose) and disaccharides (such as sucrose, lactose, and maltose) added to foods by the manufacturer, cook, or consumer, plus sugars naturally present in honey, syrups, and fruit juices". Free sugars are those sugars that have been, to some extent, refined, either by humans or by bees.

On food labels, many different names may be used for free sugars. "These include glucose, sucrose, maltose, corn syrup, honey, invert sugar, hydrolyzed starch and fructose. The higher up on the ingredients list any of these sugars are, the more abundant they are in the products." [Diabetes Ireland (2018)]

Free sugars are distinct from the non-free sugars that are naturally present in completely unrefined foods such as brown rice, whole-wheat pasta, fruit, milks and milk products.

The non-free low-fructose sugar combinations that occur in whole fruits such as citrus fruits and berries are preferable for weight loss, although as we always say, for weight loss it's preferable to eat no more than 2 - 3 pieces of fruit daily, and eat it in combination with other foods. Eat the whole fruit, as nature intended. "Sometimes sweeteners" include dates and fruit juices, honey, agave syrup, maple syrup and apple juice concentrate.

3. NATURAL FORMS OF SUGAR

Many people think that "sugar" means "refined white table sugar", whose scientific name is "sucrose".

However sugar is more than that. There are several different kinds of sugars naturally occurring in the foods we eat. Sugar comes in many chemical forms, including, but not limited to:

Glucose—also known as dextrose ("blood sugar")
Fructose ("fruit sugar")
Maltose ("malt sugar")
Lactose ("milk sugar")
Galactose (another "milk sugar")
Xylose ("wood sugar")

On food labels, sugar has many names. They can include terms such as syrup, nectar, malt, molasses, Demerara, evaporated cane juice, fruit juice, fruit juice concentrate, honey, Muscovado, panela, rapadura, treacle, and turbinado. Other compounds that act like sugar include maltodextrin and polyols.

4. WHERE IS SUGAR FOUND?

Sugars occur naturally in almost every plant-based food, in one form or another. Sugar is also a natural component of dairy products such as milk, cheese and yoghurt. When you're eating vegetables—legumes and grains, for example—you're eating sugars. Even lettuce contains sugar!

However eating trace amounts of sugars as part of a whole plant, with all the nutrients and fibers that naturally accompany those sugars, is very different from consuming the added refined sugars found in processed foods.

Sugars of all types, both natural and man-made, exist in a huge range of processed foods, including beverages (soft drinks, instant drink preparations, teas, fruit or vegetable juices / drinks), breakfast cereals and cereal bars, confectionery and chewing gum, fondants and fillings, jams and marmalades.

5. "NO ADDED SUGAR" CAN BE MISLEADING

"No added sugar" printed on food labels doesn't necessarily mean "containing no sugar".

Many sweet-tasting recipes are touted as having "no sugar" or "no added sugar". This can be misleading, because the dishes are often sweetened with fruits or honey or plant syrups which actually do contain sugar. It's not refined sugar, but it's still sugar.

6. SHOULD YOU SWAP SUGAR FOR FRUIT?

Due to the dietary trend away from sugar consumption, it is often said, "Use fruit as your sugar". In other words, some people suggest, "When you crave for something sweet, eat fruit."

While this is a good starting point, because whole fruit is better for you than refined sugar, there's a lot more to it than simply, say, swapping puréed dates for refined white sugar in your recipes.

The thing is, not all sugars have the same effect on the body. One form of sugar, in particular, may actually make you hungrier; fructose. [Luoa et al., (2015)]

Read on, to find out more about this form of sugar.

7. FRUCTOSE

Fructose, commonly known as "fruit sugar", exists in fruit, honey, high-fructose corn syrup (HFCS), agave syrup, and sucrose (table sugar). Small quantities also exist in vegetables. Fructose is often used by processed food manufacturers as a sweetener in snacks and soft drinks. It is the sweetest of all the naturally-occurring carbohydrates, being twice as sweet as table sugar.

Sucrose is commonly known as "table sugar" or simply "sugar". Sucrose molecules are made of one molecule of fructose and one molecule of glucose joined together, so it's 50% glucose and 50% fructose. After you eat sugar, your digestive system breaks it down into the separate fructose and glucose components. Fructose and glucose molecules are not made of any other molecules. They are sugar in its simplest form.

Thus, when you eat sugar, you are eating half fructose and half glucose. Glucose is the most important simple sugar in human metabolism. It circulates in your blood as "blood sugar".

"Fructose is the major carbohydrate present in fruit, and although some dietary fructose is derived from fruit, much fructose consumed in the diet is derived from sucrose (commonly known as 'sugar') and from foods containing added sucrose. This is because sucrose consists of 50% fructose and 50% glucose." [Nutrition Australia (2016)]

Your body processes sugars in different ways. Glucose is the most important simple sugar in your metabolism, supplying fuel for your muscles, and nearly all the energy needed by your brain. Almost every cell in your body is able to use glucose as an energy source.

Fructose is a different matter. Almost the only cells in your body that can break down fructose to produce energy are certain cells in your liver.

Fructose can also be generated in your body by the breakdown of fructans (another nutrient that occurs naturally in foods), which is accomplished by bacteria in the gut.

Some wholesome foods naturally contain high levels of fructose, (i.e. over 3g per serving), or of fructans, (i.e. over 0.5g/serving). Foods high in fructose and fructans include many fruits, berries, some vegetables and some cereals. Many healthful foods contain fructose or fructans, and they are an important part of a diverse, satisfying diet that can help weight loss.

Well . . . what's wrong with fructose?

Nothing is intrinsically wrong with fructose. It's the way you eat it and how much of it you eat that's the issue.

During most of human history, people existed on a diet containing very little sugar and almost no refined carbohydrates. For millennia, our forebears mainly obtained fructose by eating fruits, vegetables or honey. Honey was a scarce luxury, and the small, often sour or tart fruits eaten in bygone days were unlike the intensively hybridized fruits we know today. They were the ancestors of the huge, glowing, colorful, sugary-ripe fruits we buy from the supermarkets.

Before refined sugar began to be mass-produced, we humans rarely consumed large amounts of fructose. It's only relatively recently, as sugar cultivation and production methods have improved, that sugar has come to form a major part of our diet—in the form of candies, baked goods, sugary breakfast foods, sodas, ice creams etc. In particular, the introduction of high-fructose corn syrup and other sweeteners in the 19th and 20th centuries has impacted people's consumption of fructose, and of sugar in general.

477

In the 21st century, we have access to huge amounts of fructose and it permeates our food supply more than ever.

Not only do we have access to an endless supply of highly-bred fruits, we also consume fructose in many processed foods. As mentioned, fructose is a sugar that is sweeter and less expensive than glucose, so food manufacturers often use a processed form of pure fructose, stripped of the other nutrients, to sweeten manufactured foods. They add it to a wide variety of sodas, fruit-flavored drinks, candies and other products.

Numerous studies imply that modern advances in food processing and the marketing of food has led to people all over the world eating more sugar, with its accompanying fructose. This is believed to have contributed to the global obesity problem.

Researchers who ran a 2013 study on the effect of fructose noted that the obesity crisis ballooned at exactly the same time as people's consumption of fructose increased. " . . . high-fructose diets," they wrote, "are thought to promote weight gain and insulin resistance."

The study showed that when rats ate fructose, they produced fewer satiety hormones (leptin) than when they ate glucose. And when they were given fructose, they ate more food than when they were given glucose.

The researchers concluded that ". . . fructose possibly increases food-seeking behavior and increases food intake. . . Substantial increases in the use of fructose as a sweetener may play a role in the current obesity epidemic." [Page et al., (2013)]

Fructose and hunger.

Consuming large quantities of fructose can make you hungrier.

Fructose affects your body in a way that other sugars do not. Your body digests fructose by processing it through your liver, where it is converted to glucose or fat. It also affects hunger cues, stimulating your appetite.

Dietician Dimple Thakkar of the British Dietetic Association explains it this way: "Usually when we eat sugar, our body releases the hormone insulin, which tells the brain we've had enough to eat.

High insulin levels dampen the appetite, but fructose . . . doesn't trigger this response, so the brain doesn't get the message that you are full."

Fructose doesn't contribute to satiety. In fact, it can even make you feel hungrier. Study after study supports this.

". . . increased consumption of fructose may be detrimental in terms of body weight and adiposity. . . . the long-term consumption of diets high in fat and fructose is likely to lead to increased energy intake, weight gain, and obesity." [Elliott et al., (2002)]

"Fructose is a unique sweetener that has different metabolic effects on the body than glucose or sucrose. Fructose is absorbed further down the intestine, and whereas circulating glucose releases insulin from the pancreas, fructose stimulates insulin synthesis but does not release it. Insulin modifies food intake by inhibiting eating and by increasing leptin release, which also can inhibit food intake. Meals of high-fructose corn syrup can reduce circulating insulin and leptin levels, contributing to increased body weight. Thus, fructose intake might not result in the degree of satiety that would normally ensue with an equally caloric meal of glucose or sucrose." [Avena et al., (2008)]

". . . decreases of circulating insulin and leptin and increased ghrelin concentrations, as demonstrated in this study, could lead to increased caloric intake and ultimately contribute to weight gain and obesity during chronic consumption of diets high in fructose," wrote the authors of a 2004 study published in the *Journal of Clinical Endocrinology & Metabolism*. [Teff et al., (2004)]

A 2015 study found that, "Fructose compared with glucose may be a weaker suppressor of appetite." [Luoa et al., (2015)]

If you stop eating large amounts of fructose, you might find you're not as hungry as before.

On the other hand, glucose can promote satiety.

As discussed, the ways your body metabolizes glucose and fructose are quite different. Fructose is mostly metabolized in your liver, while glucose can be used directly by your muscles and brain, and burned for energy anywhere throughout your body. Glucose is your body's fuel. It's often called "blood sugar", because it circulates throughout your body in your bloodstream, so that it can be utilized instantly when you need energy. When you digest glucose, your body sends satiety signals to your brain.

Fructose also affects the appetite-regulating areas of the brain in different ways than glucose.

"In a study examining possible factors regarding the associations between fructose consumption and weight gain, brain magnetic resonance imaging of study participants indicated that ingestion of glucose but not fructose reduced cerebral blood flow and activity in brain regions that regulate appetite, and ingestion of glucose but not fructose produced increased ratings of satiety and fullness." [Page et al., (2013)]

For centuries, people in many parts of the world have enjoyed a sweet course or dessert after meals. Jane Lustwerk, former Chef at New England Culinary Institute says, "There are Greek writings that mention a sweet final course[41] served in Persian meals that would consist of sweet fruits, a sweet liquor, or a type of honey cake.

It is thought that eating dessert may promote satiety. For weight loss, this would be a small dessert containing minimal fructose.

"… sugars stimulate satiety mechanisms and reduce food intake in the short term…" wrote the authors of a 2003 review published in *The American Journal of Clinical Nutrition*. The reviewers proposed that when people consumed sugar as part of their meal, their satiety was boosted for up to two hours. This would leave enough time

---

41 "The word "dessert" is most commonly used for a final sweet course in the United States, Canada, Australia, New Zealand and Ireland while "pudding" is more commonly used in the United Kingdom. Alternatives such as "sweets" or "afters" are also used in the United Kingdom and some other Commonwealth countries, including Hong Kong, and India." [Wikipedia 7th Feb 2018)]

for the more slowly-digested foods in the meal to break down and prolong satiety beyond two hours. [Anderson & Woodend (2003)]

Sugar is 50% glucose and 50% fructose, so it's likely to be the glucose component that provides the satiating effect.

About fruit.

Eating fresh, whole fruit two or three times a day helps you stay healthy. Yes, you'll be eating fructose, but fructose is a nutrient, not a poison!

Fruit should be considered as a special treat. For centuries, it has been regarded as a delight to be eaten by the rich, or by the poor on special occasions. As recently as the early 20th century, there were children who looked forward to receiving an orange as a gift in their Christmas stocking.

Fruit breeding.

Our hunter-gatherer ancestors rarely consumed fruit. Ripe fruit was only available at certain seasons of the year. When they found it, they would have eaten it with relish. Fruit is naturally rich in sugar and our bodies are "wired" to seek that sweetness. Yet the wild fruits they ate would have borne little resemblance to the highly-bred fruit we see in supermarkets these days. It would have been smaller, dryer and less sweet.

Modern fruit has been bred almost beyond recognition. The original apples, pears, peaches etc. that hung on the wild ancestral trees were smaller, often less colorful and juicy, less fleshy, and generally lower in sugar content than their modern descendants. After all, in most cases their only job was to be attractive enough to be eaten by some passing bird or animal. Later, the undigested kernel of the fruit would be excreted by the wild creature in a new growing space, complete with ready-made fertilizer to nourish a new generation, thus expanding the plant's range and keeping the species going.

Humans interfered with the evolution of plants by selecting them according to preferred characteristics. The first wild apples looked more like crab apples. Peaches were small, with large kernels and not much flesh. Over the centuries apples, pears, peaches etc. became sweeter, bigger, juicier, more colorful, less fibrous. Most modern fruit has been "designed" to have a higher sugar content, because sweet fruit sells better. When you eat a peach in the 21st century, it's likely you'll be eating a lot more sugar/fructose than someone eating a peach in say, pre-Roman times.

Keep eating fruits and vegetables!

Limiting your fructose intake doesn't mean avoiding fruits and vegetables. The authors of a study on fructose and weight gain published in *The American Journal of Clinical Nutrition* say, "The consumption of fruit and vegetables should continue to be encouraged because of the resulting increased intake of fiber, micronutrients, and antioxidants. In addition, the intake of naturally occurring fructose is low . . . and is unlikely to contribute significantly to the untoward metabolic consequences associated with the consumption of large amounts of fructose." [Elliott et al., (2002)]

Endocrinologist Dr. Kathleen Page is the research leader and co-author of a glucose/fructose study published in the *Journal of the American Medical Association* (JAMA) that suggested glucose promotes satiety while fructose makes you hungrier. She says, "The best way to reduce fructose intake is to decrease the consumption of added sugar sweeteners, which are the main source of fructose in the American (and indeed most developed nations') diet."

Jonathan Purnell, MD, an endocrinologist at Oregon Health & Science University in Portland, wrote: "It would be a mistake to give up fruit, which has naturally occurring fructose. We don't recommend limiting fruit intake. Although there's fructose there, it's also present with water and fiber that alter the characteristics of straight fructose alone. We think that doesn't make fruit as much of a bad actor."

It is almost impossible to avoid eating any sugar or fructose at all, and in fact if you try to do so by cutting out fruits and vegetables, you are in danger of removing valuable, nutritious foods groups from your diet. The important thing is to be able to identify where that sugar or fructose is hiding, especially in processed foods, and then to minimise consumption of it over the long term.

How to eat fructose.

Nothing is wrong with fructose per se, as long as you consume it the way your ancestors consumed it—that is, inside whole fruits (not in fruit juices, or dried fruits, or high-fructose corn syrup, or in other processed forms). When you eat a whole fruit, the fiber content slows down your body's uptake of fructose.

For weight loss, instead of giving up fruit:

* **Reduce the total amount of fructose in your diet.** Give up or cut back on processed foods containing added fructose and other sugars.

* **Say no to HFCS.** Stay away from foods containing high-fructose corn syrup (HFCS). This processed food is hidden in many other processed foods.

* **Limit or give up refined sugar.** Like HFCS, refined sugar is hidden in many processed foods, including savory ones you wouldn't believe contain sugar. Read the labels!

* **Read the labels on processed foods.** Say "no" to any that contain lots of added sugars, especially fructose.

* **Read the labels even more closely!** Identify sugar that is lurking under other names! See our section on "Other Names For Sugar".

* **Avoid eating large amounts of fructose in one sitting**. High levels of fructose can prevent leptin and insulin from returning to normal levels after a meal, while promoting the production of ghrelin, the "hunger hormone".

* **Eat whole fruits.** Always eat fruit in its whole form, whether fresh, cooked or frozen. Of course it's okay to slice or dice fruit before you eat it, instead of chomping into a whole piece of fruit! And of course it's okay to remove inedible fruit rinds, such as the

outer coverings of bananas and citrus fruits. Just refrain from peeling apples and pears and plums and other fruits with edible skins. Eat the skins, too, whenever possible (Did you know you can eat the skin of kiwi fruit?)

Free fructose is the problem, not small portions of whole fruit. When you eat fruit in its whole, unprocessed form, with the skin on (except in the case of thick, bitter skins such as citrus rinds) you are eating the fiber that helps to slow down the digestive process and slow down the release of fructose into the liver. This gives your liver a chance to process the fructose more efficiently.

Tim Spector, professor of genetic epidemiology and author of *The Diet Myth*, says that whole fruit, containing all the natural pulp, provides excellent nutrition for us and for our microbiota.

"For high-fiber fruits, the fiber and polyphenols can balance out the effects of the fructose," says Spector. "Strawberries are good as they contain a relatively high amount of fiber and more than 95 polyphenols, which the microbes feed off and which act as antioxidants."

* **Eat fruit with other foods.** Eat fruit as part of a meal rather than a snack on its own—for example, as an ingredient in a dessert. It is best to consume fructose-containing foods at the same time as other foods, especially foods rich in protein and fiber. These are the nutrients that can help to put the brakes on sugar absorption, so that the fructose enters the bloodstream more slowly. They can also help you to reach satiety, so that cravings disappear.

* **Avoid eating sugars in conjunction with fats/oils.** This is a combination that has been called "addictive". Examples include banana splits, ice-cream, fruit-topped cheesecake, and doughnuts deep-fried in oil and sprinkled with sugar.

* **Treat fruit as a dessert or special treat.** This is how fruit was viewed in days of yore!

* **Eat fruit that's fresh or frozen, or canned in water (not syrup or juice).** It's okay to use frozen fruit if necessary, because modern methods of snap-freezing preserve almost all the nutrients in foods. Like cooking, freezing does alter some of food's qualities. It breaks down cell walls, for example.

* **Avoid eating dried fruits.** Drying removes the valuable water content from fruit and concentrates the sugars. Dried fruits contain excessive sugar, per gram, so that they are more like commercial candy than fresh fruits. Fruits in dried form, such as dates and apricots, taste deliciously sweet, which makes us tend to eat more.

* **Avoid "fruit leathers".** They are just another form of dried fruit.

* **Know that it's fine to cook your fresh, canned or frozen fruit before you eat it.** Raw fruit is best, but it's also okay to cook your fruit as long as the cooking process doesn't add fats, oils or too many extra sugars. Cooking does alter the characteristics of food—for example, heat destroys Vitamin C.

* **Don't gorge on fruit.** Know that one to three pieces of fruit per day is considered sufficient in a balanced diet.

* **Space out your fruit consumption.** Eat those pieces of fruit well-spaced throughout the day, not all together, and eat the in conjunction with other foods, preferably containing fiber and protein.

* **Choose mainly low-fructose fruits.** No fruit is off limits, but choose mainly low-fructose fruits such as citrus fruits, blueberries, strawberries and raspberries, kiwi fruits, kiwi berries, honeydew melon, cantaloupe. We encourage you to eat a variety of foods, so we're not advising you to cut out all high-fructose fruits! If you're going to eat high-fructose fruits, eat them in small portions, and observe the other fruit-eating tips we've listed here.

485

* **Be careful when using dates as a substitute for sugar.** Some people think that eating crushed dates instead of table sugar is "healthier". Indeed dates do contain more nutrients and fiber than processed sugar, but they have been referred to as "sugar bombs", for good reason. According to Food Standards Australia New Zealand, dried dates contain 33% fructose and a total sugar content of more than 60%. Fresh dates contain more water than dried dates, but their fructose content is still high.

***Avoid commercial fruit juices, smoothies, shakes etc.** The fruits have had most of the fiber removed and they've been mashed up into tiny pieces, which makes it easier for your body to extract the most Calories with the least effort. Sugary drinks and treats like fruit juices and smoothies often contain high levels of fructose and added sugars.

* **Avoid home-pressed fruit juices/smoothies/shakes.** Just avoid juice! Even when you juice fresh fruit in the home kitchen and leave all the fiber in, it's not as good for you as eating whole, fresh fruit (despite the claims of juicing-machine salespeople). Home-made juices encourage over-consumption, and their energy is absorbed more readily. And when you drink your Calories instead of eating them, you're less likely to achieve satiety.

* **Avoid "soft serve" fruits.** Fruits that have been frozen and then puréed to form a "soft serve" dessert are not quite as likely to spike blood sugars, because generally they still retain their fiber. However once again, eating fruits as a soft serve is not as beneficial for weight loss as eating them in their whole form because:

A) a machine has done all the chewing for you, so not only do your jaws do less exercise, but you're likely to consume more food in a shorter time, and your body will be able to extract Calories from the fruit more easily.

B) soft serve fruit desserts are usually eaten on their own, without other foods to slow down the rush of sugars into your bloodstream.

* **Know that some fruits can be eaten semi-ripened.** The sugar content increases in most fruits as the fruit ripens. The term "ripening" refers to the conversion of starches to sugars. Unripe fruits usually contain more complex forms of carbohydrates and sugars than ripe fruits. These complex compounds are not readily digestible which is why you can get a stomach ache after eating unripe fruit. Unripe fruits also contain resistant starches, which is why they are generally firmer in texture than ripe fruits.

If you wish to eat unripe fruits due to their lower sugar content, choose green mango, green pawpaw or even green banana. Most other unripe fruits are too hard to digest and too unpalatable. Remember to eat no more than 2 to 3 portions of any fruit per day, spaced out through the day, and eat them in conjunction with other foods.

* **Train your brain.** You can train yourself to prefer savory foods over sweet foods by gradually cutting down on sweet foods and decreasing the amount of sugar in recipes.

* **Stop consuming artificial sweeteners.** These can contribute to sugar cravings and also affect your insulin balance. One exception is possibly erythritol, a natural sugar alcohol. (Pure stevia is not an artificial sweetener.)

* **Use rice malt syrup.** This natural product is a good choice of sweetener, if you really crave something sweet. It contains no fructose. For fewer Calories, combine rice malt syrup (RMS) with stevia, half and half.

Some foods high in fructose.

apples	bananas
cherries	custard apples
dates	feijoas
figs	grapes
guavas	jackfruit
lychees	longans
loquats	mangos
nashis	papayas
persimmons	quinces
sapotes, mamey	star fruit
watermelons	

- **Dried fruits** (e.g. apple, apricot, date, fig, nectarine, peach, plum, raisin).
- **Processed fruit;** barbecue sauce, chutney, canned fruit (which is often canned in pear juice), plum sauce, sweet and sour sauce, tomato paste.
- **Sweets;** food and drinks with very high sucrose (table sugar) content and with high-fructose corn syrup (HFCS). Honey, maple syrup. Agave syrup.
- **Sweet wines,** e.g. dessert wines, muscatel, port, sherry. Beer in large amounts.
- **Many wheat-based products;** flour, pasta, bread, whole-grain breakfast cereals.

Some lower fructose foods .

Blueberries	Cantaloupe (rock melon)
Clementines	Coconuts
Cranberries	Cumquats
Grapefruits	Lemons
Limes	Mandarins

Melons, honeydew	Oranges
Raspberries	Rhubarb (technically not a fruit)
Strawberries	

8 SUGAR

In this book we use the term "sugar" to refer to white, refined, crystalline table sugar, or sucrose. As mentioned, a sucrose molecule is actually two simpler sugars stuck together; fructose and glucose. Some diet gurus advocate cutting down on refined sugar or ditching it from your diet altogether. Demonizing single foods in this way, however, is not helpful. Sugar is not "evil"—it occurs naturally in many whole foods and should be consumed as part of them, as nature intended. Over-consumption of refined sugar is, on the other hand, undesirable for many reasons.

Our bodies are "wired" to seek Calories, so many of us prefer sweet foods. Numerous processed foods such as candy, white bread, white rice, "breakfast cereals", and sugary soda drinks contain refined sugar.

Eating large amounts of (refined) sugar can:
* release huge amounts of sugar into your bloodstream
* make your blood sugar levels rapidly rise
* make your insulin levels spike
* cause your blood sugar levels to then fall quickly
* leave you feeling hungrier than before
* make you accustomed to overly-sweet foods
* encourage your body to store fat

Sugar plus fat—the dangerous combination.

Furthermore, it's been demonstrated that it's the combination of sugar and fat that's the greatest danger to our waistlines. If you continued to eat as much sugar as you normally do, but stopped eating fat, you'd probably lose weight. And if you continued to eat as much fat as you normally do, but stopped eating sugar, you'd also be likely to lose weight.

However, Dr. Alexander van Tulleken, who has a master's degree in Public Health from Harvard University, says, "Any diet that eliminates fat or sugar will be unpalatable, hard to sustain and probably be bad for your health, too."

He goes on to say, ". . . the real reason we're all getting fatter isn't fat or sugar. . . . sugar alone isn't very addictive . . . very few people gorge on boiled sweets. And fat isn't really addictive either; when did you last sneak a spoonful of butter from the fridge late at night? What we relish is fat/sugar combinations—chocolate, ice cream. . ."

Addictive foods can affect your brain in a similar way to cocaine. This is why it's so difficult for people not to over-indulge in them. Unprocessed foods, by contrast, don't have that effect.

Food manufacturers know how powerful that addictive combination of fat and sugar can be. Most of their products are both sugar-rich and fat rich—such as milk chocolate and ice cream. If you take all the sugar out of these foods and leave the fat, or remove the fat and leave the sugar, the food loses its deliciousness and addictiveness.

The answer, for people who want to lose weight, is to avoid processed foods that contain both sugar and fat. [van Tulleken. (2014)]

Should you go sugar-free?

Some people ask, "Will a completely sugar-free diet help me lose weight?"

For a start, it's close to impossible to eradicate all sugar from your diet. A diet that's rich in a wide variety of whole, unprocessed or lightly-processed foods, will contain natural sugars in various forms. This is what nature intended for us!

It's true that people living the typical western lifestyle eat too much sugar and that this is a major factor boosting the "obesity crisis". The problem lies in the fact that we have become habituated to huge sugar loads—sugar is added to the processed and junk foods we eat every day, and even to the sweet foods we bake in the home kitchen.

Yes, cutting all sugar out of your diet will help you lose weight, but this may be chiefly because you'll have to stop eating cakes, ice-cream, chocolate, cookies, sweetened yogurts and candy bars and drinking sugary drinks. It's likely that instead, you'll be eating foods that are more nutritious and satisfying.

If you choose natural, whole foods such as vegetables, that have some naturally occurring sugars in them, you will be consuming nutritious, satisfying foods that are low in Calories. Which means you're likely to be satisfied with eating fewer Calories. And after all, weight loss or gain depends on energy consumed and expended.

Quitting sugar

We talk about "quitting sugar" when it's really only quitting *added* sugar we're talking about. Anyone who eats a diverse diet of whole foods will be eating the sugars naturally found in those foods—which is a good thing, not a bad thing!

As discussed earlier, no matter whether you get a hit of sweetness from real sugar or artificial sweeteners, experiencing a sweet taste in your mouth is likely to enhance your appetite. Therefore cutting down on sweet-tasting foods is going to help curb your appetite and may promote weight loss.

As well as quitting the added sugar that's found in processed foods, it's useful to cut down on natural sugars—particularly fructose—to boost satiety and help weight loss.

Emotion-driven sugar-cravings

When you are aiming to eat less added sugar, be aware that it might be your emotions that are in command of your sugar-cravings. You're likely to give in to the desire to eat something sweet when you're at your weakest—in a negative emotional state such as sadness, loneliness, or even boredom. If you are aware of this you can prepare to fight it. Distract yourself for half an hour or so, and wait until the cravings subside. If they don't go away, have sweet, low Calorie snacks on hand and eat them mindfully.

491

Discover naturally-sweet plant foods

To lose weight, replace sugary foods with nutritious, delicious, naturally-sweet, satiating foods. Fresh vegetables can give you practically all of the same nutrients and fiber as fruits, without as much fructose. Naturally sweet vegetables include carrots and butternut squash (butternut pumpkin). Sweet plant based-foods that are slightly higher in Calories include chestnuts, sweet potatoes and coconut. Natural licorice root also tastes sweet, due to its glycyrrhizin content.

A change in your body's perception of sweetness

After a few weeks of eating less fructose and added sugar, your taste-buds will "shift". That is, they will adapt to your new way of eating and become more sensitive to sweetness than before, which means you won't need as much sweetener in your food to get the sweet taste you love.

If you fall down, get up and keep going.

If you do give in to the temptation to eat something laden with sugar, don't punish yourself mentally (with guilt, regret, or low self-esteem) or physically (by bingeing on every sweet food in sight just because "I ate a candy bar, so I might as well give up all hope of weight loss.").

Instead, just get over it. Accept that very few of us can always win against the body's strong drives. Move on and resume the Satiety Diet lifestyle.

Increase your willpower

Share your lower-sugar journey with others. Joining a community of like-minded people has been shown to help boost willpower and keep you on the path you want to travel.

Make it a habit

Cutting down in sugar becomes much easier when:
a) your taste-buds make the "shift"
b) it becomes a habit, a way of life; second nature

Author Sarah Wilson writes: "Change doesn't happen with an about-face. It happens by building up habits in our minds. Slowly, by flexing regularly, we build new neural pathways in our brains until we're doing things differently, effortlessly. So every day that we flex our 'I'm not eating sugar, thanks' muscle, the stronger we get." [Wilson (2014)]

Beware of sugar substitutes.

Some sugar substitutes are much higher in fructose than table sugar. People who want to lose weight by cutting down on table sugar (sucrose) sometimes substitute sweeteners that can be just as fattening, and loaded with even more fructose. Here are some natural but high-fructose sweeteners to eat sparingly:

- Agave syrup is mostly fructose. In fact it contains more fructose than table sugar does.
- Coconut sugar/nectar/syrup: This s almost as high in fructose as table sugar.
- Honey and maple syrup: these are nutritious foods but again, they are high in fructose.
- Dates. Many so-called sugar-free recipes call for dates to add sweetness. The fructose content of dates is around 30%, and you need to add lots of them to get a really sweet taste. On the plus side, they have a low glycemic index.

9. RICE MALT SYRUP

Rice malt syrup is also known as brown rice syrup or rice syrup. This is a traditional Japanese sweetener which is completely fructose-free. The Japanese have been making it for centuries. You could actually make it in your own home kitchen if you had the right training—it is a complex process which takes a lot of skill!

Rice malt syrup is made by culturing brown rice with amylase enzymes (obtained from sprouted barley grains) to break down the starches, then cooking it until it becomes syrup. This syrup contains a mixture of complex carbohydrates, glucose and maltose.

Maltose is the natural sugar produced when amylase breaks down starch. "It is found in germinating seeds as they break down their starch stores to use for food, which is why it was named after malt. It is also produced when glucose is caramelized." ["Maltose." Wikipedia. Retrieved Aug. 2016]

Because it contains no fructose, rice malt syrup is the sweetener of choice for many people. It is not as sweet as sugar.

10. NON-SUGAR SWEETENERS

Stevia—a natural, virtually zero Calorie sweetener that is not sugar.

Stevia has no notable effect on blood glucose levels. It's completely fructose-free.

"Stevia is a sweetener and sugar substitute extracted from the leaves of the plant species *Stevia rebaudiana*. The active, sweet-tasting compounds of stevia are **steviol glycosides**, which have up to 150 times the sweetness of sugar. These steviosides have a negligible effect on blood glucose. Stevia's taste has a slower onset and longer duration than that of sugar, and some of its extracts may have a bitter or licorice-like aftertaste at high concentrations." ["Stevia". Wikipedia. Retrieved 1st Sep. 2018.]

Stevia's after-taste can be masked if you use it in combination with rice malt syrup, or low fructose fruits such as berries, or naturally sweet vegetables. To disguise the after taste, many commercial stevia products are mixed with erythritol, which is a sugar alcohol.

About sugar alcohols.

The term "sugar alcohol" can be confusing because these reduced-Calorie sugar substitutes are neither a sugar nor an alcohol. They are not considered to be artificial sweeteners, because they're derived from natural sources.

Low Calorie sugar alcohol sweeteners include:
- E420 Sorbitol
- E421 Mannitol
- E422 Glycerol
- E953 Isomalt
- E965 Maltitol
- E966 Lactitol
- E967 Xylitol
- E968 Erythritol

Sugar alcohols are obtained from the carbohydrates in plants such as fruits. The carbohydrate is altered through a chemical process.

Sugar alcohols are popular as a sweetener in foods because they contain few Calories, minimally impact insulin levels, are safe for those with diabetes, and are better for your teeth. However, many of them also have a laxative effect.

Of all the sugar alcohols, xylitol and erythritol are considered to be the safest.

Xylitol.

Xylitol tastes like table sugar. It naturally occurs in low concentrations in the fibers of many fruits and vegetables. Xylitol can be extracted from certain berries, oats, and mushrooms, as well as fibrous material such as corn husks, birch tree bark and sugar cane bagasse.

The liver converts xylitol to glucose, which is why it is usually considered the only sugar alcohol that is 100% risk-free. However, this also means it is a source of Calories, though not many.

Table sugar: 4 Calories per gram.

Xylitol: 2.4 Calories per gram.

On the plus side, Xylitol doesn't spike blood sugar levels [Islam & Indrajit (2012)] and it is actively beneficial for the health of your teeth. On the minus side, in large doses (more than 35g per serve) it can have a laxative effect.

Erythritol.

Erythritol, which also tastes like table sugar, is found naturally in some fruits, mushrooms, and fermented foods and beverages such as sherry, wine, and soy sauce. It contains even fewer Calories than xylitol, making it popular among people who want to lose weight. In fact its Calorie content is close to zero.

Table sugar: 4 Calories per gram.

Erythritol: 0.24 Calories per gram.

It is commercially made by fermenting the natural sugar found in corn. Erythritol's sweetness intensity varies from 60% to 80% that of sucrose. [Goosens & Roper (1994)]

Safety reviews have found erythritol to be non-toxic. [Munro et al., (1998)] Like xylitol, erythritol does not raise blood sugar levels. Another benefit is that it doesn't cause tooth decay, because bacteria in the mouth are unable to feed on it. On the negative side, if you eat more than 50g of erythritol in one serving, you might become nauseous or experience laxative side effects or a headache.

Some commercially available sweeteners blend erythritol with stevia, with the idea that the sweetness of the erythritol will mask the slightly bitter after taste of the stevia.

About artificial sweeteners.

Artificial sweeteners are synthetic compounds, chemically processed to make them hundreds of times sweeter than the same weight of table sugar, with few or no Calories. When artificial sweeteners were first invented they were hailed as the miracle substances that could replace sugar, giving us all the sweetness we crave without the Calories. They've been around for a long time now, but still our waistlines are expanding. [Fowler et al., (2008)]

Artificial sweeteners—are they really helping?

Artificial sweeteners have been associated with weight gain in several studies. [Fowler et al., (2008); Swithers (2013)]

Research suggests that some people who drink artificially sweetened diet drinks and eat artificially sweetened diet foods are more likely to be overweight than people who drink sugary sodas. The San Antonio Heart Study examined 3,682 adults over eight years. It found that people who consumed diet sodas consistently had higher Body Mass Indexes (BMIs).

Another study that took place around the same time, conducted by the American Cancer Society, focused on 78,694 women for 12 months. The results? Those who habitually consumed artificial sweeteners were on average 2lb (900g) heavier than those who did not.

Why is this association showing up? Here are some possible explanations:

1) Consuming artificial sweeteners may increase appetite.

People use low Calorie sweeteners, whether artificial or natural, to keep foods tasting sweet while consuming fewer Calories. This means that the body detects sweetness in the mouth, and prepares to receive the energy that's usually associated with sweetness, but that energy is not delivered to the digestive system. Experts are concerned that this dissociation of sweetness from Calories might disrupt the body's mechanisms. [Drewnowski et al., (2012)] It could make the "Inner Guardian" think that higher and higher levels of sweetness are needed, to deliver the Calories it demands. It might have the effect of actually increasing the appetite for sweet foods.

Studies on animals have shown that artificial sweeteners can increase appetite by activating the body's hunger pathways. A study in the journal *Cell Metabolism* reported that when mice and fruit flies experienced lots of sweet-tasting food, but that food ended up delivering fewer Calories, their bodies entered "hunger mode".

"Together, our data show that chronic consumption of a sweet/energy imbalanced diet . . . increases the motivation to eat." [Wang et al, (2016)]

When the natural link between sweetness and Calories is broken, the body's food reward pathways are only partially activated. The sweetness delivers a reward that's not followed by the reward of incoming energy. This may contribute to increased appetite.

Artificial sweeteners may fool the tongue but they cannot fool the brain. "Food reward consists of two branches: sensory and postingestive"—in other words we love sweetness not just because of the taste in our mouths but because of certain signals sent to our brains by sweet foods after they arrive in our stomachs. Artificial sweeteners provide the taste, but not the follow-up.

"Increasing evidence suggests that artificial sweeteners do not activate the food reward pathways in the same fashion as natural sweeteners." [Qing Yang (2010)]

More research is needed to find out whether what holds true for animals also holds true for humans.

The Journal of Experimental Psychology reported, "… it is likely that one of the earliest associations formed by humans and other animals is that based on the signaling relationship between sweet taste in the mouth and the subsequent arrival and absorption of Calories in the gut. This type of signaling relationship is thought to enable sweet taste to evoke physiological responses that anticipate and promote the efficient utilization of the energy contained in foods and fluids. Therefore, if consuming non-caloric sweeteners weakens this relationship, the ability to regulate intake of sweet, high Calorie foods and beverages could also be degraded. [Davidson et al., (2011)]

A study published in *The British Journal of Nutrition* showed that while drinks sweetened with glucose and fructose increased satiety and decreased levels of the hunger hormone ghrelin, drinks sweetened with an artificial sweetener had no effect on satiety hormones.

2) Artificially sweetened foods may cause sweetness cravings.

People who consume artificially sweetened foods may develop a craving for sweeter and sweeter tastes, as their taste-buds become accustomed to all that sweetness.

". . . artificial sweeteners, precisely because they are sweet, encourage sugar craving and sugar dependence. Repeated exposure trains flavor preference. A strong correlation exists between a person's customary intake of a flavor and his preferred intensity for that flavor." [Qing Yang (2010)]

3) Consuming artificially sweetened drinks is linked with eating "junk" food.

People who consume highly processed artificially sweetened drinks are more likely to also consume highly processed "junk" foods.

Dr. Aseem Malhotra, a cardiologist and spokesman for The National Obesity Forum, says: "There is a health halo around these diet drinks. People think that drinking them somehow has a protective quality or lessens the damage of a generally unhealthy lifestyle when they don't."

People who eat only low-energy, whole, nutritious foods and sometimes consume diet drinks are unlikely to gain weight. The fact is, however, that the people who are most likely to drink diet sodas are the people who are most likely to consume a lot of other highly-processed fatty, salty, sugary "junk" foods.

4) "Compensating" for artificial sweeteners.

People who consume artificially sweetened foods may unconsciously compensate for it later, by consuming high Calorie foods. They eat more because they think they are entitled to more Calories. It's tempting to think, "I have been good, and only had low Calorie diet soda, so I can afford to have a doughnut or two."

5) Your body's satiety mechanisms might be disrupted.

Consuming artificially sweetened foods and drinks may disrupt your body's ability to monitor Calories and boost your risk of eating in excess. In the end you would consume more, because the satiety signals do not kick in. [Davidson et al., (2011)]

Scientists at Purdue University, USA, found that artificial sweeteners could disturb the body's innate mechanisms for measuring energy intake based on the sweetness of food and drink. This could be a clue as to why so many people in the modern world seem to have lost the capacity to regulate their body weight. [Davidson & Swithers (2004)]

"The body's natural ability to regulate food intake and body weight may be weakened when this natural relationship is impaired by artificial sweeteners," said Professor Terry Davidson, one of the researchers. "Without thinking about it, the body learns that it can use food characteristics such as sweetness and viscosity to gauge its caloric intake. The body may use this information to determine how much food is required to meet its caloric needs."

6) Your body's blood sugar mechanisms might be disrupted.

Artificial sweeteners may interfere with your body's blood sugar controls by altering your gut microbiota. This could raise blood sugar levels. Having blood sugar levels that are too high can put you at risk of diabetes. There's also a connection between high blood sugar and obesity.

A 2014 study published in *Nature* showed that artificial sweeteners alter your microbiome, the population of bacteria living in your digestive tract. Many health problems, including obesity and diabetes, have been linked to changes in the microbiome. [Suez et al., (2014)]

Dr. Michael Mosley in the episode of his TV show "Trust me, I'm a Doctor" entitled "Saccharin, stevia, and time-restricted eating", compared two sweeteners: the artificial sweetener saccharin and the natural sweetener stevia, which is derived from natural plant sources. The effects of each sweetener was tested on two groups of volunteers.

The results showed that saccharin consumption led to significant spikes in blood glucose levels while stevia had barely any effect on those levels. Saccharin increases blood sugar to unhealthy levels, with a risk of diabetes.

These effects are thought to be associated with the composition of gut bacteria, the microbiome, and the impact that sweeteners can have on it, even over a remarkably short period.

Dr. Mosley's small study indicated that unlike stevia, saccharin has adverse effects on some people, people who host a certain combination of microbes in their gut. Without a simple way to find out whether you're one of the people who is badly affected by saccharin, the best advice is to avoid it altogether.

Dr. Mosley suggested that people should avoid artificial sweeteners—not only saccharin but others such as aspartame and sucralose, which might have the same effect. Meanwhile, those who are seeking a non-sugar sweetener could try stevia.

11. SWEETNESS CRAVINGS

Deprivation can cause cravings.

When you're on a quest to lose weight you don't have to give up sweet foods altogether. In fact giving them up can put you at risk of cravings. Research shows that ignoring a food craving can lead to food bingeing.

". . . deprivation causes craving and overeating. . . " say the authors of a 2005 study published in *The International Journal of Eating Disorders*. [Polivy et al., (2005)]

When people feel deprived of a food they're hankering for, they're more likely to eventually throw caution to the winds and gorge on the craved-for food. If you experience a strong urge to eat something sweet and deny it, time after time, eventually your willpower will probably cave in and you'll find yourself bingeing on every sweet food within reach. You may win small skirmishes against your body's hunger mechanisms but its very unlikely you can win an all-out war.

The more sweet stuff you eat, the more you want!

Citing a 2007 study published in *The Journal of Food Science*, [Mahar & Duizer (2007)] the authors of a 2012 article on "Sweetness and Food Preference" wrote, "Persons who frequently consume sweet-tasting products show a preference for sweeter beverages when tested in the laboratory; this effect is the same for frequent consumers of non-nutritive and nutritive sweeteners." [Drewnowski et al., (2012)]

In other words—as we've already mentioned—it's likely that the more often you eat or drink sweet foods or beverages, the more you crave for them. And this is true, whether the sweetness is provided by low-Calorie sweeteners such as erythritol or aspartame, or Calorie-dense sweeteners such as sugar, honey, dates etc. This is perhaps why some people seem to have what is known as a "sweet tooth"!

To diminish your sweetness hankerings, gradually cut down on the sweetness of the food you eat. For example, add a little less sugar to recipes or beverages, or choose bittersweet, dark chocolate instead of super-sweet milk chocolate. Eventually your tastes will adapt.

How to deal with sweetness cravings.

* Make sure this is not just a passing urge.

When a sweetness craving hits, wait a few minutes (preferably 20 minutes if you can stand it) to see whether it subsides. If it doesn't, proceed to the next step!

* Find the true cause, and address it.

While cravings can be caused by deprivation, they can also arise from such sources as emotional states (e.g. stress), or by the body's need for nutrition. Deal with stress by giving yourself some relaxation time, or meditating, or taking a warm bath, or seeking counseling etc. More generally, give your body the nutrition it needs by regularly eating a wide range of whole foods.

502

Make sure it's not a craving for something else.

If you crave sweet snacks, try sipping some water first. If that does not assuage your craving, eat a satiating food that is not sweet, such as a Calorie-sparse food that's rich in protein and fiber. If all else fails, choose a Satiety Diet sweet snack and eat it mindfully.

Swap, downsize, be mindful.

Columbia University nutrition professor Audrey Cross, PhD recommends that instead of ignoring cravings, people should "Go for the lowest-fat, lowest-Calorie item in the category you're craving, say chocolate frozen [low-fat] yogurt for a chocolate fix." Alternatively, you could mindfully eat a small portion of actual chocolate, making sure that it's high-quality chocolate with plenty of flavor and you savor every mouthful to make the most of it. The same principles apply to cravings for other foods.

Be prepared to satisfy time-of-the-day cravings.

It's not unusual for people to get sugar cravings mid-morning and/or mid-afternoon. It's easy, at such times, to reach for the most convenient, high-energy snack such as candy or cake. The high sugar load can cause a spike in blood sugars, followed by a steep fall, with an associated increase in hunger and sweetness cravings.

Alternatively, some people try to quell those cravings by eating fruit. This is a better idea, but many fruits contain relatively high levels of fructose, which can also stimulate the appetite.

To appease your circadian sweetness cravings, carry with you and have ready at hand, a suitable Satiety Diet sweet snack.

Address cravings for sweetness after meals.

There's a good reason why sweet desserts are traditionally eaten at the end of a meal. Sweetness cravings often occur after eating. If you deny a genuine post-meal sweetness craving, you might end up either feeling miserable and deprived, or surrendering and bingeing on sugary, Calorie-dense snacks.

503

The solution is to:

- Eat a Satiety Diet meal mindfully.
- Finish meals with a Satiety Diet dessert or sweet food.

Losing weight without giving up sweet foods:

- When you can't resist having dessert at the end of a meal, have a small portion—just a few bites, eaten slowly—so that the sugars are less likely to make your blood sugar levels spike.
- Eat any sweet foods at the end of a meal, around 20 minutes after eating the protein/fat component of the meal.
- If you're craving sweetness at other times, slowly and mindfully eat a small portion of sweet food.
- Eat sweet foods only now and then.
- When you eat sweet foods, eat small portions.
- Sweet snacks and desserts should contain some protein,
- Eat sweet foods as mindfully as possible, with no distractions, chewing thoroughly and really enjoying every bite.
- Train yourself to prefer savory foods over sweet foods by gradually cutting down on sweet treats.
- When you follow a recipe for a sweet dish, use as little sweetener as possible while still making it taste good.
- When you eat fruit, choose naturally-sweet, whole, low-fructose varieties, preferably low-fructose (although no fruit is off-limits). Eat fruit in combination with other ingredients that are satiating, high in protein and fiber, low in fat or fat-free, and low GI. For example, you could eat fruit as part of a dessert recipe combined with black beans. (Of course fruit already has fiber in it, but incorporating more can help boost satiety.)
- Sweeten snacks and desserts with naturally sweet vegetables such as sweet potatoes, pumpkin or carrots.
- Alternatively, sweeten food with stevia, a small portion of rice malt syrup or a combination of the two.
- If you wish to use natural sugar alcohols as sweeteners, erythritol is arguably your best choice.

504

- Sweet snacks or desserts can be made by combining whole fruit with low-fat protein, or sweetening adzuki bean paste with a little rice malt syrup, or by creatively blending any other combination of low-fructose sweetness, protein and fiber.

Recipes for sweet dishes and snacks can be found in *Crispy, Creamy, Chewy: The Satiety Diet Cookbook* (#3 in the Satiety Diet series).

12. SWEETNESS IN THE SATIETY DIET

Sweetness Level 1

In a perfect weight-loss world, we would all be able to wean ourselves off sweetness and be content with the naturally sweet tastes found in whole, fresh foods.

Sweetness Level 2

If you want to add sweetness to your food, we recommend using whole fruit and vegetables which possess their own natural sweetness. (Sweet vegetables include sweet potato, pumpkin and carrots.) Choose mainly low-fructose fruits, but allow yourself to eat all fruits. Eat fruit in combination with other foods, especially foods with protein and fiber.

Sweetness Level 3

Now and then, when you feel you need something sweeter you could use:
- A small portion of rice malt syrup, which contains Calories but no fructose
- Stevia, which is natural, has few or no Calories and does not cause blood sugar spikes, but which may have a slightly bitter after-taste

Sweetness Level 4—the emergency sweetness plan.

If you haven't yet weaned yourself off sugary tastes, or if you are really craving for that extra sweetness, here's the emergency plan:

To your Level 3 sweeteners, add a small amount of xylitol or erythritol. These are considered to be the "safest" of the sugar alcohols. Both of them taste like table sugar, both are extracted from natural sources, and neither of them causes significant blood sugar spikes. On the negative side, they are highly processed. (See our section on Sugar Alcohols.)

Xylitol and erythritol can be mixed with rice malt syrup and/or stevia to give an extra sweetness burst. Note that some experts are concerned about non-nutritive sweeteners possibly interfering with the body's regulatory mechanisms.

Summary: How to enjoy sweet foods on the Satiety Diet

The Satiety Diet is about flexibility, satisfaction and the pleasure of food. We all know that we need to eat less sugar. We also know that processed sweeteners are not real food and have their drawbacks. However it's also okay to be kind to yourself and not too pedantic about strict rules. If you really must, you can allow yourself a little sweetener from time to time. Choose wisely, use artificial sweeteners infrequently, and if you're going to have sweet food, preferably eat it at the end of a meal.

FOODS AND DRINKS THAT CAN HINDER WEIGHT LOSS

If you eat large quantities of certain foods you are likely to put on weight. These include:

- Deep-fried foods
- Highly processed foods
- Refined and sugar-coated cereals
- Cookies, cakes, desserts, ice cream
- Candy, chocolate
- White rice, white flour
- Margarine, mayonnaise
- Colas and other sodas
- Processed meats
- Packaged foods
- Foods with artificial ingredients
- Fructose, e.g. in maple syrup, molasses, agave syrup

Foods that can sabotage weight loss.

There are, however, other foods that may appear to be healthful and even low in Calories, but which, in fact, may be sabotaging your weight loss efforts. These include fruit and vegetable juices, commercial energy/granola/muesli/health bars, and dried fruits.

Read on to discover more about these sabotaging foods.

1. HIDDEN FATS, SUGARS AND APPETITE TRIGGERS

Always read the labels of processed foods.

Many processed foods that are touted as "low-fat" can have sugar added by the manufacturer, to compensate for the loss of flavor. Peanut butter and flavored yogurts are good examples of this.

Other processed foods advertised as having "no added sugar" might be low in added cane sugar but high in other forms of sugar.

An example of this is canned fruits with "no added sugar", which may be immersed in fructose-rich fruit juices.

Some sugarless processed foods contain artificial sweeteners that can increase appetite. [Steinert et al., (2011); Swithers (2013)]

Mayonnaise, salad dressings and processed sauces can be very Calorie-dense. People tend to think that eating plenty of salads is a good way to lose weight—and it is, unless your salad dressings are sabotaging your efforts. Salad dressings also tend to "disappear" when they are mixed in, so it's easy to forget that they are still present. Read labels carefully to find out how many Calories are contained within 100g (3.5 ounces) of your chosen product. Even avocado, a natural and healthful food often used as a salad dressing, should only be used in small portions because of its Calorie-density.

2. ENERGY/GRANOLA/MUESLI/HEALTH BARS

Energy bars are extolled as being packed with nutrition, but many of them are also packed with sugars and fats—and not the "good" fats, either. These processed foods may be high in fiber, and even high in protein, but their water content is low. Any fruit in energy bars has had most of its water removed. Remember that "energy" is another word for Calories. Energy bars may seem like a good choice for a quick "pick-me-up" but they don't provide long-term satiety, and they generally contain a lot of Calories per ounce/gram.

3. SHAKES, SMOOTHIES & JUICES

Warning: drinking fruit juice is likely to undermine your weight loss! Juice is fruit in an processed form that is easy to consume rapidly and delivers a sudden sugar-hit to your body. The fiber is either mashed up or removed completely.

The Calories eaten in solid or viscous food suppress appetite more readily than the same number of Calories consumed as a drink.

Shakes, smoothies and juices don't really satisfy your hunger. What's more, all juices—even vegetable juices with all the fiber left in—slip though your digestive system more quickly than solid foods.

They don't have to be chewed, your stomach doesn't have to work hard to churn them into smaller pieces, and they land in your gut in one sudden flood of nutrients, with the potential to send blood sugars skyrocketing. It's easier to gulp down many Calories' worth of food in a liquid state than in a solid or viscous state. This is not the way nature intended for us to eat fruits and vegetables. In particular, your appetite can be stimulated when high-fructose fruits are included in shakes, smoothies and juices.

Puréeing fruits and vegetables to make them into a drinkable smoothie is not a good idea if you want to lose weight. Blending machines and other electric food processors break up much of the fiber in food. They mash it into much smaller pieces than we could create by chewing. Fiber in its natural form is important for slowing down sugar absorption. When you consume fruits and vegetables, eat them whole.

4. SODA/SOFT DRINKS & ENERGY DRINKS

Sugary soft drinks, also known as soda, soda pop, carbonated beverages, fizzy drinks, lolly water etc. are among the worst culprits in the obesity crisis. The same applies to energy drinks, fruit juices and so-called vitamin-water. (It may also apply to low-Calorie diet sodas.)

- These drinks are usually loaded with Calories that can be easily and quickly consumed, leading to excessive weight gain.
- Despite the fact that soda/soft drinks deliver lots of Calories, they leave you hungry for more.
- Some studies have shown that people who drink diet soda/soft drinks are more likely to be overweight or obese than those who drink sugary soda.
- Soda/soft drinks can be "addictive".
- Soda/soft drinks contain no vitamins, minerals, fiber or protein.
- Consumption of sugary soda/soft drinks is associated with a greater risk of diabetes.

- Studies show that tooth decay is linked with drinking either sugary or "diet" soda/soft drinks.
- Consumption of both sugary and diet soda/soft drinks is also linked with decreased bone-density.
- Both types of soda/soft drinks have been shown to be associated with heart disease and depression in women.
- Soda/soft drinks can contain high levels of chemicals such as artificial colorings and preservatives. [BBC News 23 March 2017]

Dr. Walter Willett, the chair of the nutrition department at the Harvard School of Public Health (USA) says that long-term consumption of sugary drinks can double the risk of diabetes, and part of that risk is due to the excess weight gained from sugar-Calories.

Artificially sweetened "diet" sodas.

Don't think that artificially sweetened soda/soft drinks are not fattening!

- Diet soda/soft drinks can make your blood sugar levels spike, just like the sugary versions. Sweeteners such as sucralose and aspartame are more intensely sweet than sugar. Your body responds to this intense sweetness by sending your insulin levels soaring.
- Artificial sweeteners in diet soda/soft drinks may increase your cravings for sweetness. When you drink them, your Inner Guardian expects to receive plenty of Calories after experiencing such a sweet taste in the mouth, but no Calories arrive in the gut. Your Guardian thus ends up with a sense of incompleteness, which may prompt it to send out sweet-ness-craving signals to make you seek more Calories in compensation.
- Artificial sugars and sweeteners in "diet" drinks can inflame the gut of around 50% of the human population.

How to break the soda habit.

Read the labels of soda/soft drinks and add up how many extra Calories they are giving you each day. Work out how far you'd have to run to work off the Calories you get from a single drink. You might be surprised!

If you're addicted to soda/soft drinks, wean yourself off them slowly. Have fewer drinks each day, over the course of several weeks. Over time, mix your soda drinks with plain, sparkling water to gradually get used to the lack of sweetness in natural water.

Avoid soda-drinking triggers, such as vending machines. Don't have any soda in the house.

If you feel like having a soda/soft drinks, drink a glass of water first. You might simply need hydration. After you drink some still or sparkling water the desire for a soda might pass.

Substitute other drinks for soda—such as unsweetened tea, or tea with lemon, orange, mint, or tea made with hot water and a slice of fresh root ginger. Add a slice of lemon or lime, or a dash of lemon juice, or a few frozen berries and some ice cubes to a glass of sparkling water.

When you think of drinking soda/soft drinks, remember how much they can harm your body. You can still have a soda/soft drink, if you really want to. Just save it for special occasions, or sip it once a week.

5. ALCOHOLIC DRINKS

I know, I know. Everyone always tells us to "drink in moderation" or "avoid all alcohol". We're getting so tired of hearing it that we just want to forget about it and have a beer.

But health experts tell us these things for a good reason.

Apart from other considerations, alcohol contains a lot of Calories. It's fattening.

Too much alcohol can sabotage your chances of weight-loss efforts.

- It can cause blood estrogen levels to rise. Estrogen is a hormone which, in both women and men, encourages fat storage, and reduces muscle growth.
- In the short term, alcohol is an appetite stimulant. You're more likely to eat more food when you've had a few drinks before a meal. [Hetherington et al., (2001)]
- Alcohol can also contribute to weight gain because it weakens your inhibitions. Your willpower decreases, and your intentions to mindfully eat only low Calorie, satiating foods can go straight out of the window.
- Even when you don't add high-Calorie mixers such as cream and fruit juices, alcoholic drinks contain a lot more Calories than you might think. They all contain Calories to a greater or lesser extent, and when you consume Calories in beverages, those Calories are less satiating. You hardly notice that you're pouring overloads of energy into your body. If you're going to drink alcohol, it's useful to know that plain, unmixed spirits such as vodka on the rocks are relatively low in Calories. Soda water, mineral water and water-ice have no Calories, so they are good mixers. A slice of lime of lemon adds zing with negligible Calories.

However like everything else on the Satiety Diet, alcohol is not "forbidden". If you really want to, go ahead and drink it.

In moderation!

Some tips:
- Measure how much alcohol you're pouring into your glass; don't just estimate it.
- Avoid alcoholic drinks that contain fat and extra sugar, such as most cocktails.
- Choose drinks that are relatively low in Calories.
- When you want to lose weight, you can still have alcohol in small portions. Just choose low-Calorie drinks and enjoy them sparingly.

6. PROTEIN POWDERS

Protein powders are highly processed products. While they may be useful for people with certain digestive health issues, they cannot be considered as "whole food" because unlike like the foods from which they are derived, they are not balanced.

Weight loss diets that substitute protein shakes for real meals only work because the dieter decreases the number of Calories they consume in a day. This can leave you feeling hungry.

Protein powders are monotonous, highly processed foods with a narrow range of nutrients. It's dietary *diversity* that promotes satiety.

Some people find drinking protein shakes more convenient than preparing meals, which is why they're popular. However the same amount of protein can be obtained from a whole-food diet as from protein shakes—but with other nutrients and fiber into the bargain. Dietician Julie Gilbert, of the Dieticians Association of Australia, says, "The main concern is that high-protein shakes may replace other valuable foods, such as fruit and vegetables, or other important nutrients, such as carbohydrates and fiber from the diet."

Animal-based protein powders that are derived from egg whites or whey may contain traces of antibiotics and hormones. If you do use protein powders, choose vegetable-based ones made from foods such as peas and rice. Together, pea protein isolates and rice protein isolates make a complete amino acid profile, but without the risk of those unwanted contaminants.

7. INFLAMMATORY FOODS

Inflammation plays an integral role in your body's healing system, but too much inflammation for too long can do more harm than good. Being overweight or obese is linked with chronic, low-grade inflammation in the body, which in turn is linked with atherosclerosis, depression and other health problems.

Inflammation is the body's response to a swathe of irritants such as smoking, lack of exercise, high-fat and high-Calorie meals, and highly processed foods.

Obesity can lead to chronic, low-grade inflammation and some scientists believe it might also be *caused* by inflammation.

"… inflammation may be the single-most important mechanism driving the diabesity [diabetes/obesity] epidemic," says alternative medicine guru Chris Kresser. [Kresser (2010)]

Some foods and other substances have been found to have an inflammatory effect on the body while others are anti-inflammatory.

Anti-inflammatory foods include:

- Olive oil
- Oily fish.
- Whole-grain bread, brown rice, and other whole grains
- Fresh vegetables
- Nuts
- Herbs and spices
- Green tea. (Note that the anti-inflammatory compound in green tea, EGCG, can be neutralized by eating iron-rich foods like steak.)

Smoking and excessive alcohol consumption can cause inflammation, as can:

- Artificial food additives (including artificial sweeteners)
- Meat from animals raised in feed-lots
- Most processed foods
- Saturated and trans fats
- Sugars
- Refined grains
- Omega 6 Fatty Acids. These are found in oils such corn, safflower, sunflower, grapeseed, soy, peanut, and vegetable.
- Red meat and processed meats. [Pattison et al., (2004); Ley et al., (2013)] In addition to increasing your risk of dying early, red meat consumption has also been linked to cancer. Farvid et al., (2014); Farvid et al., (2015)] Processed meat consumption has been linked to a shorter lifespan. Even small quantities of processed meats such as salami, bacon and sausages can increase the risk of an early death by as much as one fifth, according to researchers from Harvard School of Medicine (USA).

8. MASHED POTATOES

Puréeing, mashing, cooking and otherwise breaking down food, especially starchy food, can have a huge impact on how those foods affect your blood sugar levels.

When potatoes are boiled and mashed, they release 25% more of their natural sugars than they do when they're simply cut into wedges or chips, then steamed or dry-roasted. When you want to lose weight, avoid mashed potatoes and choose a baked jacket potato instead, loaded with salad vegetables.

9. FOOD ADDITIVES

Food additives are substances mixed into food to preserve it, or to improve its flavor, appearance, smell, texture or other characteristics. These substances can be natural or artificial. Some food additives have been used by humans for centuries. Vinegar, fat and salt are traditionally used for preserving food, for example.

Because consumers want the convenience of food with a long shelf-life, manufacturers have to add preservatives and/or antioxidants. Food manufacturers may also add colors, flavors, flavor enhancers, emulsifiers, stabilizers, thickeners and artificial sweeteners, to make their products more tempting.

The long-term effect of food additives on our bodies, in particular on our gut microbiota, requires further study, but some evidence of their effect has already been found.

- **Artificial sweeteners.** These have been linked to glucose intolerance and changes in the gut microbiota.
- **Emulsifiers.** Studies show that emulsifiers, which are added to most processed foods, (to help prevent oil and water blends from separating) could be associated with obesity, diabetes and inflammatory bowel disorders. Emulsifiers are common in foods such as ice cream and mayonnaise. [Chassaing et al., (2015)]

- **Monosodium glutamate (MSG).** The flavor enhancer monosodium glutamate (MSG) can make your hunger come back more quickly after a meal. According to a 1990 study published in the journal Physiology & Behavior, "…motivation to eat recovered more rapidly following a lunchtime meal in which MSG-supplemented soup was served as the first course (compared both with the effect of unsupplemented soup and no [soup])" [Rogers & Blundell (1990)]. MSG is present in virtually all fast foods, and many processed foods. The US Food and Drug Administration (FDA) has classified MSG as being "generally recognized as safe," but its use is controversial.

10. OILS

Prior to the 1960s, edible oils were generally used frugally in cooking. Cooking oils have now become so cheap that people use them liberally. Yes, some of these oils (such as olive oil) confer enormous health benefits, but all edible oils are naturally high in Calories and that should be taken into account when you want to lose weight. Oil can contain around 120 Calories per tablespoon.

It can be hidden in packaged, processed foods. It can be invisible in salad dressings. And any deep-fried foods are sure to contain a lot of oil. In fact, oil is one of the foods that provides most of the human population's Calories.

To lose weight, choose oils that are low in saturated fats (such as olive oil, flaxseed oil and grapeseed oil), and use them sparingly. Oil sprays are useful, as are "air fryer" machines that cook food using less oil (oil-free oven-roasting can work just as well). Non-stick pans work well without added oil—until their special surface wears off. You can line your frypan with baking paper, instead of using oil to cook. Some people pan-fry using a little water.

11. TOO MUCH OR TOO LITTLE FAT

Too much fat.

High-fat diets can actually work a change on your taste buds and stop you from tasting fat. When this happens, your sensitivity to fat decreases; it takes more fat to satisfy your taste buds. You might end up eating too many fatty foods without realizing it.

Researcher Professor Keast of Deakin University's Centre for Physical Activity and Nutrition Research (Australia) said that the mouth's fat-insensitivity was reflected throughout the digestive system. "If you require high concentrations to be able to identify fat in the oral cavity, the same thing is happening in your gut," he said.

In other words, if your taste buds think you haven't eaten any fat, neither does the rest of your digestive system and neither does your Inner Guardian. Your Inner Guardian is unlikely to send out satiety signals after a meal, because it is wants you to eat more fat. [Newman et al., 2016)]

Too little fat.

Too much fat makes you fat, but strangely enough, too little fat could have the same effect. Very low-fat diets don't work in the long run. Taking all, or most of, the fat out of food leaves the food tasting bland and unsatisfying. It also leaves the body craving for fat! Your mouth and tongue need to sense some fat in food in order to trigger your body's satiety response. When you eat modest amounts of fat from time to time, your taste buds stay sensitized to it. [Tobias et al., (2015)]

Fat is not as satiating as carbs.

Fat and carbohydrates do not have the same effect on satiety. A study published by The American Society for Clinical Nutrition found that dietary fat has a weak action on satiation compared with carbohydrates.

The researchers wrote, "These studies suggest that the appetite-control system may have only weak inhibitory mechanisms to prevent the passive overconsumption of dietary fat." They suggested that this weak satiating effect of fat could, over time, lead to gradual weight gain. [Blundell et al., (1993)]

PART FIVE

THE TIMING OF EATING

1. THE DAILY EATING ROUTINE

"Most animals, including humans, have habitual meal patterns, consuming approximately the same number of meals and at the same times of day each day," wrote the authors of a 2004 overview published in *The American Journal of Physiology*. [Woods (2004)]

People generally eat their meals at times that are convenient, or part of their daily routine. This means that the timing of your meals generally springs from social circumstances (e.g. you eat when your colleagues or families or friends eat) or learned factors (e.g. you eat when you know you might not have time to eat later) instead of eating to balance out the energy requirements of your body.

2. DURATION OF MEALS

The time taken to eat a meal is important. If you quickly gulp down your food, then in the ancient language of your Inner Guardian you could be signaling:

- "There's not much food, so I must quickly get my share before it's all gone", or—
- "I need to eat quickly because there's danger approaching and I'll have to fight or flee."

Eating quickly can send body-speech signals indicating either a shortage of food or a need for a surge in cortisol.

It also means that your meal spends less time in front of your eyes and in your mouth, the smells and sounds of food spend less time stimulating your senses, and the experience of food spends less time being imprinted on your memory. In the ancient body-speech of the Inner Guardian, this can mean you've had less food to eat.

If your Inner Guardian thinks that food is scarce, or you're under stress, or you have not had much to eat, then it tries to protect your energy stores by sending out hunger signals.

So, eat more slowly!

If a meal is of long duration and you feel relaxed while eating, and you eat mindfully, your Inner Guardian gets the message that, "There is plenty of food. And there is no need to panic!"

3. CIRCADIAN RHYTHM

Your body's circadian rhythm is a daily cycle that regulates its patterns of sleeping, activity, eating, metabolism, sensitivity to pain, hormone release, body temperature and many other physiological functions.

Your "biological clock" or "master body-clock" is what drives your circadian rhythms.

"The biological clocks that control circadian rhythms are groupings of interacting molecules in cells throughout the body. A 'master clock' in the brain coordinates all the body-clocks so that they are in synch."[NIGMS (2017))]

Our body-clocks get their timing cues from our environment. When the light of the rising sun peeps between the bedroom curtains and touches your eyelids in the morning, for example, your body-clock gets the message to put you into waking mode. And when the sun goes down and you no longer see daylight, it puts you into "sleep" mode.

Temperature also plays a role. Nights are usually colder than days, so your body-clock uses temperature cues to help it know when to put you into sleep mode. You tend to sleep better in a cooler environment.

Your natural circadian rhythm can be disrupted by such factors as

- artificial lighting
- airplane travel through different time zones
- shift work
- disturbed sleep patterns
- living in darkness
- living in places where smog is so thick it blots out the sky's natural light and color
- eating meals out of synch with the body-clock
- living in high latitudes where winter days are extremely short and summer days are extremely long.

Scientists have discovered that the disruption of the natural circadian rhythm can badly affect your health in many ways. It can increase the risk of such problems as:

- depression
- obesity
- diabetes
- heart disease
- bipolar disorder
- sleep disorders

The circadian rhythm & weight loss

The timing of eating plays a major role in weight loss. In particular, the circadian rhythm governs the way your body metabolizes food. [Gal & Gad (2016)]

Throughout the millennia of human existence, people have naturally fasted overnight. Our bodies, our body-clocks, our circadian rhythms are all geared towards overnight fasting while we sleep.

When you eat out of synch with your body-clock, your food may not be digested optimally. Your body is best at processing fats and sugars at certain times of the day.

This is why it's important, for weight loss, to eat at the right times.

It's not just WHAT you eat and HOW you eat that's important. It's also WHEN you eat.

Blood sugar levels and the circadian rhythm.

Your blood sugars have a distinct circadian variation, synchronized with your body-clock. [Aparicio et al., (1974); So et al., (2009); Kalsbeek et al., (2014)]

"Blood sugar regulation and the biological clock are closely entwined," says Erin Digitale, science writer for Stanford Medicine's Office of Communication and Public Affairs (USA).

Two main environmental factors send cues to your body-clock. One of these factors is light entering your eyes. Even the tiniest glimmer of light can be enough to tell your master body-clock to switch on your "wake up" functions. And conversely, darkness tells you to sleep.

522

Food intake and the circadian rhythm.

Food is an important environmental factor affecting your daily cycle. So vital are mealtimes and food nutrients to the rhythms of your body that, following a study published in the journal *Cell Reports,* Dr. Makoto Akashi of Yamaguchi University, Japan, suggested that your circadian clock can even be adjusted by manipulating your diet.

A century ago, people tended to get up around sunrise and go to bed when the sun went down. If they stayed up after sunset, their houses were lit with the warm, dim rays of firelight or candle-light.

As mentioned, light is a key player in our circadian rhythms. In a 2016 study, researchers looked at the way light affects our eating patterns, and asked how artificial light could contribute to obesity. They studied two groups of mice.

One group was allowed to live with the sun's natural cycle of 16 hours of bright daylight and 8 hours of absolute darkness.

The other group lived with 16 hours of bright daylight and 8 hours of twilight, to replicate what it's like for people living in cities, where artificial lights burn continuously all through the night.

Both groups were equally active and ate exactly the same number of Calories.

After only eight weeks, the mice whose nights were lit by twilight weighed 50% more than the mice whose nights were pitch dark. The twilight mice also had the symptoms of pre-diabetes.

The only difference between the groups was the lighting, which influenced WHEN the mice ate. The twilight mice sometimes ate during the bright-light period and sometimes ate during the twilight.

The mice who experienced the more natural rhythms of day and night ate only during the bright "daylight" hours and fasted during the pitch darkness. They had a smaller "eating window".

To make sure that it really was the eating times and not some other effect of the twilight, the researchers ran the same experiment again. This time everything was the same, except that no food was available to the twilight mice during the twilight time.

And they didn't experience that enormous weight gain!

[Lucassen et al (2016); Fonken et al., (2010)]

4. HOW OFTEN SHOULD YOU EAT?

Should you stick to three meals a day with no snacks in between?
Should you have six small meals a day?
Or should you just nibble and graze all day?
Some people are free to choose when they eat: These include people who work at home, retirees etc. Others have to conform to imposed eating times, to fit in with their work timetable, or for other reasons. Some people feel hungrier in the mornings, others get the urge to eat more in the evenings.

Every person is different, so there is probably no "one size fits all" answer to these questions. Despite that, it is possible to work out how often (ideally) you should eat.

Eat only when you're actually hungry.

Don't eat when you're not hungry or only feeling peckish. Consuming foods or Calorie-dense beverages for reasons other than hunger is the perfect way to GAIN weight. Ideally, you should eat when you experience real hunger, a level of hunger that is more intense than peckishness and less intense than ravenous hunger.

If you get really hungry between meals a satisfying satiety snack (i.e. 2-3 snacks per day) can help you avoid feeling deprived and developing cravings for Calorie-dense foods.

Avoid "grazing".

"Grazing" does not aid weight loss. Medical reporter Dr. Michael Mosley says that eating numerous small meals throughout the day as a way of losing weight is no more than a "popular diet myth". It is natural and beneficial for the digestive system to experience rest periods between meals; periods when you're not eating. According to Dr. Mosley, consuming several small meals throughout the day only serves to increase your hunger levels. [Mosley (2016)]

A 1997 review of several studies found that with the exception of only one study, there was no evidence that frequent eating of small meals throughout the day ("grazing"), helps with weight loss. [Bellisle et al., (1997)]

A 2014 study separated people with type 2 diabetes into two groups [Kahleova et al., (2014)]. Both groups consumed the same number of Calories per day, but one ate those Calories in the form of six small meals while the other ate them as two large meals; breakfast and lunch. Compared to the six-meals-a-day group, the people in the two-meals-a-day group—

- lost more weight
- felt more satisfied
- experienced less hunger

Your blood sugar levels normally rise after meals, as you digest your food and your body absorbs glucose. They fall again, back to their usual "baseline", as your cells take up the glucose and used it for energy or store it to use later.

It's normal and healthy for your blood sugar levels to gradually rise at mealtimes and gradually fall between meals. What's not healthy is if they suddenly surge to a high spike, then steeply fall below the baseline (which happens when you eat too many refined carbohydrates, such as sugar).

What is also unhealthy is always having slightly elevated blood sugar levels, due to continual eating. Frequent eating of small meals and snacks through the day keeps your blood sugar levels high.

"Increased meal frequency does not promote greater weight loss . . . " suggest the results of a study published in *The British Journal of Nutrition*. [Cameron et al., (2009)]

And if you need any more convincing—nutritionists tell those who want to GAIN weight to "aim for three meals and several snacks a day." Siobhan Harris, writing for WebMD says, "Eat often to gain weight ... eating meals or substantial snacks (think mini-meals) more often is the way to pack more Calories into the day. Maybe have six mini meals a day."

Aim for three satiating meals per day

Breakfast, lunch and dinner!

Yes, we recommend that you aim to eat three low-Calorie, high-satiety meals a day. Exactly when you eat them is your own business. Listen to your body—it will tell you.

That said, it's okay to eat satiating snacks between meals if you need them to stave off ravenous hunger.

5. BREAKFAST

What is "breakfast"? By definition it's the first meal of the day. It does not have to be a meal that's eaten in the morning. This is an important distinction! You could eat your first meal of the day in the afternoon and it could still be called "breakfast".[42]

As discussed in our section "About skipping meals, especially breakfast," you don't have to eat breakfast early in the day, if you don't feel like it. Eating only when you're hungry makes sense if you want to lose weight. So if you'd prefer to eat breakfast at 11am, or 1am (for example) instead of at 7am, there's no reason why you shouldn't—and in fact, it could help with weight loss!

The experts disagree on whether "skipping breakfast" helps people lose weight or not. This might be due to some confusion about the definition of breakfast.

When people talk about "skipping breakfast" they are usually referring to skipping a morning meal. On the Satiety Diet, it doesn't matter if you eat your first meal of the day in the morning or the afternoon. As discussed, if you're aiming to lose weight, you should eat when you're hungry, and if you're not hungry first thing in the morning, then that is a good reason to leave eating until later.

---

42 A team of scientists at the Weizmann Institute of Science (Israel) published a study suggesting that you should should eat breakfast four hours after sunrise, because that is when your body is best at turning sugars into energy. However, the sun rises at very different times, depending on the season and your geographical location. Furthermore, not all of us are exposed to sunlight as soon as it peeps over the horizon. We may sleep in dark rooms, in dark buildings. And shift workers cannot conform to this schedule.

Never eat breakfast if you're not hungry!

However, on the Satiety Diet skipping breakfast when you really ARE hungry is a bad idea. Some people don't eat breakfast in an effort to lose weight. They reason that if they miss out on breakfast they're missing out on Calories and their bodies will then burn fat.

But it doesn't work that way.

What happens inside your brain when you skip breakfast despite feeling hungry? Brain scans show that we are biologically driven to desire Calorie-dense foods when we are ravenously hungry. This is bad news for weight loss. Ravenously hunger stimulates the production of the hunger hormone ghrelin, which send powerful signals to the brain: "Consume lots of energy NOW".

This is a biological, physiological drive; a potent chemical compulsion. It is not under your conscious control. Denying the body's commands is NOT a matter of willpower

So if you're hungry, don't skip meals, because your brain will powerfully drive you towards compensatory Calorie-dense foods, and willpower may not be enough to fight it.

Conflicting research results

A study published in the American Journal of Nutrition found that people who "skip breakfast" are more likely to have a higher body weight and to suffer from:

- hypertension
- insulin resistance
- higher fasting blood-fat concentrations

The researchers suggested that the hunger people experience when they fail to eat a satiating first meal can make them more likely to eat Calorie-dense foods later in the day, which increases their chances of developing obesity-related diseases. [Mekary et al., (2013)]

A study reported in *The American Journal of Epidemiology* found that "… skipping breakfast was associated with increased prevalence of obesity…" [Ma et al., (2003)]

Children who eat breakfast at home and again at school have been shown to have healthier body-weights than students who skip the meal altogether. And overweight children are likely to grow up to be overweight adults.

A study printed in *Pediatric Obesity* suggested that for children, two breakfasts are better than one! The researchers wrote, " . . . there was an increased odds of overweight/obesity among frequent [breakfast] skippers compared with double breakfast eaters . . . " [Wang et al., (2016)]

The results of other studies appear to contradict this idea, so the jury is still out. There is some disagreement, among experts, about the breakfast issue!

Here's the solution:

To lose weight, enjoy those three meals a day, but consume them when you're hungry, make them high-satiety meals, and preferably eat them within an 8 or 12 hour eating window.

Instead of skipping breakfast, simply delay it. When you're ready to eat breakfast (i.e. your first meal of the day, which should be eaten when you feel hungry, and not before), sit down to a super-satisfying, satiating meal. Remember the saying, "Breakfast like a king, lunch like a prince and dine like a pauper"? Eating a really slap-up, satisfying breakfast will set you up for the day. It will provide fuel for your body at the beginning of the active circadian period, which is when you need it most. Your body is fine-tuned to make the best use of sugars and fats and other nutrients early in the day.

For breakfast, eat all the macronutrients. Choose real, whole foods with a wide range of colors, textures and flavors; low-fructose fruits, whole grains, lean protein, and healthful fats. If you're going to eat something sweet today, now's the time (remember the 2012 study in the journal "Steroids" that advocated eating dessert at breakfast-time?)—but eat it as the last part of the meal. Choose a sweet food that's low in fructose AND low in fat because eating fat and sugar together is more likely to promote weight gain. [Jakubowicz et al (2012)]

Set your entire meal out in front of you before you begin eating, so that your eyes can tell your brain, "This is my meal!" and help you remember it and picture it later. Eat mindfully.

6. HAVE A SMALLER EATING WINDOW

Your "eating window" helps with weight loss.

What is an eating window? It's the daily period of time in which you eat—as distinct from the period of time in which you fast. Most of your fasting period usually exists during the night, while you are asleep.

People (and mice) who have a shorter daily eating window experience a range of health benefits including:

- Less storage of fat on the body
- Lower body weight
- A decreased risk of diabetes
- A decreased risk of heart disease
- Lower cholesterol,
- Lower blood glucose,
- A decreased risk of liver damage on a high fat diet.

Mice with a smaller eating window.

In 2012 a group of researchers gave two groups of mice the same high fat diet. One group was allowed to eat whenever they wanted, day and night. The other group only had access to the food for eight hours, beginning in the afternoon and stopping at night.

The scientists from the University of California and the Salk Institute for Biological Studies found that " . . . mice fed on a high-fat diet, but only allowed to eat within an eight-hour window, were healthier and slimmer than mice that were given exactly the same food but allowed to eat it whenever they wanted." [Mosley (13 January 2016); Hatori et al., (2012)]

Biologist Dr. Satchidananda Panda said, "Surprisingly, the mice that were eating the same number of Calories, but ate only for eight hours, did not become as obese as the first group. Less than 12 percent of their body weight was fat, as opposed to 40 percent."

The mice that ate whenever they wanted not only gained fat—they also developed high cholesterol, high blood glucose and liver damage. The mice with the eight-hour eating window experienced no health problems, despite the fact that they were eating the same high-fat foods.

Dr. Panda found even when researchers tested obese mice, and even when they fed them on a high-fat, high-sugar diet, time-restricted feeding bestowed huge health benefits. A smaller eating window can even reverse obesity and diabetes! [Chaix et al., (2014)]

A later study by these scientists showed that mice who fasted for at least 12 hours per day remained healthier and slimmer than mice who ate exactly the same number of daily Calories, but spread throughout the 24-hour period.

Humans with a smaller eating window.

You might say, "But these are mice! How do these results apply to humans?"

Medical researchers use mice and rats as models in medical studies because their genetic, biological and behavior characteristics are very much like ours. That said, they are NOT identical to humans, and of course human trials are always the most accurate.

This is why Dr. Jonathan Johnston at the University of Surrey DID use humans in his 10-week "eating window" experiment.

At the beginning of the experiment, his team measured the volunteers' body fat, blood sugar levels, blood fat (triglycerides) and cholesterol levels. The team then divided up the volunteers into 2 groups choosing them at random.

One group was the "control" group, which in science-language means that they did not alter anything about the way they ate, but simply continued to eat as they had always done.

Control groups are used in experiments and studies as a benchmark, against which the researchers can measure how experimental group performs. Subjects in control groups don't receive any treatment.

Dr. Johnston's team asked the other group in the study to continue eating what they normally ate, but to eat their breakfast 90 minutes later than usual, and their dinner 90 minutes earlier. In other words, they restricted their "eating window" and made it shorter, while their "fasting window" became longer.

This shift in eating times meant that the people in the experimental group fasted for an extra three hours every day.

The test took place over 10 weeks, and at the end of it, people in both groups underwent the same blood tests they'd had at the beginning of the study.

The results were astonishing.

The group that restricted their "eating window" had:
- Significantly improved fasting blood sugar levels
- Significantly improved cholesterol levels
- Decreased their body fat.
- Developed more lean muscle mass

Remember that each day they had been eating the same number of Calories as they usually ate. They'd simply changed the times at which they consumed them. [Mosley (13 January 2016)]

Medical researchers involved with the experiment, say that these results could be due to two factors:
- Fasting has health benefits.
- Your body processes Calories better during the day than late at night.

The benefits of short periods of fasting.

Short, intermittent periods of fasting are good for your health. They have been shown to normalize insulin and leptin sensitivity, normalize ghrelin levels, boost mitochondrial energy efficiency, readjust the body to burn fat as its primary fuel, stimulate human growth hormone (HGH) production, lower triglyceride levels, permit your body's cells to repair themselves and decrease the accumulation of oxidative radicals in your cells. (Prolonged high levels of blood fat or blood sugar are bad for you.)

Be kind to yourself.

The volunteers in Dr. Johnston's experimental group were happy with the results of the test. They did, however, comment that it was hard to abstain from eating and drinking in the evenings. Some of them, for example, were accustomed to drinking a glass of wine around that time. They missed it, and found it hard to stick to the new routine. Besides, never eating after 8pm can interfere with social occasions.

If you want to use a shorter eating window as a tool for weight loss, you'll find it is highly successful. However it's also important to be kind to yourself. Cut yourself some slack.

Being too regimented and strict can have negative psychological repercussions. Some people may start to feel deprived, or resentful or guilty. Others may feel get ravenously hungry by bedtime, and feel like reaching for the most Calorie-dense snack they can find. Some people find it hard to sleep when they are very hungry—and good sleep is vital to health and weight loss.

Adopt the shorter eating window tactic whenever you can, but don't feel bad if you cannot manage it every day. Every time you do manage to experience a longer overnight fast, you are losing weight and improving your health.

The "Shorter Eating Window Tool" in a nutshell:

Aim to limit your eating window to period of 8 or 12 hours per day. Eat breakfast as late as practicable and your last meal of the day as early as practicable.

Example #1:
- Have breakfast 1 1/2 hours later than usual.
- Have dinner 1 1/2 hours earlier than usual.

Example #2:
- 8am breakfast
- 1pm lunch
- 6pm dinner

Consume most of your Calories earlier in the day. Remember, "Breakfast like a king, lunch like a prince and dine like a pauper."

Helpful tips:
- No late night snacks.
- No eating before bed.
- Eating late, starting at 8 pm, is less helpful than eating your last meal at 5 or 5:30pm

Good news: you can even have weekends off!

"Researchers gave some of the time-restricted mice a respite on weekends, allowing them free access to high-fat meals for these two days. These mice had less fat mass and gained less weight than the mice given a freely available, high-fat diet the whole time. In fact, the mice that were freely fed just on weekends looked much the same as mice given access to food 9 or 12 hours a day for seven days a week, suggesting that the diet can withstand some temporary interruptions." [Salk (2014)]

7. BEDTIME AND WEIGHT LOSS

Bedtime and your body-clock.

Metabolism is closely associated with your circadian rhythm. Your internal body-clock makes you process food differently through the day. There are times in the 24-hour day when your body processes fats and sugars better than at other times. As the sun falls, your body prepares itself for sleep, and for the fasting that occurs during sleep.

Your Inner Guardians expects you to fast at night. Your body is naturally prepared to release stores of energy while you are sleeping and fasting, to keep your brain and other organs fuelled.

Your metabolism functions at its best when you eat your last meal long before bedtime. If you eat after about 8pm, you are loading the body with nutrients it's not programmed to metabolize efficiently. In particular, eating in the evenings can have a bad effect on your blood sugar and blood fat levels.

After a meal eaten in the morning, your blood sugars return to normal in about two hours and your blood fats in three hours. Eat that same meal in the evening, and afterwards your blood sugars and fats stay high for longer.

If you eat a lot of Calories in the hours before you go to sleep, those Calories will not be used to power your activity. Instead, your body will store them as fat.

If you're not already convinced, here's another reason it's not a good idea to indulge in midnight snacks or late-night meals: After you eat, sugars from your food pass into your blood stream and your blood sugar levels rise. (There can be sugars even in foods that do not taste "sweet" or "sugary".) Your body needs to produce insulin to process these sugars.

If your body starts secreting insulin in the middle of the night, this messes with your circadian rhythms. It can also lead to a later fall in blood sugars, which can disrupt your sleep, waking you in the night or disturbing the deep sleep cycles your body needs for proper repair and restoration.

Eating too close to bedtime is bad for your health and can make you put on weight!

Don't eat a meal just before bedtime.

When you eat later, you tend to eat more. Research by Dr. Louis J. Aronne, director of the weight control program at the Weill Cornell Medical Center (USA), indicates that people who eat late consume more food than they would at a meal eaten during the day. [Ray (2008)]

Late night eating can cause health issues. It can:
- increase your risk of diabetes and heart disease
- raise your glucose and insulin levels
- affect cholesterol levels
- increase your risk of heart disease
- impair your memory and cognitive functions
- give you bad dreams
- give you acid reflux

More pertinently for those of us who want to shed excess pounds, late night eating can cause weight gain. It can disrupt your "hunger hormone" rhythms and make you feel hungrier than usual when you wake up the following morning.

Dr. Aronne says, "Eating a big meal just before going to bed has been found in studies to elevate triglyceride levels in the blood for a period of time." Triglyceride levels are associated with diabetes, metabolic syndrome, and overall weight gain [C. Claiborne Ray. Midnight meals. The New York Times. 2008 February 26.]

Dr. Ebru Özpelit, associate professor of cardiology, at Dokuz Eylül University (Turkey) says, "We must have a small dinner and it mustn't be later than 7 o'clock in the evening."

Go to bed earlier for better weight loss.

Going to bed late has a profound effect on your body weight. The results of a study from the University of California, Berkeley, USA, showed that over a five-year period, teenagers who go to bed late are more likely to gain weight than those who go to bed early. [Asarnow et al., (2015)]

Get a good night's sleep.

If you don't get enough sound, restful sleep at nights, your stress levels and cortisol levels will probably rise. The stress hormone cortisol is strongly linked with obesity. [Björntorp & Rosmond (2000)] In other words, getting a good night's sleep is vital for weight loss.

We further discuss the role of sleep in weight loss in the "Sleep Tools" section of *The Satiety Diet Weight Loss Toolkit*, book #2 in the Satiety Diet series.

Lose weight while you sleep.

When you refrain from eating (or drinking anything except water or herbal teas) close to bedtime, you're pretty much guaranteed to lose weight while you sleep—if you sleep for long enough.

Going to bed on an empty stomach means you are fasting while you sleep. Fasting is not only an excellent way to lose weight, it's also the pathway to better health.

Fasting lowers your insulin levels, and can help overcome insulin resistance. Insulin resistance goes hand-in-hand with obesity. The experts are divided as to whether insulin resistance causes weight gain and obesity, or whether weight gain causes insulin resistance, but one thing is for certain—insulin resistance can make weight loss very difficult!

To properly lower your insulin levels for long enough to make a difference, you need to fast for more than just six or seven hours.

It makes sense not to feel ravenously hungry when you're awake.

The Satiety Diet helps you feel satisfied for the greater part of the day—the part when the sun is in the sky and you are active, when your digestive system is working at its optimum, and when your brain and body need fuel. Perhaps most importantly, your awake-time is also the time when you are most conscious of any feelings of hunger or deprivation. Why endure the nagging, uncomfortable effects of hunger while you are awake? Why not experience some hunger while you are asleep and thus unaware of it?

Fasting in your sleep is a lot easier than fasting when you're awake. Arguably, it's also psychologically better for you, because you're more likely to feel deprived when you're awake and conscious that you're forbidding yourself from scoffing all those delectable goodies whose images surround you everywhere you look.

Losing weight in your sleep is not as strange as it sounds. Your digestive system was built to take a rest when you sleep. Nature doesn't expect you to be full of food when you lie down to rest.

That said—sometimes hunger can disrupt sleep, so it's a delicate balancing act.

Fasting is more efficient at night-time.

"Nighttime fasting—also known as 'closing the kitchen early'—may help you lose more weight, even if you eat more food throughout the day," say the researchers who performed the mouse study with the eight hour eating window. [Hatori et al., (2012)]

8. ABOUT FASTING

How long should you fast?

Some diet gurus tell us to fast for 24 hours or 48 hours or even longer, but most of us cannot manage such a long period. For most people, fasting isn't easy!

For the best chance at weight loss, the shortest fasting period you should aim for is 12 hours (mainly overnight). If you can fast for longer than that without suffering from cravings, irritability, hunger pangs, headaches, faintness etc.—great! Do it!

You can drink liquids while fasting.

And just because you're fasting before bedtime doesn't mean you should stop drinking liquids. It's important to remain well hydrated throughout any fast. When fasting, you can drink low-Calorie fluids such as:

- plain, still water (you can add a slice of lemon or lime, or a sprig of mint)
- plain, sparkling water (flavored as for plain, still water)
- plain, green tea (no milk or sugar)
- weak, black tea (no milk or sugar)
- herbal teas
- It's preferable to avoid coffee, because caffeine before bedtime can keep you awake.

Find out more useful facts about fasting in *The Satiety Diet Weight Loss Toolkit*, book #2 in the Satiety Diet series.

Intermittent fasting on the satiety diet.

People on the 5:2 diet often complain about hunger during their two fasting days. The Satiety Diet advocates intermittent fasting in a very different way. After all, we are about satiety, *not* deprivation!

- Aim to take your last mouthful of your final meal of the day before 7pm. See our section on "The Timing of Eating".

- Fast overnight. If you're sleeping while you fast, you won't notice that you're fasting. Also it's natural and healthy for your body to fast overnight.

- Aim to limit your eating window to a period of 8 to 12 hours per day. The smaller your eating window, the bigger the benefits—with this proviso—as long as you are not experiencing ravenous hunger!

- It has been suggested that men's eating window can be shorter than women's. So for example:
  * Men: fast for 16 hours, eat during an 8 hour period
  * Women: fast for 14 hours, eat during a 10 hour period
  These are rough guidelines only, and should vary according to your individual needs. Hunger is fine, but don't allow ravenous hunger to set in.

- During the fasting period, you can drink unlimited quantities of water, sparkling water and herbal teas. Be warned that black coffee or black tea might interfere with your sleep. Staying well hydrated makes fasting easier.

- As much as possible, keep to a regular schedule. Give your body a consistent rhythm to which it can adapt. Once your digestive system, satiety hormones and other processes start to follow a regular cycle, it will become easier for you to stick to the schedule.

- Use the power of your mind to visualize all the amazing health benefits of fasting. Think of overnight fasting as *getting good things*, not giving them up. Think of it as *repairing and energizing your body* (which is exactly what it is doing). Think of overnight fasting not as self-denial—quite the opposite! It is as a positive and wonderful gift you are giving to yourself.

Don't Panic.

Be kind to yourself. Don't put yourself through ravenous hunger. Words that refer to the complete cessation of eating, such as "fast" and "fasting", give many people a sense of dread.

Chris Clark says, "The mere mention of the words *fast* or *fasting* make me hungry. Those terms on their own make me feel deprived. They send me scurrying to find food and squirrel it away somewhere in case of 'emergencies'.

"I've tried fasting, like I've tried every other diet method known to man. I've tried long-term fasting and intermittent fasting. I have been for as long as three days without eating anything at all. I have tried skipping the evening meal and going to bed feeling ravenous. I've tried skipping breakfast and only eating one or two small meals per day. Every time I fast, I feel deprived, sick, exhausted, hungry, desperate, depressed, and utterly terrible. I am barely able to function, because all I do is think of food. I always *hated* fasting.

"Until I found out that a) there's an easier way to do it and b) it's actually the reverse of deprivation. If you approach it the right way it's giving you bonus after bonus.

"The easier way? Sleep through it! Stop eating well before bedtime. Sleep through your fast. Next morning, eat a late breakfast.

"And how is it the reverse of deprivation? Think of fasting this way: 'Fasting is not taking anything away from me—it is actually *giving* to me. It is giving me health, strength, rejuvenation; it is taking another step on the road to slenderness and vigor.'"

9. THE TIMING OF EATING: DAYS OF THE WEEK

Take the weekend off!

As discussed, the "circadian rhythm" refers to a daily cycle measured by your body-clock. There are also other cycles.[43]

According to a 2013 study undertaken at Cornell University (USA), our body-weight fluctuates according to a regular weekly rhythm. We gain a small amount of weight over the weekend and lose a little during the week.

This means that most people are at their highest weight on Sunday nights and at their lowest on Friday mornings. Perhaps this is because we are more likely to indulge ourselves with eating and drinking on the weekends. [Orsama et al., (2013)]

The researchers who performed this study were interested to note that it was the people who lost the most weight between Sunday night and Friday morning who were most likely to become slimmer over a the course of a year.

The long-term weight losers started compensating for their weekend splurge as soon as the working week began, on Monday mornings. And they continued their weight loss, but by bit, throughout the working week.

So you don't have to see the number on the scales go down every day of the week to be successful in your weight loss journey!

In fact, it's the people who let themselves have a bit of a fling once a week who are most likely to lose weight and keep it off!

These results indicate not only that you can get away with weekend food flings if you go back to your Satiety Diet during the week—it also suggests (hooray!) that you are more likely to lose weight and keep it off in the long term, if you permit yourself to have weekend splurges.

---

43   "The study of biological temporal rhythms, such as daily, tidal, weekly, seasonal, and annual rhythms, is called chronobiology." *Wikipedia, "Circadian rhythm." Retrieved 5th Feb 2017*

10. THE TIMING OF EATING AND EXERCISE

Scientific research suggests that men should exercise *before* eating and women *after,* to burn the most fat. [Fuchs et al., (2011)]

The study found that men who exercised before eating burned up to 8% more fat. Women, on the other hand, burned 22% more fat if they exercised after eating a meal. It is thought that this is because men's more muscular bodies burn more carbohydrates, while women's bodies are wired to burn fat and save carbs.

The Satiety Diet suits both men and women. During the day you'll have a period of eating until you are full. Women can exercise after that, to promote faster fat loss. You'll also have short periods of fasting—one first thing in the morning on waking and another late in the afternoon. Men can use these fasting periods to exercise, promoting quicker fat loss.

PART SIX

MIND TRICKS FOR WEIGHT LOSS

1. YOUR MIND IS A POWERFUL TOOL

Your mind is incredibly powerful. It has profound effects on your body, and on your general wellbeing. In this section you'll find some methods of harnessing the power of your mind to help with weight loss.

Healthy bodies have a natural tendency to progress towards balance, called "homeostasis". For example, when you are deprived of Calories (an energy deficit), your Inner Guardian sends signals to make you hungry, so that you will consume more Calories. Theoretically, if you already have enough Calories on board in your digestive system and stored as fat (an energy surplus), homeostasis should make you stop eating. This would keep your energy in balance. You would eat more food after skipping a meal, and less food after eating an extra meal.

If the amount of food you eat depended only on homeostatic processes, then you would simply eat when you felt hungry, and you would never eat when you were full or overweight.

However, it doesn't always work that way.

This is because so many other variables are at play; variables that affect how much you eat. Cues you receive from your environment, as well as eating patterns you have learned as you grew up, can override your hunger and satiety signals.

Overeating can have genetic causes, but it can also can be influenced by your mind. In fact your mind plays a vital role in your eating habits. You may not be able to control your genetic heritage, but in many ways you can take control of your thoughts to help you lose weight.

The psychological tactics described here are easy. Practise as many of them as you can, in conjunction with the other advice in this book, and you will find they can be surprisingly powerful weight loss tools.

2. MIND TRICKS FOR WEIGHT LOSS: POSITIVE THINKING

Reframe your attitude towards your weight loss journey. "Reframing" refers to a technique of replacing negative attitudes with positive ones. It's about changing your point of view. The original situation remains the same, but when you change the way you perceive it, you can respond in a new and better way. To help yourself become slimmer, change the way you think.

The very term "weight loss" is a negative one, because "loss" is a negative concept. "Loser" is an insulting term, a negative term. Loss, in its various forms, can be hard to bear.

Human beings generally prefer to accumulate, gather, amass, and collect. If we are to survive, we must collect food and obtain shelter. After that, we are often driven to pursue the getting of wealth, and sex and happiness. Survival is all about gain, not loss, and we are hard-wired to think this way. Your Inner Guardian is prompting you to *get* energy stores, not to strip them away. It aims to *gain* and *keep*. Unfortunately, the *getting* of food-energy can easily spin out of control and cause weight gain.

We're primed more to "get" than to "discard". Most people find it harder to let go, to give things away, to scatter and disburse the things they have worked so hard to obtain. Some find it so difficult to let go that they live a cluttered lifestyle or become hoarders.

One of the reasons it can be hard to shed unwanted fat is because of this negative connotation. Subconsciously, you may be averse to "losing". If you think of your journey to a slimmer body as "weight loss" you could be making the process harder for yourself.

Flip this around to a positive mindset which can motivate you. Motivation springs from thinking of your journey to slenderness not as a way of "losing", but as "gaining". View your journey as *adding* something to your well-being instead of taking something away from you.

Visualize the shedding of excess fat as "throwing off a burden" or "gaining a stronger, more slender body".

545

Alternatively, compose your own positive phrase. Find the words that suit you best and repeat them to yourself at those times when you need motivation.

When you follow the Satiety Diet, what exactly are you *getting*?

- Nutrition, to heal and repair your body; to make it vibrant and strong.
- The lifting of that heavy burden of unwanted fat which has been dragging you down.
- The feeling of lightness and well-being that accompanies being a normal weight.
- Pleasure. A wide variety of foods provides enjoyment in the form of tastes, aromas, textures and colors etc.
- Relaxation, when you eat mindfully.
- Guiltlessness about eating.
- Comfort, fullness, satiation, and *satiety*.

* Note that in this book we still use the term "weight loss" because it is familiar to most readers.

Reassure your Inner Guardian

Reassure your Inner Guardian that you're not being deprived. Receiving signals that your body is being denied sustenance can make your Inner Guardian panic. After all, its top priotity is to make sure you're getting enough energy to survive. If it gets the message that for some reason you don't have access to plentiful food, it can start sending out those dratted weight-loss-sabotaging hunger signals to make you eat more. Some of those deprivation signals can be generated by your thoughts, beliefs and emotions.

Studies show that when people feel food-deprived, they are more likely to gain weight. [Markowitz et al., (2008)]

One way of changing your thoughts is to use positive affirmations. For example, you could repeat to yourself, "I can eat anything I like, any time I like."

This is not untrue—on the Satiety Diet you can eat anything you like, any time you like, as long as you:

- Eat anything you *really* feel like eating, not just some food you merely fancy, or that you've been triggered to want by seeing images of it on TV or elsewhere.
- Eat any time you *really* feel hungry—not just when you feel peckish or tired or thirsty or stressed or bored.
- Eat energy-dense foods mindfully and in small, balanced portions.

Use your thoughts to convince yourself that you're not being deprived, and you might also convince your Inner Guardian.

Think positively about food.

Be positive in your attitude to those nutritious, Calorie-sparse foods that won't sabotage your goals.

Remind yourself that your healthy body seeks foods that "love you". When you re-learn to listen to your body's natural signals, you'll find that your body really wants foods that nourish you and help you become leaner. Your Inner Guardian does not *really* want "unloving" foods, those Calorie-dense foods that easily turn into fat that clamps onto your stomach and hips and thighs, and drags you down and smothers your vital organs, ruining your health!

We should not label foods "good" or "bad", but concentrate your thoughts on the enormous health benefits those nutritious, Calorie-sparse foods are giving you. They are helping you become healthier and slimmer.

Your attitude to food affects how much you eat.

If your attitude to a certain food is positive, because the food is familiar or because you think the food is healthful, you are more likely to want to eat that food.

* **Familiarity:** Studies show that preschool children are more likely to eat foods that are already familiar to them. People in western cultures tend not to like certain foods of eastern cuisine that have a slimy or spongy texture, because such textures are unfamiliar. Asian people often dislike the unfamiliar sensory characteristics of cheese.

* **Attitude:** Having a negative attitude to food can make you eat less of it. Researchers who conducted a 2015 study published in *Appetite* taught volunteers to match food-words such as pizza, chips and chocolate with negative terms such as sickness, fear and pain. The volunteers' attitudes to those foods changed, becoming less positive. Those of the volunteers who were generally susceptible to the lure of junk food ate less of it after they had participated in the word-matching exercise! [Calitri et al., (2010)]

Think about the nourishment.

Other perceptions of foods can also affect food intake; for instance, if you think a food is low in Calories, you're more likely to subconsciously believe you need to eat more of it in order to feel satisfied. In one study, women were given two tubs of yoghurt, one labeled "low-fat" and the other labeled "high-fat." The subjects ate significantly more at lunch shortly after consuming the yogurt labeled "low-fat" than after consuming the yogurt labeled "high-fat." [Rolls, et al., (1992)]

How can you use this subconscious bias to your advantage? You can play mind-tricks with yourself, savoring the richness of flavor and visualizing the nutrient density of the low-Calorie foods you eat. Then, that instead of perceiving the foods as "less satisfying" you may begin to perceive them as "highly satisfying".

548

Develop a positive attitude towards all food.

While it's true that some foods are more nutritious than others, and some are lower in Calories and better for your waistline, this doesn't mean the less nutritious, more fattening food ("junk food") is "evil".

It's all just food.

The danger with thinking of some foods as "evil" is that when you eat them you might feel like a bad person, and hate yourself. Call them or "sometimes foods" instead.

If you really want those sugary, fatty foods, give yourself permission to eat small portions of them—not every day, but from time to time. And really enjoy every bite!

Thoughts affect appetite.

The way you think of food influences how attractive it is to you.

A review paper published in *The American Journal of Clinical Nutrition* examined what happens when food manufacturers develop a new product. The review's authors wrote, "New product development requires the integration of sensory attributes including product taste, texture, and appearance with consumer attitudes and health biases. Both sensory and attitudinal variables determine food preferences, product purchase and food consumption."

In other words, in order to get people to buy more of a certain product, food manufacturers do a great deal of research into two areas:

- Sensory variables—that is the taste intensity, flavor profile, texture, consistency, smell and appearance of foods.
- Attitudinal variables—that is, the way people think of different foods; the way they perceive them, the emotions they associate with them. "Sometimes it is not enough to know that a stimulus has a particular sweetness intensity: what matters more is whether it is perceived as too sweet or not sweet enough," say the researchers. "Factors other than food taste, texture or appearance can contribute significantly to the willingness to eat a given food."

Here's an example. Many people want to reduce the amount of sugar or salt in their diet, for health reasons. They would probably perceive very salty or very sweet foods as being bad for their health, which might make them view the taste as unpleasant. This is a case of people's attitudes influencing their sensory assessment. It is their beliefs and thoughts that make the food taste unpleasant, not necessarily the characteristics of the food itself.

Our thoughts have been shown to affect our sensory perceptions. In a 2008 study, when people were given a taste of a food paired with the words "rich delicious flavor", they said it tasted more pleasant than the same taste paired with the words "boiled vegetable water". Not only that, but when the food was associated with the words "rich delicious flavor", tasting that food stimulated the reward-related areas of the brain more strongly. This is convincing evidence that using words to describe food can make those foods actually seem to have a better or worse flavor. [Grabenhorst et al., (2008); Johnson & Wardle (2014)]

Some of the factors that may influence how much a food attracts you include:

- how much satiety you expect the food will provide
- how many Calories you think are in the food
- how healthful you believe the food to be
- how rich in nutrients you suppose the food to be

Any one, or any combination of these could sway your opinion of a food and make you want to eat more or less of it.

You can use this to your advantage when you want to achieve slenderness, by becoming aware of the nutritional levels of foods and the Calories they contain, as well as learning how to choose low Calorie foods with the greatest power of satiety. Here are some suggestions:

- Buy a Calorie-counter booklet
- Use a free online Calorie-counter or an app
- Read the labels on food products
- Visit reputable websites that offer free nutritional information
- Borrow a book on nutrition from your local library

3. THE POWER OF VISUALIZATION

Visualization, also known as mental imagery, is a powerful mind technique. When you imagine that you're doing something or experiencing something, the same parts of your brain are activated as when you really are doing or experiencing that thing. As proof of this there is, for example, the famous "imaginary lemon" trick. Picture a slice of freshly cut lemon, zinging with sour and tangy juices. Now imagine yourself popping that slice into your mouth and sucking it. The odds are that your mouth will fill with saliva. Your lips might even pucker. The visualization of sucking on lemon has made your salivary glands start pumping, even without the presence of an actual lemon.

Visualization has been used by sports psychologists for years to improve athletic performance on the playing field. Athletes and players picture the outcome they want, just before they perform the action needed to obtain that outcome.

Weightlifters use the technique to actually strengthen their muscles. Merely picturing the muscles working sends electrical signals to those muscles, which enables them to lift more weight.

Professional musicians often supplement actual rehearsals by performing musical passages in their minds.

Negative imagery.

And in a negative way, people sometimes use mental imagery to stop themselves from eating. They may look at, or imagine, an image of something that they find unattractive and gross, such as rotting food, or surgical procedures. Some people engage in a task that disgusts them, such as cleaning the toilet or the cat's litter box, to turn off their hunger. Or they might use disgusting smells to kill their appetite, such as the stench from a garbage can or even a strong, sickly perfume (the latter are not really image-based techniques).

We're not saying this is a good idea—we're merely reporting that it happens!

Food cravings and vivid imaginings.

When you crave a food, you tend to imagine it vividly. Studies show that it is possible to induce food cravings in people by telling them to imagine seeing, smelling or eating that food. [Green et al., (2000)]

The more vividly you picture a food, the more you crave it. (This is why seeing images of food on TV or in magazines etc. can awaken an appetite for that food.)

When people describe how they feel when they are experiencing a food craving, most of them mention that they strongly imagine seeing and eating the food. [Tiggemann & Kemps (2005)]

Imagery interruption techniques.

This is why some researchers have tried to curb people's food cravings by "interrupting" that mental imagery. The concept of Dynamic Visual Noise (DVN) has been discussed earlier in this book. The idea is that if people's mental images of food can be disrupted by "competing cognitive activities in the same sensory modality", such as watching a flickering pattern of black and white dots (DVN) the vividness of the mental food images will be reduced. People's brains can only cope with a certain amount of information, and the disruptive visual image or dots competes with the food image, making it fade or even disappear. [Kemps & Tiggemann (2014)]

This technique of using competing cognitive tasks to interrupt mental imagery and curb food cravings does work, but only for a short while. After the disruptive images cease, the cravings return.

So what's the best way to use mental imagery to curb cravings?

Visualization to curb cravings.

Strangely enough, the visualization technique that seems to work better than disruption and blocking out pictures of that craved-for food is imagining yourself eating it!

As part of his TV show *Trust Me I'm a Doctor*, Dr. Michael Mosley conducted a test to find out whether people's chocolate cravings could be curbed by the power of visualization. He and his team of researchers found out that while this technique didn't work for everyone, it did help to curb the chocolate cravings of many volunteers who participated in the test. The researchers believe that this method can also help quell cravings for other things. Indeed, it has been successful in dampening the desire for cheese!

What does the technique involve?

If you're craving a food that's Calorie-rich, imagine eating 30 pieces of that food, one at a time. As in, "I am putting the first piece of chocolate in my mouth now. I am feeling the smooth texture in my mouth, swirling it with my tongue, slowly chewing it and tasting the sweet, chocolaty flavor. Now I am swallowing the chocolate and feeling it slip down my throat. Now I am putting the second piece of chocolate in my mouth . . ." and so on, taking around 7 seconds to savor each imaginary mouthful, so that the whole process takes at least 20 minutes.

After you've eaten the imaginary food, allow yourself to eat some of the real food and you could find that you want to eat less of it. It appears that imagining yourself eating the food you crave tricks your Inner Guardian into believing you've already eaten some, and this helps to significantly reduce your cravings.

These results have been supported in at least one other study. [Morewedge et al., (2010)]

Two kinds of visualization.

Scientists recognize two kinds of visualization:
- Internal imagery. Also known as first-person imagery, this is a technique that involves imagining how the physical sensation of performing some action actually feels. You imagine the sensations within your body.
- External imagery. Also known as third-person imagery, this involves picturing yourself performing the action as if you were watching yourself on stage. You're imagining yourself as being outside your body.

For the purposes of weight loss, the most effective kind is internal imagery. It can produce real chemical and electrical responses in the body, even changing your heart rate and blood pressure.

Use visualization to extend satiety.

Staring to feel peckish? Recalling your last meal can curb your appetite. Visualize the last meal you ate. Picture it as you saw it on the plate—all the colors and shapes of the food, accompanied by the delicious aroma. Remember how it tasted, looked smelled. Remember how replete you felt after you had eaten it. Think: "That food is inside me right now, nourishing my body."

Studies show that this kind of imagery can help keep you going till the next meal. It's like food for the mind. [Higgs et al., (2008)]

"Memory plays an important role in appetite control," concluded scientists from the University of Birmingham. The researchers conducted a study in which three groups of volunteers ate the same food, in the same quantities, for lunch.

- The "food focus" group were asked to eat their lunch mindfully, concentrating on the sensory characteristics of the food.
- The "food thoughts control" group ate lunch while reading a newspaper article about food.
- A third group—the "neutral control group"—simply ate lunch.

Later that same day the volunteers were asked how hungry they felt, and how well they remembered their lunch. Those in the mindful-eating group rated their appetite as lower than the others. They also recalled their experience of eating lunch more vividly.

All volunteers were then given access to snacks—namely, cookies. The researchers measured how many cookies the volunteers ate.

The people in the mindful-eating "food focus" group consumed significantly fewer cookies than those in the other two groups!

"These results suggest," wrote the researchers, "that enhancing meal memory by paying attention to food while eating can reduce later intake..." [Higgs & Donohoe (2011)]

Other studies support this conclusion. [Higgs (2002); Higgs (2005)]

Use visualization to help weight loss.

Dr. Michael Kaplan, Founder and Chief Medical Officer of The Center for Medical Weight Loss (USA) advocates the power of the subconscious mind. He recommends visualizing yourself at your goal weight, for a few minutes every day. You could do this with External Imagery—for example by picturing yourself in your new, smaller-sized clothes looking good and effortlessly jogging—or you could use Internal Imagery—imagining what it would feel like to be lighter and more energetic, more confident. He adds that it is preferable to place your visualizations in the present time, not as something that is going to happen in the future.

4. MIND TRICKS TO MAKE YOU WANT LESS JUNK FOOD

It might be possible for you to use your conscious thoughts to train yourself to make better unconscious responses to food. An example of unconscious responses to food happens when you are trying to lose weight but you are offered some Calorie-dense food. You know that food will be rewarding *while you are eating it*, because it tastes good. However it's the opposite of rewarding *after you've eaten it* and can no longer taste it, and its Calories, now turned to fat, are sitting on your hips!

Consciously, you understand that the food will sabotage your weight-loss efforts, but an unconscious desire seems to take control of you, driving you to pick the short-term reward of flavor, mouthfeel and other sensory delights over the long-term reward of a slim figure.

Visualize the happiest possible future event.

A 2013 study published in *Psychological Science* suggests that you can train yourself to have better unconscious responses. It's a technique called "episodic future thinking". Researchers asked overweight adults to vividly imagine a pleasurable event taking place in the future, such as a celebration, or falling in love, while simultaneously considering whether to accept $10 in cash on the spot right now or $100 at some time in the future.

Overweight people in a control group were not asked to imagine this.

When volunteers imagined their wonderful future, they were more likely than the control group to choose the delayed reward of $100 to be paid to them later.

Some time afterward, all the volunteers were invited to enjoy a smorgasbord for 15 minutes while they listened to a recording of their own voice describing their personal happy future. Amazingly, episodic-future-thinking volunteers consumed almost 20% fewer Calories than did volunteers in the control group!

Psychologist Bärbel Knäuper surmises that this technique might work because it makes a distant, abstract future reward seem more concrete (solid and real), and closer in time.

This would suggest that if you're the kind of person who usually chooses short term rewards over long-term ones, vividly visualize the happiest future possible and see whether this helps you stick to your weight loss plan. [Daniel et al., (2013)]

5. MIND TRICKS USING VISUAL CUES

5.1 Plate size, portion size, bite size.

We want more. It's a natural human tendency to want to eat larger amounts of food. This is part of your Inner Guardian's strategy to give you lots of energy and nutrition.

Bite size: chop it up.

People tend to take larger bites when they are served with large pieces of food. When you take larger bites of food you tend to consume more food in less time, which can lead to overeating. The mind trick solution?

Cut your food into multiple smaller pieces and spread it out over your plate. A researcher at Arizona State University found that when people ate food that had been chopped into multiple smaller portions, they achieved better satiety than when they ate the same amount of food as one large piece.

A similar satiety-effect was observed when portions of food were served scattered over a wide area on the plate, instead of being clustered into a pile.

Not only did people who ate food cut into pieces and spread over the plate's surface achieve better satiety than those who ate one large piece of food or multiple portions piled in one spot; they also consumed fewer Calories at their subsequent meal!

Most people instinctively prefer to eat more food rather than less. Cutting food up into pieces can make it appear as if there's more of it. The researchers wrote: " . . . multiple pieces of food may appear like more food because they take up a larger surface area than a single-piece portion. . . . these studies show that number and surface area occupied by food pieces are important visual cues determining … both food choice and intake in humans."

In other words, by cutting up your food and spreading it out on the plate you're likely to get more satiation and eat fewer Calories. What a handy mind-trick! [Bajaj (2013); English et al., 2014)]

A 1972 study found that when people are offered four sandwiches cut into quarters (i.e. 16 pieces) they tend to eat more food than when they are offered four identical sandwiches cut into eighths (i.e. 32 pieces). [Nisbett & Storms (1972)]

And a 2011 study found that when people were offered 10 big pieces of candy they ate more than when they were offered the same candy sliced into 20 pieces. [Marchiori et al., (2011)]

Several other studies also support the premise that when food is served to you in a larger number of small pieces you are likely to eat less of it than when you're served fewer, larger pieces. So cut up your food into smaller, more numerous portions! Give yourself four small sandwiches instead of one large one, or two thin slices of cake instead of one wide one, for example.

Portion size: serve less.

People of all ages tend to be more attracted to large food portions than small ones, and if they are served with large portions they will eat more. [Burger et al., (2011a); Ello-Martin et al., (2005); Rolls (2003)].

It's not only in laboratory studies that this happens, but also in real life. When you are given larger portions of food, you eat more. The mind trick solution? Have smaller portions!

But it's not as simple as that—there's more.

Plate size: use smaller tableware.

Seeing a tiny amount of food sitting in the middle of your plate with a large expanse of empty space around it can make you feel deprived. Psychologically, it's not very satisfying to perceive your meal as being tiny. You're likely to want to compensate for such a tiny meal by snacking later on.

The mind trick solution? Use smaller tableware. Arrange your food on smaller plates and spread it out.

Using smaller plates and bowls creates the illusion of having bigger portions. Even when you are fully aware that there is less food served up to you, the fact that it's on a smaller plate can actually lull your Inner Guardian into a sense that you're surrounded by abundance and getting plenty of food, so there's no need to send out more hunger signals.

"When food is served on plates, people tend to focus on the diameter of the plate to determine food amounts." [Bajaj (2013)]

Study after study shows that our minds are easily tricked by the relationship between plate size and how much the food is spread out on the plate. When food is spread out, it looks like a larger serving. The closer food is spread to the edges of the plate or bowl, the bigger the serving appears to be. (This is called "the Delbouef illusion".) Because of this visual illusion, people are more likely to serve themselves smaller portions of food when they have to use small bowls and plates.

Serving food on smaller plates help you stop eating. If you use smaller plates you're more likely to eat less food but feel just as full.

"… the food portion served on a plate may serve as a visual benchmark or guide to determine the appropriate amount of food to consume." [Bajaj(2013)]

Without thinking about it, most people tend to keep eating until their plates are empty, or almost empty. The amount of food served up in front of you at mealtimes can determine the amount you eat. As mentioned earlier in this book, this was demonstrated spectacularly in an experiment where people were given "bottomless" bowls of soup. The bowls were secretly self-refilling, at a rate so slow as to be undetectable. No matter how much soup the volunteers ate, there was always a bit more left in their bowls.

The study's authors wrote, "Participants who were unknowingly eating from self-refilling bowls ate more soup than those eating from normal soup bowls. However, despite consuming 73% more, they did not believe they had consumed more, nor did they perceive themselves as more sated than those eating from normal bowls. This was unaffected by BMI the (Body Mass Index of the diners)." [Wansink et al., (2005)]

This supports the idea that when there is more food on a plate or bowl, people eat more. Seeing food on your plate makes you feel you should eat it—even if you are not hungry and even if you have already eaten a lot. This leads to unintentional overeating.

"It seems that people use their eyes to count Calories and not their stomachs," wrote the researchers.

The other bonus that comes from eating smaller portions is that your stomach adapts to not being over-stretched. This means that your body becomes more sensitive to satiety signals when you're eating a meal. When you feel satiated earlier, you tend to eat less.

5.2 Visual mind tricks: Eat off a plate!

Speaking of tableware, when you eat off a plate you're likely to feel satisfied with eating less. When your food is spread out on a plate you can see it all. On the other hand, when you eat from a takeaway food box or bag, or from a disposable plastic package or container off the supermarket shelf, it's harder to judge how much you've eaten. It can look (to your Inner Guardian)as if you've eaten less. If you had spread out that same amount of food on a plate, it would have looked like more.

5.3 Visual mind tricks: Plate color.

Choose plates whose color contrasts highly with the color of your food. Scientists have found that when the color of your plate has a high contrast with the color of the food on that plate, you're likely to feel satisfied with eating less!

For example, you'd probably be satisfied with eating fewer blueberries off a white plate than off a dark blue plate. And you'd be more likely to eat less white rice off a dark blue plate than off a white plate.

5.4 Visual mind tricks: The size of cups and glasses.

The size of drinkware can influence how much liquid you consume.
- Drink from smaller cups, and you're likely to drink less.
- Use small, short, squat glasses when your drink is Calorie-dense (e.g. milkshakes, creamy cocktails).
- Use tall, narrow glasses or large glasses when you're drinking Calorie-free or low-Calorie liquids such as sparkling water or green tea.

5.5 Visual mind tricks: Use smaller eating utensils.

Silverware, flatware, tableware, cutlery—call it what you will. These terms refer to our eating utensils such as knives, forks and spoons. Most researchers report that using smaller eating utensils makes people eat less food.

5.6 Visual mind tricks: Low light and soft music.

Dine by candlelight—or with the lights turned down low. In a 1970 thesis published by Columbia University L. D. Ross, reported that people ate less food when dining in dimly lit surroundings than when eating under bright lights. [Ross (1970)]

Soft background music has also been shown to decrease the amount of food people eat. [Spence et al., (2012); Linne et al., 2002); Wansink (2004)]

5.7 Visual mind tricks: Leave inedible leftovers on view.

When you're chowing down, being able to get an idea of how much food you've already eaten can affect how much you consume.

A 2011 study found that when people were eating pistachio nuts from the shells, they ate fewer nuts when the empty shells were allowed to remain and pile up in front of them. [Kennedy-Hagan et al., (2011)].

Seeing the empty shells acted as a reminder to them of how many nuts they had eaten. When the shells were routinely taken away, they ate more!

The same thing happened in 2007, when people were given a meal of chicken wings. They ate less when the bare bones remained in sight on the table than when the bones were removed. [Wansink & Payne (2007)]

5.8 Visual mind tricks: Move away from food.

When it's not time for a meal, or when you've just finished a meal, remove yourself from the proximity and sight of food.

When people are physically close to food and can easily see the food, they are likely to eat more than when they are further away and the food is hidden from view.

If there's a bowl of free candy in the office, place yourself as far away from it as you can. Make sure you can't see it as you go about your work! Don't leave food out on your kitchen counter—even bowls of fruit. Yes fresh fruit is good for you, but over-consumption can pile on the pounds. If you're at a restaurant with a buffet, take the table furthest from the food on display and sit with your back to it.

Serve your meals from the stove instead of from the table. You'll eat less if your meal is served onto a (small) plate from the cooking pots, rather than poured into serving dishes and placed on the table for everyone to take as much as they like.

This has been supported in numerous studies. [Vanata et al., (2011); Meyers & Stunkard (1980); Engell et al., (1996); Meiselman et al., (1994); Musher-Eizenman et al., (2009); Wansink et al., (2006)]

5.9 Visual mind tricks: Make healthful foods look as good as possible.

When food looks good, people tend to think it tastes good, too. Studies into food labels and packaging have confirmed this—which is why food manufacturers spend millions of dollars making sure their labeling and packaging appeals to the consumer.

In an unpublished study [Kramer et al., (1989)], researchers gave volunteers the same puddings in three different styles of packaging:
- commercial packaging, with bright colors and attractive pictures
- military packaging, colored brown, black or khaki, generally with only words, not pictures, and a stark, functional design
- neutral, or generic packaging, with a limited range of colors and a few pictures

The volunteers were not told that all the puddings were the same. They reported that the puddings in the military packaging did not taste as good as those in the other types of packaging. They ate less of the food in the military packaging.

"These studies," wrote the researchers, "demonstrate that perceptions of foods can affect food intake." [Marriott 1995)]

When you prepare your meals, make a little extra effort to present them attractively. Add a sprig of parsley to garnish a savory meal, for example, or drizzle a glossy sauce in a spiral pattern around the edges of the plate, as many chefs do.

6. MORE BRILLIANT MIND TRICKS FOR WEIGHT LOSS

6.1 Avoid word triggers.

Words are powerful. For example, even reading the words "hunger" or "hungry" can make you feel hungry. Simply reading or hearing the word "chocolate' can trigger chocaholics' cravings.

6.2 Identify over-eating triggers.

1. Identify whether you "comfort-eat" (e.g. to relieve stress, to overcome anxiety etc) and work out non-food ways to comfort yourself and regulate your emotions. You could join a support group, or pamper yourself in an inexpensive way (take a bubble bath, for example), or make sure you look your best each day, or remind yourself of how far you've come, not how far you've got to go.

2. Identify which foods may trigger binges, and don't even take the first bite. Some people, for example, find that single mouthful of candy, or cake, or ice-cream, can trigger an overeating binge.

6.3 Choose your unit of measurement.

Some people say that weighing themselves in pounds instead of kilograms helps them lose weight. This is because it's easier to lose a pound of fat than a kilo of fat, and therefore they feel as if they are achieving more, which gives them incentive to continue.

6.4 Adjust your expectations.

Train yourself to expect to lose a small amount of weight each week. (Some people choose to tell themselves they expect no weight loss at all, and simply hope that they didn't gain weight that week.)

Keeping your expectations modest can have many advantages. If you expect to lose a huge amount of weight each week, you're likely to feel dispirited if it does not happen.

563

Tell yourself you might only lose a small amount each week, and when you weigh yourself on the seventh day you will:

- Avoid feeling disappointed and discouraged if you've only lost a few ounces/grams, or
- Enjoy a pleasant, motivating surprise if you've lost more weight than you expected.

6.5 Don't try to stave off real hunger.

It's almost impossible to defeat your Inner Guardian. When it sends out genuine hunger signals, you'd better do something about it. Some people, knowing that they are going to have a big night out at a party or restaurant, deliberately eat very little during the day. They try to "save up" their daily ration of Calories so that they can overindulge later on, without feeling guilty.

This is not a good move, as it can lead to weight gain.

If you are ravenously hungry when you arrive at the eatery, your Inner Guardian will have already turned up your hunger signals to full volume. In this state, you are likely to choose higher-Calorie foods, and to eat a greater quantity than you'd have eaten if you arrived feeling less hungry. Staving off hunger can lead to overeating.

Instead, have a small, healthful high-satiety snack before you go out to a function.

6.6 Love your shape.

Celebrities and models pictures in glossy magazines and on TV generally flaunt bodies that are considered to be the current ideal of beauty. They may have achieved these body-shapes, or the appearance of these shapes, by :

- genetic inheritance
- constant exercise
- rigorous dieting
- cosmetic surgery
- body makeup
- photographic manipulation

Many people compare themselves to these ideals and feel miserable when, no matter how much they diet and exercise, they cannot emulate them. Some people simply cease trying and abandon themselves to weight gain.

Stop reading those magazines!

Instead, get online or go to a library or an art gallery and look at some paintings of women from the 15th and 16th centuries (before the era of corsets!). Examples include Titian's Venus of Urbino or Botticelli's Birth of Venus. Painters chose models they considered beautiful, and they painted what they saw. The ideal of beauty then was much closer to the natural shape of a healthy woman.

The same goes for men. Instead of comparing your body to the covers of men's fitness magazines, go and watch some footage of old Batman, Superman, James Bond or Tarzan movies from the 'sixties. Note the complete lack of sculpted muscles; the dearth of six-packs and bulging biceps; the body hair... in some cases these superheroes even had small paunches. These were healthy men in their natural state!

6.7 Keep moving, keep busy.

The busier you are exercising, working or having fun with hobbies or friends, the less time you're likely to spend eating, or thinking about eating. Your mind will be occupied with non-food thoughts.

6.8 Weigh yourself every day.

Scientists used to assume that weighing yourself every day was counter-productive for weight loss. That way of thinking has now changed, due to some interesting studies.

Tracking your weight by weighing yourself every day is considered a useful tool for losing weight and—most importantly— keeping it off. [Steinberg et al., (2015); Steinberg et al., (2013); Pacanowski et al., (2014)]

6.9 Mind tricks to help you deal with hunger.

Mind tricks to help you love peckishness and mild hunger.

When you feel somewhat hungry, say to yourself, "I love this feeling. It reassures me, because I know I'm likely to see a lower number on the scales."

Mind tricks to distract yourself from peckishness.

Peckishness can be a prelude to real, physical hunger or it can be reaction to boredom or some other trigger. Either way, peckishness is not hunger, and if you can wait until you are really hungry before you eat, you're more likely to lose weight. So to distract yourself from peckishness, find something immersive and interesting to do for around 20-30 minutes. Remove yourself physically from food triggers such as vending machines, cafes and the kitchens. Your peckishness might fade during that time.

Mind tricks to help you beat cravings.

When you experience a craving to cram your mouth with some Calorie-dense food, repeat to yourself, "If I gorge on this I will feel sad. And I don't want to feel sad."

Or, "If I eat that fattening comfort food to distract me from my problem, I will have two problems instead of one."

Mind tricks to help you dampen hunger.

We've already mentioned using vizualization, but here's a recap. When you start to feel hungry, stop and picture the last meal you ate. Visualize it as if it's in front of your eyes. Remember that all that food is now inside you, nourishing you.. Remember how it tastes, how it felt in your mouth, how it smelled. Recall how replete you felt after you'd eaten it. In this way you can remind your Inner Guardian that you have received energy and nutrition recently and therefore it does not need to send our hunger signals just yet.

6.10 Treat all meals like a special occasion.

Many of us gulp down our food in as short a time as possible so that we can get on with other tasks. Surveys show that as many as 70% of American office-workers eat lunch at their desk.

In countries where obesity is less of a problem, meals are eaten in a dedicated eating space, with no other distractions. Plenty of time is allotted for the eating and full enjoyment of meals.

Japanese schoolchildren, for example, are encouraged to enjoy eating as an essential and pleasurable daily activity, rather than as an intrusive nuisance impinging on more important tasks. From a very early age they are taught, in school, how to choose healthful foods, serve meals, and eat mindfully. Some schools have vegetable patches tended and harvested by the students. Before meals in many Japanese schools, the children welcome the food with a song.

When you respect your meals, giving yourself enough time and mindfulness to appreciate them, treating them as daily events to look forward to, you are letting your Inner Guardian know that you are receiving proper, regular nourishment and there is no need for it to panic and send out hunger signals!

6.11 Recognize procrastinatory eating.

Do you find yourself reaching for a snack instead of knuckling down to a task you don't particularly relish? Perhaps there's a difficult email you have to write, or a chore you've been putting off. Suddenly the idea of having a snack pops into your mind. Some inner voice is telling you that if you go and have a snack you can put off the task for a bit longer. It feels like peckishness, but it's really procrastination.

Be aware of this little trick your mind can play on you.

Instead of either giving in or denying yourself, tell yourself that you will have a small portion of your desired food and/or beverage at a specified time of the day. Then when that time rolls around, if you still want the snack, go ahead and have it. It's possible that you might have lost the desire for the snack by then.

6.12 Use the "If-Then" technique to change habits.

The "If-Then" technique was developed by Peter Gollwitzer of New York University. It's a way of training yourself to have new and better habits. With regard to weight loss, it teaches you to associate food cues (such as being tempted by junk food) with an alternative, more healthful reaction that is also rewarding. It's based on the proven fact that people are two to three times more likely to succeed in achieving their goals if they use an "if-then" plan than if they don't.

Having a pre-planned alternative to eating junk food is a lot easier than simply resisting the temptation to eat it. It's a positive action instead of a negative one. It's like saying "Yes, I will do something else instead of eating that," rather than, "No, I won't eat that."

This is how it works. You say to yourself, "If X happens, then I will do Y."

X can be:
- an event, like being offered a slice of cheesecake at a party
- a time, for example 3:30 pm when your blood sugars are low and you crave sweet food
- a place, such as the supermarket
- a time and place, such as morning tea time at work

Y is the thing you will do whenever X happens.

Using the "If-Then" technique helps you to narrow down general goals (such as "lose weight", or "don't eat junk food") to make them more specific and do-able. Instead of these general goals, you could say, for example:

X: Someone offers me dessert at a party. Y: I will politely decline and have salad or coffee instead.

X: It's 3:30 pm and I am craving for sweet food. Y: I will slowly and mindfully eat my pre-prepared creamy Satiety Diet snack sweetened with rice malt syrup or stevia/erythritol.

X: I am about to go to the supermarket, where I will see shelves laden with tempting Calorie-dense, highly processed foods. Y: I will have a drink of water/tea and a healthful, satiating snack, so that I don't feel hungry when I go grocery-shopping.

X: It's morning-tea time at work and everyone else is having cake and cookies. Y: I will remove myself from the sight of that food and mindfully enjoy the Satiety Diet snack I brought with me. Or, without paying attention to all that food I will eat no more than two cookies, and I will eat them slowly and mindfully.

When you have these contingency plans in place already, you don't need as much willpower to resist temptation when it comes along. And the more you use this technique the easier it becomes, as your mind naturally becomes more aware of the X-cues and responding with Y-behavior becomes second nature.

[Gollwitzer (1999); Gollwitzer & Oettingen (2011); Gollwitzer & Sheeran (2006); Oettingen (2012); Oettingen & Gollwitzer (2010)]

6.13 Eat alone, or in the company of strangers.

Studies show that we're likely to eat more when we dine in the company of family and friends. This might be because we eat less mindfully when we are distracted by conversation. [de Castro (1990); de Castro (1994); Herman et al., (2003)]

But what if you have to eat with other people?

Aim to choose dining companions who are health-conscious.

Studies have shown that people eat less food when they eat alone. However it's good for your health to be in happy groups; we all need positive social interactions to help boost our mood. Besides, when you dine in pleasant social groups you're more likely to take longer over a meal and not bolt your food. So what's the solution?

People tend to eat the same type and amount of food as their dining companions, so if the friends and family who share your dinner table eat a lot of Calorie-dense foods, or eat very quickly, you're likely to do the same.

569

This tendency to "mirror" your dining companions can work to your advantage, however. If you eat a meal with health-conscious people who want to lose weight, who choose Calorie-sparse foods and eat them at a leisurely pace, you too are more likely to eat in a way that helps your weight loss.

6.14 Don't eat too late in the day.

We're all likely to consume more food when we eat later in the day, closer to bedtime [de Castro (2004)].

Read more in our section "The Timing of Eating."

6.15 Eat pungent, aromatic, scented food.

The more strongly you can smell your food, the more satisfied it can make you feel, even with small bites. Researchers found that people took smaller bites of desserts with added odors than of desserts with little or no odor. Smell is a huge sensory component of flavor. Intense sensory experiences of food can help you eat more mindfully. It sends the message to your Inner Guardian that you really have consumed food, and now it's okay not to feel hungry. So perfume your desserts with fragrant rose water or orange blossom water or sweet spices, and throw pungent garlic into your savory dishes. [de Wijk et al., (2012)]

6.16 Hypnosis may help you lose weight.

The reasons behind gaining too much weight are many and varied, which is why we need many tools in our "Weight Loss Toolkit". Hypnosis is one such tool. It has been shown to help some people, although it does not work for everyone.

Virtual lap-banding.
One form of weight loss hypnosis is called "virtual lap-banding".
Actual lap-banding is a procedure in which surgeons wrap an adjustable silicone belt around the upper portion of the stomach. The belt can be tightened by filling it with saline solution. This brings about weight loss by reducing the stomach's capacity. People simply

cannot fit as much food into their stomachs and theoretically this means they will consume fewer Calories. In practice, this does not always work, as some people compensate by eating foods that are more Calorie-dense.

With virtual lap-banding, patients are hypnotized into believing they have had a lap-band surgically inserted.

The Transtheoretical Model.

Other forms of hypnosis used for weight loss include the "Transtheoretical Model", which involves changing people's habits. This can be used for such purposes as to help people eat less chocolate, or exercise more often. It involves re-programming the subconscious; for example, making people associate exercise with feeling great instead of associating it with hard work.

Visualization.

Another method used by hypnotists is visualization. The hypnotist asks hypnotized clients to imagine themselves with a slim, toned body. The hypnotist might even place clients in front of a mirror to help with the visualization.

How does hypnosis work best for weight loss?

A 2014 review published in the International Journal of Clinical and Experimental Hypnosis [Entwistle et al., (2014)] found that hypnosis works best—

- on people who are more open to hypnotic suggestion
- when it's undertaken over a period of time, not just in a single, one-off session
- when it's used in conjunction with other weight-loss aids such as exercise and good nutrition

7. TIPS TO COMBAT EMOTIONAL/COMFORT EATING.

We've discussed "comfort eating" earlier in this book, but it's worth mentioning it again because it is such a powerful driver of overeating and obesity.

People often eat when they're not physically hungry. Tune in to your body's signals and you'll be more able to diagnose whether your desire for food is driven by physical need or by some other motivator. That other motivator could be anything from thirst, boredom, habit, or tiredness, to a need for comfort.

Eating, (particularly eating certain things such as sweet or crunchy foods), is a method many people use to divert or deflect psychological and emotional needs that are not being met. Change the way you view food. Instead of it being something you turn to for comfort, think of it as your body's fuel.

Food-free comfort.

If it's comfort you're seeking, find sources other than food. Soothe and pamper yourself in a way that doesn't involve weight gain. Be kind to yourself in other ways—ways that make you feel better without putting extra Calories into your body. The first step is to give yourself permission to take time to care for yourself. The second step is to choose a no-Calorie feel-good, low-cost technique that suits you, for example:

- Take off your shoes. Wear comfortable slippers or go barefoot.
- Wear soft, comfortable clothes.
- Have a bath, complete with the trimmings such as scented bath oils and bubbles.
- Sip some hot tea or iced tea or sparkling water flavored with lemon mint or orange.
- Listen to your favorite music. Sing along, if you like!
- Take a walk in the park.
- Phone an understanding friend and have a chat about what's on your mind.

The book *The Satiety Diet Weight Loss Toolkit*, #2 in the Satiety Diet series, has a section that includes strategies to reduce stress.

8. MIND TRICKS FOR WEIGHT LOSS: MEDITATION

Meditation is an excellent weight loss tool.

Meditation is free, it's easy and you can do it almost anywhere. It's also very powerful—it can even generate an increase in the amount of "gray matter" in your brain! [Lazar at al., 2005)]

Meditation can be profoundly relaxing and energizing. It has been proven to lower stress levels. Lowering stress levels also decreases cortisol levels, which can help dampen appetite.

A 2014 review of fourteen studies investigating the effect of mindfulness meditation concluded that ". . . mindfulness meditation effectively decreases binge eating and emotional eating in populations engaging in this behavior . . ." [Katterman et al., (2014)]

So, how do you meditate?

There are in-depth meditation courses available in the real world and online, including guided audio meditations, books and videos. Here's a broad outline of how it's done. You don't have to set aside hours every day to meditate. Even fifteen minutes a day, or ten, or five, or even two minutes daily can make a difference! The more you meditate, the easier it becomes.

- Find a quiet place with few sensory distractions.
- Sit or lie down comfortably on the floor or in a chair.
- Relax your muscles.
- Close your eyes or unfocus your gaze.
- Pay attention to your natural breathing without trying to direct it.
- Acknowledge your feelings and thoughts, and then let them go.
- Allow yourself to release any tensions in your body.
- Focus on feeling calm, and breathing slowly and regularly.
- Allow your thoughts to come and go without holding on to any of them.
- Some people like to focus on peaceful imagery to help them meditate.

9. LEARN TO LOVE MORE FOODS

Foods taste different to different people.

Science has revealed that there are some food characteristics that all human beings love or loathe.

- We are all born with an innate liking for sweetness in foods
- We are all born with an innate *dis*like of bitterness in foods

Beyond this, there is a huge variation in people's opinion of what foods taste delicious and what foods taste disgusting! There are many reasons why the same food tastes different to different people. They include our genes, our experience/upbringing, our culture, and our gender.

Fortunately we can change many of our food preferences. Almost all food-dislikes can be turned into food-likes if you go about it the right way. Even your inborn preferences can be shaped by environmental factors as you grow up. For example, tiny babies instinctively spit out bitter-tasting foods, yet by the time they are adults many of them enjoy the bitter flavors of coffee, dark chocolate and bitter greens.

Why we should learn to like more foods.

To lose weight on the Satiety Diet, we recommend that you eat a wide variety of foods. But what if you just don't like the taste or texture of some foods?

Aside from giving you more opportunities to savor more fresh, natural flavors and textures, being able to consume a wide range of foods can make life more enjoyable. It can also make it easier for you to:

- consume a wider range of nutrients
- join in and eat what other people are eating at social occasions
- experience the cuisine of other cultures
- find something convenient to eat

574

How many of the recipes you cook/eat contain the same ingredients prepared in different ways? Many people eat the same "trusted" ingredients day in and day out. In First World countries these are likely to include foods such as carrots, potatoes, pumpkin/squash, salad leaves, muscle meats, eggs, cheese, tomatoes, eggplants, bell peppers, green beans, wheat flour, apples, pears, bananas etc. These are all good foods, but there are thousands of other edible plants, fruits and vegetables available on Planet Earth.

What about the pomegranates, the teff and einkorn and amaranth, the lupins, the jaboticaba and dragon fruit? The goji berries and tigernuts, the oca and kohlrabi? The seaweed, salsify and celeriac? The samphire, nopales and manioc?

Many people walk past the unusual fresh food section of their supermarket, thinking, "Those weird foods are nothing to do with me".

But they are.

Those 'weird' foods contain a wealth of micronutrients your body might be needing.

"But," I hear you say, "I don't like those foods."

You might also be surprised how easy it is to learn to really love the deliciousness of a huge variety of foods. Many people think they don't like a food simply because they are unfamiliar with it, or because the texture surprised them when they first tried it, or because as a child they had an unpleasant experience with it.

By following our tips on learning to like different foods, you'll be opening the door to a vast range of amazing flavors and culinary delights you never dreamed were out there waiting for you.

We're going to look at the reasons why some people don't like certain foods. Then we are going to give you a "tool kit" of ways to learn to enjoy a lot more foods than you do already. And the reward? A whole new world of flavors and textures will open up to you!

How to learn to like more foods.

Think back to when you were a child. The odds are that you like eating a lot more foods now, than you did back then. Our tastes tend to change during our teenage years. And when we become adults, we often teach ourselves to like certain flavors and textures, for one reason or another.

Very few of your food partialities are determined by your genes. Most have been learned—developed throughout your life, beginning before you were born. It's pretty difficult to change food preferences that are encoded in your DNA, but you CAN change food preferences that you have learned.

By knowing what elements determine your food preferences, you can deliberately increase the range of foods you enjoy.

All you need is a sense of adventure, a desire to enjoy novel experiences, persistence, and a list of psychological tools.

Tool #1: Become familiar with the food you want to like.

In the words of Joseph Bennington-Castro, a freelance science journalist, "We don't just eat foods because we like them, we like them because we eat them."

People have a natural distaste for foods that are unanticipated. For example if you've never eaten okra before, you might think, by the look of it, that it ought to have a texture similar to zucchini. You'd be startled when you realize how mucilaginous cooked okra is, with a texture that's quite unusual in a vegetable.

Psychologists report that when people encounter something new and strange in a food, they often identify their discomfort at the unexpected oddness as dislike of that food.

When you taste a food repeatedly, it's very likely that you'll gradually come to like that food better than you did to begin with. A study of schoolchildren showed that when they were offered certain vegetables once a week for 10 weeks, their liking for almost all of those vegetables increased significantly. [Lakkakula et al., (2010)]

Children are born with very few taste preferences. For the first two years of life most children are happy to eat almost any foods, whether they are familiar with them or not. Around the age of two they start to refuse foods they have not tasted before. That is why it's important to let children try a lot of different foods before the age of two.

It's important, too, to show them that their carers/parents enjoy eating a wide range of foods. Children tend to follow the examples of the adults who raise them. [Harper & Sanders (1975)]

If your child refuses to eat a new food, simply continue to briefly offer them that food once or twice a week, without forcing them to eat it. Chances are that they will become so familiar with the new food that they will venture to taste it. If they keep tasting it, it's likely they will enjoy it more and more.

The same may apply to adults.

> Chris Clark says: "Raw fish? Seaweed salad? The leaves of some weird Vietnamese plant called laksa leaf? [*Persicaria odorata*] I was brought up in a middle class family, surrounded by Western culture. As a child, I had very little exposure to Asian foods. The first time I tried those three foods aforementioned, I hated them. In particular I loathed the flavor of laksa leaf. But everyone else seemed to be eating these foods, and I kept seeing them for sale in shops, and I knew they were full of nutrition. So, without deliberately trying to make myself like them, I just kept nibbling at them from time to time. Lo and behold, all three of them are now among my favorite foods. (I'm still working on celeriac.)"

In studies involving children, the participants are often given a small reward for tasting the new food—a reward such as a sticker. As an adult teaching yourself to like a new food, your reward could be simply knowing that you're a step closer to enjoying a food that's good for you.

How many test-tastes does it take before you start to like a new food? A 2004 study suggests 10 to 14 (tasting it daily for up to 14 days). [Wardle et al., (2003)]

That said, forcing yourself to eat the new food against your own will could be counter-productive. Keep in mind the positive characteristics of the food and the reasons why you want to learn to like it.

Tool #2: Learn to like a food by association.

If you are really repelled by a food, then even nibbling a tiny scrap of it may be too hard. It may even make you gag. Clearly you're not going to be able to taste-test such a food repeatedly. But there is a way around this setback. It's called "associative learning".

This term refers to what happens over time when you associate the disliked food with a food you really like.

Association with another taste.

Sweetness, for example, lures us into liking flavors associated with that sweetness. Some parents have been known to get their children to like cruciferous vegetables, such as Brussels sprouts, by adding sugar to the vegetables. The children liked the sweetened vegetables. Then gradually, meal by meal, the parents lowered the amount of added sugar until there was no sugar added at all. The result was that the children ended up liking the vegetables, even without sugar.

When you want to lose weight, adding sugar to your food is not a good idea!

Associative learning by food combination.

Chris Clark says, "I hated licorice as a child, and the herb "dill" has a licorice/aniseed flavor so in adulthood I decided I didn't like anything aniseed-flavored, including dill. A local bakery started selling fish pies with the most delectable pastry and luscious fillings of fish pieces, leeks and dill in a creamy sauce. So tasty were these pies that I took the plunge and tried them. And kept trying them. And began to associate the dill flavor with all the other deliciousness. Now I enjoy the flavor of dill so much that I cook with it in my home kitchen."

People who once hated tomatoes may learn to love them after eating them on pizza or in a tomatoey risotto. Other, who may despise peas, can mix them with something they love, such as toasted almonds and rice. You don't like corn but love mashed potatoes? Try combining them.

In order to learn to eventually like the flavor of a disliked food, you can mix it with any food that you do like, with two provisos:

- Obviously you wouldn't mix two foods that really don't go together, such as onions and ice cream!
- You must be able to detect the flavor of the dislike food. Don't smother it completely and block it out.

Association with a thought or mental image of a texture.

This method works well with foods whose texture you don't like.

When we think of textures, we frequently link them with other textures that seem to be in the same category—for example,

- The texture of the aptly-named sponge cake may remind you of clouds and other light, fluffy and airy things.
- The mouthfeel of creamy foods might remind you of silk or velvet.
- The gelatinousness of cooked or soaked chia seeds might evoke images of snot or mucus.
- Some people say that mushrooms and offal have a "slug-like" or "rubbery" texture.

The last-mentioned comparisons are, of course unappetizing, but once your mind has associated certain foods with repulsive images, it's hard to shake them off. The sense of "disgustingness" masters and subdues any enjoyable characteristics the food has.

579

You can turn this mind-trick of association to your advantage. When you want to learn to like a food, think of another food you enjoy, that has the same texture as the disliked food.

One of the comfort foods many mothers used to cook for their families during the period after the Second World War was sago pudding or tapioca pudding. Sago dessert is also a traditional dish in South East Asian cuisine, and it's delicious. If you like sweet sago/tapioca puddings, then thinking of them could help you learn to like other gelatinous foods, such as soaked chia seeds.

Associative learning by verbal links.

Even the name of a food can evoke an image that may enhance or detract from the food's appeal.

> Chris Clark says: "When I was a child, eggplants (aubergines) were rare. The first time my mother served up this vegetable as part of a meal, I was about nine years old. She told my siblings and me that it was called eggplant. We looked at the slimy, gray mass on the plate and thought of it as "eggs gone bad". After that we refused to touch the stuff. It was years before we ventured to try it again! Having learned her lesson from this episode, Mum used a different tactic to get us to eat tripe. Instead of telling us outright that it was the lining of a sheep's stomach, she kind of hinted that it was a type of fish. Mum never lied to us, but on this occasion she prevaricated. It worked. We didn't mind eating fish, so we ate the tripe."

Even a tiny alteration in how you view a food can make a huge difference.

Tool #3: Eat the food in different surroundings.

When you dine in unfamiliar surroundings, you're more likely to try foods you don't usually eat. This may because when your environment is unfamiliar, the unfamiliarity of a food's taste or texture is less apparent. Often when people travel abroad and are exposed to the cuisine of foreign cultures, they find themselves eating foods that they would never dream of eating at home. And if they eat them often enough, they can end up liking them.

Tool #4: Prepare the food in a different way.

Chris Clark says: "My mother, though loving and very well-meaning, was not a natural-born cook. When I was a child she used to cook Brussels sprouts in a pressure cooker until they were soggy, watery and bland. I grew up loathing Brussels sprouts, and for years I refused to eat them. In later life a friend served me with a small portion of Brussels sprouts that were, to my surprise, delicious. She had selected fresh, young sprouts and cooked them lightly, so that they retained their crispness. They were a small portion of a recipe that included foods I loved, and they were also topped with some kind of delicious sauce. I've liked Brussels sprouts ever since."

Cooking food in a different way can alter the texture, and texture is a very important food characteristic.

Another example involves eggplant (aubergine). If you cook it with some oil in a frypan it can end up with a slimy texture. If you roast it instead, its texture becomes drier and chewier, which is more appealing to many people. After people become used to the flavor of this vegetable by eating the roasted version, they are more likely to appreciate the fried version.

Adding other ingredients to change the texture can work as as well. Some people add fruits or seeds or nuts to cooked chia seeds, to give the gelatinous texture some added crunch.

Chris Clark writes: "Tofu was always on my 'I never eat that' list, because I disliked the rubbery texture of tofu in stir-fries and the slippery, slimy texture of it in soups. I wanted to like it, but I couldn't. Then I discovered silken tofu. Whipped up in a food processor, it has the exact texture and mouthfeel of cream. That made all the difference! Now

581

I make lemon and lime 'cheesecakes' with silken tofu, and flavor it with spices to make creamy dessert toppings, and use it as a base for mayonnaise. It has endless possibilities and it's full of protein, iron, and calcium. It's also naturally gluten-free and relatively low in Calories (much better for weight loss than cream!)."

Nutritional content of silken tofu vs. heavy cream.
- Silken Tofu: (8 oz/230g.) 112.5 Calories, 5 g of fat, 2.5 g of carbs, 10 g of protein.
- Heavy Cream: (8 oz/230g.) 821 Calories, 88 g of fat, 6.5 g of carbs, 4.8 g of protein.

In conclusion; look for some good recipes that include your "disliked" food, or order it when you eat out. Different preparation methods can really win you over to liking foods you've previously avoided.

Tool #5: Learn about the nutrient value.

Here's another mind-trick to help you love more foods; learn more about the nutrient value of the food you want to like. Tthe more you become aware of a food's nutritional benefits, the more you will be influenced to like it—especially if you are the kind of person who cares about good nutrition. [Alford & Tibbets (1971); Eertmans, et al., (2001); Engell et al., (1998)]

Find out as much as you can about the nutrient content of your disliked food. Learn about the health benefits of those nutrients, and you're more likely to want to eat that food!

Tool #6: Feel the benefits of the food you want to like.

Feeling good after eating or drinking something is a form of reward. It can reinforce your behavior. When you feel good after consuming a food or beverage, you're more likely to want to eat it again—even if you're not too keen on its flavor, texture or aroma.

When you eat sugary foods your blood sugars rise and the glucose sends "feel-good" signals to the brain. The brain's main energy source is glucose, so the brain gets happy! However, when you want to control your weight, guzzling sugary foods is a bad idea.

There are other, more nutritious foods that can give you an after-eating "buzz". They usually contain complex carbohydrates. Some people get that good feeling after eating brown rice, or soaked chia seeds. One person who is not keen on the gelatinous texture of chia seeds began by mixing a small amount of chia in water, so that it was still quite liquid. When she drank it, she imagined the nutrients flowing into her body and making her feel good. Over time, she would mix a thicker and thicker solution, until she was enjoying it at "pudding" consistency. At this point she barely noticed the texture.

This is an example of combining Tool #6 with Tool #1.

Tool #7: Make vegetables lovable.

Here are some ways to make yourself (and your family) love to eat vegetables.

Secret vegetables.

Purée cooked vegetables and hide them in patties or rissoles or Bolognese sauce. Veggies that work well include broccoli, carrots, courgettes (zucchinis) and bell peppers (capsicums). Pumpkin scones and pumpkin pie are good examples of how to incorporate puréed vegetables into delicious dishes. If the purée is very fine, the vegetables become, visually, almost unnoticeable. Use small portions to begin with, until you come to really appreciate the flavors, then add more. Obviously it's best to incorporate the natural textures of veggies into your food, but a purée is a good way to introduce them and get used to them.

Grated vegetables.

Grating vegetables is another good way to re-introduce them into your diet and get used to them. You can use grated vegetables not only in savory dishes but also in sweet ones such as carrot cake, muffins, red velvet cupcakes or brownies (use beetroot) or banana-and-courgette (zucchini) bread.

Spiralized vegetables.

Use a spiralizer to make "vegettie" and vegetable noodles. Many vegetables are suitable—notably carrots and courgettes. Also take a look at our section on combating food cravings.

Wrapped vegetables.

For some reason vegetables tend to be more appealing when they are wrapped in flat breads, mountain breads, pitas, parathas, burritos, tacos, rice-paper wrappers etc. Mix raw or cooked veggie fillings with other tasty ingredients.

For more information on how to make vegetables taste better, see our section under "Food and Drink" entitled "Vegetables".

10. LEARN TO UNLOVE CALORIE-DENSE FOODS

Cravings for high Calorie foods can ruin your weight-loss efforts. Here are some methods to help you get over your cravings for chocolate, sugar, fat, salt, alcohol etc.

Tool #1: Gradually reduce.

Gradually reduce the level at which the taste of the Calorie-dense food satisfies you. For example, some people stir several teaspoons or sugar into their cup of coffee or tea, while others find their beverages sweet enough with no added sugar at all. Everyone has different levels at which a certain taste makes them feel satisfied. This is not only because we all have different combinations of DNA, and different numbers of taste buds with different sensitivities; it's also because as time goes by, we become accustomed to a particular level of a taste.

It's pretty hard to change your physiology, but you can more easily change the taste levels of, say, sugar or fat, that you're used to.

The important thing is, do it gradually. Going "cold turkey" and switching from full-fat to no fat, or super-sweet to sweetener-free, can make you dislike the new taste so that, in the end, you're likely to reject it and return to high Calorie foods. So, to return to our example, over a period of weeks or even months, lower the levels of sugar in your coffee bit by bit. Or if you're into dairy products and used to eating full-fat yoghurt, mix full-fat with low-fat for a while, gradually decreasing the proportion of full-fat and increasing the proportion of low-fat.

Tool #2: Switch to healthier versions.

Switch to more healthful forms of foods you already like. This may not be easy at first, but it pays off in the long run. It can take 10 - 14 days to learn to like a new or previously disliked food, but it takes longer to switch to a different form of a food you already love.

If you want to like low-fat or low salt or low sugar versions of the foods that are already in your diet, it can take between two and four months before the adaption is complete. This is because your physiology, especially your taste buds, has become accustomed to the levels of salt or fat or sugar you normally eat.

Once you have weaned yourself off the unwanted foods, a marvellous thing happens to your senses.

- High-fat foods taste too rich and greasy.
- Very salty foods have a taste that resembles sea-water.
- Sugar-rich foods taste almost sickeningly over-sweet.

If this happens—congratulations! You have adapted to a healthier way of eating!

Tool #3: Keep satiating snacks on hand.

Keep lower calorie snack alternatives handy throughout the day.

To help you kick the desire for fatty, sugary snacks, make sure you have plenty of healthful lower Calorie snacks within reach, ready for when the craving hits. When you're at home, store peeled, raw vegetables and low Calorie dips in the refrigerator. When you're travelling, take raw vegetables or high satiety snacks with you. Include foods that contain protein, complex carbs and resistant starch to help stave off hunger pangs.

Carry a small plastic plate with you, if possible. Then, when you're about to have your snack, set out three small high-satiety snacks on the plate; preferably of three different colors. Allow your eyes to see what you're about to eat, so that your brain will remember it later.

585

Why three foods in three colors? Because it's more likely to satisfy you on a subconscious level—that is, if you're an adult! A 2012 study reported that adults are most attracted to food plates loaded with three items in three colors. (Children preferred seven different items and six colors.) [Zampollo et al., (2011)]

Tool #4: Change your food habits.

Change your high-calorie food habits. It's often habits that keep people from losing weight. You might associate eating an energy-dense food with a particular time of day, or a certain location. Perhaps it's having sweet cookies during your morning coffee-break every day, or buying a doughnut every time you're near your favorite bakery. The trick is to become aware of these habits and replace them with better alternatives, such as drinking some soda water or going for a short walk. Exercise and re-hydration can help you curb those cravings.

Tool #5: Learn to unlove a food by association.

Just as you can learn to like foods by association, so you can teach yourself to *unlike* foods. Here are some mind-tricks to achieve this:

- Mentally associate high-fat foods with greasiness, blubber and feeling queasy from eating over-rich foods.
- Associate sugary foods with feeling nauseous after eating too much of something sickeningly sweet.
- Learn about the ingredients of processed foods. Once you associate soft-serve ice-cream with a mixture of emulsifiers and chemical preservatives and other chemical ingredients which may be carcinogenic, you might feel less inclined to put it into your body. The same goes for soda drinks, processed meats, packaged ready-meals and almost every other processed food.

11. WILLPOWER AND CREATING GOOD HABITS

Let's face it—it's probably your habits that made you put on excess weight in the first place. Day by day, year after year, your habits of eating and exercising (or not exercising) eventually determine your body shape.

You might have developed habits of:

- drinking large quantities of soda
- eating late at night
- eating while watching TV or reading
- always eating a cookie or two whenever you drink a cup of coffee or tea
- eating a limited range of foods
- avoiding exercise

Many people begin weight loss diets, then relapse. They reach for high Calorie snacks, instead of eating nutrient-rich, Calorie-sparse foods, even though they know they'll put on more weight. They buy a gym membership, then cease going to the gym after a week or two.

When it comes to weight loss we all know what we should be doing on a regular basis—eating well and exercising. It's actually sticking to this regime for longer than a couple of weeks that's the hard part.

Why do we give up trying to change our bad habits? There are many reasons, such as:

- Because it's more convenient to eat processed and fast "junk" food than to prepare our own "real food" meals
- Because it's easier to be inactive than active
- Because we get distracted from our weight loss goals

The hardest thing about losing weight and becoming healthier isn't knowing what to do…

It's actually doing it.

After that, it's sticking to it!

"It's too hard to break bad food habits and replace them with good ones!"

Or is it?

It may be easier than you think!

Here's your new-habits-for-old tool-kit.

Tool #1: Community support.

Community support can help you create good weight loss habits. It's social connection, support and even pressure that helps people stick to resolutions.[44]

For some people, this involves *cooperation*.

For others it's *competition*.

David Desteno, PhD, author and professor of psychology at Northeastern University in Massachusetts (USA), proposes that some of our innate emotional responses may be the most powerful tools we have to strengthen our willpower. He suggests that social emotions such as sympathy, gratitude, love, empathy and compassion can improve self-control.

Being part of a supportive weight-loss community can keep you motivated and powerfully boost your weight loss. It can even lend a much-needed element of fun to the weight loss experience; losing weight is not easy, and sharing a few laughs can only help!

That community can consist of people you know in the real (offline) world—family, friends and workmates, for example. Or it can be an online community.

A group of people whose shared goal is weight loss can offer encouragement by means of cooperation or competition or both. It's up to you to choose which tactic works best for you.

Cooperation.

The sense of helping others has been shown to actually boost willpower. It keeps you accountable to others, not just to yourself. Group exercise can be very encouraging. Getting together for such events as a walk, a jog, a bicycle ride, a swim, a ball game can improve everyone's motivation and add a sense of fun. Cooperation can also involve such activities as:

- Sharing of recipes
- Sharing of weight loss tips

---

44   Note: As a bonus, feeling socially connected has been shown to be good for your general physical and mental health. People who lack community support and connection have decreased immune function. [Holt-Lunstad et al., (2015)]

- Sharing of exercise tips
- Commiseration for any setbacks and "falling off the wagon"
- Congratulations for any goal reached, such as weight loss or an exercise goal
- Sharing of solutions to problems
- Connection with people who are going through the same experience as you
- Connection with people who are happy and willing to listen to you

Competition.

Weekly group weigh-ins can make you work harder, so that you don't lag behind. Keeping tabs on other people's weight-loss progress and/or exercise achievements gives you incentive to compete with them in a friendly way.

Online weight-loss communities.

Some people prefer to join real-world weight-loss groups while others choose to join an online weight-loss community. Online groups offer different benefits; for example, if you choose to publish your weight online, you can do so anonymously.

If you suffer from a condition that limits your mobility (and thus your ability to exercise), an online community is perhaps more likely to put you in contact with others who face similar difficulties.

You can also form your own online weight-loss group with friends or people living in your neighborhood.

Tool #2: Use a positive replacement behavior.

It is much easier to break a habit when you replace it with another behavior. The idea is to replace a bad habit with a good habit. The new behavior begins to grow stronger than the old behavior, and eventually overpowers it altogether. Instead of drinking soda, for example, drink water or tea. Instead of eating late at night, go to bed earlier. Instead of watching TV or reading while you are eating, look at your plate and take delight in your food.

Tool #3: Believe and remember.

Believe in your personal motivation for change. If you want to break bad food habits because losing weight and becoming more healthy really matters to you, you will probably be successful a a lot faster than people who have been told to change by other people—such as doctors, or family members. As you keep practising the new, good habit, keep remembering what motivated you to break the old habit in the first place.

Tool #4: Persevere.

Habits that have existed for a long time have actually become embedded into the neural pathways of the brain. This is why they influence your behavior so strongly. They are, however, able to be changed.

Researchers from University College London investigated habit formation in 96 people over a period of 12 weeks. Specifically, they looked at changing an eating, drinking or activity behavior. The researchers reported that the average time it took for a new behavior to become a real habit is 66 days, although individual times ranged from 18 days to as much as 254 days (approx. 36 weeks)!

The longer you've had a habit, the longer it takes to break it. Some people have had the same habits for years!

So if you really want to change a habit, just keep repeating the new behavior, without giving up, for at least two months. You will be rewarded by the realisation that the new behavior is becoming easier and easier as the habit forms and becomes "second nature". [Lally et al., (2010)]

12. DE-STRESSING HELPS WEIGHT CONTROL

Stress is associated with obesity. [Björntorp (2001)] Feeling good is one of the important keys key to weight control—feeling happy, content and relaxed. One of the aims of the Satiety Diet is to help you achieve a positive mental state—a bright outlook on life.

Happier people make healthier choices. Take care of yourself from the inside out; feeling good can really help you lose weight.

12.1 About stress.

Stress can be good for you. Short term stress can actually boost your brain power. It's chronic stress that can be harmful, particularly when you have no control over the stressor. What causes stress?

External stressors.

Relationships, money problems, socioeconomic handicaps, health problems, the pressures of work, a poor diet, physical abuse, emotional abuse, pollutants, extreme weather and so on—many external factors can cause stress in our lives. The effects of stress can be increased by smoking, drinking, other forms of substance abuse, and over-eating.

Internal stressors.

You don't even have to be in a stressful situation to experience stress. It can also come from within you—from our thought patterns and from the physiological chemicals in your brain. Depressive and anxiety traits can cause stress.

12.2 Stress can weaken self-control.

Research reveals that stress is a major cause of junk food eating. Relaxed people are more likely to have the self-control to say "no" to unhealthful food.

In 2015, Swiss researchers subjected young, health-conscious, diet-conscious volunteers to the stress of plunging their hands into an ice-bath for three minutes. Immediately afterwards they were asked to choose what foods to eat, from a range of healthful and "junk" foods offered. They were much more likely to select the more delicious and tempting "junk" foods than a control group of similar volunteers who did not undergo the stress.

The volunteers who said they felt the most stressed were also the ones who made the quickest choice to eat the "junk" food. [Maier et al., (2015)]

The volunteers also underwent brain scans, which showed that it was not only the stress hormone cortisol that was to blame for their weakened self-control. There were other physiological factors at work in the brain, too.

As a result of their study, the researchers concluded that even low-level, moderate stress can weaken self-control.

Surveys have found that most of us suffer from low-level stress around 20 percent of the time. The American Psychological Association reported in 2011, "Most Americans are suffering from moderate to high stress, with 44 percent reporting that their stress levels have increased over the past five years..." [Clay (2011)]

In 2016 market research company OnePoll conducted a survey of 2,000 people. When asked to rate their stress levels out of 10, with 1 being the lowest and 10 being the highest, most respondents said that when they were at home their levels rated about 5, while their stress levels at work averaged about 6½.

This could indicate that most people—at least in the USA—are experiencing moderate to high levels of stress on a regular basis.

Why do you lose self-control when under stress?

When you experience stress, your Inner Guardian (who is always trying to look after you) tries to give you all the tools you need to get out of the stressful situation. It stimulates cortisol production, and it sends signals to your brain, saying, "Focus on the moment!"

By focussing your attention on the here and now, you are more likely to be able to figure out how to remedy the stressful situation. Dealing with the stressor becomes a priority.

Under stress, long-term goals such as weight loss and good health are relegated to secondary status. Under stress, dieters often reach for chocolate bars, gamblers take more risks and substance addicts may use larger doses.

Aside from making you over-eat and choose Calorie-dense foods, stress can contribute to weight gain in other ways, too. People experiencing stress often exercise less, have problems sleeping, and drink more alcohol. These three factors can all exacerbate weight gain.

12.3 Stress, cortisol and weight gain.
Stress triggers the release of cortisol.

When you experience stress, your body responds by producing more of the hormone cortisol. Your Inner Guardian floods your body with this cortisol, in case you need to fight or run away from whatever is causing the stress.

Cortisol primes your body for fighting or fleeing by inundating it with glucose, which delivers an instant energy supply to your large muscles (the muscles you need for running or fighting!). It also curbs insulin production, so that the glucose can be used by your muscles, instead of stored. Your Inner Guardian sends signals to your brain and the adrenal glands, telling them to get ready to make a dash for safety or pick up the nearest spear, ready defend your body from some stressful enemy. This is a healthy, natural response to stress.

Temporary high levels of cortisol are useful for helping you deal with stress. In the short term, stress can even dampen or even wipe out your appetite. Eating and appetite get postponed for the time being.

However, that state of affairs doesn't last.

If you experience prolonged stress, and are thus exposed to high levels of cortisol over a longer period of time, the consequences can be dire.

Cortisol and weight gain.

Constant or repeated elevation of cortisol levels can lead to weight gain. [Epel et al., (2000)]

How does this happen?

- The way cortisol works, it can move your fat stores from just beneath your skin to deeper inside your body, so that they accumulate around your internal organs. This "visceral fat" is directly associated with insulin resistance, as well as with higher LDL (bad) cholesterol levels.
- Cortisol helps your adipocytes (baby fat cells) develop into mature fat cells.

Cortisol stimulates appetite.

By flooding the body with glucose and suppressing insulin, cortisol gives you high blood sugar levels. This can lead to insulin resistance, which is associated with type 2 diabetes. It also leads to your body's cells being starved of glucose, since it's all flowing past in your bloodstream. Those cells, however, desperately need energy, which is why your Inner Guardian subsequently pumps out hunger signals and sends them to your brain. Levels of ghrelin, the hunger hormone, soar. When you are under stress you are often driven to overeat. Any leftover glucose you don't use for fighting or fleeing gets stored as body fat. And let's face it, in the modern world how often can you resolve stress by running away or coming to blows with an enemy? All that glucose is unlikely to be used up. Thus you gain weight.

Cortisol has numerous other appetite-stimulating properties, too. It can bind to hypothalamus receptors in the brain, and it can influence other hormones and physiological systems that arouse the appetite.

"... psychophysiological response to stress may influence subsequent eating behavior. Over time, these alterations could impact both weight and health." [Epel et al., (2001)]

Cortisol makes you crave for Calorie-dense foods.

The higher your cortisol levels, the more strongly you desire sugary, fatty, high-energy foods. [Epel et al., (2001)]

A 2000 study published in the journal Psychosomatic Medicine found that "... stressed emotional eaters ate more sweet high-fat foods and a more energy-dense meal than unstressed and non-emotional eaters." [Oliver et al., (2000)]

After you eat these Calorie dense (and usually extremely delicious) foods, they give you a rush of flavor and blood sugar and mood-lifting other rewarding effects.

Sometimes people talk about "comfort eating", and these fatty, sugary foods really can provide pleasurable comfort—at least while they are being eaten and for a short time afterwards.

Eating highly-rewarding foods could help decrease physiological stress responses. Consuming them can also provide a brief distraction from the stressful situation. If you find that Calorie dense foods provide some stress relief, you are likely to turn to them every time you feel stressed.

Excessive cortisol can impair proper digestion.

Cortisol activates your sympathetic nervous system (SNS), whose primary function is to stimulate your body's fight-or-flight response.

The parasympathetic nervous system (PNS) is responsible for stimulation of "rest-and-digest" or "feed and breed" activities that occur when your body is at rest, especially after eating, during digestion. [Wikipedia (15th February 2017)]

In your body, the SNS and the parasympathetic nervous system cannot work at the same time, so when you are stressed, the PNS is suppressed.

This means that if you eat when stressed, the performance of your hormones and enzymes regulating your digestion and absorption of nutrients is impaired. You don't digest properly when you are under stress. In the long term, poor digestion can have adverse effects on the lining of your digestive tract. When you don't absorb enough of a wide range of nutrients, your Inner Guardian sends out demands for "more food". And of course, eating more food can lead to weight gain.

12.4 Tips on stress reduction.

Dealing with stress helps with weight loss. For essential tips on how to reduce stress in your life, see *The Satiety Diet Weight Loss Toolkit*, #2 in the Satiety Diet series of books.

13. DEPRESSION AND WEIGHT MANAGEMENT

Weight problems often accompany depression. Some people pile on the extra pounds when they feel depressed, while others can't help shedding weight to an extent that may harm their health.

In 2010 a scientific review of 15 studies concluded that depression is associated with a greater chance of becoming obese—and that becoming obese is linked with a higher probability of developing depression. [Luppino et al., (2010)]

Experts are unsure about the reasons behind these associations. Depression might lead to obesity because people suffering from depression:

- tend to lack the energy and motivation to move around and exercise
- may self-medicate with alcohol
- may prefer Calorie-dense "comfort foods"

Treatment of depression can involve counseling and/or anti-depressant medications. Some natural methods of countering depression have been discussed earlier in this book. They include getting daily exercise, having a supportive social network, laughing, listening to music, dancing, experiencing the natural environment, enriching the microbiome with foods containing prebiotics and probiotics, and getting a good night's sleep.

13.1 The antidepressant effects of cold water.

One treatment for depression that has been gaining attention recently is the use of "cold hydrotherapy"—that is, immersing your body in cold water. On his TV show "The Doctor Who Gave Up Drugs", celebrity doctor Chris Van Tulleken treated a depressed woman with cold water swimming. She swam in a lake for one hour, three times a week, and felt so good that she could be weaned off her antidepressants.

"The theory is that repeated exposure to cold water improves your response to the stress that often accompanies depression," writes Dr. Van Tulleken.

Adapted cold shower.

You may not have a handy lake nearby to swim in, but you can still enjoy the antidepressant benefits of cold hydrotherapy. A 2008 study published in Medical Hypotheses suggests that you might be able to achieve similar effects using the "adapted cold shower" technique.

Volunteers showered once or twice a day. Each time, they began by standing beneath a stream of lukewarm water for an adaption period of 5 minutes, during which time they gradually turned off the hot water, until only the cold was running. The temperature of the cold water measured at 20° C (68°F). They stayed in the cold water for 2-3 minutes.

The researchers concluded that " . . . the cold hydrotherapy can relieve depressive symptoms rather effectively. The therapy was also found to have a significant analgesic effect and it does not appear to have noticeable side effects or cause dependence. ...The proposed duration of treatment is several weeks to several months." [Shevchuk (2008)]

Cold therapy and weight loss.

Cold water therapy may also promote weight loss. Exposure to very low temperatures activates the body's "brown fat". Unlike white fat, which stores Calories, brown-fat cells *burn* Calories, a process that produces heat to warm you up when you're cold.

14. SOCIAL CONNECTION

Social connection can help you lose weight. When you are part of a group of like-minded people, instead of being isolated, you may feel accountable to the other people in the group. You might also feel encouraged to pursue a common goal. If you join a weight loss group you're are more likely to succeed with losing weight than people who go it alone.

14.1 Real life social connection.

Studies show that people who participate in weight loss programs in the company of their real-life friends tend to lose weight and keep it off. [Wing & Jeffery (1999); Verheijden et al., (2005)]

14.2 Online social connection.

According to a 2015 study, people who use online programs to lose weight get a much better result when they join an online social support group. [Poncela-Casasnovas et al., (2015)] There are plenty of weight loss groups/forums available on the World-Wide Web.

Advantages: When you join an online weight loss support group, you can be anonymous. When nobody knows who you are, you can be completely honest without fear of being judged in real life. You can confess your weird eating habits, for example, without worrying that friends or family will disparage you.

Disadvantages: Sometimes there are people who post negative comments online. These are sometimes called "Internet trolls". Fortunately, forums that have volunteer human moderators, or paid ones (these forums naturally cost money to join), are less likely to be plagued by "trolls".

14.3 Types of support often shared in social groups

- Photographs of meals
- Photos of daily exercise such as landscapes seen on a walk, or a pet accompanying a walk
- Meal plans (daily or weekly)
- Statistics from fitness tracking devices
- Exercise tips and tricks
- Success stories (these can be inspiring)
- Failure stories (sympathy helps, as does encouragement to leave the failure behind and keep going)
- Weight loss strategies
- Recipes
- Sources of hard-to-find ingredients
- Local eateries that offer healthful dishes
- Sympathy and commiseration for emotional distress

PART SEVEN

THE SATIETY DIET LIFESTYLE

ABOUT THE SATIETY DIET

1. A way of life.

The Satiety Diet is not really a diet. It's a way of life.

You've probably heard that before, but this time it's true.

Why? Because on the Satiety Diet, you're listening to your body's signals, instead of fighting against them.

The Satiety Diet is built around the way Mother Nature intended you to live—the way human beings lived and ate before the "obesity crisis". And that is a method of weight control that has been proven over countless millennia of history!

Although this is a way of life, we've simply called it a "diet" because many people think of a diet as the only way they can lose weight.

You can't lose weight without altering something about your current lifestyle. After all, it's what youve been doing every day until now that has shaped your body.

2. Types of weight-loss regimes:

Weight loss regimes generally fall into one of the following categories—

- **Restricted food groups**: You are allowed to eat as much as you like, but only within certain food groups or macronutrient groups.
- **Restricted eating times**: You are allowed to eat as much as you like of any food in any quantity as long as you only eat within certain hours of the day ("eating windows") and fast for the rest of the time.
- **Restricted food portions**: You are allowed to eat any food you like, at any time, but portions of certain foods are limited.

Restricted food groups: Virtually the entire scientific community agrees: Diets that omit whole food groups are bad for your health and not tenable in the long term. They are also likely to give rise to the "rebound effect"—that is, when you stop following the "restricted food groups" diet and finally give in to your body's demands for the "forbidden" foods, you're likely to regain all the weight you lost, and sometimes more.

Restricted eating times: Fasting may also increase the risk of bingeing, for similar reasons. [Stice et al., (2008)]

A diet that forbids certain food groups or certain eating times can trigger cravings and lead to compensatory overeating. When this happens most people assume its their fault for not having enough willpower. It is not their fault—it's the diet's fault for demanding that they fight against their body's own needs and their Inner Guardian's insistent survival signals.

Restricted food portions: In order for you to lose weight, something has to change. Changing the size of your Calorie-dense food portions is the best way to lose weight without adverse effects on your physical or mental well-being. You never need to feel deprived when you know you can eat any food at all (in small portions) and *unrestricted* amounts of NTS foods, any time you truly feel hungry.

3. On the satiety diet, no food is off limits.
When we say you can eat all foods, we really mean ALL foods—even high-fat high-sugar highly-processed foods, which many people call "bad" or "junk" foods. On the Satiety Diet you can go ahead and eat these "sometimes" foods, but only if—
- you are really, really craving for them
- you are aware that the more Calorie-dense food you eat, the less likely you'll be to lose weight
- you choose a small portion size and eat it mindfully

This is why the Satiety Diet falls into the "restricted food portions" category. Many foods however, such as Nourishing, Tasty, Slimming (NTS) vegetables, can be eaten freely in any amount. You can eat at any time of the day, but for more effective weight loss it is recommended that you have a relatively small eating windoe and don't consume a heavy meal just before bedtime.

The Satiety Diet also teaches you how to avoid eating triggers and craving triggers. It teaches your body how to decrease its desire for Calorie-dense foods—for example, when you switch to eating low-fat foods, your sensitivity to fat becomes amplified and you perceive even small amounts of fat in your mouth as being super-rich and creamy.

Willpower can be used up!

Even though willpower is a renewable resource, it can be finite in a given time period. The more you exercise self-control in the face of temptation, the harder it can become to maintain that self-control.

Calling upon willpower to fight against the drives of your Inner Guardian can be exhausting.

Using willpower to stop yourself from eating can be compared to firing a cannon. There is a recoil effect. The more willpower you exert now, the more cravings may plague you later—possibly leading to bingeing. This is exemplified by some of the "dieting memes" doing the rounds of the Internet, for example this one:

> **"Breakfast**: kale smoothie with a banana.
> **Lunch**: Avocado toast and quinoa salad.
> **Dinner**: 57 bagel bites, 13 donuts, 2 buckets of fried chicken, 1 bottle of wine."

It's almost impossible to fight the recoil effect of exerting willpower and self-control to curb eating. Trying to do so can result in:

- feelings of failure and low-self esteem
- eating disorders

With the Satiety Diet, a minimum of willpower is necessary. You need a small amount of willpower to plan meals ahead of time, and organize nutritious meals for yourself, but if you follow our guidelines you should not need to exert enormous willpower to restrain hunger or cravings.

SATIETY DIET GENERAL GUIDELINES

1. Food

These days there is a bewildering barrage of conflicting advice about what you should be eating if you want to lose weight and be healthy. Yet the latest research into what foods are best for weight loss and good health confirms the fact that human beings are generally healthier, fitter and slimmer when they:

- Eat minimally processed, whole foods that are close to nature
- Eat mainly plant-based foods
- Eat a wide variety of foods, encompassing all nutrients, without singling out any particular nutrient as being in some way "evil".
- Limit refined starches and added sugars
- Limit the intake of certain fats
- Aim to reach satiety at every main meal
- Eat foods that give you the highest nutritional content for the lowest Calorie count, so that you'll feel fuller (and be healthier) even while you're consuming fewer Calories.

Plan, plan, plan!

Always have your next meal and snack ready to go. "Being organised" is the small price you pay for becoming slimmer. This means taking the time to shop more often and more wisely, and preparing your own meals more often. Plan your meals ahead of time. Have fresh ingredients on hand ready to go—ready, that is, to be either cooked (in the case of most dishes) or tossed together (in the case of raw dishes such as salads).

People who plan their Satiety Diet meals are less likely to fall for snacking on the kinds of food that pack on the pounds.

Planning also means convenience. One day a week of cooking and freezing meals can provide reheatable meals throughout the week. Two well-organized shopping trips per week can provide you with fresh food for minimum bother.

When you take the time to plan, you will find that instead of panicking and feeling deprived, you will feel relaxed knowing your next meal is organized and that you have the right—indeed, almost the obligation—to sit down and really enjoy it.

Take the stress out of your life with planning, and you can lower your cortisol levels. Lower levels of cortisol can help dampen hunger.

> Chris Clark says, "For me, the second hardest thing about the Satiety Diet was planning and organizing healthful, delicious, varied meals in advance. I was not in the habit of doing this. My daily routine included very little thought about future meals. This meant that when I got hungry I would grab whatever food was conveniently on hand. Food that's conveniently on hand is generally Calorie-dense, low-nutrition food such as cookies and cake."

Swap, swap, swap!

Switch Calorie-dense foods for Calorie-sparse foods that can provide similar textures, colors and flavors. This can give you satiety with a lower energy intake and help to stop feelings of deprivation.

Track, track, track!

Keep track of all the snacks you nibble on throughout the day.

A cookie here, a candy bar cake there—extra Calories you snack on without thinking as you go about your daily business can soon add up to surplus fat stored on your waistline. It is easy to forget how many snacks you've eaten, especially if you eat "on the run".

Every mouthful counts.

Your brain might develop convenient amnesia but your Inner Guardian knows exactly how many Calories you've ingested. And it's probably stored them on your hips....

Nourish your gut microbes.

Feed your microbiome with assorted fibers, the right kinds of probiotics, and food variety.

Choose wisely

In general, favor foods that are unprocessed or lightly-processed, low in *Calories,* low in *saturated* and *trans fats,* low in *sugar (especially fructose),* high in *fiber* and rich in *protein.*

Choose natural.

Eat mainly whole foods, not processed foods or smoothies and juices. Aim to eat only "real" or "natural" foods—that is, avoid additives as much as possible but don't worry if you can't avoid them altogether; just do the best you can and remain calm.

Veggies, veggies, veggies!

NTS (Nourishing, Tasty, Slimming) veggies generally have a high water content and a high fiber content, as well as being packed with nutrients. It helps to think of all non-vegetable foods as existing simply to make veggie recipes taste delicious! For example sauces, gravies, relishes and tasty starchy or low-fat foods exist to be mixed with non-starchy vegetables. The more NTS vegetables you eat, the more satisfied you'll feel, without all the Calories. It's likely, nonetheless, that you'll only eat them if they taste good. Examples of tasty vegetable dishes include silver beet/spinach quiche, stir-fried vegetables, vegetables in white sauce sprinkled with nutritional yeast, zucchini slice.

Prefer low GI.

Favor low GI foods, and foods containing resistant starch.

Food: Macronutrients and fiber.

- Consume all the macronutrients in a balanced ratio—including the "good" fats.

- In your daily diet, include approximately 10-35% protein, 20-35% unsaturated ("good") fats, 10-15% starchy carbs, 35% non starchy carbs, 15% low fructose fruit and 25-38 grams (1- 1 ¼ oz) of mixed dietary fiber.

- approximately 25% protein, 10% starchy carbs, 30% non starchy carbs, 15% low fructose fruit and 20% unsaturated ("good") fats.

- Your diet should contain a small amount of "healthful" fat. The Satiety Diet is neither a no-fat regime nor a high-fat regime. Everyone needs to eat some fat for satiety. A low-fat diet is recommended for weight loss, since it helps boost both satiety and good health. Preferably eat foods containing fats at the beginning of meals. Fat occurs naturally in many foods, so be aware of it and track it. Apart from coconuts and avocados, most fruits and vegetables in their natural form contain little to no fat. Count all the fats in your diet; you may not have to add extra fat to be getting your quota. Avoid trans fats (hydrogenated fats) and saturated fats.

- Aim to eat some protein with every meal, as it promotes satiety. Protein does not automatically mean meat. Vegetable protein comes naturally packaged with fiber, which helps promote satiety.

- Become more easily satiated by eating more fiber of all kinds.

- Incorporating soluble and insoluble fiber into meals helps you achieve both satiation and satiety.

Keep these foods to a minimum.

You can eat anything on the Satiety Diet, but it's wise to cut down on the following foods or even avoid them altogether if you wish.

Sugar

Sugar is a food that is present in most other foods. In itself it is not a "poison" but in affluent societies it is sometimes visualized as a bane, not a boon.

As mentioned, it is wise to avoid consuming large quantities of fructose, which can be an appetite stimulant. Fructose is available in foods in "free" form or it can be bound up in sucrose (table sugar), which the body breaks down into fructose and glucose. Fructose can also be found in foods containing fructans; it can be generated by the breakdown of fructans by bacteria in the gut. (People with fructose intolerance are advised to avoid foods containing fructans.)

Fat

Choose small portions of the right kinds of fat. It is important to include some fat in your diet, but it's Calorie-dense, so when you want to lose weight its best to avoid eating it in large quantities. The CSIRO recommends, "When choosing fats, unsaturated sources that are softer or liquid at room temperature are best choices." As we've mentioned, avoid foods containing trans fats (hydrogenated fats) and saturated fats.

Sugar combined with fat

Sugar + Fat = the most tempting, unnatural, addictive, delicious, fattening food combination! One of the few natural sources of this combination is breast milk and other milks/dairy products. In other words, nature intended [sugar + fat] to be consumed by growing infants, not by adults.

Most other natural, unprocessed foods contain either sugars or fats, but not both. People who cut sugar and other carbs out of their diet but keep eating fat, generally lose weight. People who cut fat out of their diet but keep eating sugars/carbs, generally lose weight too. It's the combination of the two that makes it harder to get rid of excess fat. And it's no coincidence that some of the most addictive junk foods are loaded with both fats and sugars—think cheesecake, donuts, milkshakes and even burgers with their carb-laden buns.

Refined carbs

Stop eating refined carbs. White flour is an example of a food high in refined carbs. It is found in many products, including white bread, pastries, tortillas, and most pasta. Swap white flour products for a variety of nutritious foods such as brown rice, whole-wheat bread, pulse or buckwheat pasta, corn tortillas and nuts, especially almonds.

Good Food Habits: Protein.

Include protein in your meals. It doesn't have to be animal protein. Plant-based proteins have the added benefit of being naturally packaged with fiber, which boosts satiation and satiety.

Good Food Habits: Portion size.

Your food portion sizes should be close to the sizes recommended by the Satiety Diet, but don't stress if they're not precise. Use your hands, or your plate, or everyday objects as a rough guide to portion sizes.

Good Food Habits: Sweetness.

- For weight loss, eat no more than 2 to 3 servings of fruit per day. Treat fruit as if it were dessert, or candy. Choose whole, fresh fruits, and eat them in conjunction with other foods.
- Train yourself to enjoy foods that are low in sweetness. Sweeten your food with low-fructose fruits or a small amount of rice malt syrup (which is fructose-free) or stevia, and/or erythritol.
- Eat sweet foods *separately* from fatty foods. Sugar plus fat is an addictive combination.
- A small amount of sweet food is fine but try to avoid refined white sugar. Raw sugar contains more nutrients.
- Stevia and erythritol don't make your blood sugars spike.

Good Food Habits: Variety.
* Eat a variety of food types, colors, shapes, textures, sounds, smells etc. presented in a variety of ways.
* Train yourself to like foods that you've previously dismissed as "foods I don't eat" (unless you've been diagnosed with a food allergy or intolerance, of course).
* Choose food that is as tasty, as multi-textured and as highly flavored as possible. Really *know* you are eating and enjoy it. Strong smelling foods and strong tasting foods are more satisfying. They appeal to your senses.
* No food is "forbidden". The Satiety Diet strongly encourages you to eat a wide variety of natural, unprocessed foods.

In an ideal world, you'd aim to eat different foods without repetition, for at least 7 days in a row. Then repeat the exercise for another 7 days, and so on. This can be hard to achieve! Seven different breakfasts in a row, seven different lunches and seven different dinners... and only *one* of those meals can contain, for example, wheat-based food.

Most of us gravitate towards our favorite foods and our familiar recipes. Aiming to break free of these restrictions will encourage you to eat foods you would not usually consider. Variety is good for you, and a variety of nutrients can contribute to better satiety!

Here are some examples of a week's worth of breakfasts and lunches[45]:

BREAKFASTS
1. Scrambled tofu on whole wheat toast, garnished with fresh parsley or arugula (rocket). A side of cooked tomatoes and spinach. (Vegan)
2. Half a cup of cooked brown rice mixed with tuna and a spoonful of plain, low-fat Greek yoghurt.
3. Buckwheat pancakes with almond butter and blueberries. (Vegan)

---

45   See the Satiety Diet Cookbook for more recipe ideas!

4. 1/3 cup teff porridge with raspberries, drizzled with a little rice malt syrup and topped with a dollop of low-fat labne or creamy silken tofu (blitz it in a food processor).

5. Chia pudding: 2 tbsp chia seeds soaked overnight in 1 cup unsweetened almond milk with added blackberries or sliced mandarins, topped with 1 tbsp of either chopped almonds, sunflower seeds or pumpkin seeds. (Vegan)

6. Taco "boats" with a filling of minced beef or marinated tofu, with Mexican spices, bell peppers and mushrooms.

7. Cannelloni beans in tomato sauce on toasted rye bread. (Vegan)

LUNCHES
1. Prawn rice-paper rolls with salad and dipping-sauce.
2. Vegetable stew with barley and chickpeas. (Vegan)
3. Quinoa lentil salad. (Vegan)
4. Sun-dried tomato, mushroom, and spinach tofu quiche. (Vegan)
5. Stir fried vegetables with fish on a bed of steamed freekeh.
6. Baked jacket potato with coleslaw, chopped tomato and spring onions/scallions/salad onions, grated low-fat cheese and a dollop of low-fat hummus.
7 Mexican bean enchilada bake. (Vegan)

Good Food Habits: The timing of eating.

- Eat breakfast as late as possible and your last meal of the day as early as possible.
- Preferably don't eat between meals. It takes about three hours for your body to finish digesting a meal. If you eat every two or three hours, your body will constantly be in what nutritionists call the "fed state." This simply means that you are always in the process of digesting food.
- Nutritionists advise those who want to *gain* weight to snack frequently; eat small amounts often, throughout the day. To *lose* weight aim to eat fully satiating meals, three times a day.

Good Food Habits: Sensory characteristics.

Choose flavorful, colorful, Calorie-sparse, nutrient-dense foods with a variety of textures and temperatures. Add herbs, spices or a sprinkle of citrus juice for extra flavor and zing.

Good Food Habits: Starters

A "starter" is a smaller dish served before the main meal. In French cuisine, as well as in the English-speaking world (save for the US and parts of Canada) it is also called an entrée. Include a starter of a Calorie-sparse, nutrient-dense soup or salad at the commencement of your meal. Not only will this help to reduce your hunger, it will also help to prolong and extend the duration of the meal. Eating slowly, over a longer period, contributes to satiation and satiety.

DRINK

- Drink between meals is a good idea. Thirst can be mistaken for hunger.
- Drink unsweetened black tea or coffee, herbal teas, still or sparkling water, or other natural, low Calorie fluids.
- Avoid juices, smoothies, shakes and sodas. Nutritionists recommend drinking smoothies and juices to pile on the weight. Therefore those who wish to lose weight should do the opposite.
- Sip some water at the commencement of meals.

EXERCISE

* Raise your heart-rate for a minimum of 20 minutes daily. Don't overdo it.

* The secret to getting regular exercise is enjoying it. Pick something you enjoy, and schedule it into your week. You can, for example take a brisk walk, dance, ride a bicycle, do some gardening or engage in any other relatively vigorous activity you enjoy.

* Incidental exercise can help a lot, so for example, when you're talking on the phone, walk around.

* Dr Mosley's research indicates that women should exercise after eating, while men should exercise on an empty stomach.

YOUR MIND

- Your mood is important to your weight loss.
- Sing. It can make you happy.
- Speaking of worry—don't! Aim for calm and contentment in your whole life. Stress can contribute to weight gain.
- Sleep well.
- For motivation, join or form a weight-loss group to help boost your motivation through cooperation and/or competition. This can be as informal as a group of friends. Or join the free forums on our website.
- Avoid visual eating triggers. Keep food out of sight, and only shop for food when you're not hungry. Don't watch TV shows about food, or if you do watch them, make sure you're not hungry. The same goes for reading magazines containing images of food, or food-themed movies.
- Avoid other appetite triggers, such as reading words about food, or going to places where there are food smells.
- In between meals, do not be reminded of food. Stay out of the kitchen or canteen. See no food ads or pictures, or written words. Smell no food smells.

1. Dealing with hunger

- Listen to your body. Are you really hungry, or just peckish or thirsty? Is it really potato crisps/chips you're craving, or is it protein?
- Between meals, allow yourself to become hungry but not starving.
- Use mental imagery of your last meal to curb hunger.
- Optionally, use placebo weight loss pills.
- Never make yourself eat if you are not hungry.
- Befriend hunger. *Know* that hunger is safe. It is not only safe but *good*. Don't panic. Feel your hunger and *relax*. Remember that the hunger you feel between meals is actually a sign your body is burning fat. You don't have to panic, because you have planned your next meal. You can be sure that before

your hunger becomes ravenous, you are going to eat your pre-planned fully satisfying and nutritious meal.

- Try not to snack between meals, but do snack if you feel desperate. Eat healthful, satiating snacks only. Satisfying your cravings can prevent you from feeling deprived.
- Between meals, visualizing your body assimilating the nutrition from your last meal can help curb hunger.

2. How to deal with cravings

- If you feel an urgent craving to eat something sweet after a meal or between meals, then do so. Fighting cravings is a sure way to end up losing the war with weight loss. Ghrelin, the hunger hormone, is more powerful (in healthy people) than willpower.
- When cravings hit, eat a little of what you crave even if it's Calorie-dense. Or eat a lower-Calorie version of what you crave.

3. Non-food nourishment.

Nourish yourself in ways that don't necessarily involve food. Food is not always nourishment and nourishment is not always food.

Sometimes when you think you are hungry and need food, what you really need is a positive feeling such as comfort, tranquillity, reassurance, joy. People can be nourished by things that promote happiness, such as pampering and creature comforts. A massage, a chat with a good friend, the scent of a (cruelty-free) perfume, a peaceful walk along the beach or through the park, reading a good book, listening to music, flying a kite... living well is nourishment for the body, mind and spirit.

When you don't live well, when you are not kind to yourself by occasionally pursuing activities that promote relaxation, joy and healing, you might seek nourishment in food instead. This is when you might choose to eat too much food, or the wrong kinds of food—the foods that can bring a rush of instant pleasure, such as the combination of sugar and fat.

4. Affirmations.

Affirmations are simple, proven psychological methods of changing your mindset and lifting your mood. Research has shown that they actually have the power to rewire the brain! Affirmations can be thoughts, or words spoken out loud. Merriam-Webster dictionary defines an affirmation as "a positive assertion." When you repeat affirmations, you boost your body's feel-good hormones (such as dopamine) and encourage the brain to grow new neuronal clusters that promote positive thinking.

Your actions and behavior are influenced by the words you say, which in turn are influenced by your thoughts. When you think positive thoughts you are more likely to say positive things, such as, "I can do this." And since your Inner Guardian tends to believe what you say about yourself, the more you repeat, "I can do this" the more you are likely to be able to do it! Affirmations can break negative thought-speech-behavior cycles. They should be repeated often, to have the best effect.

The power of thought.

Your thoughts influence your whole life. They influence your attitude, thereby affecting your behavior. Not only your "big" actions are influenced by your thoughts but also your "small", almost undetectable actions, such as a fleeting smile instead of a fleeting frown. That smile on your face affects not only your own biochemicals, but also the reactions of the people around you. Something so seemingly minor can snowball, resulting in positive consequences.

You have the power to change your thoughts. Changing them can help improve your life. Affirmations may not make you the richest, healthiest, most successful person in the world, but they can definitely help you. Affirmations in the form of thoughts can be repeated in your head whenever you don't have to focus on something else.

Speaking aloud.

Eastern philosophers have used the power of one's own voice for thousands of years, in the form of mantras. The Oxford Dictionary defines these as "a word or sound repeated to aid concentration in meditation". The sound of your own voice has an enormous effect on you. You hear your own voice every day, usually without consciously thinking about it. It is your constant companion. In fact, so powerful is the sound of your own voice that when you speak in a happy way, you can actually become happier—and vice versa. [Aucouturier et al., (2016)]

As mentioned, affirmations can be silently thought, or spoken aloud. They can be repeated as often as you like. It's up to you. Some people repeat their affirmations while driving, or walking the dog, or taking a coffee break.

It's preferable to compose your own affirmations, because they are the most meaningful for you. However if you're stuck for ideas, here are some examples of pre-constructed weight-loss affirmations from www.self-help-and-self-development.com:

- Life is beautiful and I enjoy life by staying fit and maintaining my ideal weight.
- Every physical movement that I make burns the extra fat in my body and helps me to maintain my ideal body weight.
- Every cell in my body is healthy and fit and so am I.
- I easily control my weight through a combination of healthy eating and exercising.

Some Satiety Diet affirmations include:
- "I can eat anything I want, any time I want. I am surrounded by the foods I like." (Note that the definition of "want" refers to "genuine wanting", as signaled by your Inner Guardian. Your Inner Guardian knows what nutrients your body really needs.)
- "I can relax, knowing that I don't have to store food as fat on my body. Food is all around me all the time, and whenever I feel real hunger I can reach out and get it." (Note that most people in societies with an obesity problem have access to a wide variety of foods in local markets and supermarkets.)

5. Your mood while eating.

Eat happily, slowly, mindfully and calmly. Most importantly, eat until you are satisfied.

Seeing other people calmly eating while you are eating can also send beneficial signals to the Inner Guardian. "There is plenty of food for everyone," is one subconscious message. This can indicate to the Inner Guardian that it does not need to store extra fat on your body. "These other diners are relaxed, therefore there's probably no danger about," is a cortisol-lowering message.

6. Seeing the whole meal all at once

Whenever you prepare your dinner table for a meal, try to ensure that all the food you are about to eat is displayed before your eyes, simultaneously. When your eyes see your entire meal, instead of just one course at a time, your mind can absorb the sight of that food, and your Inner Guardian will remember how much was available for you to eat.

Appreciatively looking at the food you are eating, and recognizing that you are eating it, is very important for your sense of satiety. If, for example, you are watching a movie and eating popcorn without looking at the popcorn, or even registering how many mouthfuls you've consumed, you're more likely to feel hungry soon afterwards. Your Inner Guardian may have received a fullness signal from your popcorn-filled stomach, but it did not receive a visual image of the food, or a cognitive appreciation of it. Without those missing signals, your Guardian cannot be certain that you've had enough to eat, so it prompts you to feel hungry again.

Similarly, seeing one course at a time set before you, (*service à la russe*) instead of the whole meal at once (*service à la française*), can mean your Inner Guardian fails to recognize the quantity of food you've eaten. Serve your meals in the French style, instead of the Russian style!

7. Mindfulness

Eat meals slowly and mindfully, paying attention to all the sensory attributes of your food.

Mindful dining companions

Have you ever eaten in the company of people who stuff food into their mouths unmindfully, as if eating is merely a task that must be finished as quickly as possible? This can make you feel a need to eat more quickly, to match that person's pace. It may also trigger stress hormones such as cortisol. Moreover, it can also send subconscious signals to your ever-vigilant Inner Guardian, telling it that "food is scarce". If people around you are wolfing down food as fast as possible, this seems to indicate there is a need to panic about food shortages. This is the way your primitive, protective Inner Guardian interprets the world.

8. Background sounds while you eat

While you're dining, it's important for you to be able to hear the sounds of your food—sounds your mouth makes, such as crunching and slurping; sounds your cutlery makes, such as scraping or clinking. There can be some background sound, as long as it's not loud or stressful. Pleasant relaxing music is fine, or the softly murmuring, ambient susurrus of a well-run eatery, or birdsong, or the sound of water falling. Peaceful silence is also fine!

9. Allow yourself joy.

Be kind to yourself. The Satiety Diet is about pure joy, relaxation and contentment.

It is a joy to sit down to a delicious, nutritious meal and slowly eat until you feel satiated—not forcing yourself to hold back, and not hankering after a little more food when the meal is over.

It is a joy not to feel "stuffed to the gills".

Gradually over time, as you follow the Satiety Diet—pampering yourself with relaxation and food variety and mindful eating and enjoyable movement—the excess fat stores will slip away easily... with no rebound effect and no repercussions aside from contentment!

10. Stop looking at pictures and words about food.

As a general rule, never read cookbooks or look at any written descriptions or pictures of food unless you are already feeling full and have reached satiety. Images and descriptions of food can make you feel hungry! Your brain signals to the Inner Guardian that "food is nearby," and therefore it must be time to eat, so the digestive juices start flowing in preparation. Yet no food arrives in the stomach, because there WAS no food, only words and pictures...

11. Keep food and food-related items out of sight.

The design and layout of your home can affect your weight loss. The best kitchen or eating area is a secluded one which can be sealed off from the rest of the house. Open plan kitchens are a recipe for weight gain, because the appliances and instruments of cookery (such as the refrigerator, the stove) are always visible from the living areas. Even if you're not consciously aware of it, your eyes are seeing these reminders and your brain is constantly receiving food cues.

MEDICATIONS

If you are taking medications whose side effects include weight gain, ask your doctor how you can wean off them or swap them for other medications.

HOW TO EAT AN IDEAL SATIETY DIET MEAL

- Start by sipping your sparkling water, or your miso soup.

- Eat off smaller plates. As we've already mentioned, when you eat food off a smaller plate, you'll tend to feel fuller than when you eat the same amount of food off a big plate. If you pile food right to the edges of a small plate, your Inner Guardian gets the visual message that there's a lot of food on offer. In contrast, if you put that same amount of food on a large plate, with empty space left around the edges of the plate, your Inner Guardian thinks you're not getting as much to eat! [Wansink et al., (2005)]

- Set out all your dishes of food in front of you at the beginning of each meal and really look at them. Know how much you're going to eat, and afterwards, be fully aware of how much you've eaten. As you eat, let your eyes linger on the array of colorful, diverse foods in front of you. "Photograph" the entire meal with your mind. Recall this "photograph" later, to stave off hunger between meals.

- Dine in a relaxed, mindful way. Eat slowly, until you feel satisfied. Take at least half an hour to eat the meal from the first bite to the last. Make it an hour, if possible. Admire the food. Savor it, smell it, taste it. In a leisurely way, enjoy the different tastes and textures of the meal. Take it slowly, but only as slowly as feels natural for you. Don't worry about whether you are eating too fast or too slow. Just relax.

- When you eat a meal don't read, or watch TV, or otherwise be distracted while eating. You could listen to soft, relaxing music, as long as it does not drown out any crunching, slurping sounds you may hear while eating your food.

- Use small, many-colored tableware in a variety of shapes and sizes. Use plates and dishes whose color contrasts with the food.

- Preferably place different foods in different bowls. Separate each type of dish.

- Eat mostly non-starchy vegetables, with some protein, a little unsaturated fat and a few carbohydrates.

- The three most relished texture notes are crispy/crunchy, creamy and chewy. Include these in every meal if possible.

- Eat something red or purple.

621

- And preferably eat something green as well.

- Take mouthfuls from different bowls/dishes, alternately, to surprise your mouth.

- Sip a pleasant, low Calorie liquid during meals if you wish.

- Preferably use chopsticks or heavy cutlery.

- Use mental imagery to picture the nutrients you're consuming, instead of picturing a lack of Calories. Think of low-Calorie meals as giving you more, not less— more health, more energy.

- Sit down to eat every meal; don't eat "on the run".

- Chew thoroughly.

- During meals take small sips of warm tea or other Calorie-sparse liquid from time to time, when you feel like it. "There's no concern that water will dilute the digestive juices or interfere with digestion. In fact, drinking water during or after a meal actually aids digestion. Water and other liquids help break down food so that your body can absorb the nutrients." [Mayo Clinic (2017)]

A DAY IN THE SATIETY DIET LIFESTYLE

Here's an example of the ideal daily regime for people following the Satiety Diet. Note that this is an IDEAL Satiety Diet day. In the real world, circumstances will not always permit ideal situations, but each day, try to get close. If you can't follow it exactly, that's fine. Just do the best you can, and be kind and forgiving to yourself!

AT THE COMMENCEMENT OF EACH WEEK

Plan your meals at the beginning of each week. Do your planning after you've eaten a satisfying meal, when you are not feeling hungry! Why? Because planning menus involves thinking about food, which is an eating trigger!

Go shopping when you're not hungry. Don't over-shop. Buy only as much as you need for the next few days, and only buy foods you won't regret eating.

A WORK DAY

A work day breakfast.

In the morning, wake up in your calm, clean, uncluttered house with an enclosed kitchen and no food on display. You might rise a little earlier than you used to, to make sure you have time for a leisurely breakfast,

If you're male, before breakfast is the ideal time to go for an early morning run or bicycle-ride, or engage in a floor workout at home, or go for a workout at the gym. According to research, if you're female, you should exercise after breakfast instead.

If you are not hungry yet, don't force yourself to eat breakfast. Instead, pack your breakfast in appropriately insulated containers and take it with you to work. Try to find a calm space where you can mindfully eat breakfast (or "brunch") later in the morning, when you are experiencing real hunger.

If you are hungry *before* you leave for work, read on . . .

Yesterday evening you prepared the breakfast table in advance. You laid out—
- A pretty tablecloth
- Condiments—sauces, spices, pepper etc. are encouraged
- Tall, slim tumblers
- Small plates and dishes in an assortment of shapes and colors
- Serviettes (table napkins)
- Heavy eating utensils (silverware) or chopsticks
- Ideally, even a small vase of fresh flowers!

623

Last night you may have even cooked some Satiety Porridge and stored in in the refrigerator in a non-plastic container, to allow it too cool overnight and build up resistant starch. You might also have set out any cooking utensils you need.

Now, prepare every part of your delicious, colorful, variety-rich, nutritious breakfast. Lay out all the food and drinks you are going to consume, all together on the table so that your eyes can see the total quantity of food you are about to incorporate into your body—for example:

- A tall, narrow tumbler containing your pre-meal 2 cups of carbonated water,
- A cup of coffee, green tea, or miso soup,
- A small bowl of "textured" creamy/crunchy porridge with nuts and legumes for protein, or a small plate of cooked free-range eggs on whole grain bread,

- A side-plate containing cooked tomatoes, spinach and mushrooms sprinkled with freshly-ground black pepper and chopped parsley,
- And perhaps a small portion of sweet-tasting low fructose "dessert" such as a wholegrain muffin with fresh or frozen blueberries, to finish the meal.

Such a breakfast consists of all the necessary macronutrients, 20%-25% protein, whole, complex carbohydrates, a small amount of "good" fat, plenty of colors and textures that are crunchy, chewy, crispy, creamy.

We know that soups and salads as starters can help boost satiety. However, you might not feel like eating a starter of soup or salad at breakfast time. That's fine. There's no need to force yourself.

All meals are an occasion. As late as possible before leaving for work, eat your leisurely breakfast taking a minimum of 30-45 minutes. Preferably an hour. Yes, this is new to you isn't it . . . ☺

You can, if you wish, play soft, relaxing music in the background as you sit down to enjoy your breakfast.

As you eat your breakfast, the main factors to aim for are:
- Eating while in a relaxed state
- Really appreciating the look and taste of the food (mindful eating). Focus on the food. Do not pick up a newspaper, phone or devices, do not have the TV switched on. Even if you eat one single dish/course/food item mindfully, it's better than nothing!
- Taking time over the meal
- Reaching satiation. If you reach satiation you shouldn't start to feel hungry again for a few hours.
- Allow at least 30-45 minutes to actually eat the food. An hour to an hour and a half is better. (This doesn't include preparation time.)
- Request that the people around you respect your time for eating and do not interrupt or make demands on you. In the best scenario, they would join you at the table, the conversation would be relaxed and topics would be pleasant.

After breakfast, pack the lunch and healthful snacks you prepared yesterday, ready to take with you to work (unless you choose to buy your lunch pre-prepared). Your portable food is packed in bags made of cotton or brown paper, or in plastic-free insulated containers made of stainless steel. If there are no small plates and dishes available at work, bring your own.

Walk to work or ride a bicycle if possible.

If you take public transport to work, distract yourself from looking at colorful, visually-appealing food advertisements along the way.

At work, take the stairs instead of the lift.

If your job is sedentary and involved long periods of sitting down, get up and move as often as possible—at least every half an hour. Consider setting a discreet alarm on your smartphone or watch or clock or computer, to remind you to stand up and walk around for at least few minutes.

A work day mid-morning.

In the middle of the morning, if you've tuned in to your body and you're sure you are REALLY hungry, eat a healthful snack. Don't eat just because everyone else is eating, or because you looked at the food vending machine, or because you smelled someone else's food, or because you feel bored or peckish.

Still want more food after eating your snack? Pull out your Weight Loss Toolkit and use anything you find useful. Practise some of the mind games you've learned in this book, too.

A work day lunch.

Eat lunch as late as possible—try for around 2pm. If your hunger is threatening to become ravenousness, or if your schedule is not flexible, by all means eat lunch a lot earlier. Don't let yourself get over-hungry. That's dangerous! It sends the wrong messages to your Inner Guardian.

Like your breakfast, your Satiety Diet lunch should consist of "whole foods" unprocessed or lightly-processed, containing all the macronutrients, with no artificial additives, with strong, appealing flavors, and with bright colors and interesting textures.

If you feel you need something sweet to reach satiation, finish your lunch with a small, sweet, low-fructose high-fiber, protein-rich treat.

And if you buy your lunch from a café , deli, or food store, choose to eat something different each day. Bored by your usual eatery's menu? Try another eatery. Ditch your preconceived notions that "I don't eat that"! Scared of eating something different? Take a deep breath and order it anyway. You never know—you might discover you like it after all.

If you have brought your home-made lunch to work, go somewhere pleasant and calm to eat it. If the weather suits, find a place outdoors, such as a park. Go alone or in the company of delightful people. Set out every course of your lunch in front of you before you eat. Mentally photograph the colors, the shapes, so that you can recall them later and remind your Inner Guardian of how much nutritious food you ate.

Lay out every course in front of you before you start. Take at least half an hour to eat it. Enjoy every bite slowly and mindfully, chewing it thoroughly, but not counting every chew or worrying about how you're chewing, or doing anything else that's annoying. Food is for enjoyment.

Reach satiation! If you do, you shouldn't feel hungry until at least mid-afternoon.

After lunch, continue to take regular breaks from sitting. Walk, fidget, climb stairs, and move as much as possible throughout the day. But don't make it a stressful obligation! Always be kind to yourself.

A work day mid-afternoon.

In the middle of the afternoon ask yourself if you feel genuinely hungry. If the answer is "yes", then eat a healthful Satiety Diet snack. Measure your hunger and aim to only eat when you are actually "hungry"—not simply "peckish" and not yet "ravenous".

Still thinking yearningly about food after your snack? Practise some of the mind tricks you've learned in this book. Use some of the strategies in *The Satiety Diet Weight Loss Toolkit* (book #2 in the Satiety Diet series), if you have access to this publication.

Around this time of day, stop consuming caffeine. Instead of drinking coffee or cola, go for herbal tea, weak black tea, water, or plain, unsweetened, carbonated water, perhaps with a twist of lemon or a sprig of mint. (Of course you've already cut out all soda drinks, including caffeine-laden ones, haven't you?) This will help ensure you get the good night's sleep that is so important for weight loss.

A work day evening.

The working day is over, and let's hope you've made it home without being bombarded with vivid images of food on advertising banners along the way.

Before the evening meal is a good time for men to take a brisk walk or engage in some other form of exercise. After the evening meal is a good time for women to take a brisk walk or do some other light exercise, be it ever so simple.

627

Eat dinner, the last main meal of the day, as early as you can. That is, as early as you feel genuinely hungry. Reach satiation! If you do, you shouldn't feel hungry for a few hours, at least.

While you're still feeling satiated, plan your breakfast for the following day (you might even make some porridge in advance), make sure all the ingredients and utensils are at hand, and set the breakfast table ready for tomorrow morning.

You might also prepare your lunch for the following day and store it in plastic-free containers in the refrigerator.

Then get out of the kitchen!

A work day later in the evening.

For many people, it is later in the evening that the danger period begins—the time for peckishness and nibbling; the time for watching TV and being bombarded with food ads.

And cooking shows. Turn off those cooking shows!

This is the time of day when your body should be peacefully digesting the last of your nutritious food, in readiness for powering down into sleep mode. It is NOT a time for loading up on more food.

If you feel peckish, distract yourself. Or clean your teeth, or rinse your mouth with mouthwash as a way of toning down your peckishness. Use the tools in *The Satiety Diet Weight Loss Toolkit* (book #2 in the Satiety Diet series).

Plan on going to bed with a fairly empty stomach. Don't go to bed feeling ravenous, however, or you're likely to sleep poorly, and poor sleep hinders weight loss.

Hungry before bed?

Gauge your feelings and aim to only eat when you are actually "hungry"—not simply "peckish" and not yet "ravenous".

If you really feel hungry just before bed, slowly eat a couple of low Calorie wholegrain crispbreads or some other form of energy-sparse carbohydrate. Carbs help you sleep. Studies show that "Dietary carbohydrate intake has been shown to increase the plasma concentration of tryptophan, a precursor of serotonin and sleep-inducing agent." [Afaghi et al., (2007).]

A work day—at bedtime.

Make your the bedroom perfect place for a good nights sleep. You've learned how to do that in this book.

Meditate for at least one minute.

Sleep well!

A NON-WORK DAY—VACATIONS, WEEKENDS ETC.

You have more options for a flexible schedule on days when you're not working. You can follow the Satiety Diet just as you would on a work day, but without the time restrictions. Being off work allows you free time to incorporate more movement and relaxation into your day. You could make time to:

- Meditate for a few minutes
- Go for a brisk walk in "nature".
- Sing
- Dance
- Visit friends
- Pursue your favorite hobbies
- Stay out of the kitchen unless you are actually preparing, storing or eating food!

As always, at each meal:

- Aim to include a variety of food textures (crispy chewy creamy etc), flavors (salty sweet etc.) and colors.
- Sit down at the table and look at all your food in dishes and plates laid out together.
- Relax, take time, chew, see the food, enjoy it fully, eat slowly so that food has time to be absorbed. Don't watch TV or read.
- Preferably begin meals with a starter of low-Calorie soup or salad. For convenience, soups can be made in advance and frozen in meal-sized portions.
- Include all the macronutrients—carbs, protein, fat—in the right proportions.
- Include 20%-25% protein, preferably plant-based.

- Include whole, complex carbohydrates, such as brown rice. Note that foods that combine carbs and protein include beans and lentils.
- Include as many NTS vegetables as you can manage. About 50% of your smaller-sized plate should be covered with NTS. vegetables. Remember the saying, "All non-vegetable foods exist to make vegetables taste good." Don't overdo your portions of starchy vegetables such as potatoes and corn.

PART EIGHT

EXERCISE

THE BENEFITS OF EXERCISE

EXERCISE IS MEDICINE

What if you could take a pill that, used regularly, gave you a slimmer, more toned body, an endorphin rush, an uplifted mood, better sleep and a longer, healthier life? It sounds like a miracle drug! What would you pay for something like that?

Well, it's free.

And, if taken the right way, it doesn't deliver any unwanted side effects.

"Exercise is medicine and physicians need to prescribe it!" proclaims the headline of a 2009 article in *The British Journal of Sports Medicine*. [Sallis (2009)]. The Academy of Medical Royal Colleges (UK) stated in its report, "Exercise: The Miracle Cure", that if physical activity was a drug, it would be classed as a wonder drug, so numerous are its positive effects on the body. [AMRC (2015)]

Scientific research shows that regular physical activity confers a huge range of health benefits. It's an essential tool for weight control, but it can also help protect against diabetes, hypertension, cancer, depression, osteoporosis and dementia. People who exercise regularly tend to live longer.

Physical exercise encourages the generation of new brain cells, slows down brain cell aging, improves the flow of nutrients to the brain and increases levels of dopamine and the other "feel good" neurotransmitters serotonin and norepinephrine. [Warburton et al., (2006)]

In 2007, the "Exercise Is Medicine" (EIM) initiative arose in the medical community. Supported by the American Medical Association and the American College of Sports Medicine, their initial aim was to "make the scientifically proven benefits of physical activity the standard in the U.S. health-care system." It has grown beyond the borders of the USA, however, and has become an international network.

Reframing: "Movement is medicine".

Some people associate the term "exercise" with arduous, painful routines such as lifting heavy weights in the gym, or running a marathon. Yet exercise can be pleasant, gentle, and part of daily life. Instead of saying "exercise is medicine" we can simply say "movement is medicine". Any movement you make is doing you good.

MOVEMENT IS A POWERFUL WEIGHT LOSS TOOL

Exercise is a great weight loss tool because it can:
- Curb your appetite
- Distract you from thoughts of food
- Alleviate stress, thus bringing down cortisol levels
- Reduce food cravings
- Prime your body to burn more Calories even when you're not exercising

Burn fat, not just food.

"Most people who are obese are metabolically inflexible," said Dr. Collins of the University of Surrey, in an 2016 interview with *The Daily Mail*. "They are constantly burning glucose and never make the switch to fat. Exercise is healthy because it stresses the muscles and forces them to become better at managing fuels, and switching between fuels. You can manage your food and nutrients better because you've got the ability to switch between carbohydrate and fat." [Davies (2016)]

Note that working out is essential for good health, and it can help with weight loss, but it cannot make you lose weight if your diet is too rich in Calories.

Movement helps regulate appetite.

When you exercise, you can use up the Calories from your fat stores. Regular exercise primes your bodys to become more efficient at using those fat stores, which in turn can help curb hunger. Physical activity also exerts an effect on your appetite by influencing your body's levels of leptin, ghrelin and insulin.

Vigorous movement.

Intense exercise, such as heavy weight training or high-intensity interval training (HIT), can curb your appetite.

As part of a 2013 study published in *The American Journal of Clinical Nutrition*, volunteers in a laboratory jogged for an hour on a treadmill. Before and straight afterwards, the researchers measured their levels of ghrelin (the hunger hormone) and peptide YY (a hormone associated with decreased appetite). Running caused a reduction in ghrelin and a surge in peptide YY. [Crabtree et al., (2014)]

The more vigorously you work out, the longer the benefit of appetite suppression tends to last. Generally, this satiating effect lasts for about an hour, but the good news is that moving frequently throughout the day ". . . appears to help restore sensitivity to brain neurons that control satiety," according to Neil King, Ph.D., professor of human movement studies at Queensland University of Technology. This means that the more often you move, the better you are able tune in to your natural satiety signals.

Low-intensity cardiovascular movement.

Low-intensity cardiovascular exercise includes such activities as jogging, rowing or swimming. You know you are engaging in low intensity exercise if you can still talk comfortably with your exercise partners. Some people mistakenly avoid low intensity cardiovascular exercise, because they have heard it rumored that "it won't make you thin because it makes you hungry."

Studies show that it tends to be only lean people whose appetite increases after cardiovascular exercise, because their low-fat stores need to be re-stocked with energy. On the other hand, obese people, whose fat stores are excessive, don't automatically get hungrier after exercise. They don't spontaneously seek for Calories to replace the ones they've just used up. Their Inner Guardians seem to know that those Calories can easily be spared!

"… in the long term there appears to be no automatic increase in energy intake to compensate for an exercise induced energy deficit in overweight and obese individuals," say the authors of a review published in *Current Obesity Reports*. [Caudwell et al. (2013)]

A 2013 study in the journal Appetite found that when workers went for a 15-minute walk, rather than taking a 15 minute sedentary break, they ate 50% fewer snacks during the working day. [Oh et al., (2013)]

In a 2010 research article published by the Public Library of Science, it was found that exercise can increase your brain's sensitivity to the hormones, insulin and leptin, which help to regulate appetite. This increases the likelihood of satiety, which leads to lower food consumption. [Ropelle et al., (2010)]

Regular exercise can prevent weight regain.

After weight loss, ". . . regular exercise counters some of the biological responses to dieting that drive weight regain," say the authors of a 2011 study published in The American Journal of Physiology. ". . . regular exercise remains the most potent strategy for successful long-term weight maintenance after Calorie-restricted weight loss." [Steig et al., (2011)]

When you want to maintain your new, trim figure after losing weight, exercise is an important key.

Exercise burns fat even while you sleep

Exercise not only makes you feel good, it also helps you burn carbohydrates and fat. It's mainly carbs that fuel you while you're working out, and your body doesn't replace those carbs for around 22 hours. Meanwhile, it continues to burn fat after you finish exercising. Exercise's fat-burning effect lasts for around 24 hours, and keeps going when you are at rest, or even asleep.

Having said that, it is important to note that this fat-burning after-effect works best after really vigorous exercise, rather than light activity such as strolling or gardening.

Exercise alone is not enough for weight loss.

It's been said that losing weight is 90% due to diet and 10% due to exercise—and this is pretty accurate! Exercise is vital for good health and it does contribute to weight loss, but it's important to remember that for weight loss you should not only exercise but also eat wisely.

TIPS FOR MOVING YOUR BODY

EXERCISE CAN BE GENTLE AND FUN!

According to fitness advocate Leslie Sansone, reality television shows give the impression that the only way to get fit is to undergo an exhausting and painful workout session. She says, "There's this Biggest Loser idea out there that if you're not throwing up and crying you're not getting fit."

Exercise doesn't have to involve strenuous exertion, so stop panicking and read on!

START WITH A WARM-UP

A warm-up is a short session of light physical activity, gradually increasing in intensity. You should always do a warm-up before an exercise session. Its purpose is to elevate your heart rate and breathing rate, to prepare your body for activity, and to warm up your muscles, which can be more susceptible to injury when cold. The warm-up should never be missed. It is an essential part of any exercise program.

Some exercises appropriate for warm-ups include walking, slow jogging, relaxed swimming, cycling on a stationary bike, or low-intensity aerobic dance. How long your warm-up session lasts depends on how fit you are, but in general it should take about five to ten minutes. After your warm-up your skin should be moist with a light sweat.

The Australian Institute of Sport recommends, "For most athletes, 5 to 10 minutes [for a warm-up] is enough. However in cold weather the duration of the warm-up should be increased."

After you've warmed up, do your stretching exercises before your exercise session.

636

BEGIN YOUR PROGRAM MODERATELY

If you're new to physical exertion, start exercising gently and gradually increase the intensity over time. When people decide to start exercising, sometimes they can get over-enthusiastic and overdo it. If you're a couch potato and you decide to go for a long, fast run, you're going to feel sore and exhausted afterwards. This is likely to put you off exercising. Your mind will associate exercise with pain!

What's more, if you're unfit and begin exercising vigorously you might strain your muscles or cause injuries. More pain is the result. And again, this can put you off exercising.

Begin any new exercise routine with "baby steps'. Start with short, gentle workouts. Over a period of weeks, make each session longer and more vigorous. Give your body time to adapt. It's worth it!

MOVE OFTEN

Current research suggests that moving more often, even if it's gentle movement, is far more beneficial for weight loss and good health than being sedentary for long periods alternating with bouts of extremely vigorous exercise.

The body's systems thrive on constant motion.

In other words, the houseperson/housewife who moves about all day cooking, cleaning, shopping and child-minding but never goes to the gym is getting more health benefits than the office worker who sits at a desk all day then engages in a punishing gym workout/bike ride/boxing session three times a week.

Furthermore, five minutes of High Intensity Interval Training (HIIT) exercise once a day is better for health and weight loss than doing the same exercise once a week for 45 minutes. (That said, a vigorous workout three times a week is way better than no exercise at all!)

Sitting for long periods combined with being inactive carries the greatest risk of dying early! People who sit for eight hours a day, but are physically active the rest of the time, have a much lower risk of premature death compared with generally inactive people who sit for fewer hours per day. Exercising briskly every day can reduce the risks of having a sedentary job. [Ekelund et al. (2016)]

637

Break up periods of protracted sitting.

What if your job involves a lot of sitting? How can you stop all this inactivity from messing with your blood sugars and increasing your appetite?

There is a solution.

Studies have found that breaking up protracted sitting by getting up and moving around every 20-30 minutes can decrease blood sugar spikes after meals.

Obese adult volunteers took part in a 2012 study published in the journal *Diabetes Care*. They were divided into three group, all of whom sat around, inactive for several hours.

- A "control" group of people simply continued to stay seated for a long time, without taking any breaks.
- The people in a second group got up every 20 minutes and went for a walk of "light intensity" for 2 minutes before sitting down again.
- A third group got up every 20 minutes and went for a walk of "moderate intensity" for 2 minutes before sitting down again.

After measuring the volunteers' blood sugar and insulin levels both before and after the trial, the researchers concluded that "Interrupting sitting time with short bouts of light- or moderate-intensity walking lowers postprandial [after-meal] glucose and insulin levels in overweight/obese adults. This may improve glucose metabolism…"

Biochemist Katy Bowman, author of the book "Move Your DNA: Restore Your Health Through Natural Movement", writes, "'Actively Sedentary' is a new category of people who are fit for one hour but sitting around the rest of the day. You can't offset 10 hours of stillness with one hour of exercise."

Chris Clarke says, "I work at a desk job that involves a lot of sitting. I can sit for hours uninterrupted, because I get so involved with what I am doing that I don't notice time passing. I now set the alarm on my smartphone or computer, so that it goes off every 30 minutes, reminding me to stand up and walk around a bit. Maybe it's all in my mind, but since I started doing this, I don't feel as ridiculously hungry after meals as I used to."

The dangers of being a "couch potato".

Being a couch potato can mess with your body's chemistry. Sitting or lying around for long periods, barely moving, can play havoc with your blood glucose levels.

A 2011 study published in *Medicine & Science in Sports & Exercise* showed that prolonged physical inactivity can lead to a spike in blood sugar levels after meals.

The blood sugar levels of healthy active young adults were monitored continuously while they ate their meals as usual but changed their activity levels. For a few days they were as active as usual, then for another few days they sat around relaxing on a couch and barely moving.

After the sessions of lazing around, when they ate their normal meals their blood sugar rose significantly higher. [Mikus et al., (2012)]

High blood sugar levels can trigger the release of floods of insulin. In turn, this can increase hunger.

So . . . keep moving as much as possible, as you go about your daily activities!

WHAT IF YOU DON'T HAVE TIME TO EXERCISE?

Many people say they don't exercise because they don't have time for it. But is that just an excuse?

Chris Clark writes, "My grandmother used to say, "We make time for the things that really matter to us". In other words—no-one is really "too busy" it's all about priorities.

We've discussed this topic earlier in this book, but it's worth repeating for readers who prefer to "browse" rather than reading from beginning to end.

Even if you are time-poor, there are ways you can get enough exercise to lose weight and become healthier. Small changes during your day can add up to big benefits.

Examples:

- When talking on the phone, walk around the room instead of sitting down.
- Walk to the local shops, or ride a pushbike, instead of driving. If you live close to your workplace, walk or cycle to work.
- Invest in a mini-cycling machine. You can sit in your chair and use it while you watch TV.
- If your knees and hips are up to it, use the stairs instead of elevators.
- Even when you're sitting in a chair, you can still perform buttock clenches!
- Practise high-intensity interval training (HIIT). More about HIIT later. Read on!

DON'T SABOTAGE YOURSELF!

Don't sabotage your exercise regime by giving yourself food "rewards". Diet and exercise work together to enable weight loss. Some people exercise vigorously for hours, but then "reward" themselves by consuming food that contains more Calories than they just expended. As a result, they fail to lose weight. Running two miles burns about 240 Calories. That's the same number of Calories you'd get from eating a small chocolate bar. Rewarding yourself with junk food is self-defeating. Use non-food rewards instead.

BEWARE OF UNDOING THE BENEFITS OF EXERCISE

Exercise is an incredibly valuable weight loss tool but like all weight loss tools, it's not the one and only solution.

If you've been jogging and skipping and boxing for hours every week with very little noticeable effect on your waistline, the problem might be that:

- You're overestimating the number of Calories and the amount of fat you can burn through exercise. Fat is very energy-dense! To burn off a single pound of fat you'd have to run for approximately 30 miles (48 km).
- You're "rewarding" yourself for your workouts by eating Calorie-rich foods. It may only take a candy bar and a milkshake to restore the Calories you burned during a hard, half-hour run. Yes, you've speeded up your metabolism and burned Calories and worked hard, but if you want to lose weight, don't undo all the good you've done.
- You're cutting down on normal everyday activity because you've worked out. For example, if you've just been to the gym you might decide you deserve to take the elevator instead of the stairs.

DIFFERENT FORMS OF MOVEMENT

AEROBIC EXERCISE

Aerobic exercise, otherwise known as "cardio" exercise, is any movement that significantly boosts your heart rate, thus improving the body's use of oxygen[46]. It suppresses appetite by influencing appetite hormones.

In 2008, researchers found that aerobic exercise dampened the appetite more effectively than nonaerobic exercise.

"A vigorous 60-minute workout on a treadmill affects the release of two key appetite hormones, ghrelin and peptide YY, while 90 minutes of weight lifting affects the level of only ghrelin. The research shows that aerobic exercise is better at suppressing appetite than nonaerobic exercise and provides a possible explanation for how that happens.

---

46 Originally the word "aerobic" was coined in 1863 by Louis Pasteur, from the Greek aero, meaning "air" and bios, meaning "life". Back then, it meant "living only in the presence of oxygen." It still means that in scientific terms, but in 1968 by a U.S. doctor by the name of Kenneth H. Cooper added a new meaning. It now refers to sustained activities that require moderate to high oxygen intake.

This line of research may eventually lead to more effective ways to use exercise to help control weight." [Broom et al., (2008)]

This doesn't mean that you should drop non-cardio exercise! Any form of exercise aids weight loss, and non-cardio exercise such as weight-lifting increases muscle mass, which helps you use up Calories even while you're at rest.

WEIGHT-LIFTING

Weight-lifting can counteract the effects of menopause and aging.

As you grow older it usually becomes harder to lose weight. Both men and women experience loss of muscle tissue as they age. The energy the body would have used to build muscle may instead be turned into fat. It takes more energy for your body to maintain muscle than fat, so people with more muscle tend to have a faster metabolic rate, which is the rate at which it converts food into energy..

It is thought that the decreased levels of estrogen in the female body after menopause might causes weight gain. Lower levels of estrogen may decrease the body's metabolic rate.

The solution for both women and men is to regularly lift heavy objects. Weight-lifting (be it only a heavy bag of groceries, a toddler, a large pot plant or a basket of wet laundry) helps you maintain your muscles, and helps speed up your metabolism. As always, start with a light weight and gradually progress to heavier weights.

MOTIVATION TO EXERCISE

TECHNOLOGY CAN MAKE YOU LAZY

Why don't we exercise as much as our ancestors?

There's a pretty good chance that up until the beginning of the 20th century, none of your ancestors owned a car. Even until the later half of the 20th century, in the Western world, if people privately owned a means of transport there was generally no more than one car per family.

Chris Clarke writes: "I was a child in the 1960s. My grandparents did not own a car, so they walked everywhere or used public transport. My parents did not own a car either, until I was about eight or nine years old. Everyone walked to the shops to buy food. We walked to the railway-station or the bus stop. We walked to school and back, and to and from the public library. We walked to our friends' houses to visit them, even if they lived in a distant suburb. And as we walked, we often carried heavy loads of shopping or school books. We thought nothing of it, because that's how it had always been.

"My parents saved up and eventually bought a family car, but they did not have the time to be unpaid cab-drivers and deliver their children all over town whenever we wanted to visit friends or go shopping. Thus my generation continued to do a lot of walking.

"I remember that in those days, suburban sidewalks and footpaths were busy with people of all ages, walking up and down, carrying bags, or stopping to chat to neighbours over the fence. Kids would ride bicycles. (Dogs and cats roamed freely, too!) Occasionally a lone car or truck would go humming up the road, or (and this was very exciting) a motorcycle. These days, those same footpaths I trod during my childhood are deserted, and the roads are swarming with vehicles."

In modern, technologically advanced societies, people move around a lot less than their ancestors did. They own household appliances to save them from doing vigorous activities such as doing the laundry by hand, squeezing the water out of washed garments by turning the handle of a mangle, or beating the dust out of carpets.

Our activity levels are lower but our appetites have stayed the same, and the food available to us—while it might be just as Calorie-dense—is easier to obtain, more attractively packaged, and often enlivened with artificial additives to make it taste better.

Thus in general, we're fatter than our forebears were.

"Technological changes associated with cultural evolution almost exclusively reduce the energy requirements of human labor. In general, cultural evolution has meant the harnessing of greater amounts of energy through technology (one aspect of the mode of production). In order to prevent obesity, people in developed societies must burn energy through daily workouts rather than daily work." [Brown (1991)]

HOW CAN YOU STOP HATING EXERCISE?

Exercise really does make you feel good, but there are people who don't believe that. Many people hate exercise. If you do too, there are many reasons why this could be so:

- Your body may have grown used to inactivity, so that it hurts to move vigorously. *The solution:* Begin with a short, gentle exercise routine and gradually increase the duration and intensity over the following weeks.

- You might find it boring. *The solution:* Choose a form of exercise that interests you and stimulates your mind. Bicycling outdoors, for example, can give you lots to look at.

- You might find it exhausting. *The solution:* Eat well, drink enough water, get enough sleep, start with gentle exercises, and be kind to yourself.

- You could feel that society expects impossibly high standards of fitness. *The solution:* Remind yourself that those images of buff bodies are unrealistic.

- You might have watched those "reality" TV shows in which obese people are put through grueling exercise routines to the point of fainting or vomiting. This shows exercise in a bad light. *The solution:* Remind yourself that those shows are constructed with maximum drama to attract viewers, not to give a realistic formula for weight loss. Exercise should never make you sick.

- If you are overweight, you might feel ashamed of your body and be reluctant to exercise in public. *The solution:* Exercise in the privacy of your home or join a small, private workout group of like-minded people.

- You might have overdone a work-out in the past, and suffered from aching muscles and exhaustion. *The solution:* Remind yourself that exercise done the right way makes you feel GOOD in the long run. A little muscular stiffness is a great sign that you are getting results, but exercise should never be really painful.

- If you choose to work out in a way you find unenjoyable you are unlikely to continue exercising. *The solution:* Choose an activity that you enjoy—for example, dancing to music.

- Pain can put you off exercising. *The solution:* See your doctor, visit a physical therapist or join a "clinical Pilates" class.

- Some people think it costs too much money to exercise. *The solution:* Exercise is free. Wherever you are, your body is there too; you don't have to go to a special place, such as a gym, to exercise it. You can do gym-free, equipment-free workouts in your own home. Simply walking around is one of the best exercises, too.
- The most common excuse for not exercising is lack of time. *Time-saving solutions can include:*
  - HIIT (High Intensity Interval Training)
  - Fidgeting more often throughout the day
  - Incidental exercise as part of your day

TIPS TO MOTIVATE YOU TO MOVE MORE OFTEN:

- Think positively. When you exercise, think positive thoughts such as, "The more I do this the easier it gets." Which is actually true!

- Know you're doing yourself good. Keep in mind the fact that every time you move, you're benefiting your body.

- Know that you're also benefiting your own mental health! Exercise can lift your spirits and help combat depression and anxiety.

- Choose exercises you enjoy. The best exercise is one that gives you some pleasure. If you enjoy it, you're more likely to keep doing it regularly.

- Move to pleasant music and feel the rhythm. You think you hate moving? No you don't! You probably love to dance when no one is watching! We all love moving to the beat of good music. So turn up your favorite music and dance!

- Be kind to yourself. Don't beat yourself up if you don't do your exercises every single day. Just do the best you can.

- Invest in a group fitness tracker. A fitness tracker is a wearable device that monitors your movements. It records your daily physical activity, such as the number of steps you take, or the altitude to which you climb. It may also record your heart rate and other health indicators. Group fitness trackers can be linked, via an app on your computer, phone or other device, to fitness trackers belonging to your friends and family. In this way you can compare, compete with and encourage each other.

- Exercise in nature. Whether you hike through wilderness, or walk in the park, go paddle-boarding or surfing at the beach, or simply do some yoga in the garden, surrounding yourself with nature and The Great Outdoors has been shown to have multiple health benefits. The joy of immersing yourself in the natural world can also be very motivating.

- Revel in feeling good! Believe it or not, the more you move, the better you'll start to feel! And feeling good can be a great reason to move even more.

- Take pride in feeling strong! As you exercise you'll feel changes in your body. It will become firmer as your muscles become toned. Your shape will change (for the better!) Things that used to be hard for you to do will become easy. You'll enjoy feeling strong, capable and confident.

- Take part in group exercise activities led by an instructor.

Group exercise
Types of group exercise.
Group exercise classes can include activities such as:
- Pilates®
- Aerobics
- Spinning (stationery bicycling)
- Weight lifting to music (sometimes called "pump" or "resistance training".)
- Air-boxing (also known as shadow boxing)
- Dance
- Yoga
- Step aerobics (stepping up and down on a small platform, in time to music)

Benefits of group exercise.

The American College of Sports Medicine advises that, "Group exercise offers a variety of benefits you might miss out on if you choose to work out on your own."

These benefits can include:

- Having fun.
- Social interaction and encouragement from fellow participants
- Performing a safe workout designed by professionals. "An appropriately designed class includes warm-up, cool-down and flexibility in addition to the conditioning section," according to the American College of Sports Medicine.
- Performing an effective workout.
- Motivation to exercise regularly. "…the consistency in scheduling offered by group exercise programs allows participants to choose a time and schedule it in their planner as they do other daily activities."
- Feeling accountable to others to turn up at classes (another form of motivation).
- There's no need for you to learn in advance how to exercise—your instructor teaches you.
- There's less likelihood of your omitting your least favorite exercises
- And there's more likelihood that you'll increase the intensity of your workout (through competition with others, or a sense of accountability)
- The opportunity to network with like-minded people who are keen on health and fitness
- The opportunity to tailor exercise times according to your daily schedule. Classes may be available before or after work, for example.
- A wide choice of different types of exercise.
- A variety of movements within the exercise type. Professional class instructors generally change or vary their routines from week to week, to make sure that classes remain interesting to participants.

EXERCISE WITHOUT A "WORKOUT SESSION"

Working out at the gym for an hour or so 3 to 4 times a week is one way to get fit and burn fat. But if for some reason you can't get to the gym, or you can't afford it, or you hate gyms, there are other ways to exercise that really don't need a lot of willpower or gym membership fees!

FIDGETING

To lose weight, stay active. Organized workouts are not the only way your body expends Calories. Even simple, light exercise does the job. Research shows that small, frequent movements can actually burn as many Calories as vigorous, infrequent exercise.

Mayo Clinic scientists have a term for burning Calories without consciously doing exercise. They call it "non-exercise activity thermogenesis", or NEAT.

People who fidget a lot are burning Calories without being aware of it. Fidgeting seems like a very minor way of moving the body, but any movement uses Calories and if you fidget enough, you could use up quite a lot of energy!

What is fidgeting?

Some examples include:
- foot-tapping
- finger-drumming
- pacing
- changing position
- crossing and re-crossing your legs when sitting
- toe-wriggling
- jiggling

"Eight hours of vigorous foot-tapping in the office, for instance, may equal one work-out session in the gym, or 30 minutes of squash. And involuntary foot-tappers have been known to keep going for such long periods without even being aware of what they are doing." [Dobson (1999)]

INCIDENTAL ACTIVITY

All movement burns Calories, whether you recognize that movement as exercise or not! You can really boost your weight loss and movement levels by adding "incidental" activity to your daily routine.

Incidental activity is any activity accumulated bit by bit over the course of the day, as part of your normal daily routine. It's unplanned exercise. Examples include such simple activities as strolling around while you're talking on the phone instead of sitting down; climbing up stairs; walking between stores at a shopping center; getting up from your desk to make a cup of coffee; maintaining posture when sitting; or simply standing in one place. Like fidgeting, these can be classified as NEAT activities—Non Exercise Activity Thermogenesis

Every movement adds to your daily total. The more often you move and elevate your heart rate, the more energy your body burns.

People who naturally perform frequent, low-intensity movements dispersed over the course of the day are better off than those who remain still for long periods.

Each time you move, you encourage your bodys' vascular systems to deliver nutrients to your cells and carry away waste from those cells. [Biswas et al., (2015)]

Adding incidental activity to your day.

To exercise more without workout sessions, you can do the following for free:

- Instead of trying to park your car as close as possible to your destination, park further away and walk.
- Think of housework as exercise. That way you get a clean house as well as burning up Calories!
- Play games with your kids or the dog, indoors or outdoors.
- Walk somewhere that you'd normally drive to. Instead of taking the car, walk or ride a pushbike to close-by venues such as the local store, post office or library. Walk or cycle to work,

or take public transport.

- Walk around while you're talking on the phone.
- Keep a pair of walking shoes in your car. That way, you can use them to take a walk whenever the opportunity arises.
- You can do a lot of miles when you're forced to wait for something—for example, if you're in an airport waiting for a plane to arrive.
- Use the stairs instead of the elevator or escalator.
- On work days, instead of sitting around at lunchtime take a 20 minute walk.

For more suggestions, look under the heading, "Thrifty exercising outside the home".

FOUR TYPES OF EXERCISE

Exercise can be roughly grouped into four categories:

A) CARDIOVASCULAR EXERCISE

The word "cardiovascular" means "relating to the heart and blood vessels." Among fitness fans it's often referred to as "cardio", and it is also known as aerobic exercise. Cardiovascular exercise not only burns Calories, it is also good for your heart. It includes high intensity interval training, low intensity "steady state" cardio exercise, dancing, cycling, running, fast swimming, brisk hiking, in-line skating, aerobics, jumping rope etc. Anything that gets your heart beating faster!

B) RESISTANCE TRAINING

Also known as "weight training", this form of exercise involves lifting or pressing weights such as dumbbells. Particular muscle groups are targeted, such as the muscles in the upper arms or the thighs. Weight-lifting stimulates your body's production of more metabolically active tissue. When your muscle-mass increases, your metabolism gets moving too. This means that even when you're at rest, your body is burning Calories.

It is best to do resistance training at least three days a week, allowing a day of rest for each muscle group between sessions, so that muscles can recover. According to exercise physiologist and dietician Joanne Turner, every kilo of extra muscle you develop by doing resistance training will burn off an extra kilo's worth of fat per year.

Technique is everything. Doing weight training exercises correctly with light weights is better than doing them badly with heavy ones.

You can do this type of exercise at home.

- Buy a set of dumbbells or resistance bands. (You can substitute plastic bottles filled with water if this equipment is beyond your budget.)
- Choose a dumbbell weight or resistance level that you find really hard to manage after eight repetitions of an exercise.
- Using these tools, press-up, pull-up, squat, and lunge eight times on each side of your body.
- Repeat three times.

C) CORE STRENGTHENING

The "muscular core" of the body is located in your midsection. It includes every muscle in your front, back and sides. Muscles include the *transverse abdominis* (TVA), the *erector spinae*, the obliques and the lower *latissimi dorsi* muscles ("lats"). These muscles are your body's stabilizers. You can strengthen these muscles and improve your balance with core training workouts such as yoga, Pilates, stand-up paddle-boarding and balancing on an unstable surface.

D) STRETCHING

Yes, stretching can be considered an exercise even though it's slow and gentle. Stretching your muscles is essential for keeping them flexible, strong, and healthy. You need to be supple to maintain a good range of motion in your joints. Without stretching, your muscles can shorten and tighten. The best time to stretch is when your body has warmed up and your muscles are pliable. Do some light "warm up" exercises before any training session, followed by some gentle stretches. Then repeat the stretches just after exercising, when the body is still warm.

Here's another benefit of stretching—it can actually help you burn Calories! The BBC TV show "Trust Me, I'm A Doctor," in conjunction with Dr. Ian Lahart of Wolverhampton University, asked ten volunteers to take part in a stretching study. The researchers found that "passive stretching" (i.e. having your muscles stretched by someone else) lowered their blood sugar levels by 23%! It boosted their heart rates by 17% and increased the number of Calories they were burning by 126%. Just by getting someone else to stretch their limbs for them, they used up almost 100 extra Calories per hour. [BBC Two (2016)]

Dr. Lahart suggests that if people did their own stretches, they would get an even greater benefit. Who'd have thought that simply stretching could use up Calories and improve blood glucose levels? Stretching is easy to do and can be performed almost anywhere— even while sitting down and reading this book!

Note that it's important to warm up your muscles before you stretch. This makes them more elastic and less likely to tear. As mentioned earlier, warm-ups are gentle exercises that raise your heart rate and get your blood flowing.

The ideal exercise routine includes daily activities from all four of these categories. The ideal exercise routine also begins with gentle exercises of a short duration, particularly if you're unfit. Don't start exercising vigorously if you're not used to it—you could hurt yourself! Gradually increase the intensity and duration of exercise as your fitness increases.

THE BENEFITS OF SIMPLY WALKING
Walking? Just do it!

WALK OFF THAT WEIGHT

You don't have to push yourself to the limit working out at the gym to lose weight. You don't have to do High Intensity Interval Training either. HIIT is suggested for people who don't have much time to exercise, or who prefer HIIT for other reasons.

However if you can spare 20 minutes a day to get slimmer and fitter, take a walk! You don't even have to go outdoors. Many people with wearable fitness trackers say they simply walk around the house to get their "step count" up, if the weather is inclement, or if darkness has fallen, or if they're simply having a bad hair day!

If you choose to do only ONE exercise, make it walking. Walking is the defining movement of being human. Cardiovascular exercises like running, and resistance training exercises like weightlifting can help you reach specific goals, but their effects on the body are not as broad as walking.

Walking is one of the best exercises for weight loss because:
- It can be done almost anywhere, almost anytime
- It can be calming and reduce stress
- It allows you time to reflect and be mindful
- It improves insulin sensitivity
- It burns Calories and helps with weight control
- While you're walking you're less likely to be eating
- Like any other exercise, it can lift your mood
- Like any other exercise, it can improve your sleep
- You can do it at any fitness level
- It makes you feel great
- You can walk sociably, with friends, pets, family or co-workers
- You don't need special gym clothes or equipment for it
- It improves your circulation
- It is easier on the joints than high-impact exercise like running
- You can do it no matter how old you are (health permitting!)

WALKING REALLY DOES USE UP CALORIES!

Many people think that walking doesn't burn many Calories. It's true that it doesn't use up energy at the rate of, say, running, or playing squash, or jumping rope; but if it's done daily, briskly and for at least 20 minutes at a time, it can, over time, make a significant difference to your waistline. [Ludlow & Weyand (2015)]

HOW TO MOTIVATE YOURSELF TO WALK REGULARLY

Unless you are fairly self-disciplined you may not walk every day. Social motivation is a powerful force, so join a walking group, or walk with a friend, or take your dog for a walk. You could also join an online weight loss community to share your walking experiences, milestones and photographs.

USING A TREADMILL FOR WEIGHT LOSS

In 2015, 27-year-old Alasdair Wilkins lost 100 pounds (45kg) just by walking. Alasdair was a student of science and medical journalism at the University of North Carolina, USA. His weight was 285 pounds when he decided to start walking on a treadmill every day, by himself at home, while watching streamed TV shows on a portable device to pass the time. He would walk uphill, at a brisk pace, for about an hour every day. Every day without fail, for nine months! Aside from the walking, he did not do much else to help his weight loss. The only adjustment he made to his diet was that he simply ate smaller portions of the same foods he had always enjoyed.

The point is, walking helped Alasdair lost weight because he liked it.

"I just found something that I enjoyed doing and that worked for me," said Alasdair. "What works for some won't work for others. The big mistake people make is assuming that there is one right way for everyone to lose weight. It varies from person to person."

He says he did not have to restrain himself from eating and he never felt deprived.

"I didn't lose 100 pounds because I have amazing willpower," he says. "There's 26 years of evidence to show that I have very mediocre willpower. I just found a routine that I actually enjoyed and stuck with it." [Wilkins (2016)]

THE MANY HEALTH BENEFITS OF WALKING

Walking for at least half an hour every day is associated not only with weight loss but also with many health other benefits, including:

- Improved insulin sensitivity [Audelin et al., (2012)]
- Decreased body weight and fat mass, and increased cardio-respiratory fitness [Riesco et al., (2010)]
- Lowered blood pressure and triglycerides (blood fats) [Miyashita et al., (2008)]
- Extended longevity. [Harmon (2011)]

FOR HOW LONG SHOULD YOU WALK, AND HOW OFTEN?

On his TV show "The Doctor Who Gave up Drugs", Dr. Chris van Tulleken recommends taking a brisk walk five times a week for a minimum of 30 minutes to improve general health.

Weight Watchers™ also recommends walking for a minimum of 30 minutes per day, starting with shorter, gentler walks.

"If you've been inactive," they say on their website, "fifteen minutes of walking three to four times a week may be plenty for your first few weeks … Then increase the frequency, aiming for a 30-to 60-minute walk each day of the week. Gradually raise your intensity level by walking on inclines, with hand weights or on wet sand."

HOW BRISKLY SHOULD YOU WALK?

As your fitness levels increase, gradually build to a pace as fast as you can manage without discomfort. This is the best level for burning Calories efficiently. You should be breathing faster, but not so fast that you would not be able to hold a conversation with a walking companion. By the time you finish the walk you should feel tired and be perspiring a little. You shouldn't feel worn out.

HOW MANY STEPS SHOULD YOU TAKE PER DAY?

Now that relatively low-cost, wearable fitness trackers are readily available, it's possible to count how many steps you take per day. Many fitness and weight loss gurus recommend taking 10,000 steps every day. But where does this number come from?

"In the 1960s, a researcher in Japan discovered that most people took fewer than 4,000 steps per day. He found that increasing those steps to 10,000 could improve overall health. It was a nice, round number; it gained momentum and before long 10,000 steps became a worldwide phenomenon. The issue is that 10,000 steps is often mistaken as a magic number—the key to staving off diseased caused by inactivity—when, in actual fact, it's a basic guideline." [White (2017)]

The step-count evidence is conflicting. A 2017 study in the *International Journal of Obesity* examined postal employees in Scotland. Comparing the wellbeing of those who delivered letters and packages by walking the streets from house to house, with that of staff who sat at desks to perform their duties, they found that there was a significant difference in waist circumference and risk of heart disease. The walkers were—as expected—healthier and slimmer than the sedentary workers. This research also uncovered an interesting statistic—the optimum number of steps per day for best health and fitness appeared to be 15,000. [Tigbe et al., (2017)]

Do you really have to walk 10,000 steps a day?

TV journalist and presenter Dr. Michael Mosley is not a big fan of trying to take at least 10,000 steps per day. He makes allowances for the frailty of human willpower. Late in 2017 he teamed up with Professor Rob Copeland from Sheffield Hallam University to perform a small experiment on volunteers fitted with fitness tracking devices. They wanted to see how walking 10,000 steps per day compared to a regime called "Active 10". "Active 10" involves doing three 10-minute bouts of heart-rate-raising exercise each day. The exercise can be as simple as a brisk walk, as long as it gets your heart pounding. You count the minutes, but not the number of steps you take.

The researchers found that:

- It was easier for people to achieve three brisk, 10 minute walks per day than 10,000 steps.
- Despite the fact that the volunteers doing "Active 10" spent less time walking than the 10,000-step-volunteers, they did better at making their hearts beat faster. They did 30% more moderate-to-vigorous physical activity, which was a better health outcome.

GET GOOD WALKING SHOES

Have your walking shoes properly fitted to the size and shape of your feet. Good walking shoes include features that may not be built into running shoes or other sports shoes.

The Mayo Clinic recommends the following features for the ideal pair of walking shoes [Mayo Clinic (2017)]:

- **Achilles tendon protector**. Reduces stress on the Achilles tendon by locking the shoe around the heel.
- **Heel collar**. Cushions the ankle and ensures proper fit.
- **Upper**. Holds the shoe on your foot and is usually made of leather, mesh or synthetic material. Mesh allows better ventilation and is lighter weight.
- **Insole**. Cushions and supports your foot and arch. Removable insoles can be laundered or taken out to dry between walking sessions.
- **Gel, foam or air mid-sole**. All of these materials cushion and reduce impact when your foot strikes the ground.
- **Out-sole**. Makes contact with the ground. Grooves and treads can help maintain traction.
- **Toe box**. Provides space for the toes. A roomy and round toe box helps prevent calluses.

WALK IN NATURAL SURROUNDINGS

In our section on Stress Reduction we discuss "forest bathing"—the therapy of simply being in a forest.

Walking in any peaceful natural environment, not just forests, can do more than just relieve stress and provide fat-burning exercise. Being outdoors is good medicine.

A 2012 study published in *The Proceedings of the National Academy of Sciences* showed that 90 minutes of walking through a natural environment had quite an amazing physiological and psychological effect on a group of volunteers. Brain scans showed that there was decreased blood flow to the area of their brains associated with sadness, worry and depression. The participants also reported feeling less worried after their walk. [Bratman et al., (2015)]

Walking or hiking in natural surroundings can also help you focus, improve your memory, and boost your self-esteem.

A 2012 research article showed that people's creative and problem-solving abilities soared to new heights after a four-day hike in the wilderness, away from technology. [Atchley et al., (2012)]

Some examples of natural environments in which you could walk include:

- Forests and woodlands
- Suburban gardens
- Public parks and gardens
- Seaside reserves
- Mountains and hills
- Lake-sides, river-sides, stream-sides
- Village greens
- Walking tracks

659

THE MINIMUM AMOUNT OF EXERCISE

What is the minimum amount of time you should spend exercising, for weight control and good health? This is something of a controversial topic, upon which there are several opinions.

OFFICIAL RECOMMENDATIONS

The US Department of Health and Human Services recommends that for optimum health, healthy adults 18 to 64 years old should do at least two types of physical activity each week to improve their health—aerobic [cardiovascular] and muscle-strengthening.

They say the time spent on these exercises should be as follows:
- 2 hours and 30 minutes (150 minutes) of moderate-intensity aerobic activity (such as brisk walking) every week, and
- Muscle-strengthening [resistance training] activities on two or more days a week that work all major muscle groups (legs, hips, back, abdomen, chest, shoulders, and arms)."

Working out every day.

For cardiovascular activity, this averages out at around 20 minutes per day, seven days a week. If you add 10 minutes of weight training, that would make it around 30 minutes per day.

Working out three times a week.

For cardiovascular activity, this boils down to around 50 minutes three times per week. Adding 10 minutes of weight training makes it around 60 minutes of exercise three times per week. Health experts recommend that you leave a day or two between workouts on the same part of the body, to allow muscles to repair.

The best amount of exercise for fat-burning.

A 2009 study published in *Exercise and Sport Sciences Reviews* found that "Exercise increases the capacity of muscle to oxidize fat, but moderate duration exercise (less than or equal to one hour) does not impact 24-hour fat oxidation or fat balance." [Melanson et al., (2009)] This indicates that if you want to burn fat without exercising vigorously, you should exercise moderately for longer than an hour at a time.

HIGH-INTENSITY INTERVAL TRAINING (HIIT)

In the latter part of the 20th century another view emerged concerning the minimum amount of exercise required for good health and weight loss. It's called "High-intensity interval training (HIIT)"

Other names for this type of exercise include High-Intensity Intermittent Exercise (HIIE) and Sprint Interval Training (SIT). Sometimes it's also abbreviated to HIT.

HIIT is cardiovascular exercise technique which repeatedly alternates short bursts of intense exercise with less intense recovery periods. "Intense exercise" in this case means moving at the utmost of your ability, with your heart rate racing at 90% or more of its capacity.

HIIT has been shown to lower insulin resistance and help with weight loss. "HIIT significantly lowers insulin resistance compared to continuous training or control conditions and leads to modestly decreased fasting blood glucose levels and weight loss compared to those who do not undergo a physical activity intervention," according to researchers. [Jelleyman et al., (2015)].

HIIT is useful for people who are time-poor, but want to keep fit and lose weight.

HIIT MAY CURB YOUR APPETITE

Engaging in HIIT has a significant effect on how many Calories you eat during the 24 hours after the workout.

A 2012 study published in *The International Journal of Obesity* found that overweight men in their 20s and early 30s ate fewer Calories after doing very high-intensity exercise sessions (594 Calories) than after moderate workouts (710 Calories). Those same men reported that they ate fewer Calories on the day following the HIIT session than after a session of conventional, moderate exercise. [Sim et al., (2013)]

HIIT MAY BURN FAT

Another 2012 study, published in *The Journal of Obesity*, found that for young, overweight males, "Twelve weeks of high intensity intermittent exercise (HIIE) resulted in significant reductions in total, abdominal, trunk, and visceral fat and significant increases in fat free mass and aerobic power." [Heydari et al., (2012)]

Studies from many institutions, including the University of Guelph in Canada and the University of NSW in Australia suggest that when cyclists or runners add bursts of speed to their workout, they burn more fat than travelling over the same distance at a steady, moderate rate.

Other researchers are more cautious about touting the fat-burning effects of HIIT. "The effects of HIIE on subcutaneous and abdominal fat loss are promising but more studies using overweight individuals need to be carried out." [Boutcher (2011)]

SIX MINUTES A WEEK? REALLY?

High-intensity interval training takes a lot of motivation. It's unlikely that the general population will do it for 30 minutes every day for the rest of their lives!

Fortunately, science suggests that doing HIIT for just a few minutes a week may have huge benefits too!

"Get Fit in Six Minutes a Week" is the title of an episode of *Catalyst*, the highly acclaimed science show on ABC television (Australia).

The show's presenters talk about mitochondria—tiny structures that inhabit the cells of our bodies. They play a huge role in your health and longevity. They also regulate your body's ability to burn fat.

Have you ever wondered how the energy gets from your food (or your fat stores) into your body? Your mitochondria use oxygen to harvest electrons from your food or from your fat stores, to create energy. That is why they are known as the powerhouses of the living cell. They power every living thing, from the tiniest plant to the biggest animal.

Most people have billions of mitochondria in their muscles. In fact, those tiny little mitochondria make up around 10% of your body mass. Highly trained athletes have even more. As you age, your mitochondrial function gradually declines. You can, however, slow this decline.

The more rapidly and intensely you exercise, the more your mitochondrial function improves and your numbers of mitochondria multiply.

"Firing up your mitochondria can transform your health and fitness," according to *Catalyst*, "and the evidence is mounting you can do it incredibly fast."

The more oxygen your mitochondria can consume when you push yourself as hard as you can go, the better is your measure of your aerobic fitness.

Professor Martin Gibala, a professor and chair of the kinesiology department at McMaster University in Hamilton, Canada, found that as long as your exercise intensity is high enough, you can get significant improvements to your mitochondria numbers and function in less than 150 minutes a week.

In fact, you might be able to do it in *six minutes* a week!

How to improve your aerobic fitness in 6 minutes.

How can you build up your mitochondria numbers and function when you're time-poor? Just go for four 30-second sprints three times a week. You must sprint as fast as you can possibly go. And preferably run uphill, to increase the intensity of the exercise.

Between each sprint, rest for four and a half minutes. During this time your heart rate will slow down. All counted, your session will last for 20 minutes, during which you'll be resting for 18 minutes.

However, running at your top speed for 30 seconds is not as easy as you might think. And if you're unfit to begin with, it's best to gradually work up to your top speed over a period of about two weeks. Otherwise you risk straining your muscles.

Professor Martin Gibala's studies show that after only four weeks of training like this, people develop lower body fat and higher lean (muscle) mass. [Gibala et al., (2012)]

There is a rapid increase in the number and function of mitochondria following flat-out sprints. Professor David Bishop, professor and research leader (Sport Science) at the Institute of Sport, Exercise and Active Living (ISEAL), Australia—found that with the 6-minutes-per-week method, the mitochondrial function of a group of volunteers improved by up to 30% in just four weeks. There was no significant change in mitochondrial function in a second group of people who practised more traditional endurance training for four weeks.

High-intensity exercise demands that your body must produce large amounts of energy very rapidly. Your body responds by creating more mitochondrial powerhouses to meet the demand, and by making the existing mitochondria more efficient at drawing oxygen out of the blood into the muscles and using it to generate energy.

Professor David Bishop says, "What we think is that with the high-intensity training, we're probably replacing some of the older mitochondria with new, better-functioning mitochondria, and we think that may not be happening as much with the low-intensity exercise."

It's moving FAST that makes you burn fat better! Lifting heavy weights or jogging for long distances are also excellent forms of exercise which can help you lose weight, but they don't make your mitochondria go into fat-burning overdrive like sprinting flat-out does.

Perhaps when you move fast, your Inner Guardian gets the message that you are either running away from a deadly enemy or running towards your prey as you hunt for food. Either way, your Guardian responds by flooding your body with hormones such as adrenalin and noradrenaline. Receptors for these hormones exist on fat cells—especially on the cells of visceral fat, which is the most dangerous kind. (It's the fat that clings around many of your important internal organs deep inside your abdomen.) Scientists think that HIIT may be able to reduce visceral fat more efficiently than other types of exercise.

The jury is still out …

Whether HIIT provides substantial benefits for weight loss is still being studied. One study showed that it was ineffective in improving aerobic capacity, glucose metabolism or inflammatory profile within an overweight and obese group of men. [Kelly et al., (2017)]

If you do decide to take up HIIT, make sure you:
- Visit your doctor for a check-up before you start.
- Warm up and stretch before a sprinting session.
- Start gently. With each session, gradually work up to your top speed, over a period of about two weeks.

If you love the challenge and the benefits of doing HIIT for six minutes a week, you're more likely to keep doing it.

No matter how much time you have, the exercise you enjoy will be the one you stick to, and that's the best exercise for you.

WHAT ABOUT THREE MINUTES A WEEK?

If you're *really* time-poor, you could try exercising at high intensity for an even shorter period.

Jamie Timmons, professor of systems biology at Loughborough University in the UK, has done a great deal of research into the way HIIT improves the health of normal people.

He explains that " …three minutes of HIIT a week have been shown to improve the body's ability to cope with sugar surges (i.e., your metabolic fitness), and how good the heart and lungs are at getting oxygen into the body (your aerobic fitness)." [Mosley (2014)]

In 2013, medical journalist and author of "Fast Exercise" Dr. Michael Mosley engaged in three 1-minute sessions of high intensity exercise per week on a stationary exercise bike for four weeks, making 12 minutes of HIIT in total.

This is how he did it:

The one-minute flat-out HIIT workout.

- A 2-minute warm-up of gentle cycling at low resistance for a couple of minutes.
- Cycling as hard as possible for 20 seconds with the bike set to the highest resistance.
- A 2-minute recovery period of gentle cycling at low resistance.
- Cycling as hard as possible for another 20 seconds with the bike set to the highest resistance.
- Another 2-minute recovery period of gentle cycling at low resistance.
- A third and final bout of cycling as hard as possible for another 20 seconds with the bike set to the highest resistance.
- It's advisable to cycle gently for a few minutes to cool down after a workout like this. (Yes I know, this does add a few minutes to your exercise routine, but it's worth it!)

The total amount of high-intensity exercise per session, (not including the warm-up) was one minute.

After four weeks of doing this 3 times a week, Dr. Mosley's insulin sensitivity had improved by 24%—an outstanding result! In fact, it's doubtful that even doing hours of standard/typical exercise would give such a significant outcome.

As discussed earlier in this book, insulin resistance can make it harder to lose weight. The opposite of insulin resistance is insulin sensitivity, and anything that can improve your insulin sensitivity may also improve your chances of losing weight more easily.

Dr. Mosley says that he continues to practice HIIT because it measurably improves his glucose sensitivity, lifts his mood and controls his appetite.

. . . AND BACK TO SIX MINUTES A WEEK . . .

In a 2014 Daily Mail article, Dr. Mosley describes a "gentler version" of his HIIT workout, which should also be performed three times a week.

Dr Mosley's two-minute 90% HIIT workout.

This is how to do it, using cycling or uphill running:

- A 2-minute warm-up of gentle cycling at low resistance (or light jogging on a level surface).
- For 60 seconds, cycling at about 90% of your best effort with the bike set to the highest resistance, or running uphill at about 90% of your best effort. Aim to elevate your heart rate to around 150 beats per minute.
- A 90 second (1½-minutes) recovery period of gentle cycling at low resistance (or light jogging on a level surface).
- For 60 seconds, cycling at about 90% of your best effort with the bike set to the highest resistance, or running uphill at about 90% of your best effort. Aim to elevate your heart rate to around 150 beats per minute.
- It's advisable to cycle or jog gently for a few minutes to cool down after a workout like this.

The total amount of vigorous exercise per session is two minutes. Including the warm-ups and recoveries, it's around eight to ten minutes.

The important difference is that you don't push yourself quite as hard as you would in the one-minute flat-out HIIT workout. Instead of exercising as vigorously as possible, you move at about 90% of your maximum capacity.

This gentler version of HIIT can be intensified as your fitness improves. Beginners should commence with two bursts of one minute, three times a week. People who are very fit can then increase to ten bursts of one minute.

COMBINING HIIT WITH OTHER TYPES OF EXERCISE

You can enhance your fitness by combining your One-Minute Flat-Out HIIT Workout with a simple, 10-minute strength and flexibility regimen (such as yoga or Pilates), which you would practice three times a week.

Before you start:

Before you commence any new exercise regime, it's prudent to ask your doctor for a general check-up—especially if you are frail or very unfit.

THE BEST TIME OF DAY TO EXERCISE

For weight loss, when is the best time of day to exercise? This varies between men and women. As mentioned elsewhere in this book, to burn the most fat men should exercise *before* eating and women *afterwards*.

An experiment run by Dr. Adam Collins, of the University of Surrey found that when women exercised during the hour after eating a meal their bodies burned 22% more fat. By contrast, the bodies of men who exercised before eating burned as much as 8% more fat.

"For women, most fat-burning occurs in the three hours after they stop exercising," said Dr. Collins. "Women who eat during the 90 minutes after they exercise could actually be impeding their fat-burning." [BBC Two (2016)]

To improve insulin sensitivity, the best time for males to exercise is in the morning, on an empty stomach according to a 2010 study published in the Journal of Physiology. [Van Proeyen et al., (2010)]

THRIFTY EXERCISING

Some people spend a lot of money on workout gear, gym memberships and personal trainers. That's fine, and has the added benefit of helping with motivation—but you don't *need* to spend money in order to exercise. After all your body is right with you 100% of the time. All it needs is some space to move. That space can be as big as a marathon track, a beach or a sports oval, or as small as the space your body occupies. Doing isometric exercises, for example, requires barely any space at all! (By way of illustration, put your hands together as if you were praying, and press them together as hard as you can for as long as you can. That is an isometric strength-building exercise.)

HOME WORKOUT CIRCUIT

If you don't have the time, money or inclination to regularly exercise at your local gym, you can get a great whole-body workout at home. There are plenty of fun, free, no-special-equipment, no-gym workouts you can do without even stepping outside your front door.

It's quick and easy to create a "workout circuit" for yourself. This consists of a series of "stations"—places in your house or backyard at which you perform a certain exercise.

At each exercise session, switch on your favorite motivational music on your portable music player, and move around the circuit, repeating each exercise at each station the required number of times. You can set up as many stations as you like, but it's best to include at least:

- one that works out the arms
- one for the legs
- one for the core and abdomen
- one for the back
- one cardio fitness station.

Each time you arrive at a station, do one set of exercises in time to the music before you move on to the next station. Start with a gentle 4 reps (repeats) of each exercise on each side of the body and, over the next 2 weeks, work up to 8 or 10.

Notes:

- If you're not used to exercising, get checked out by your doctor before you start. Begin your circuit work very gently and gradually work up to a more strenuous level, over a few weeks.
- Correct technique is WAY more important than the number of reps you manage to pump out, or the heaviness of the weights you're using. Incorrect technique can not only make your body recruit other muscles to help the ones you want to tone (decreasing the effectiveness of the exercise); it can also cause injury.
- Always warm up before you start your exercises. A good way to warm up is to go for a brisk, 5 minute walk or do 5 to 10 minutes of vigorous housework!
- Enjoy a home workout session 3 to 4 times a week, spread out over the seven days.

Home workout circuit stations.

Here are some suggestions for your Home Workout Circuit Stations. Choose what suits you!

- **The arms station:** This is the place where you perform bicep curls, push-ups, reverse push-ups (dips), push-downs, and tricep extensions. All you need is some hand-held dumbbells and a place to stand or lie down. If you don't own any dumbbells, use some of the low-tech equipment suggested below.

- **The legs, hips and butt station:** Here's where you do lunges, deadlifts, standing calf raises, and squats (wide and narrow). All you need is the floor. Hand-held dumbbells are optional.

- **The core/abdomen station:** This is the place for abdominal crunches, Russian twists, planks, single-leg circles, criss-cross, and sideways planks. Again, all you need is the floor.

- **The back and shoulders station:** To work your back and shoulders, do bent-over rowing, pull ups, back extensions, Pilates "darts", and the "bridge" (otherwise known as "bottom lifts". If you're not sure what these exercises are, do an Internet search or look on YouTube.

- **The cardio workout station:** To raise your heart rate, run up and down the stairs, perform some fast "step-ups" on a low, firm platform, or do some rapid air-boxing.

- **The stretching station:** While you're cooling down after each workout session, gently stretch your muscles; shoulders, triceps, lower back, hip flexors, hamstrings, quadriceps, calves etc.

Low-tech equipment.

All you need to set up your home workout circuit is:
- A rubber Pilates/yoga mat; or even a long piece of carpet or a thick bath-sheet. Something comfortable but firm, to lie on when you perform sit-ups, bridges, planks etc.
- Hand-weights/dumbbells—either store-bought ones, or plastic bottles of water or shopping bags containing a few grocery products, such as bags of rice. Hold these in your hands when you perform such exercises as bicep curls or walking lunges.
- A flat, firm cushion or pillow to put under your head when you do abdominal crunches.
- A heavy book or other weight to hold against your chest when you perform wide squats.
- A fitness stick such as a Gymstick®. A perfect substitute is a broom, or the handle of a rake. This can be lightly held across the back of your shoulders when you do narrow squats.

THRIFTY EXERCISING OUTSIDE THE HOME

We've covered a lot of these suggestions already, but here's a recap. To exercise thriftily outside the home:

- Go for a run at a nearby park or through your local streets.

- For extra motivation, join a running or walking club. Social groups can provide great motivation, as well as friendship and fun, and it's usually free or very low-cost. To find one near you, telephone your local council or search the Internet for "running clubs", "jogging clubs" or "walking clubs" in your vicinity.

- Join an amateur sporting team or club. Football, tennis, netball etc. are enjoyable games to play, with the added bonus of fitness and sociability. Teams are often eager for new members, no matter what your skill level.

- Ride a bicycle. It doesn't have to be a top-of-the-range machine with 27 speeds and a carbon-fiber frame. In fact the heavier your bicycle is, the harder you have to work when you ride it! Just make sure your saddle and handlebars are set at the correct position for your body.

- Engage in Pilates or Yoga or other fitness classes that are demonstrated for free on websites such as Vimeo or YouTube.

CREATE GOOD EXERCISE HABITS

Schedule workouts.

Instead of just telling yourself that you'll "exercise more often", put your calendar in front of you and schedule your workouts. Remind yourself that workouts don't have to involve special clothing and gyms—they can be as easy as going for a brisk walk, or riding your bicycle. Set aside specific dates and times, at least three times a week, and do something that raises your heart rate.

Get more incidental movement.

Move more often.

Movement is your miracle medicine. Every time you move, you're doing yourself good. Even incidental movement is stimulating your body to become a little bit fitter and burn more fat. You can even exercise when you're seated. Tap your fingers or wiggle your feet when you're sitting down at your desk, or extend each leg alternately and move it gently up and down while keeping your abdominal muscles tight. If you're watching free-to-air TV, stand up during the ads. Engaged in a long telephone conversation? Walk around while you're talking.

Walk, walk, walk.

Whenever possible, walk instead of driving, and take the stairs instead of the elevator/escalator. Park your car further away from your destination and walk a extra few steps. All these steps add up, and if you buy a wearable fitness tracker you'll be able to count them more easily!

PART NINE:

SLEEP

BETTER SLEEP = BETTER WEIGHT LOSS.

To achieve better weight loss, sleep longer and more soundly. Sleep is absolutely crucial for optimal health and weight control. There's a direct association between how much good quality sleep people get, and the amount they eat. Study after study confirms that a lack of sleep can make you eat more and gain weight. People who regularly get plenty of sound, restful slumber are, in general, slimmer than people who get less sleep or poor quality sleep.

Decreased sleep times are linked with higher BMI levels and increased fat stores. Circadian neuroscientist Russell Foster, of Oxford University, says that those who sleep five hours or less a night have a 50% greater chance of being obese. Results from the *US Nurses' Health Study*, which reported on 68,000 women, showed that women who got less sleep were more likely to become obese. [Patel et al., (2006)]

Poor sleep increases the risk of overeating and obesity, so it follows that weight loss efforts can be boosted by getting a good night's sleep.

WHAT CAN CAUSE POOR QUALITY SLEEP?

The invention of artificial lighting, particularly electric lighting, meant that sunrise and sunset no longer ruled people's circadian (daily) rhythms. These days, we humans are more likely than our ancestors to be suffering from a shortage of sleep. On average, our forebears enjoyed more sleep each night than we do. Digital devices with screens—such as tablets, televisions, computers and smart-phones—have us staring at blue light wavelengths for extended periods. This, combined with the anxieties often generated by the frantic pace of modern life, has led to many of us being chronically sleep-deprived. Other health factors can contribute to sleep-disruption, such as sleep apnea, restless leg syndrome, narcolepsy, polyuria and nocturia.

HOW SLEEP AFFECTS BODY-WEIGHT REGULATION

Lack of sleep is known to affect cognitive function, concentration, memory, cellular repair, immune function, sex drive, skin tone and more. Disrupted sleep increases the risk of high blood pressure and strokes. Getting enough sleep is important in so many ways, not least of which is to keep the brain functioning at optimum levels and to balance hunger and satiety hormones. Most importantly for dieters, lack of sufficient sleep can also contribute to weight gain.

Sleep affects hormones.

Poor sleep affects a number of hormones produced by your body, including leptin, ghrelin and cortisol. Sleep deprivation gives rise to the release of ghrelin—the "hunger hormone"—which signals the brain to desire carbohydrates and sugars.

When you don't get enough sleep, your levels of leptin—the "satiety hormone"—drop, which increases the appetite. According to Seth Santoro, a Los Angeles based health and nutrition coach, people who don't get enough sleep ". . . burn fewer Calories, lack appetite control and experience an increase in cortisol levels, which stores fat."

676

In short, a lack of sleep causes cortisol and ghrelin levels to rise which makes you hungry, while levels of leptin, the satiety hormone, fall.

When you're tired, as opposed to feeling rested, you're likely to feel hungrier. Sleeping for fewer than 7 hours per night is associated with increased ghrelin levels and reported hunger, and higher body weight.

A study conducted at the University of Chicago found that short-term sleep deprivation altered the way the brain controlled appetite in healthy young men. Deprived of sleep the men experienced ". . . decreased leptin levels, increased ghrelin levels, and markedly elevated hunger and appetite ratings. The subjects were found to particularly crave sweets, starch, and salty snacks after being deprived of sleep." [Hogenkamp et al., 2013)]

Sleep-deprivation affects insulin response.

A lack of sleep can also alter insulin sensitivity. Sleep deficiency is associated with decreased glucose tolerance, which in turn leads to a greater risk of obesity.

One study found that healthy men whose were only allowed to sleep for 4 hours every night for 6 nights suffered a 30% reduction in insulin response to glucose. [Spiegel et al., (1999)]

A study undertaken at Leiden University Medical Center in The Netherlands found that as little as one single night of sleep deprivation (only 4 hours of sleep instead of 8 hours) was enough to significantly disrupt people's insulin sensitivity. [Donga et al., (2010)]

The brain can interpret fatigue as hunger.

Fatigue itself can also encourage overeating and less physical activity. An over-tired body can send signals that it needs energy in the form of food when in fact, it simply needs sleep. When you think you're feeling hungry, you might actually be feeling tired. It might simply be a nap you're in need of, not a donut.

When people don't get enough sleep they tend not only to eat more food, but also to choose food that is more Calorie-dense. [Hogenkamp et al., (2013)]

677

Poor sleep can lead to poor decisions.

People who get plenty of sleep are also more mentally alert. They are likely to make better food choices, and follow a more nutritious diet. A study published in *The American Journal of Clinical Nutrition* found that people who sleep for longer are inclined to consume less saturated fat than people who have fewer hours of sleep. [Dashti et al., (2015)]

"... insufficient sleep may lead to the development/maintenance of obesity through [changes in brain functions], resulting in the selection of foods most capable of triggering weight-gain." [Greer et al., (2013)]

Poor sleep makes people more likely to choose bigger food portions than they really need. While the links between poor sleep and weight gain are becoming clear, another study looked at the effect of sleep loss on appetite; in particular, the size of portion choice in the sleep deprived. In a 16-men study, those with total sleep deprivation had higher ghrelin levels and chose larger portions. They also reported feeling hungrier. [Hogenkamp et al., (2013)]

Alissa Rumsey, Registered Dietitian and Spokesperson for the *Academy of Nutrition and Dietetics*, says, ". . . when we're sleep-deprived, our brains respond more strongly to junk food and have less of an ability to practice portion control."

Researchers agree on the importance of sleep for weight management. "If metabolic changes resulting from sleep deprivation contribute to weight gain, then interventions designed to increase the amount and quality of sleep could potentially augment the most common clinical interventions of increasing physical activity and improving nutrition." [Gangwisch et al., (2005)]

In other words, weight control can be much easier if you get plenty of good, sound sleep every night.

SLEEP SHORTAGE INCREASES OBESITY RISK

A shortage of sleep puts both adults and teenagers at risk of obesity.

Adults.

An analysis of data from the Wisconsin Sleep Cohort Study found that fewer hours of sleep were associated with lower leptin levels, higher ghrelin levels, and increased Body Mass Index (BMI) in people between the ages of 30 and 60 years. For people who slept for less than 8 hours per night, those who slept least had the highest BMI. [Taheri et al., (2004)]

Teenagers.

Not getting enough sleep affects obesity in teens. Between the ages of 14 to 17 they need about eight to ten hours of sleep. According to a study published in *The American Journal of Human Biology,* ". . . obese adolescents experienced less sleep than non-obese adolescents . . . For each hour of lost sleep, the odds of obesity increased by 80%."

Sleep disturbance also influenced physical activity level. The study of teens aged between 11-16 found that " . . . daytime physical activity diminished by 3% for every hour increase in sleep disturbance." Another study reported that six nights of sleep loss caused a 30% reduction in the insulin response in young men. In short, not getting enough sleep can make teens obese and less active during the day, and as they get older, lack of sleep can cause a pre-diabetic condition. [Gupta et al., (2002)]

HOW TO GET A BETTER NIGHT'S SLEEP

If you want to "sleep your way slim," but find it hard to come by a good night's sleep, science can offer some helpful tips. There are many natural sleep aids that are drug-free and Calorie-free! We have so many tools and tips for better sleep that we could not fit them into the pages of this book. See *The Satiety Diet Weight Loss Toolkit,* book #2 in the Satiety Diet series.

Good night!

. . . and thank you for reading this book.

AFTERWORD

The first volume of the Satiety Diet series ends here, due to limitations on the number of pages in the printed edition. Other books in this series include Book #2: *The Satiety Diet Weight Loss Toolkit* and Book #3: *Crispy, Creamy, Chewy: The Satiety Diet Cookbook*.

In this current volume we have offered readers the full outline of the Satiety Diet.

Book #2 expands upon Book #1. It contains tricks and tips to make it easier for you to live your happy, healthy, satisfying weight-loss lifestyle. The contents include information on how to get a better night's sleep, decreasing your child's obesity risk, stress reduction, how to increase dopamine naturally. more mind tricks for weight loss, addictive foods and drinks, how to combat the effects of obesogens, tips about gluten, choosing the best tableware for weight loss, thrifty weight loss, keeping hunger at bay and eating out.

Book #3 gives you a selection of recipes designed for the Satiety Diet.

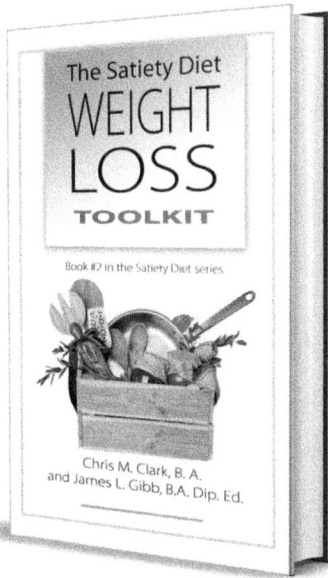

The Satiety Diet
Weight Loss Toolkit
Chapters include:
* Why Is Everyone on a Diet?
* Food Tools
* Tableware Tools
* Meal Preparation Tools
* Mealtime Tools
* Breakfast Tools
* More Tips for Satiety
* Tools for Keeping Hunger at Bay
* Planning Tools
* Sweetness and Sweeteners
* Dining-out Tools
* Children and Obesity
* Stress Reduction Tools
* Sleep Tools
* Brown Fat Tools
* Fasting Tools
* Weight Loss Mind Tricks
* A Bag of Assorted Weight-Loss Tools
* Tools for Creating Better Habits
* Obesogens
* Thrifty Weight Loss
* About Dietary Supplements

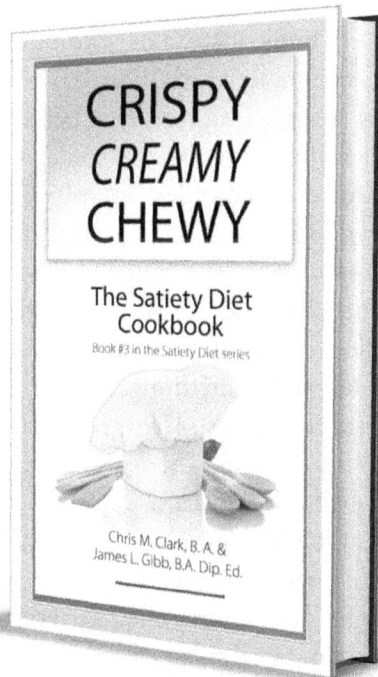

DEFINITIONS

Amino Acids:
Amino acids are compounds that join together to form proteins. Hundreds of different amino acids exist. Your body uses them to build the proteins necessary for survival.

Calories:
In this book, instead of "kilojoules" we will use the term "Calories", with a capital letter, to mean units of food energy.

The term "Calorie" has been superseded in the International System of Units by the joule, with one food Calorie equivalent to about 4.2 kilojoules. In spite of its non-official status, the term "Calorie" for a unit of food energy is still popular around the globe, which is why we've decided to use it.

"The only valid use of the Calorie is in common speech and public nutrition education," says James L. Hargrove, Associate Professor of Foods and Nutrition at the University of Georgia, referring to "Calorie confusion". [Hargrove (2007)]

Strictly speaking there are two types of calories:

* Small calories (cal).

* Large Calories, also known as kilocalories (kcal). These are the units of energy in food, the "dietary Calories".

Large Calories are officially written with a capital letter, to distinguish them from small calories.

"The terms 'large Calorie' and 'small calorie' are often used interchangeably. This is misleading. The calorie content described on food labels refers to kilocalories. A 250-Calorie chocolate bar actually contains 250,000 calories." [Nordqvist (2017)]

Energy-dense:
Energy density is the amount of energy (or Calories) per gram of food. "Energy dense" is a term used to describe foods with high levels of Calories, as distinct from "energy sparse".

GI tract:
Gastrointestinal tract. Part of the digestive system.

Glycemic Index (GI):
"… a relative ranking of carbohydrate in foods according to how they affect blood glucose levels. Carbohydrates with a low GI value (55 or less) are more slowly digested, absorbed and metabolized and cause a lower and slower rise in blood glucose and, therefore usually, insulin levels." [Glycemic Index Foundation, retrieved August 2017]

Hunger:
The British Nutrition Foundation defines hunger as "A compelling need or desire for food; the painful sensation or state of weakness caused by the need of food."

Microbiome:
The collective genomes of the microorganisms that reside in an environmental niche. The human body is host to numerous micro-organisms both inside the gut and on the skin.

Microbiota:
The microorganisms that inhabit the microbiome.

Nourishing, Tasty, Slimming (NTS) Vegetables:

As advertisers and menu-writers know so well, the way we perceive food is incredibly important to our appreciation of that food.

It's even more important for weight loss.

If you're just about to tuck in to a plate of "nourishing, tasty, slimming vegetables" you're much more likely to feel indulged, pampered, eager, and ready to be satisfied than if you're sitting at a table in front of a plate of "low-Calorie vegetables". And yet it's the same meal!

Words frame our emotions and beliefs. When you know that your plateful of colorful, flavorsome vegetables is not only nourishing your body with vitamins and minerals, it is also contributing to your feelings of satiation, you are likely to love those foods more. After all, they are helping you to achieve your goal of a slimmer, fitter self.

NTS vegetables are those which contain fewer Calories (chiefly in the form of starches and/or sugars) than other vegetables. For a given number of Calories, you can eat larger quantities of these low-Calorie NTS vegetables than you could eat of starchy/sugary vegetables.

As a rule of thumb, NTS vegetables exclude grains, seeds, and legumes. Some examples of starchy/sugary non-NTS vegetables include corn, peas, sweet potatoes, yams, parsnips and potatoes.

Real food:

Food that is minimally processed and retains its natural integrity.

Satiety vs Satiation:

There is a subtle but important difference between Satiation and Satiety. The British Nutrition Foundation defines these terms as:

* Satiation—the feeling that prompts us to stop eating a meal. It refers to the end of the desire to eat, and it is governed by hormones and stretch receptors in the stomach. Satiation controls the amount we eat at one sitting.

* Satiety—the feeling of fullness and satisfaction and repleteness that persists after we have finished eating. Satiety controls the length of time until we next have the desire to eat. In healthy individuals, satiety diminishes as our bodies use up the nutrients we ate. When those nutrients are at low levels, hunger returns.

Both are important in controlling energy intake.

Service à la française / à la russe:

"Service à la française (French: 'service in the French style') is the practice of serving various dishes of a meal at the same time, in contrast to service à la russe (in French, 'service in the Russian style'), where the dishes are brought sequentially and served individually." [Wikipedia (October 2017)]

"Sometimes food":

Words are powerful. If we are to have a healthy relationship with food it is best not to attach emotional labels such as "good" or "evil". Instead of describing sugary, fatty, highly processed food as "bad" or "junk", call it "sometimes food". For weight loss, we only eat this kind of food sometimes (in small portions) and not every day.

Western Dietary Pattern:

A diet consisting of food which is most commonly consumed in developed countries. Examples include meat, white bread, milk and puddings. [BBC News (2007)]

The name is a reference to Western culture or civilization, "a term used very broadly to refer to a heritage of social norms, ethical values, traditional customs, belief systems, political systems, and specific artefacts and technologies that have some origin or association with Europe. The term is applied to European countries and countries whose history is strongly marked by European immigration, colonization, and influence, such as the continents of the Americas and Australasia, whose current demographic majority is of European ethnicity, and is not restricted to the continent of Europe." [Wikipedia 6th Sep. 2016]

ABOUT THE AUTHORS

James L. Gibb, B.A. Dip. Ed.

James L. Gibb is an educator, writer and health researcher. A university graduate with a diploma of education, Gibb is interested in the relationship between nutrition and health. He is the author of the best-selling book *Is Food Making You Sick? The Strictly Low Histamine Diet.*

Chris M. Clark, B. A.

Chris Clark is a tertiary qualified professional who, throughout her life, has conducted extensive research into weight loss. She collected the results of thousands of peer-reviewed studies on obesity published over the last couple of decades, and devised a weight management lifestyle that actually works.

She used her research collection as a basis for this book and the other titles in the Satiety Diet series.

BIBLIOGRAPHY

ABC Catalyst (2016) "Gut Reaction." Catalyst special edition Gut Reaction: Could food be making us sick - very sick? ABC television, Thursday 21 August 2014

Abraham & Beaumont (1982). "How patients describe bulimia or binge eating." Abraham SF, Beaumont PJV Psychological Medicine 1982 12: 625-635

ACCP (2008). "Smoking Linked To Sleep Disturbances." American College of Chest Physicians. ScienceDaily. ScienceDaily, 7 February 2008. <www.sciencedaily.com/releases/2008/02/080204172250.htm>

Acheson (1993). "Influence of autonomic nervous system on nutrient-induced thermogenesis in humans." Acheson KJ, Nutrition 1993, 9(4):373-80

AHA (2016). "Fats 101". American Heart Association, Apr 28, 2016

Akabas et al., (2012). "Textbook of Obesity: Biological, Psychological and Cultural Influences." Edited by Sharon Akabas, Sally Ann Lederman, Barbara J. Moore. April 2012, ©2012, Wiley-Blackwell

Alang & Kelly (2014). "Weight Gain After Fecal Microbiota Transplantation." Neha Alang and Colleen R. Kelly. Department of Internal Medicine, Newport Hospital, and Division of Gastroenterology, Center for Women's Gastrointestinal Medicine at the Women's Medicine Collaborative, The Miriam Hospital, Warren Alpert School of Brown University, Providence, Rhode Island. November 28, 2014.

Alford & Tibbets (1971). "Education Increases Consumption of Vegetables by Children." Alford, B. B. and Tibbets, M. H. (1971) Journal of Nutrition Education 3: 12-14

Alleaume (2014). "Food bashing: Why we are more confused about what to eat than ever before." Alleaume, Kathleen News.com.au November 15, 2014

Almiron-Roig et al., (2013). "Factors that determine energy compensation: a systematic review of preload studies." E. Almiron-Roig, L. Palla, K. Guest, C. Ricchiuti, N. Vint, S.A. Jebb, et al. Nutrition Reviews, 71 (7) (2013), pp. 458–473

Alper & Mattes (2002). "Effects of chronic peanut consumption on energy balance and hedonics." Alper CM, Mattes RD. Int J Obes Relat Metab Disord. 2002 Aug;26(8):1129-37

AMRC (2015). "Exercise—the Miracle Cure." 13th February 2015. The Academy of Medical Royal Colleges. Available at http://www.aomrc.org.uk/wp-content/uploads/2016/05/Exercise_the_Miracle_Cure_0215.pdf

An Pan et al., (2012). "Red Meat Consumption and Mortality: Results from Two Prospective Cohort Studies." An Pan, PhD, Qi Sun, MD, ScD, Adam M. Bernstein, MD, ScD, Matthias B. Schulze, DrPH, JoAnn E. Manson, MD, DrPH, Meir J. Stampfer, MD, DrPH, Walter C. Willett, MD, DrPH, and Frank B. Hu, MD, PhD. Arch Intern Med. 2012 Apr 9; 172(7): 555–563. doi: 10.1001/archinternmed.2011.2287. PMCID: PMC3712342. NIHMSID: NIHMS462637

Anderson & Woodend (2003). "Consumption of sugars and the regulation of short-term satiety and food intake." Anderson GH, Woodend D. Am J Clin Nutr. 2003 Oct;78(4):843S-849S.

Anderson et al., (2010). "Relation between estimates of cornstarch digestibility by the Englyst in vitro method and glycemic response, subjective appetite, and short-term food intake in young men." Anderson GH, Cho CE, Akhavan T, Mollard RC, Luhovyy BL, Finocchiaro ET. Am J Clin Nutr. 2010 Apr;91(4):932-9. doi: 10.3945/ajcn.2009.28443. Epub 2010 Feb 17

Andrade et al., (2008). "Eating Slowly Led to Decreases in Energy Intake within Meals in Healthy Women." Ana M. Andrade, Geoffrey W. Greene, Kathleen J. Melanson. Journal of the American Dietetic Association. 2008, Vol.108, No.7, p.1186

Andrews (2016). "All About Appetite Regulation Part 1." Ryan Andrews, for Precision Nutrition, www.precisionnutrition.com Retrieved 5th June 2016

Angelopoulos et al., (2013). "The effect of slow spaced eating on hunger and satiety in overweight and obese patients with type 2 diabetes mellitus." Theodoros Angelopoulos, Alexander Kokkinos, Christos Liaskos, Nicholas Tentolouris, Kleopatra Alexiadou,1 Alexander Dimitri Miras, Iordanis Mourouzis, Despoina Perrea, Constantinos Pantos, Nicholas Katsilambros, Stephen R Bloom, and Carel Wynard le Roux. BMJ Open Diabetes Res Care. 2014; 2(1): e000013. doi: 10.1136/bmjdrc-2013-000013. PMCID: PMC4212566

Anthony (2014). "Understanding Satiation and Satiety". Mark Anthony, Ph.D., Technical Editor, Food Processing 2014.

Aparicio et al., (1974). "Circadian Variation of the Blood Glucose, Plasma Insulin and Human Growth Hormone Levels in Response to an Oral Glucose Load in Normal Subjects." Néstor J Aparicio, MD, Félix E Puchulu, MD, Juan J Gagliardino, MD, Maximino Ruiz, MD, Jóse M Llorens, MD, Jorge Ruiz, MD, Aldo Lamas, Biochem and Raul De Miguel, Biochem. doi: 10.2337/diab.23.2.132. Diabetes February 1974 vol. 23 no. 2 132-137

Asarnow et al., (2015). "Evidence for a Possible Link between Bedtime and Change in Body Mass Index." Lauren D. Asarnow, Eleanor McGlinchey, Allison G. Harvey. SLEEP, 2015; 38 (10): 1523 DOI: 10.5665/sleep.5038

Astrup et al., (2000). "The role of low-fat diets in body weight control: a meta-analysis of ad libitum dietary intervention studies." A. Astrup, G.K. Grunwald, E.L. Melanson, W.H. Saris, J.O. Hill. International Journal of Obesity, 24 (12) (2000), pp. 1545–1552

Atchley et al., (2012). "Creativity in the Wild: Improving Creative Reasoning through Immersion in Natural Settings." Ruth Ann Atchley, David L. Strayer, Paul Atchley. PLOS. Published: December 12, 2012. http://dx.doi.org/10.1371/journal.pone.0051474

Aucouturier et al., (2016). "Covert digital manipulation of vocal emotion alter speakers' emotional states in a congruent direction." Jean-Julien Aucouturier, Petter Johansson, Lars Hall, Rodrigo Segnini, Lolita Mercadié, Katsumi Watanabe. Proceedings of the National Academy of Sciences, 2016; 201506552 DOI: 10.1073/pnas.1506552113

Audelin et al., (2012). "Change of energy expenditure from physical activity is the most powerful determinant of improved insulin sensitivity in overweight patients with coronary artery disease participating in an intensive lifestyle modification program." Audelin MC, Savage PD, Toth MJ, Harvey-Berino J, Schneider DJ, Bunn JY, Ludlow M, Ades PA. Metabolism. 2012 May;61(5):672-9. doi: 10.1016/j.metabol.2011.10.001. Epub 2011 Dec 5

Aune et al., (2016). "Whole grain consumption and risk of cardiovascular disease, cancer, and all cause and cause specific mortality: systematic review and dose-response meta-analysis of prospective studies." Aune D, Keum N, Giovannucci E, Fadnes LT, Boffetta P, Greenwood DC, Tonstad S, Vatten LJ, Riboli E, Norat T. BMJ 2016; 353 doi: http://dx.doi.org/10.1136/bmj.i2716 (Published 14 June 2016) BMJ 2016;353:i2716

Austad (2006). "Why women live longer than men: Sex differences in longevity." Gender Medicine Volume 3, Issue 2, June 2006, Pages 79-92. PhD Steven N. Austad. https://doi.org/10.1016/S1550-8579(06)80198-1

Australian Bureau of Statistics (2008). "Overweight and Obesity in adults, Australia, 2004-05." Australian Bureau of Statistics. Cat No. 4719.0. 2008, Canberra.

690

Ayers (2008). "Lectins - Heat'em and Eat'em" Dr. Art Ayers, Cooling Inflammation Blogspot, Monday, December 15, 2008

Azadbakht & Esmaillzadeh (2010). "Dietary diversity score is related to obesity and abdominal adiposity among Iranian female youth." Azadbakht L, Esmaillzadeh A. Public Health Nutr. 2011 Jan;14(1):62-9. doi: 10.1017/S1368980010000522. Epub 2010 Mar 31

Baillie-Hamilton (2002). "Chemical toxins: a hypothesis to explain the global obesity epidemic." Baillie-Hamilton, P. F. J Altern Complement Med 8, 185–192 (2002)

Bajaj (2013). "Effect of Number of Food Pieces on Food Selection and Consumption in Animals and Humans. A Dissertation Presented in Partial Fulfillment of the Requirements for the Degree Doctor of Philosophy." Devina Bajaj, Arizona State University, 2013.

Barry et al., (2009). "Obesity and Its Relationship to Addictions: Is Overeating a Form of Addictive Behavior?" Barry D, Clarke M, Petry NM. The American journal on addictions / American Academy of Psychiatrists in Alcoholism and Addictions. 2009;18(6):439-451. doi:10.3109/10550490903205579

BBC News (2007). "Dog-owners 'lead healthier lives.'" BBC News. Jan. 21, 2007. (March 21, 2008) http://news.bbc.co.uk/2/hi/health/6279701.stm

BBC News (2007). "Western diet risk to Asian women". 10 July 2007.

BBC News (2017). "Is it safe to drink Fanta and Sprite in Nigeria?" BBC News 23 March 2017

BBC Two (2016). BBC Two—Trust Me, I'm a Doctor, Series 4, Episode 1, 2016

BBC Two (2016). "Could having my muscles stretched have health benefits?" BBC Two—Trust Me, I'm a Doctor, Summer Special 2016

Beil (2014). "Ancient famine-fighting genes can't explain obesity: Scientists look beyond calorie-hoarding genes to understand widening waistlines". Laura Beil, Science News, September 5, 2014

Bellisle et al., (1997). "Meal frequency and energy balance." Bellisle F, McDevitt R, Prentice AM. Br J Nutr. 1997 Apr;77 Suppl 1:S57-70. PMID: 9155494

Bennett (1987). "Dietary Treatments of Obesity." Bennett, W. Human Obesity, 1987. Annals of the New York Academy of Sciences 499:250-263.

Béquet et al., (2001). "Site-dependent effects of an acute intensive exercise on extracellular 5-HT and 5-HIAA levels in rat brain." Béquet F, Gomez-Merino D, Berthelot M, Guezennec CY. Neurosci Lett 2001;301:143-6

Bernstein & Nash (2006). "Essentials of Psychology." Douglas Bernstein, Peggy W. Nash. Wadsworth Publishing; 4 edition, December 18, 2006.

Bertenshaw et al., (2009). "Dose-dependent effects of beverage protein content upon short-term intake." E.J. Bertenshaw, A. Lluch, M.R. Yeomans. Appetite, 52 (3) (2009), pp. 580–587.

Bertenshaw et al., (2013). "Perceived thickness and creaminess modulates the short-term satiating effects of high-protein drinks." E.J. Bertenshaw, A. Lluch, M.R. Yeomans. British Journal of Nutrition, 110 (3) (28 2013) 578–586.

Berthoud (2011). "Metabolic and hedonic drives in the neural control of appetite: who is the boss?" Hans-Rudolf Berthoud, Current opinion in neurobiology, 2011, volume 21 6, pages 888-96

Berthoud et al., (2016). "Blaming the Brain for Obesity: Integration of Hedonic and Homeostatic Mechanisms." Hans-Rudolf Berthoud, Heike Münzberg, Christopher D. Morrison. Pathogenesis of Obesity. https://doi.org/10.1053/j.gastro.2016.12.050

Biegler (2016). "Free will, food and obesity: do we really have a choice?" Paul Biegler, Cosmos Magazine, 15 June 2016.

Biswas et al., (2014). "Something to Chew On: The Effects of Oral Haptics on Mastication, Orosensory Perception, and Calorie Estimation." Biswas, Dipayan and Szocs, Courtney and Krishna, Aradhna and Lehmann, Donald R., (January 3, 2014). Journal of Consumer Research, 2014; Columbia Business School Research Paper No. 15-13.

Biswas et al., (2015). "Sedentary Time and Its Association With Risk for Disease Incidence, Mortality, and Hospitalization in Adults: A Systematic Review and Meta-analysis." Aviroop Biswas, BSc; Paul I. Oh, MD, MSc; Guy E. Faulkner, PhD; Ravi R. Bajaj, MD; Michael A. Silver, BSc; Marc S. Mitchell, MSc; David A. Alter, MD, PhD. 20 January 2015 Annals of Internal Medicine

Bjerregaard et al., (2003). "Low incidence of cardiovascular disease among the Inuit–what is the evidence?" Bjerregaard P, Young TK, Hegele RA. Atherosclerosis 2003;166:351-7.

Björntorp & Rosmond (2000). "Obesity and cortisol." Björntorp P, Rosmond R. Nutrition. 2000 Oct;16(10):924-36

Björntorp (2001). "Do stress reactions cause abdominal obesity and co-morbidities? Björntorp P. Obes Rev. 2001 May;2(2):73-86. PMID: 12119665

Blake (nd). Joan Salge Blake, MS, RD, Academy of Nutrition and Dietetics.

Blaut & Klaus (2012). "Intestinal microbiota and obesity." Blaut M, Klaus S. Handb Exp Pharmacol. 2012;(209):251-73. doi: 10.1007/978-3-642-24716-3_11

Bloomfield et al., (2016). "Effects on Health Outcomes of a Mediterranean Diet With No Restriction on Fat Intake: A Systematic Review and Meta-analysis." Bloomfield HE, Koeller E, Greer N, MacDonald R, Kane R, Wilt TJ. Ann Intern Med. 19 July 2016. doi:10.7326/M16-0361

Blundell & Bellisle (2012). "Satiation, Satiety and the Control of Food Intake: Theory and Practice." edited by John E Blundell, France Bellisle. Elsevier, 30 Sep. 2013

Blundell & Bellisle (2013). "Satiation, Satiety and the Control of Food Intake: Theory and Practice." Edited by John E Blundell, France Bellisle. Elsevier, 30 Sep. 2013

Blundell & Macdiarmid (1997). "Fat as a risk factor for overconsumption: satiation, satiety, and patterns of eating." J.E. Blundell, J.I. Macdiarmid. Journal of the American Dietetic Association, 97 (7) (1997), pp. S63–S69

Blundell (1986). "Macronutrients and satiety: the effects of a high-protein or high-carbohydrate meal on subjective motivation to eat and food preferences. Blundell, J.E. Hill, A.J. AGRIS: International Information System for the Agricultural Science and Technology 1986

Blundell et al., (1993). "Dietary fat and the control of energy intake: evaluating the effects of fat on meal size and postmeal satiety. "Blundell JE, Burley VJ, Cotton JR, Lawton CL. Am J Clin Nutr. 1993 May;57(5 Suppl):772S-777S; discussion 777S-778S

Blundell et al., (1994). "Carbohydrates and human appetite." J.E. Blundell, S. Green, V. Burley. American Journal of Clinical Nutrition, 59 (3) (1994), pp. 728S–734S

Bobroff & Kissileff (1986). "Effects of changes in palatability on food intake and the cumulative food intake curve in man." Bobroff, E. M., & Kissileff, H. R. (1986). Appetite, 7(1), 85-96. Doi: 10.1016/S0195-6663(86)80044-7

Bodinham et al., (2009). "Acute ingestion of resistant starch reduces food intake in healthy adults." Bodinham CL, Frost GS, Robertson MD. Br J Nutr. 2010 Mar;103(6):917-22. doi: 10.1017/S0007114509992534. Epub 2009 Oct 27

Bolhuis et al., (2014). "Slow Food: Sustained Impact of Harder Foods on the Reduction in Energy Intake over the Course of the Day." Dieuwerke P. Bolhuis, Ciarán G. Forde, Yuejiao Cheng, Haohuan Xu, Nathalie Martin, and Cees de Graaf. PLoS One. 2014; 9(4): e93370. Published online 2014 Apr 2. doi: 10.1371/journal.pone.0093370 PMCID: PMC3973680

Bootle (2014). "The medicine in our minds." Olly Bootle. BBC's Horizon programme, 17 February 2014. From the section "Health"

Boschmann et al., (2003). "Water-induced thermogenesis." Boschmann M, Steiniger J, Hille U, Tank J, Adams F, Sharma AM, Klaus S, Luft FC, Jordan J. J Clin Endocrinol Metab. 2003 Dec;88(12):6015-9

Boschmann et al., (2007). "Water Drinking Induces Thermogenesis through Osmosensitive Mechanisms." Michael Boschmann Jochen Steiniger Gabriele Franke Andreas L. Birkenfeld Friedrich C. Luft Jens Jordan. The Journal of Clinical Endocrinology & Metabolism, Volume 92, Issue 8, 1 August 2007, Pages 3334–3337, https://doi.org/10.1210/jc.2006-1438. Published: 01 August 2007

Bossert-Zaudig et al., (2016) "Hunger and appetite during visual perception of food in eating disorders." Bossert-Zaudig, Laessle, Meiller, Ellgring, & Pirke, 1991. Brain and Cognition Volume 110, December 2016, Pages 53–63.

Boubekri et al., (2014). "Impact of Windows and Daylight Exposure on Overall Health and Sleep Quality of Office Workers: A Case-Control Pilot Study." Boubekri M, Cheung IN, Reid KJ, Wang C-H, Zee PC. Journal of Clinical Sleep Medicine : JCSM : Official Publication of the American Academy of Sleep Medicine. 2014;10(6):603-611. doi:10.5664/jcsm.3780

Boutcher (2011). "High-Intensity Intermittent Exercise and Fat Loss. Journal of Obesity. Boutcher SH. 2011;2011:868305. doi:10.1155/2011/868305

Bowden (2016). "The Risks Of Removing Entire Food Groups From Your Diet. Jennifer Bowden, The New Zealand Listener, Nutrition 7th July, 2016

Boyland, et al., (2011). "Food Commercials Increase Preference for Energy-Dense Foods, Particularly in Children Who Watch More Television." Emma J. Boyland, Joanne A. Harrold, Tim C. Kirkham, Catherine Corker, Jenna Cuddy, Deborah Evans, Terence M. Dovey, Clare L. Lawton, John E. Blundell, Jason C. G. Halford. Pediatrics. June 2011. From the American Academy of Pediatrics.

Bracco et al., (1995). "Effects of caffeine on energy metabolism, heart rate, and methylxanthine metabolism in lean and obese women." D. Bracco, J. M. Ferrarra, M. J. Arnaud, E. Jequier, Y. Schutz. American Journal of Physiology - Endocrinology and Metabolism Published 1 October 1995 Vol. 269 no. 4, E671-E678

Bradman, et al., (2015). "Effect of Organic Diet Intervention on Pesticide Exposures in Young Children Living in Low-Income Urban and Agricultural Communities." Asa Bradman, Lesliam Quirós-Alcalá, Rosemary Castorina, Raul Aguilar Schall, Jose Camacho, Nina T. Holland, Dana Boyd Barr, and Brenda Eskenazi. Environ Health Perspect; DOI:10.1289/ehp.1408660. October 2015 Volume 123 Issue 10

Brandhorst et al., (2015). "A Periodic Diet that Mimics Fasting Promotes Multi-System Regeneration, Enhanced Cognitive Performance, and Healthspan." Brandhorst S, Choi IY, Wei M, Cheng CW, Sedrakyan S, Navarrete G, Dubeau L, Yap LP, Park R, Vinciguerra M, Di Biase S, Mirzaei H, Mirisola MG, Childress P, Ji L, Groshen S, Penna F, Odetti P, Perin L, Conti PS, Ikeno Y, Kennedy BK, Cohen P, Morgan TE, Dorff TB, Longo VD. Cell Metab. 2015 Jul 7;22(1):86-99. doi: 10.1016/j.cmet.2015.05.012. Epub 2015 Jun 18. PMID: 26094889

Bratman et al., (2015). "Nature experience reduces rumination and subgenual prefrontal cortex activation." Gregory N. Bratman,1, J. Paul Hamilton, Kevin S. Hahn, Gretchen C. Daily and James J. Gross. Proceedings of the National Academy of Sciences, vol. 112 no. 28. 8567–8572, May 28, 2015. doi: 10.1073/pnas.1510459112

Bray et al., (2004). "Consumption of high-fructose corn syrup in beverages may play a role in the epidemic of obesity." George A Bray, Samara Joy Nielsen, Barry M Popkin. The American Journal of Clinical Nutrition, Volume 79, Issue 4, 1 April 2004, Pages 537–543, https://doi.org/10.1093/ajcn/79.4.537

Březinová (1974). "Effect of caffeine on sleep. EEG study in late middle age people." Vlasta Březinová. Br J Clin Pharmacol. 1974 Jun; 1(3): 203–208. PMCID: PMC1402564

Brimelow (2014). "Mediterranean diet is best way to tackle obesity, say doctors". By Adam Brimelow, Health Correspondent, BBC News, 17 November 2014, writing about a study published by Professor Terence Stephenson, chair of the Academy of Medical Royal Colleges and Dr Mahiben Maruthappu, a senior figure at NHS England.

British Nutrition Foundation (2016). "A Healthy Varied Diet." British Nutrition Foundation. www.nutrition.org.uk/healthyliving/healthyeating/healthyvarieddiet (nd) Retrieved 17th Sept 2016

Brooks (2019). "What evolution tells us about sex, slimming and selfies." Brooks, Rob (Professor of Evolution at the University of N.S.W, Australia). ABC Radio, "On Drive with Richard Glover." Broadcast: Wed 15 May 2019

Broom et al., (2008). "The influence of resistance and aerobic exercise on hunger, circulating levels of acylated ghrelin and peptide YY in healthy males." Broom DR, Batterham RL, King JA, Stensel DJ. AJP Regulatory Integrative and Comparative Physiology, December 19, 2008; DOI: 10.1152/ajpregu.90706.2008

Brown (1991). "Culture and the evolution of obesity." Peter J. Brown. Human Nature 2 (1):31-57 (1991) DOI 10.1007/BF02692180

Browne (2015). "Can you really juice your way to good health? From Nutribullet to Vitamix, we look at the pros and cons of juicing at home" Kate Browne, Choice Magazine. 23rd September 2015

Brundige & Noll (2009). "The Science of Food Cravings".Brundige, Wendy; Noll, Eric. ABC News Network, via Good Morning America. Nov. 14, 2009

Brunstrom et al., (2008). "Measuring 'expected satiety' in a range of common foods using a method of constant stimuli." J.M. Brunstrom, N.G. Shakeshaft, N.E. Scott-Samuel. Appetite, 51 (3) (2008), pp. 604–614

Brunstrom et al., (2011). "'Expected satiety' changes hunger and fullness in the inter-meal interval." J.M. Brunstrom, S. Brown, E.C. Hinton, P.J. Rogers, S.H. Fay. Appetite, 56 (2) (2011), pp. 310–315]

Buchowski et al., (2007). "Energy expenditure of genuine laughter." Buchowski MS, Majchrzak KM, Blomquist K, Chen KY, Byrne DW, Bachorowski JA. Int J Obes (Lond). 2007 Jan;31(1):131-7

Burger et al., (2011a). "Assessing food appeal and desire to eat: the effects of portion size & energy density." Burger, K.S., Cornier, M.A., Ingebrigsten, J., & Johnson, S.L. (2011). International Journal of Behavioral Nutrition and Physical Activity, 8, 101-109. Doi: 10.1186/1479-5868-8-101

Burke, LK et al., (2017). "mTORC1 in AGRP neurons integrates exteroceptive and interoceptive food-related cues in the modulation of adaptive energy expenditure in mice." Burke LK, Darwish T, Cavanaugh AR, Virtue S, Roth E, Morro J, Liu SM, Xia J, Dalley JW, Burling K, Chua S, Vidal-Puig T, Schwartz GJ, Blouet C. Elife. 2017 May 23;6. pii: e22848. doi: 10.7554/eLife.22848

Burton-Freeman (2000). "Dietary fiber and energy regulation." B. Burton-Freeman, Journal of Nutrition, 130 (2) (2000), p. 272.

BVA (2007). "Benefits of dog ownership to human health." Journal of the British Veterinary Association. Feb. 17, 2007, Vol. 160 Issue 7, p208-208, 1/4p.

Calder (2006). "n–3 Polyunsaturated fatty acids, inflammation, and inflammatory diseases." Philip C Calder. Am J Clin Nutr June 2006. vol. 83 no. 6 S1505-1519S

698

Calitri et al., (2010). "Cognitive Biases to Healthy and Unhealthy Food Words Predict Change in BMI." Calitri, R., Pothos, E. M., Tapper, K., Brunstrom, J. M. and Rogers, P. J. (2010), Obesity, 18: 2282–2287. doi:10.1038/oby.2010.78

Cameron et al., (2009). "Increased meal frequency does not promote greater weight loss in subjects who were prescribed an 8-week equi-energetic energy-restricted diet." Cameron JD, Cyr MJ, Doucet E. Br J Nutr. 2010 Apr;103(8):1098-101. doi: 10.1017/S0007114509992984. Epub 2009 Nov 30

Carson et al., (2002). "Mindfulness-based relationship enhancement. James W. Carson, Kimberly M. Carson, Karen M. Gil, Donald H. Baucom. Behavior Therapy Volume 35, Issue 3, Summer 2004, Pages 471–494 Received 7 November 2002

Cashin-Garbutt (2013). "Diets and the famine reaction: an interview with Associate Professor Amanda Salis, University of Sydney." Associate Professor Amanda Salis, Boden Institute of Obesity, Nutrition, Exercise & Eating Disorders. Interview conducted by April Cashin-Garbutt, BA Hons (Cantab). News Medical, www.news-medical.net November 7, 2013

Cassady et al. (2012). "Beverage consumption, appetite, and energy intake: what did you expect?" B.A. Cassady, R.V. Considine, R.D. Mattes. American Journal of Clinical Nutrition, 95 (3) (2012), pp. 587–593

Cassady et al., (2009). "Mastication of almonds: effects of lipid bioaccessibility, appetite, and hormone response." Cassady BA, Hollis JH, Fulford AD, Considine RV, Mattes RD. Am J Clin Nutr. 2009 Mar;89(3):794-800. doi: 10.3945/ajcn.2008.26669. Epub 2009 Jan 14

Caudwell et al. (2013). "Physical Activity, Energy Intake, and Obesity: The Links Between Exercise and Appetite." Caudwell, P., Gibbons, C., Finlayson, G. et al. Curr Obes Rep (2013) 2: 185. doi:10.1007/s13679-013-0051-1

Cecil et al., (1998). "Relative contributions of intestinal, gastric, oro-sensory influences and information to changes in appetite induced by the same liquid meal." Cecil J E, Francis J, Read N W. Appetite 1998; 31: 377–390.

Chaix et al., (2014). "Time-restricted feeding is a preventative and therapeutic intervention against diverse nutritional challenges." Chaix A, Zarrinpar A, Miu P, Panda S. Cell Metab. 2014 Dec 2;20(6):991-1005. doi: 10.1016/j.cmet.2014.11.001

Chambers et al., (2013). "Can the satiating power of a high energy beverage be improved by manipulating sensory characteristics and label information?" L. Chambers, H. Ells, M.R. Yeomans. Food Quality and Preference, 28 (1) (2013), pp. 271–278.

Chambers et al., (2015). "Optimising foods for satiety." Lucy Chambers, Keri McCrickerd, Martin R. Yeomans. Trends in Food Science & Technology, Volume 41, Issue 2, February 2015, Pages 149–160. http://dx.doi.org/10.1016/j.tifs.2014.10.007

Chandon & Wansink (2012). "Does food marketing need to make us fat? A review and solutions." Chandon P, Wansink B. Nutrition Reviews. 2012;70(10):571-593. doi:10.1111/j.1753-4887.2012.00518.x.

Chaouloff et al., (1985). "Effects of conditioned running on plasma, liver and brain tryptophan and on brain 5-hydroxytryptamine metabolism of the rat." Chaouloff F, Elghozi JL, Guezennec Y, Laude D. Br J Pharmacol. 1985 Sep; 86(1):33-41

Chassaing et al., (2015). "Dietary emulsifiers impact the mouse gut microbiota promoting colitis and metabolic syndrome." Benoit Chassaing, Omry Koren, Julia Goodrich, Angela Poole, Shanthi Srinivasan, Ruth E. Ley, and Andrew T. Gewirtz. Nature. 2015 Mar 5; 519(7541): 92–96. doi: 10.1038/nature14232. PMCID: PMC4910713. NIHMSID: NIHMS656221

Chaudhri et al. (2006). "Gastrointestinal hormones regulating appetite". Chaudhri, Owais; Small, Caroline; Bloom, Steve (2006-07-29). Philosophical Transactions of the Royal Society of London. Series B, Biological Sciences. 361 (1471): 1187–1209. doi:10.1098/rstb.2006.1856. ISSN 0962-8436. PMC 1642697 free to read. PMID 16815798.]

Choi et al., (2014). "Eat, cook, grow: Mixing human–computer interactions with human–food interactions." [J.H.-J. Choi, M. Foth, G. Hearn (Eds.), MIT Press, Cambridge, MA (2014)]

Chopan & Littenberg (2017). "The Association of Hot Red Chili Pepper Consumption and Mortality: A Large Population-Based Cohort Study." Mustafa Chopan, Benjamin Littenberg. PLOS. Published: January 9, 2017. http://dx.doi.org/10.1371/journal.pone.0169876

CIA (2016). "The World Factbook Country Comparison: Obesity—Adult Prevalence Rate." Central Intelligence Agency (USA) World Factbook 2016

Clark & Slavin (2013). "The effect of fiber on satiety and food intake: a systematic review." M.J. Clark, J.L. Slavin. Journal of the American College of Nutrition, 32 (3) (2013), pp. 200–211]

Clay (2011). "Stressed in America." R.A. Clay. January 2011, Monitor on Psychology. Vol 42, No. 1. Print version: page 60

Clegg et al., (2013). "Soups increase satiety through delayed gastric emptying yet increased glycemic response." M E Clegg, V Ranawana, A Shafat and C J Henry. European Journal of Clinical Nutrition 67, 8-11 (January 2013) | doi:10.1038/ejcn.2012.152

Cooling & Blundell (2001). "High-fat and low-fat phenotypes: Habitual eating of high- and low-fat foods not related to taste preference for fat." Cooling J, Blundell JE. Eur J Clin Nutr. 2001;55:1016–1021.

Copinschi (2005). "Metabolic and endocrine effects of sleep deprivation." Copinschi G. PMID:16459757. Laboratory of Physiology, Université Libre de Bruxelles, Brussels, Belgium. Essential Psychopharmacology 2005, 6(6):341-347

Corwin & Babbs (2012). "Rodent models of binge eating: are they models of addiction?" Corwin RL, Babbs RK. ILAR J. 2012;53(1):23-34

Corwin & Grigson (2009). "Symposium Overview—Food Addiction: Fact Or Fiction?" Corwin, R. L., and P. S. Grigson. Journal of Nutrition 139(2009): 617-619

Cox & Blazer (2015). "Antibiotics in early life and obesity." Laura M. Cox and Martin J. Blaser. Nat Rev Endocrinol. 2015 Mar; 11(3): 182–190. PMCID: PMC4487629 NIHMSID: NIHMS703258

Crabtree et al., (2014). "The effects of high-intensity exercise on neural responses to images of food. Crabtree DR, Chambers ES, Hardwick RM, Blannin AK." Am J Clin Nutr. 2014 Feb;99(2):258-67. doi: 10.3945/ajcn.113.071381. Epub 2013 Dec 4.

Crisinel & Spence (2009). "Implicit Association Between Basic Tastes and Pitch." Anne-Sylvie Crisinel, Charles Spence. Neurosci Lett 464 (1), 39-42. 2009 Aug 11.

Crisinel & Spence (2010a). "A Sweet Sound? Food Names Reveal Implicit Associations Between Taste and Pitch." Anne-Sylvie Crisinel , Charles Spence. Perception 39 (3), 417-425. 2010.

Crisinel & Spence (2010b). "As Bitter as a Trombone: Synesthetic Correspondences in Nonsynesthetes Between Tastes/Flavors and Musical Notes." Anne-Sylvie Crisinel, Charles Spence. Atten Percept Psychophys 72 (7), 1994-2002. 10 2010.

Crisinel et al., (2012). "A bittersweet symphony: Systematically modulating the taste of food by changing the sonic properties of the soundtrack playing in the background." Crisinel A.-S., Cosser S., King S., Jones R., Petrie J., Spence C. Food Quality and Preference. 2012;24:201–204. doi: 10.1016/j.foodqual.2011.08.009.

Critchley & Rolls (1996). "Hunger and satiety modify the responses of olfactory and visual neurons in the primate orbitofrontal cortex." H. D. Critchley and E. T. Rolls. J Neurophysiol. 1996 Apr;75(4):1673-86.

Crum et al. (2011). "Mind over milkshakes: mindsets, not just nutrients, determine ghrelin response." A.J. Crum, W.R. Corbin, K.D. Brownell, P. Salovey. Health Psychol, 30 (4) (2011), pp. 424–429 discussion 430–421.

Daniel et al., (2013). "The Future Is Now: Reducing Impulsivity and Energy Intake Using Episodic Future Thinking." Daniel TO, Stanton CM, Epstein LH. Psychological science. 2013;24(11):2339-2342. doi:10.1177/0956797613488780

Dashti et al., (2015). "Short Sleep Duration and Dietary Intake: Epidemiologic Evidence, Mechanisms, and Health Implications." Hassan S Dashti, Frank AJL Scheer, Paul F Jacques, Stefania Lamon-Fava, and José M Ordovás. doi: 10.3945/an.115.008623. Adv Nutr November 2015 Adv Nutr vol. 6: 648-659, 2015

Daubenmier et al., (2011). "Mindfulness Intervention for Stress Eating to Reduce Cortisol and Abdominal Fat among Overweight and Obese Women: An Exploratory Randomized Controlled Study." Jennifer Daubenmier, Jean Kristeller, Frederick M. Hecht, Nicole Maninger, Margaret Kuwata, Kinnari Jhaveri, Robert H. Lustig, Margaret Kemeny, Lori Karan, and Elissa Epel. Journal of Obesity, Volume 2011 (2011), Article ID 651936, 13 pages. http://dx.doi.org/10.1155/2011/651936

David et al., (2014). "Diet rapidly and reproducibly alters the human gut microbiome." David LA, Maurice CF, Carmody RN, Gootenberg DB, Button JE, Wolfe BE, Ling AV, Devlin AS, Varma Y, Fischbach MA, Biddinger SB, Dutton RJ, Turnbaugh PJ. Nature. 2014 Jan 23;505(7484):559-63. doi: 10.1038/nature12820. Epub 2013 Dec 11

Davidson & Swithers (2004). "A Pavlovian approach to the problem of obesity." Int J Obes Relat Metab Disord 2004 Jul;28(7):933-5. T L Davidson, S E Swithers DOI: 10.1038/sj.ijo.0802660

Davidson et al., (2011). "Intake of High-intensity Sweeteners alters the Ability of Sweet Taste to Signal Caloric Consequences: Implications for the Learned Control of Energy and Body Weight Regulation." Terry L. Davidson, Ashley A. Martin, Kiely Clark, and Susan E. Swithers. Q J Exp Psychol (Hove). 2011 Jul; 64(7): 1430–1441. doi: 10.1080/17470218.2011.552729. PMCID: PMC3412685 NIHMSID: NIHMS373389

Davies (2016). "Men should exercise BEFORE eating and women AFTER to burn the most fat, scientists reveal." Madlen Davies for Mail Online. 8 January 2016

Davis (1928). "Self selection of diet by newly weaned infants: an experimental study." Davis CM. Am J Dis Child 1928;36(4):651-79 [Reprinted as a Nutrition Classics article in Nutr Rev 1986;44:114-6]

Davis et al., (2004). "Sensitivity to reward: implications for overeating and overweight." Davis C, Strachan S, Berkson M. Appetite 2004, 42: 131-138. 10.1016/j.appet.2003.07.004

de Castro et al., (2000). "Palatability and intake relationships in free-living humans: measurement and characterization in the French." de Castro, J. M., Bellisle, F., & Dalix, A. M. (2000). Physiology & Behavior, 68(3), 271-277. doi: 10.1016/S0031-9384(99)00166-3

de Castro, J. M. (2004). "The time of day of food intake influences overall intake in humans." The Journal of Nutrition, 134(1), 104-111

de Castro, J.M. (1990). "Social facilitation of duration and size but not rate of the spontaneous meal intake of humans." Physiology & Behavior, 47(6), 1129-1135. doi: 10.1016/0031-9384(90)90363-9

de Castro, J.M. (1994). "Family and friends produce greater social facilitation of food intake than other companions." Physiology & Behavior, 56(3), 445-455. 10.1016/0031-9384(94)90286-0

de Craen et al., (1996). "Effect of colour of drugs: systematic review of perceived effect of drugs and of their effectiveness." A. J. de Craen, P. J. Roos, A. Leonard de Vries, and J. Kleijnentries. BMJ. 1996 Dec 21; 313(7072): 1624–1626. PMCID: PMC2359128

De Filippo et al., (2010). "Impact of diet in shaping gut microbiota revealed by a comparative study in children from Europe and rural Africa." Carlotta De Filippo, Duccio Cavalieri, Monica Di Paola, Matteo Ramazzotti, Jean Baptiste Poullet, Sebastien Massart, Silvia Collini, Giuseppe Pieraccini, and Paolo Lionetti. 2010 Proceedings of the National Academy of Sciences of the United States of America vol. 107 no. 33. 14691–14696, doi: 10.1073/pnas.1005963107

de Graaf (2019). "Texture and satiation: the role of oro-sensory exposure time." Physiol Behav. 2012 Nov 5;107(4):496-501. doi:10.1016/j.physbeh.2012.05.008. Epub 2012 May 15. de Graaf C.

de Graaf et al., (1999). "Palatability affects satiation but not satiety." de Graaf C, de Jong LS, Lambers AC. Physiol Behav 1999; 66: 681–688.

de Lauzon-Guillain et al., (2006). "Is restrained eating a risk factor for weight gain in a general population?" Blandine de Lauzon-Guillain, Arnaud Basdevant, Monique Romon, Jan Karlsson, Jean-Michel Borys, M Aline Charles, and The FLVS Study Group. Am J Clin Nutr January 2006 vol. 83 no. 1 132-138

de Matos Feijó et al., (2011). "Serotonin and hypothalamic control of hunger: a review." Fernanda de Matos Feijó; Marcello Casaccia Bertoluci; Cíntia Reis. Rev. Assoc. Med. Bras. vol.57 no.1 São Paulo Jan./Feb. 2011. http://dx.doi.org/10.1590/S0104-42302011000100020

De Palma et al (2015). "Microbiota and host determinants of behavioural phenotype in maternally separated mice." De Palma G, Blennerhassett P, Lu J, Deng Y, Park AJ, Green W, Denou E, Silva MA, Santacruz A2, Sanz Y, Surette MG, Verdu EF, Collins SM, Bercik P. Nat Commun. 2015 Jul 28;6:7735. doi: 10.1038/ncomms8735.]

de Wijk et al., (2012). "Food aroma affects bite size." René A de Wijk, Ilse A Polet, Wilbert Boek, Saskia Coenraad and Johannes HF Bult. Flavour 2012 1:3. DOI: 10.1186/2044-7248-1-3. © De Wijk et al; licensee BioMed Central Ltd. 2012. Published: 21 March 2012.

Dennis, et al., (2010). "Water Consumption Increases Weight Loss During a Hypocaloric Diet Intervention in Middle-aged and Older Adults." Elizabeth A. Dennis, Ana Laura Dengo, Dana L. Comber, Kyle D. Flack, Jyoti Savla, Kevin P. Davy, and Brenda M. Davy. Obesity (Silver Spring). 2010 Feb; 18(2): 300–307.Published online 2009 Aug 6. doi: 10.1038/oby.2009.235 PMCID: PMC2859815 NIHMSID: NIHMS194440

DeNoon (2013). "A dog could be your heart's best friend." Daniel DeNoon, Executive Editor, Harvard Heart Letter. Harvard Medical School, Harvard Health Publishing. May 22, 2013, Updated October 29, 2015.

Dhurandhar et al., (2014). 'The effectiveness of breakfast recommendations on weight loss: a randomized controlled trial." Emily J Dhurandhar, John Dawson, Amy Alcorn, Lesli H Larsen, Elizabeth A Thomas, Michelle Cardel, Ashley C Bourland, Arne Astrup, Marie-Pierre St-Onge, James O Hill, Caroline M Apovian, James M Shikany, and David B Allison. First published June 4, 2014, doi: 10.3945/ajcn.114.089573. Am J Clin Nutr. ajcn.089573

Diabetes Ireland (2018). "What are free sugars?" Diabetes Ireland. https://www.diabetes.ie/what-are-free-sugars Retrieved 24th February 2018

DiBaise et al., (2012). "Impact of the Gut Microbiota on the Development of Obesity: Current Concepts." John K DiBaise MD, Daniel N Frank PhD and Ruchi Mathur MD, FRCPC. Am J Gastroenterol Suppl (2012) 1:22–27; doi:10.1038/ajgsup.2012.5

Dobson (1999). "If you want to get fit, get fidgeting." Roger Dobson, Wednesday 24 February 1999, The Guardian Health & wellbeing

Doheny (2012). "The secret to a longer life? Children." Kathleen Doheny, Reviewed by Louise Chang, MD . The Atlanta Journal-Constitution. Thursday, Dec. 6, 2012 Atlanta health, diet and fitness news.

Donga et al., (2010). "A Single Night of Partial Sleep Deprivation Induces Insulin Resistance in Multiple Metabolic Pathways in Healthy Subjects." E. Donga, M. van Dijk, J. G. van Dijk, N. R. Biermasz, G. J. Lammers, K. W. van Kralingen, E. P. M. Corssmit, J. A. Romijn. Journal of Clinical Endocrinology & Metabolism (2010)

Drewnowski (1998). "Energy Density, Palatability, and Satiety: Implications for Weight Control." Drewnowski, A. (1998) "Nutrition Reviews, 56: 347–353. doi:10.1111/j.1753-4887.1998.tb01677.x]

Drewnowski et al., (2012). "Sweetness and Food Preference. "Adam Drewnowski, Julie A. Mennella, Susan L. Johnson, and France Bellisle © 2012 American Society for Nutrition

Dulloo et al., (1989). "Normal caffeine consumption: influence on thermogenesis and daily energy expenditure in lean and postobese human volunteers." Dulloo AG, Geissler CA, Horton T, Collins A, Miller DS. Am J Clin Nutr. 1989 Jan;49(1):44-50

Duncan et al., (1983). "The effects of high and low energy density diets on satiety, energy intake, and eating time of obese and nonobese subjects." Duncan KH, Bacon JA, Weinsier RL. Am J Clin Nutr. 1983 May;37(5):763-7

Eastwood (2013). "Principles of Human Nutrition." Eastwood, Martin John Wiley & Sons, 5 Jun. 2013

Ebbeling et al., (2012). "Effects of Dietary Composition on Energy Expenditure During Weight-Loss Maintenance." Ebbeling CB, Swain JF, Feldman HA, Wong WW, Hachey DL, Garcia-Lago E, Ludwig DS. JAMA. 2012;307(24):2627-2634. doi:10.1001/jama.2012.6607

Eertmans, et al., (2001). "Food likes and their relative importance in human eating behavior: review and preliminary suggestions for health promotion." A. Eertmans, F. Baeyens and O. Van den Bergh. Health Education Research, Vol.16 no.4 2001 Theory & Practice. Pages 443–456

Ehrlich et al (2014). "Handling of Thermal Receipts as a Source of Exposure to Bisphenol A." Shelley Ehrlich, MD, ScD, MPH; Antonia M. Calafat, PhD; Olivier Humblet, ScD; Thomas Smith, PhD; Russ Hauser, MD, ScD, MPH.] [Research Letter. February 26, 2014. JAMA. 2014;311(8):859-860. doi:10.1001/jama.2013.283735

Eisenhofer et al., (1997). "Substantial production of dopamine in the human gastrointestinal tract." Eisenhofer G, Aneman A, Friberg P, Hooper D, Fåndriks L, Lonroth H, Hunyady B, Mezey E. J Clin Endocrinol Metab. 1997 Nov; 82(11):3864-71

Ejaz et al., (2009). "Curcumin Inhibits Adipogenesis in 3T3-L1 Adipocytes and Angiogenesis and Obesity in C57/BL Mice." Ejaz A, Wu, D, Kwan P, and Meydani M. Journal of Nutrition. May 2009; 139 (5): 1042-1048. 919-925

Ekelund et al. (2016). "Does physical activity attenuate, or even eliminate, the detrimental association of sitting time with mortality? A harmonised meta-analysis of data from more than 1 million men and women." Ekelund U, Steene-Johannessen J, Brown WJ, Fagerland MW, Owen N, Powell KE, Bauman A, Lee IM; The Lancet , Volume 388 , Issue 10051 , 1302 - 1310

Elliott et al., (2002). "Fructose, weight gain, and the insulin resistance syndrome." Sharon S Elliott, Nancy L Keim, Judith S Stern, Karen Teff, and Peter J Havel. Am J Clin Nutr November 2002, vol. 76 no. 5 911-922

Ello-Martin et al., (2005). "The influence of food portion size and energy density on energy intake: implications for weight management." Ello-Martin, J. A., Ledikwe, J. H., & Rolls, B. J. (2005). The American Journal of Clinical Nutrition, 82(1), 236S-241S

Elsevier (2016). "Reduction in Dietary Diversity Impacts Richness of Human Gut Microbiota." Elsevier Research And Journals, Berlin, March 15, 2016

Engell et al., (1996). "Effects of effort and social modeling on drinking in humans." Engell, D., Kramer, M., Malafi, T., Salomon, M., & Lesher, L. (1996). Appetite, 26(2), 129-138. doi: 10.1006/appe.1996.0011

Engell et al., (1998). "Effects of information about fat content on food preferences in pre-adolescent children." Engell, D., Bordi, P., Borja, M., Lambert, C. and Rolls, B. (1998) Appetite, 30, 269 – 282

English et al., (2014). "Mechanisms of the portion size effect. What is known and where do we go from here?" Laural English, Marlou Lasschuijt, Kathleen L. Keller. Appetite 3 November 2014. DOI: 10.1016/j. appet.2014.11.004

Entwistle et al., (2014). "Unconscious agendas in the etiology of refractory obesity and the role of hypnosis in their identification and resolution: a new paradigm for weight-management programs or a paradigm revisited?" Entwistle PA, Webb RJ, Abayomi JC, Johnson B, Sparkes AC, Davies IG. Int J Clin Exp Hypn. 2014;62(3):330-59. doi: 10.1080/00207144.2014.901085

Eördögh et al., (2016). "Food Addiction as a new behavioral addiction." Eördögh E, Hoyer M, Szeleczky G. Psychiatr Hung. 2016;31(3):248-255 (Article in Hungarian)

Epel et al., (2000). "Stress and body shape: Stress-induced cortisol secretion is consistently greater among women with central fat." Epel ES, McEwen B, Seeman T, Matthews K, Castellazzo G, Brownell KD, Bell J, Ickovics JR. Psychosom Med. 2000;62(5):623-632

Epel et al., (2001). "Stress may add bite to appetite in women: a laboratory study of stress-induced cortisol and eating behavior". Elissa Epel, Rachel Lapidus, Bruce McEwen, Kelly Brown. Psychoneuroendocrinology Volume 26, Issue 1, January 2001, Pages 37–49 doi:10.1016/S0306-4530(00)00035-4

Epperson et al., (2004). "Randomized clinical trial of bright light therapy for antepartum depression: preliminary findings." Epperson CN, Terman M, Terman JS, Hanusa BH, Oren DA, Peindl KS, Wisner KL. J Clin Psychiatry. 2004 Mar; 65(3):421-5

Epstein et al., (2007). "Food Reinforcement, the Dopamine D2 Receptor Genotype, and Energy Intake in Obese and Nonobese Humans." Leonard H. Epstein, PhD, Jennifer L. Temple, PhD, Brad. J. Neaderhiser, PhD, Robbert J. Salis, MD, Richard W. Erbe, MD, and John J. Leddy, MD, Behavioral Neuroscience, Vol. 121, No. 5. 2007

Evans et al., (2014). "Exercise Prevents Weight Gain and Alters the Gut Microbiota in a Mouse Model of High Fat Diet-Induced Obesity." Christian C. Evans, Kathy J. LePard, Jeff W. Kwak, Mary C. Stancukas, Samantha Laskowski, Joseph Dougherty, Laura Moulton, Adam Glawe, Yunwei Wang, Vanessa Leone, Dionysios A. Antonopoulos, Dan Smith, Eugene B. Chang, Mae J. Ciancio. PLOS. Published: March 26, 2014. http://dx.doi.org/10.1371/journal.pone.0092193

Everard, et al., (2013). "Cross-talk between Akkermansia muciniphila and intestinal epithelium controls diet-induced obesity." Amandine Everard, Clara Belzer, Lucie Geurts, Janneke P. Ouwerkerk, Céline Druart, Laure B. Bindels, Yves Guiot, Muriel Derrien, Giulio G. Muccioli, Nathalie M. Delzenne, Willem M. de Vos, and Patrice D. Cani. Biological Sciences—Microbiology: PNAS 2013 110 (22) 9066-9071; published ahead of print May 13, 2013, doi:10.1073/pnas.1219451110

Eweis et al., (2016). "Carbon dioxide in carbonated beverages induces ghrelin release and increased food consumption in male rats: Implications on the onset of obesity." Dureen Samandar Eweis, Fida Abed, Johnny Stiban. Department of Biology and Biochemistry, Birzeit University, P.O. Box 14, Ramallah, West Bank 627, Palestine. Received 7 September 2016, Revised 15 January 2017, Accepted 2 February 2017, Available online 20 February 2017. Obesity Research & Clinical Practice, Volume 11, Issue 5, September–October 2017, Pages 534-543

Farvid et al., (2014) "Dietary protein sources in early adulthood and breast cancer incidence: prospective cohort study." Maryam S Farvid, Eunyoung Cho, Wendy Y Chen, A Heather Eliassen, Walter C Willett. BMJ 2014;348:g3437

Farvid et al., (2015). "Adolescent meat intake and breast cancer risk." Farvid, M. S., Cho, E., Chen, W. Y., Eliassen, A.Heather. and Willett, W. C. (2015), Int. J. Cancer, 136: 1909–1920. doi:10.1002/ijc.29218

Fernstrom & Wurtman (1971). "Brain serotonin content: increase following ingestion of carbohydrate diet." D. Fernstrom & R. J. Wurtman (1971). Science 174, 1023–1025

Ferrero (2017). "The Kinder Story". Kinder Surprise® ©2017 Ferrero®. www. kinder.com/au/en/the-kinder-story/04

Ferriday et al., (2015). "Effects of eating rate on satiety: A role for episodic memory?" Danielle Ferriday, Matthew L. Bosworth, Samantha Lai, Nicolas Godinot, Nathalie Martin, Ashley A. Martin, Peter J. Rogers, Jeffrey M. Brunstrom. Physiology & Behavior, Volume 152, Issue null, Pages 389-396. 2015

Field et al., (2005). "Cortisol decreases and serotonin and dopamine increase following massage therapy." Field T, Hernandez-Reif M, Diego M, Schanberg S, Kuhn C. Int J Neurosci. 2005 Oct;115(10):1397-413

Fiese et al., (2015). "Family mealtime dynamics and food consumption: An experimental approach to understanding distractions." Fiese, Barbara H.; Jones, Blake L.; Jarick, Jessica M. Couple and Family Psychology: Research and Practice, Vol 4(4), Dec 2015, 199-211

Flint et al., (1998). "Glucagon-like peptide 1 promotes satiety and suppresses energy intake in humans." A Flint, A Raben, A Astrup, and J J Holst. J Clin Invest. 1998 February 1; 101(3): 515–520. doi: 10.1172/JCI990 PMCID: PMC508592.

Flood & Rolls (2007). "Soup preloads in a variety of forms reduce meal energy intake." Flood JE, Rolls BJ. Appetite. 2007;49(3):626-634. doi:10.1016/j.appet.2007.04.002

Fogel and Blisset (2017). "Past exposure to fruit and vegetable variety moderates the link between fungiform papillae density and current variety of FV consumed by children." Fogel, Anna and Blissett, Jackie. Physiology & Behavior 177. April 2017 DOI: 10.1016/j. physbeh.2017.04.015

Fonken et al., (2010). "Light at night increases body mass by shifting the time of food intake." L. K. Fonken, J. L. Workman, J. C. Walton, Z. M. Weil, J. S. Morris, A. Haim, R. J. Nelson. Proceedings of the National Academy of Sciences (2010) 107 (43) 18664-18669

Forde et al., (2013). "Oral processing characteristics of solid savoury meal components, and relationship with food composition, sensory attributes and expected satiation." C.G. Forde, N. van Kuijk, T. Thaler, C. de Graaf, N. Martin. Appetite, 60 (0) (2013), pp. 208–219

Foroni et al., (2016). "Food color is in the eye of the beholder: the role of human trichromatic vision in food evaluation." Francesco Foroni, Giulio Pergola & Raffaella Ida Rumiati. Scientific Reports volume 6, Article number: 37034 (2016). doi:10.1038/srep37034. Accepted: 11 October 2016

Fowler et al., (2008). "Fueling the Obesity Epidemic? Artificially Sweetened Beverage Use and Long-term Weight Gain." Fowler, Sharon P. and Williams, Ken and Resendez, Roy G. and Hunt, Kelly J. and Hazuda, Helen P. and Stern, Michael P. Obesity vol. 16, number 8, Blackwell Publishing Ltd, issn 1930-739X, dx.doi.org/10.1038/oby.2008.284, doi 10.1038/oby.2008.284, pp.1894--1900, 2008, @article OBY:OBY1097]

Franco et al., (2012). "The sedative effects of hops (Humulus lupulus), a component of beer, on the activity/rest rhythm." Franco L, Sánchez C, Bravo R, Rodriguez A, Barriga C, Juánez JC. Acta Physiol Hung. 2012 Jun;99(2):133-9. doi: 10.1556/APhysiol.99.2012.2.6

Free Dictionary (2018). "Homoeostasis." The Free Dictionary by Farlex. Retrieved 30th April 2018 http://medical-dictionary.thefreedictionary.com/Homoeostasis

Free Dictionary (2018). "Placebo." The Free Dictionary by Farlex. Retrieved 1st June 2018

Fuchs et al., (2011). "Investigation into gender differences in the effects of feeding around exercise on energy expenditure and substrate utilization." Abigail Fuchs, H. Young, H. Booth, F. Armitage, Adam L Collins. Proceedings of The Nutrition Society (Impact Factor: 5.27). 01/2011; 70(OCE6). DOI: 10.1017/S0029665111004654

Fujioka et al., (2006). "The effects of grapefruit on weight and insulin resistance: relationship to the metabolic syndrome." Fujioka K, Greenway F, Sheard J, Ying Y.] [J Med Food. 2006 Spring;9(1):49-54

Fukuda et al., (2013). "Chewing number is related to incremental increases in body weight from 20 years of age in Japanese middle-aged adults." Fukuda, H., Saito, T., Mizuta, M., Moromugi, S., Ishimatsu, T., Nishikado, S., Takagi, H. and Konomi, Y. (2013), Gerodontology, 30: 214–219. doi:10.1111/j.1741-2358.2012.00666.x

Gaesser (2007). "Carbohydrate quantity and quality in relation to body mass index." G.A. Gaesser. Journal of the American Dietetic Association, 107 (10) (2007), pp. 1768–1780

Gaesser (2007). "Carbohydrate quantity and quality in relation to body mass index." G.A. Gaesser. Journal of the American Dietetic Association, 107 (10) (2007), pp. 1768–1780

Gal & Gad (2016). "The Circadian Nature of Mitochondrial Biology." Manella Gal, Asher Gad. Frontiers in Endocrinology, Vol 7, 2016. Page 162. DOI=10.3389/fendo.2016.00162. ISSN=1664-2392

Gallagher (2018). "More than half your body is not human." James Gallagher Presenter, The Second Genome, BBC News health BBC Radio 4. 10th April 2018

Gangwisch et al., (2005). "Inadequate sleep as a risk factor for obesity: analyses of the NHANES I." Gangwisch JE; Malaspina D; Boden-Albala B et al. SLEEP 2005;28(10): 1289-1296

GB HealthWatch (2016). "Overeating? Blame your FTO gene." GB Health-Watch. www.gbhealthwatch.com/HotTopic-Overeating-FTO.php. Retrieved 21 November 2016

Gearhardt et al., (2009). "Preliminary validation of the Yale Food Addiction Scale." Gearhardt, AN, Corbin, WR, and Brownell, KD. Appetite 52(2009): 430-436

Gearhardt et al., (2011). "Binge Eating Disorder and Food Addiction." Gearhardt AN, White MA, Potenza MN. Current drug abuse reviews. 2011;4(3):201-207

Geier et al., (2012). "Red potato chips: segmentation cues can substantially decrease food intake." A. Geier, B. Wansink, P. Rozin. Health Psychology, 31 (3) (2012), pp. 398–401

Gholipour (2014). "5 Ways Fatherhood Changes a Man's Brain." Bahar Gholipour. Live ScienceHealth, June 14, 2014. www.livescience.com]

Gibala et al., (2012). "Physiological adaptations to low-volume, high-intensity interval training in health and disease." Gibala MJ, Little JP, MacDonald MJ, Hawley JA. The Journal of Physiology. 2012;590(Pt 5):1077-1084. doi:10.1113/jphysiol.2011.224725

Giles (nd). "How The Kitchen Became The Hub Of The Home." Alexandra Giles. (nd) Written for Origin Global (UK). https://origin-global.com/advice-centre/how-the-kitchen-became-the-hub-of-the-home

Giugliano et al., (2006). "The effects of diet on inflammation: emphasis on the metabolic syndrome." Giugliano D, Ceriello A, Esposito K. J Am Coll Cardiol. 2006 Aug 15;48(4):677-85. Epub 2006 Jul 24

Golden et al., (2005). "The efficacy of light therapy in the treatment of mood disorders: a review and meta-analysis of the evidence." Golden RN, Gaynes BN, Ekstrom RD, Hamer RM, Jacobsen FM, Suppes T, Wisner KL, Nemeroff CB. Am J Psychiatry. 2005 Apr; 162(4):656-62.

Gollwitzer & Oettingen (2011). "Planning promotes goal striving." Gollwitzer, P. M., & Oettingen, G. (2011). In K. D. Vohs & R. F. Baumeister (Eds.), Handbook of self-regulation: Research, theory, and applications (pp. 162-185). New York, NY, US: Guilford Press.

Gollwitzer & Sheeran (2006). "Implementation intentions and goal achievement: A meta-analysis of effects and processes." Gollwitzer, P. M., & Sheeran, P. (2006). Advances in Experimental Social Psychology, 38, 69–119

Gollwitzer (1999). "Implementation intentions: Strong effects of simple plans." Gollwitzer, P. M. (1999). American Psychologist, 54(7), 493-503. http://dx.doi.org/10.1037/0003-066X.54.7.493

Goodwin et al., (1975). "Drinking amid abundant illicit drugs: the Vietnam case." Goodwin, D. W., Davis, D. H. & Robins, L. N. (1975) Archives of General Psychiatry, 32, pp. 230-233

Goosens & Roper (1994). "Erythritol: a new sweetener." J. Goosens and H. Roper. Food Science and Technology Today, vol. 8, pp. 144–149, 1994

Grabenhorst et al., (2008). "How cognition modulates affective responses to taste and flavor: top-down influences on the orbitofrontal and pregenual cingulate cortices." Grabenhorst F, Rolls ET, Bilderbeck A. Cereb Cortex 2008;18:1549–59

Green et al., (2000). "Dietary restraint and addictive behaviors: the generalizability of Tiffany's cue reactivity model." Green MW, Rogers PJ, Elliman NA.. Int J Eat Disord (2000) 27:419–27.10.1002/(SICI)1098-108X(200005)27:4<419::AID-EAT6>3.0.CO;2-Z

Greer et al., (2013). "The impact of sleep deprivation on food desire in the human brain." Stephanie M. Greer, Andrea N. Goldstein & Matthew P. Walker. 2013/08/06. Nature Publishing Group. http://dx.doi.org/10.1038/ncomms3259

Grice & Segre (2012). "The Human Microbiome: Our Second Genome." Elizabeth A. Grice and Julia A. Segre. Annu Rev Genomics Hum Genet. 2012; 13: 151–170. doi: 10.1146/annurev-genom-090711-163814. PMCID: PMC3518434. NIHMSID: NIHMS424103. PMID: 22703178. 2012

Grün (2006). "Environmental Obesogens: Organotins and Endocrine Disruption via Nuclear Receptor Signaling." Grün, F. Endocrinology 147, s50–s55 (2006)

Grün et al., (2006). "Endocrine-disrupting organotin compounds are potent inducers of adipogenesis in vertebrates." Grün, F, Watanabe H, Zamanian Z, Maeda L, Arima K, Cubacha R, Gardiner DM, Kanno J, Iguchi T, Blumberg B. Mol. Endocrinol. 20, 2141–2155 (2006)

Gupta et al., (2002). "Is obesity associated with poor sleep quality in adolescents?" Neeraj K. Gupta, William H. Mueller, Wenyaw Chan andJanet C. Meininger. Article first published online: 24 OCT 2002. DOI: 10.1002/ajhb.10093. Wiley-Liss, Inc. American Journal of Human Biology Volume 14, Issue 6, pages 762–768, November 2002

Habera et al., (1977). "Depletion And Disruption Of Dietary Fibre: Effects On Satiety, Plasma-Glucose, And Serum-Insulin." Habera GB, Heaton KW, Murphy D, Burroughs LF. Lancet. 1977 Oct 1;2(8040):679-82.

Halford & Harrold (2012). "Satiety-enhancing products for appetite control: science and regulation of functional foods for weight management." J.C. Halford, J.A. Harrold. Proceedings of the Nutrition Society, 71 (2) (2012), p. 350

Hall et al., (2019). "Ultra-Processed Diets Cause Excess Calorie Intake and Weight Gain: An Inpatient Randomized Controlled Trial of Ad Libitum Food Intake." Hall KD, Ayuketah A, Brychta R, Cai H, Cassimatis T, Chen KY, Chung ST, Costa E, Courville A, Darcey V, Fletcher LA, Forde CG, Gharib AM, Guo J, Howard R, Joseph PV, McGehee S, Ouwerkerk R, Raisinger K, Rozga I, Stagliano M, Walter M, Walter PJ, Yang S, Zhou M. Cell Metab. 2019 May 16. pii: S1550-4131(19)30248-7. doi: 10.1016/j.cmet.2019.05.008.

Halton & Hu (2004). "The Effects of High Protein Diets on Thermogenesis, Satiety and Weight Loss: A Critical Review." Thomas L. Halton & Frank B. Hu MD, PhD. Journal of the American College of Nutrition, Volume 23, Issue 5, 2004. DOI: 10.1080/07315724.2004.10719381

Hargrove (2007). "Does the history of food energy units suggest a solution to 'Calorie confusion'?" Nutr J. 2007; 6: 44. doi: 10.1186/1475-2891-6-44. PMCID: PMC2238749

Harmon (2011). "Walking Speed Predicts Life Expectancy of Older Adults." Katherine Harmon, January 4, 2011 14 Scientific American

Harper & Sanders (1975). "The Effect of Adults' Eating on Young Children's Acceptance of Unfamiliar Foods." Harper, L. V. and Sanders, K. M. (1975) Journal of Experimental Child Psychology 20: 206-214

Harris et al., (2009). Health Psychol. 2009 Jul; 28(4): 404–413. doi: 10.1037/a0014399. PMCID: PMC2743554. NIHMSID: NIHMS121043. Priming Effects of Television Food Advertising on Eating Behavior. Jennifer L. Harris, John A. Bargh, and Kelly D. Brownell

Harvard (2008). "Sleep and Health" January 16, 2008. the Division of Sleep Medicine at Harvard Medical School.

Harvard (2017). "Fiber." Harvard T.H. Chan School of Public Health, The Nutrition Source, (nd) Retrieved 29th November 2017

Harvard Health (2012). "Blue Light Has A Dark Side." Harvard Health Letter 37.7 (2012): 4. Consumer Health Complete - EBSCOhost. Web. 14 Feb. 2016

Harvey et al., (2005). "The nature of imagery processes underlying food cravings." Harvey, Kirsty, Kemps, Eva, Tiggemann, Marika. British Journal of Health Psychology, February 2005. DOI: 10.1348/135910704X14249

Hatori et al., (2012). "Time-Restricted Feeding without Reducing Caloric Intake Prevents Metabolic Diseases in Mice Fed a High-Fat Diet." Megumi Hatori, Christopher Vollmers. Amir Zarrinpar, Luciano Di Tacchio, Eric A. Bushong, Shubhroz Gill, Mathias Leblanc, Amandine Chaix, Matthew Joens, James A.J. Fitzpatrick, Mark H. Ellisman, Satchidananda Panda.] [Cell Metabolism Volume 15, Issue 6, 6 June 2012, Pages 848-860. https://doi.org/10.1016/j.cmet.2012.04.019

Hattesohl et al., (2008). "Extracts of Valeriana officinalis L. s.l. show anxiolytic and antidepressant effects but neither sedative nor myorelaxant properties." Hattesohl M, Feistel B, Sievers H, Lehnfeld R, Hegger M, Winterhoff H. Phytomedicine. 2008 Jan;15(1-2):2-15

Heiman & Greenway (2016). "A healthy gastrointestinal microbiome is dependent on dietary diversity." Mark L. Heiman, and Frank L. Greenway. Mol Metab. 2016 May; 5(5): 317–320. Published online 2016 Mar 5. doi: 10.1016/j.molmet.2016.02.005. PMCID: PMC4837298. PMID: 27110483

Herman et al., (2003). "Effects of the presence of others on food intake: a normative interpretation." Herman, P., Roth, D.A., & Polivy, J. (2003). Psychological Bulletin, 129 (6), 873-886

Hetherington et al., (2001). "Stimulation of appetite by alcohol." Hetherington MM, Cameron F, Wallis DJ, Pirie LM. Physiol Behav. 2001 Oct;74(3):283-9

Heydari et al., (2012). "The Effect of High-Intensity Intermittent Exercise on Body Composition of Overweight Young Males." M. Heydari, J. Freund, and S. H. Boutcher, Journal of Obesity, vol. 2012, Article ID 480467, 8 pages, 2012. doi:10.1155/2012/480467

Higgs & Donohoe (2011). "Focusing on food during lunch enhances lunch memory and decreases later snack intake." Higgs S, Donohoe J E. Appetite. 2011 Aug;57(1):202-6. doi: 10.1016/j.appet.2011.04.016. Epub 2011 May 4

Higgs (2002). "Memory for recent eating and its influence on subsequent food intake. "Higgs S. Appetite. 2002 Oct;39(2):159-66

Higgs (2005). "Memory and its role in appetite regulation." Higgs S. Physiol Behav. 2005 May 19;85(1):67-72. Epub 2005 Apr 25

Higgs et al., (2008). "Recall of recent lunch and its effect on subsequent snack intake." Higgs S, Williamson AC, Attwood AS. Physiol Behav. 2008 Jun 9;94(3):454-62. doi: 10.1016/j.physbeh.2008.02.011. Epub 2008 Mar 4

Hill (2007). "The psychology of food craving." Hill AJ. Proc Nutr Soc. 2007 May; 66(2):277-85

Hlebowicz et al., (2007). "Effect of cinnamon on postprandial blood glucose, gastric emptying, and satiety in healthy subjects." Joanna Hlebowicz, Gassan Darwiche, Ola Björgell, and Lars-Olof Almér. Am J Clin Nutr June 2007, vol. 85 no. 6 1552-1556

Hogenkamp et al., (2011). "Texture, not flavor, determines expected satiation of dairy products." P.S. Hogenkamp, A. Stafleu, M. Mars, J.M. Brunstrom, C. de Graaf. Appetite, 57 (3) (2011), pp. 635–641

Hogenkamp et al., (2013). "Acute sleep deprivation increases portion size and affects food choice in young men." Pleunie S. Hogenkamp, Emil Nilsson, Victor C. Nilsson, Colin D. Chapman, Heike Vogel, Lina S. Lundberg, Sanaz Zarei, Jonathan Cedernaes, Frida H. Rångtell, Jan-Erik Broman, Suzanne L. Dickson, Jeffrey M. Brunstrom, Christian Benedict, Helgi B. Schiöth. Psychoneuroendocrinology Volume 38, Issue 9, September 2013, Pages 1668–1674 doi:10.1016/j. psyneuen.2013.01.012

Holt & Miller (1994). "Particle size, satiety and the glycaemic response." Holt SH, Miller JB. Eur J Clin Nutr. 1994 Jul;48(7):496-502

Holt et al., (1996). "Interrelationships among postprandial satiety, glucose and insulin responses and changes in subsequent food intake." Holt SH, Brand Miller JC, Petocz P. 1996 Eur J Clin Nutr.

Holt et al., (1997). "An insulin index of foods: the insulin demand generated by 1000-kJ portions of common foods." Holt, S.H., Miller, J.C., & Petocz, P. (1997). American Journal of Clinical Nutrition. 66, 1264-1276

Holt et al., (1999). "The effects of high-carbohydrate vs high-fat breakfasts on feelings of fullness and alertness, and subsequent food intake." Holt SH , Delargy HJ, Lawton CL, Blundell JE. Int J Food Sci Nutr. 1999 Jan;50(1):13-28.

Holt-Lunstad et al. (2010). "Social Relationships and Mortality Risk: A Meta-analytic Review" Julianne Holt-Lunstad, Timothy B. Smith, J. Bradley Layton. PLOS. Published: July 27, 2010. https://doi. org/10.1371/journal.pmed.1000316.

Holt-Lunstad et al., (2015). "Loneliness and Social Isolation as Risk Factors for Mortality: A Meta-Analytic Review." Julianne Holt-Lunstad, Timothy B. Smith, Mark Baker, Tyler Harris, David Stephenson. Perspectives on Psychological Science, March 11, 2015

Holtcamp (2012). "Obesogens: An Environmental Link to Obesity." Wendee Holtcamp. Environ Health Perspect. 2012 Feb; 120(2): a62–a68. Published online 2012 Feb 1. doi: 10.1289/ehp.120-a62 PMCID: PMC3279464

HospiMedica (2013). "Waist-Height Ratio Better Than BMI for Gauging Mortality". HospiMedica International staff writers, 18 Jun 2013.

Howarth et al., (2001). "Dietary fiber and weight regulation." N.C. Howarth, E. Saltzman, S.B. Roberts. Nutrition Reviews, 59 (5) (2001), pp. 129–139

Huss-Ashmore (1980). "Fat and Fertility: Demographic Implications of Differential Fat Storage." Huss-Ashmore, R. Yearbook of Physical Anthropology 23:65-91.

Hutchins et al., (2012). "Phaseolus beans: impact on glycaemic response and chronic disease risk in human subjects." Hutchins AM, Winham DM, Thompson SV. Br J Nutr. 2012 Aug;108 Suppl 1:S52-65

Inoue et al., (2007). "Enhanced energy expenditure and fat oxidation in humans with high BMI scores by the ingestion of novel and non-pungent capsaicin analogues (capsinoids)." Inoue N, Matsunaga Y, Satoh H, Takahashi M (2007) Biosci Biotechnol Biochem 71: 380–389

Islam & Indrajit (2012). "Effects of xylitol on blood glucose, glucose tolerance, serum insulin and lipid profile in a type 2 diabetes model of rats." Islam MS, Indrajit M. Ann Nutr Metab. 2012;61(1):57-64. doi: 10.1159/000338440. Epub 2012 Jul 20

Jakubowicz et al (2012). "Meal timing and composition influence ghrelin levels, appetite scores and weight loss maintenance in overweight and obese adults." Jakubowicz D, Froy O, Wainstein J, Boaz M.] [Steroids. 2012 Mar 10;77(4):323-31. doi: 10.1016/j.steroids.2011.12.006. Epub 2011 Dec 9

Janssens et al., (2013). "Acute Effects of Capsaicin on Energy Expenditure and Fat Oxidation in Negative Energy Balance." Janssens PLHR, Hursel R, Martens EAP, Westerterp-Plantenga MS. Tomé D, ed. PLoS ONE. 2013;8(7):e67786. doi:10.1371/journal.pone.0067786

Jelleyman et al., (2015). "The effects of high-intensity interval training on glucose regulation and insulin resistance: a meta-analysis." Jelleyman C, Yates T, O'Donovan G, Gray LJ, King JA, Khunti K, Davies MJ (November 2015). Obes Rev (Meta-Analysis). 16 (11): 942–61. doi:10.1111/obr.12317. PMID 26481101

Johnson & Clydesdale (2006). "Perceived Sweetness and Redness in Colored Sucrose Solutions." Johnson, J.L. Clydesdale, F. 2006/08/25. Journal of Food Science. Doi 10.1111/j.1365-2621.1982.tb12706.x

Johnson & Kenny (2010). "Addiction-like reward dysfunction and compulsive eating in obese rats: Role for dopamine D2 receptors." Paul M. Johnson and Paul J. Kenny. Nat Neurosci. 2010 May; 13(5): 635–641. Published online 2010 Mar 28. doi: 10.1038/nn.2519. PMCID: PMC2947358. NIHMSID: NIHMS181674. PMID: 20348917

Johnson & Kenny, (2014). "Dopamine D2 receptors in addiction-like reward dysfunction and compulsive eating in obese rats." Johnson, Paul M, and Kenny, Paul J. Nature Neuroscience 13 (2010): 635-641.18 July 2014. http://www.nature.com/neuro/journal/v13/n5/full/nn.2519.html]

Johnson & Wardle (2014). "Variety, Palatability, and Obesity". Fiona Johnson and Jane Wardle, Department of Epidemiology and Public Health, University College London, London, United Kingdom. doi: 10.3945/an.114.007120 Adv Nutr November 2014 Adv Nutr vol. 5: 851-859, 2014

Johnston et al., (2010). "Resistant starch improves insulin sensitivity in metabolic syndrome." Johnston, K. L., Thomas, E. L., Bell, J. D., Frost, G. S., Robertson, M. D. First published: 7 April 2010. DOI: 10.1111/j.1464-5491.2010.02923.x

Josse et al., (2011). "Increased Consumption of Dairy Foods and Protein during Diet- and Exercise-Induced Weight Loss Promotes Fat Mass Loss and Lean Mass Gain in Overweight and Obese Premenopausal Women." R. Josse, S. A. Atkinson, M. A. Tarnopolsky, S. M. Phillips. Journal of Nutrition, 2011; 141 (9): 1626

Juvonen et al., (2009). "Viscosity of oat bran-enriched beverages influences gastrointestinal hormonal responses in healthy humans." K.R. Juvonen, A.-K. Purhonen, M. Salmenkallio-Marttila, L. Lähteenmäki, D.E. Laaksonen, K.-H. Herzig, et al. Journal of Nutrition, 139 (3) (2009), pp. 461–466

Kahleova et al., (2014). "Eating two larger meals a day (breakfast and lunch) is more effective than six smaller meals in a reduced-energy regimen for patients with type 2 diabetes: a randomised crossover study." Kahleova H, Belinova L, Malinska H, Oliyarnyk O, Trnovska J, Skop V, Kazdova L, Dezortova M, Hajek M, Tura A, Hill M, Pelikanova T. Diabetologia. 2014 Aug;57(8):1552-60. doi: 10.1007/s00125-014-3253-5. Epub 2014 May 18

Kahn & Flier (2000). "Obesity and insulin resistance." Barbara B. Kahn and Jeffrey S. Flier. J Clin Invest. 2000;106(4):473–481. doi:10.1172/JCI10842. Volume 106, Issue 4 (August 15, 2000). Copyright © 2000, The American Society for Clinical Investigation.

Kaidar-Person et al., (2008). "Nutritional deficiencies in morbidly obese patients: a new form of malnutrition?" Kaidar-Person O, Person B, Szomstein S, Rosenthal RJ. Obes Surg. 2008 Jul;18(7):870-6. doi: 10.1007/s11695-007-9349-y. Epub 2008 Mar 4. Part A: vitamins. PMID: 18465178

Kalsbeek et al., (2014). "Circadian control of glucose metabolism." Andries Kalsbeek, Susanne la Fleur, and Eric Fliers. Mol Metab. 2014 Jul; 3(4): 372–383. Published online 2014 Mar 19. doi: 10.1016/j.molmet.2014.03.002. PMCID: PMC4060304

Kam-Hansen et al., (2014). "Altered Placebo and Drug Labeling Changes the Outcome of Episodic Migraine Attacks." Slavenka Kam-Hansen, Moshe Jakubowski, John M. Kelley, Irving Kirsch, David C. Hoaglin, Ted J. Kaptchuk, and Rami Burstein. Science Translational Medicine 08 Jan 2014: Vol. 6, Issue 218, pp. 218ra5. DOI: 10.1126/scitranslmed.3006175

Kannan et al., (2010). "Organotin compounds, including butyltins and octyltins, in house dust from Albany, New York, USA." Kannan K, Takahashi S, Fujiwara N, Mizukawa H, Tanabe S. Arch Environ Contam Toxicol. 2010 May;58(4):901-7. doi: 10.1007/s00244-010-9513-6. Epub 2010 Apr 9

Kaptchuk et al., (2008). "Components of placebo effect: randomised controlled trial in patients with irritable bowel syndrome." Ted J Kaptchuk, John M Kelley, Lisa A Conboy, Roger B Davis, Catherine E Kerr, Eric E Jacobson, Irving Kirsch, Rosa N Schyner, Bong Hyun Nam, Long T Nguyen, Min Park, Andrea L Rivers, Claire McManus, Efi Kokkotou, Douglas A Drossman, Peter Goldman, Anthony J Lembo. 5 BMJ 2008;336:999

Katcher, et al., (2008). "The effects of a whole grain–enriched hypocaloric diet on cardiovascular disease risk factors in men and women with metabolic syndrome." Heather I Katcher, Richard S Legro, Allen R Kunselman, Peter J Gillies, Laurence M Demers, Deborah M Bagshaw, and Penny M Kris-Etherton. Am J Clin Nutr January 2008. vol. 87 no. 1 79-90

Katterman et al., (2014). "Mindfulness meditation as an intervention for binge eating, emotional eating, and weight loss: a systematic review." Katterman SN, Kleinman BM, Hood MM, Nackers LM, Corsica JA. Eat Behav. 2014 Apr;15(2):197-204. doi: 10.1016/j.eatbeh.2014.01.005. Epub 2014 Feb 1

Keesman et al., (2016) "Consumption Simulations Induce Salivation to Food Cues." Mike Keesman, Henk Aarts, Stefan Vermeent, Michael Häfner, Esther K. Papies. PLOS Research Article. Published: November 7, 2016. https://doi.org/10.1371/journal.pone.0165449

Kelly et al., (2017). "An evaluation of low volume high-intensity intermittent training (HIIT) for health risk reduction in overweight and obese men." Kelly, Benjamin M. Xenophontos, Soteris. King, James A. Nimmo, Myra A. Loughborough University Institutional Repository (2017). https://dspace.lboro.ac.uk/2134/24614

Kemps & Tiggeman (2007). "Modality-specific imagery reduces cravings for food: an application of the elaborated intrusion theory of desire to food craving." Kemps E, Tiggemann M. J Exp Psychol Appl (2007) 13:95–104.10.1037/1076-898X.13.2.95

Kemps & Tiggeman (2013). "Hand-held dynamic visual noise reduces naturally occurring food cravings and craving-related consumption." Kemps E, Tiggemann M. Appetite. 2013 Sep;68:152-7. doi: 10.1016/j.appet.2013.05.001. Epub 2013 May 14

Kemps & Tiggemann (2014). "A Role for Mental Imagery in the Experience and Reduction of Food Cravings." Eva Kemps and Marika Tiggemann. Front Psychiatry. 2014; 5: 193. Published online 2015 Jan 6. Prepublished online 2014 Nov 24. doi: 10.3389/fpsyt.2014.00193. PMCID: PMC4284995

Kemps & Tiggemann (2017). "Modality-specific imagery reduces cravings for food: an application of the elaborated intrusion theory of desire to food craving." Kemps E, Tiggemann M.. J Exp Psychol Appl (2007) 13:95–104.10.1037/1076-898X.13.2.95

Kemps et al., (2007). "Concurrent visuo-spatial processing reduces food cravings in prescribed weight-loss dieters." Kemps E, Tiggemann M, Christianson R. J Behav Ther Exp Psychiatry. 2008 Jun;39(2):177-86. Epub 2007 Mar 24

Kennedy (2004). "Dietary Diversity, Diet Quality, and Body Weight Regulation." Eileen Kennedy D.Sc. DOI: http://dx.doi.org/10.1111/j.1753-4887.2004.tb00093.x S78-S81 First published online: 1 July 2004

Kennedy-Hagan et al., (2011). "The effect of pistachio shells as a visual cue in reducing caloric consumption." Kennedy-Hagan, K., Painter, J.E., Honselman, C., Halvorson, A., Rhodes, K., & Skwir, K. (2011). Appetite, 57(2), 418-420. doi: 10.1016/j.appet.2011.06.003

Kenny (2010). "Dopamine D2 receptors in addiction-like reward dysfunction and compulsive eating in obese rats." Paul M Johnson & Paul J Kenny. Nature Neuroscience pp 635 - 641. Published online: 28 March 2010. doi: 10.1038/nn.2519

Kerr et al., (2011). "Effects of mindfulness meditation training on anticipatory alpha modulation in primary somatosensory cortex." Kerr CE, Jones SR, Wan Q, Pritchett DL, Wasserman RH, Wexler A, Villanueva JJ, Shaw JR, Lazar SW, Kaptchuk TJ, Littenberg R, Hämäläinen MS, Moore CI. Brain Res Bull. 2011 May 30;85(3-4):96-103. doi: 10.1016/j.brainresbull.2011.03.026. Epub 2011 Apr 8

Kessel et al., (2011). "Sleep disturbances are related to decreased transmission of blue light to the retina caused by lens yellowing." Kessel L; Siganos G; Jørgensen T; Larsen M. Sleep (2011) 34(9):1215-1219

Kim & Camilleri (2000). "Serotonin: a mediator of the brain-gut connection." Kim DY, Camilleri M. Am J Gastroenterol. 2000 Oct;95(10):2698-709. PMID: 11051338. DOI: 10.1111/j.1572-0241.2000.03177.x

Kim et al, (2016). "Effects of dietary pulse consumption on body weight: a systematic review and meta-analysis of randomized controlled trials." Kim SJ, de Souza RJ, Choo VL, Ha V, Cozma AI, Chiavaroli L, Mirrahimi A, Blanco Mejia S, Di Buono M, Bernstein AM7, Leiter LA, Kris-Etherton PM, Vuksan V, Beyene J, Kendall CW, Jenkins DJ, Sievenpiper JL. Am J Clin Nutr. 2016 May;103(5):1213-23. doi: 10.3945/ajcn.115.124677. Epub 2016 Mar 30

Kim et al., (2008). "Meal replacement with mixed rice is more effective than white rice in weight control, while improving antioxidant enzyme activity in obese women." Kim JY, Kim JH, Lee DH, Kim SH, Lee SS. Nutr Res. 2008 Feb;28(2):66-71. doi: 10.1016/j.nutres.2007.12.006

Kim et al., (2016). "Calorie-induced ER stress suppresses uroguanylin satiety signaling in diet-induced obesity." GW Kim, JE Lin, AE Snook, AS Aing, DJ Merlino, P Li and SA Waldman. Nutrition & Diabetes (2016) 6, e211; doi:10.1038/nutd.2016.18 Published online 23 May 2016.

Kissileff et al., (1984). "The satiating efficiency of foods." Kissileff, H.R., L.P. Gruss, J. Thornton, and H.A. Jordan 1984. Physiol. Behav. 32:319-332. [PubMed]

Knäuper et al., (2011). "Replacing craving imagery with alternative pleasant imagery reduces craving intensity." Knäuper B , Pillay R, Lacaille J, McCollam A, Kelso E. Appetite. 2011 Aug;57(1):173-8 doi: 10.1016/j.appet.2011.04.021. Epub 2011 May 4

Kobayashi 2014). "Effect of measurement duration on accuracy of pulse-counting." Kobayashi H. Ergonomics. 2013;56(12):1940-1944. do i:10.1080/00140139.2013.840743

Kohatsu et al. (2006). "Sleep Duration and Body Mass Index in a Rural Population." Kohatsu ND, Tsai R, Young T, Vangilder R, Burmeister LF, Stromquist AM, Merchant JA. Archives of Internal Medicine. 2006 Sep 18; 166(16): 1701.

Koopman et al., (2016). "Brain dopamine and serotonin transporter binding are associated with visual attention bias for food in lean men." Koopman KE, Roefs A, Elbers DC, Fliers E1, Booij J, Serlie MJ, la Fleur SE. Psychol Med. 2016 Jun;46(8):1707-17. doi: 10.1017/ S0033291716000222. Epub 2016 Mar 17

Koot & Deurenberg (1995). "Comparison of changes in energy expenditure and body temperatures after caffeine consumption." Koot P, Deurenberg P. Ann Nutr Metab. 1995;39(3):135-42

Korb (2011). "Boosting Your Serotonin Activity." Alex Korb, Ph.D. Psychology Today. Nov 17, 2011

Korpela, K. et al., (2016). "Intestinal microbiome is related to lifetime antibiotic use in Finnish pre-school children." Nat. Commun. 7:10410 doi: 10.1038/ncomms10410 (2016).

Kramer et al., (1989). M. Kramer, J. Edinberg, S. Luther, and D. Engell, U.S. Army Natick Research, Development and Engineering Center, Natick, Mass., unpublished data, 1989

Krassner et al., (1979). "Cleaning the plate: Food left over by overweight and normal weight persons." Krassner, H.A., K.D. Brownell, and A.J. Stunkard 1979. Behav. Res. Ther. 17:155–156. PubMed

Kratina (2016). "Orthorexia nervosa". Karin Kratina, PhD, RD, LD/N. National Eating Disorders website, (nd) retrieved 23rd July 2016

Kresser (2010). "How inflammation makes you fat and diabetic (and vice versa). www.chriskresser.com September 15, 2010 Chris Kresser

Lager & Torssander (2012). "Causal effect of education on mortality in a quasi-experiment on 1.2 million Swedes." Anton Carl Jonas Lager and Jenny Torssander. PNAS May 14, 2012. 201105839; https://doi.org/10.1073/pnas.1105839109

Lakkakula et al., (2010). "Repeated taste exposure increases liking for vegetables by low-income elementary school children." Lakkakula A, Geaghan J, Zanovec M, Pierce S, Tuuri G. Appetite (2010) Oct;55(2):226-31 doi: 10.1016/j.appet.2010.06.003. Epub 2010 Jun 10

Lally et al., (2010). "How are habits formed: Modelling habit formation in the real world." Phillippa Lally, Cornelia H. M. Van Jaarsveld, Henry W. W. Potts and Jane Wardle. University College London, London, UK. European Journal of Social Psychology. Eur. J. Soc. Psychol. 40, 998–1009 (2010) DOI: 10.1002/ejsp.674

Lambert et al., (2002). "Effect of sunlight and season on serotonin turnover in the brain." Lambert GW, Reid C, Kaye DM, Jennings GL, Esler MD. Lancet. 2002 Dec 7; 360(9348):1840-2

Lamont et al., (2016). "A low-carbohydrate high-fat diet increases weight gain and does not improve glucose tolerance, insulin secretion or ß-cell mass in NZO mice." B J Lamont, M F Waters and S Andrikopoulos. Nutrition & Diabetes (2016) 6, e194; doi:10.1038/nutd.2016.2.

Lancet (2002). "Healthwise: Seasonal Affective Disorder (SAD)" The Lancet, Dec. 7, 2002

Larson et al., (2014). "Satiation from sensory simulation: Evaluating foods decreases enjoyment of similar foods." Jeffrey S. Larson, Joseph P. Redden, Ryan S. Elder. Journal of Consumer Psychology Volume 24, Issue 2, April 2014, Pages 188–194

Lazar at al., (2005). "Meditation experience is associated with increased cortical thickness." Sara W. Lazar, Catherine E. Kerr, Rachel H. Wasserman, Jeremy R. Gray, Douglas N. Greve, Michael T. Treadway, Metta McGarvey, Brian T. Quinn, Jeffery A. Dusek, Herbert Benson, Scott L. Rauch, Christopher I. Moore, and Bruce Fischl. Neuroreport. 2005 Nov 28; 16(17): 1893–1897. PMCID: PMC1361002. NIHMSID: NIHMS6696

Le Chatelier et al., (2013). "Richness of human gut microbiome correlates with metabolic markers. Emmanuelle Le Chatelier, Nielsen T, Qin J, Prifti E, Hildebrand F, Falony G, Almeida M, Arumugam M, Batto JM, Kennedy S, Leonard P, Li J, Burgdorf K, Grarup N, Jørgensen T, Brandslund I, Nielsen HB, Juncker AS, Bertalan M, Levenez F, Pons N, Rasmussen S, Sunagawa S, Tap J, Tims S, Zoetendal EG, Brunak S, Clément K, Doré J, Kleerebezem M, Kristiansen K, Renault P, Sicheritz-Ponten T, de Vos WM, Zucker JD, Raes J, Hansen T; MetaHIT consortium, Bork P, Wang J, Ehrlich SD, Pedersen O. Nature 500, 541–546 (29 August 2013) doi:10.1038/nature12506 26 July 2013

Leathwood et al., (1982). "Aqueous extract of valerian root (Valeriana officinalis L.) improves sleep quality in man." Peter D.Leathwood, Françoise Chauffard, Eva Heck, Raphael Munoz-Box. Pharmacology Biochemistry and Behavior Volume 17, Issue 1, July 1982, Pages 65-71https://doi.org/10.1016/0091-3057(82)90264-7

Leddy et al., (2008). "The Impact of Maternal Obesity on Maternal and Fetal Health." Meaghan A Leddy, Michael L Power, PhD, and Jay Schulkin, PhD. Rev Obstet Gynecol. 2008 Fall; 1(4): 170–178. PMCID: PMC2621047

Lederberg & McCray (2001). "'Ome sweet 'omics—a genealogical treasury of words." Lederberg J, McCray AT.Scientist. 2001;15:8

Ledochowski et al., (2015). "Acute Effects of Brisk Walking on Sugary Snack Cravings in Overweight People, Affect and Responses to a Manipulated Stress Situation and to a Sugary Snack Cue: A Crossover Study." Larissa Ledochowski, Gerhard Ruedl, Adrian H. Taylor, Martin Kopp. PLOS One. Published: March 11, 2015. http://dx.doi.org/10.1371/journal.pone.0119278

Leidy et al., (2007). "Higher Protein Intake Preserves Lean Mass and Satiety with Weight Loss in Pre-obese and Obese Women." Leidy, H. J., Carnell, N. S., Mattes, R. D. and Campbell, W. W. (2007). Obesity, 15: 421–429. doi:10.1038/oby.2007.531

Leidy et al., (2010). "The Influence of Higher Protein Intake and Greater Eating Frequency on Appetite Control in Overweight and Obese Men." Leidy, H. J., Armstrong, C. L.H., Tang, M., Mattes, R. D. and Campbell, W. W. (2010), Obesity, 18: 1725–1732. doi:10.1038/oby.2010.45

Leidy et al., (2011). "The Effects of Consuming Frequent, Higher Protein Meals on Appetite and Satiety During Weight Loss in Overweight/Obese Men." Leidy, H. J., Tang, M., Armstrong, C. L.H., Martin, C. B. and Campbell, W. W. (2011), Obesity, 19: 818–824. doi:10.1038/oby.2010.203

Leinninger et al., (2009). "Leptin acts via leptin receptor-expressing lateral hypothalamic neurons to modulate the mesolimbic dopamine system and suppress feeding." Leinninger GM, Jo YH, Leshan RL, Louis GW, Yang H, Barrera JG, Wilson H, Opland DM, Faouzi MA, Gong Y, Jones JC, Rhodes CJ, Chua S Jr, Diano S, Horvath TL, Seeley RJ, Becker JB, Münzberg H, Myers MG Jr. Cell Metab. 2009 Aug;10(2):89-98. doi: 10.1016/j.cmet.2009.06.011

Lerman et al., (2004). "Changes in food reward following smoking cessation: a pharmacogenetic investigation." Lerman C, Berrettini W, Pinto A, Patterson F, Crystal-Mansour S, Wileyto EP, Restine SL, Leonard DG, Shields PG, Epstein LH. Psychopharmacology (Berl) 2004, 174: 571-577. 10.1007/s00213-004-1823-9

Lesser et al., (2013). "Outdoor advertising, obesity, and soda consumption: a cross-sectional study." Lenard I Lesser, Frederick J Zimmerman and Deborah A Cohen. BMC Public Health 2013 https://doi.org/10.1186/1471-2458-13-20

Leung (2014). "Capsaicin as an anti-obesity drug. In Capsaicin as a Therapeutic Molecule." Leung, F. W. (2014). (pp. 171-179). Springer Basel

Levine & Billington (1994). "Dietary fiber: Does it affect food intake and body weight?" Levine, A.S., and C.J. Billington 1994. Pp. 191–200 in Appetite and Body Weight Regulation: Sugar, Fat, and Macronutrient Substitutes, J. Fernstrom, editor; and G. Miller, editor. eds. Boca Raton, Fla.: CRC Press.

Levine et al., (2014). "Low Protein Intake Is Associated with a Major Reduction in IGF-1, Cancer, and Overall Mortality in the 65 and Younger but Not Older Population" Morgan E. Levine, Jorge A. Suarez, Sebastian Brandhorst, Priya Balasubramanian, Chia-Wei Cheng, Federica Madia, Luigi Fontana, Mario G. Mirisola, Jaime Guevara-Aguirre, Junxiang Wan, Giuseppe Passarino, Brian K. Kennedy, Min Wei, Pinchas Cohen, Eileen M. Crimmins, Valter D. Longo. Cell Metabolism. Volume 19, Issue 3, p407–417, 4 March 2014. DOI: http://dx.doi.org/10.1016/j.cmet.2014.02.006

Levitsky & Pacanowski (2013). "Effect of skipping breakfast on subsequent energy intake." Levitsky DA1, Pacanowski CR. Physiol Behav. 2013 Jul 2;119:9-16. doi: 10.1016/j.physbeh.2013.05.006. Epub 2013 May 11

Levitsky, et al., (2012). "Number of foods available at a meal determines the amount consumed." David Levitsky, Sunil Iyer, Carly R Pacanowski. Eating behaviors 13(3):183-7 August 2012. DOI: 10.1016/j.eatbeh.2012.01.006

Ley et al., (2013). "Associations between red meat intake and biomarkers of inflammation and glucose metabolism in women." Sylvia H Ley, Qi Sun, Walter C Willett, A Heather Eliassen, Kana Wu, An Pan, Fran Grodstein, and Frank B Hu. November 27, 2013, doi: 10.3945/ajcn.113.075663. Am J Clin Nutr.ajcn.075663

Li et al., (2012). "Triflumizole is an obesogen in mice that acts through peroxisome proliferator activated receptor gamma (PPARy)." Li, X., Pham, H. T., Janesick, A. S. & Blumberg, B. Environ. Health Perspect. 120, 1720–1726 (2012)

Li et al., (2014). "Dietary pulses, satiety and food intake: A systematic review and meta-analysis of acute feeding trials." Li, S. S., Kendall, C. W.C., de Souza, R. J., Jayalath, V. H., Cozma, A. I., Ha, V., Mirrahimi, A., Chiavaroli, L., Augustin, L. S.A., Blanco Mejia, S., Leiter, L. A., Beyene, J., Jenkins, D. J.A. and Sievenpiper, J. L. (2014), Obesity, 22: 1773–1780. doi:10.1002/oby.20782

Liao et al., (2007). "Effectiveness of a soy-based compared with a traditional low-calorie diet on weight loss and lipid levels in overweight adults." Fang-Hsuean Liao, M.S., Ming-Jer Shieh, Ph.D., Suh-Ching Yang, Ph.D., Shyh-Hsiang Lin, Ph.D., Yi-Wen Chien, Ph.D., R.D., Nutrition, Volume 23, Issues 7–8, July–August 2007, Pages 551–556

Lillard & Panis (1996). "Marital Status and Mortality: The Role of Health." Lee A. Lillard and Constantijn W.A. Panis. Demography, 33(3):313-327, 1996

Linne et al., 2002). "Vision and eating behavior." Linne, Y., Barkeling, B., Rossner, S., & Rooth, P. (2002). Obesity Research, 10(2), 92-95. doi: 10.1038/oby.2002.15

Littel et al., (2016). "Desensitizing Addiction: Using Eye Movements to Reduce the Intensity of Substance-Related Mental Imagery and Craving." Marianne Littel, Marcel A. van den Hout and Iris M. Engelhard. Front. Psychiatry, 08 February 2016. http://dx.doi.org/10.3389/fpsyt.2016.00014

Liu et al., (2003). "Relation between changes in intakes of dietary fiber and grain products and changes in weight and development of obesity among middle-aged women." Simin Liu, Walter C Willett, JoAnn E Manson, Frank B Hu, Bernard Rosner, and Graham Colditz. Am J Clin Nutr November 2003. vol. 78 no. 5 920-927

Loos & Yeo (2014). "The bigger picture of FTO: the first GWAS-identified obesity gene". Loos RJ, Yeo GS (2014). Nat Rev Endocrinol. 10 (1): 51–61. doi:10.103 8/nrendo.2013.227. PMC 4188449 Freely accessible. PMID 24247219

Lowe, et al., (2013). "Dieting and restrained eating as prospective predictors of weight gain." Michael R. Lowe, Sapna D. Doshi, Shawn N. Katterman, and Emily H. Feig. Front Psychol. 2013; 4: 577. Published online 2013 Sep 2. Prepublished online 2013 Jun 24. doi: 10.3389/fpsyg.2013.00577 PMCID: PMC3759019

Lowette et al., (2015). "Effects of High-Fructose Diets on Central Appetite Signaling and Cognitive Function." Katrien Lowette, Lina Roosen, Jan Tack, and Pieter Vanden Berghe. Front Nutr. 2015; 2: 5. Published online 2015 Mar 4. doi: 10.3389/fnut.2015.00005. PMCID: PMC4429636

Lucassen et al (2016). "Environmental 24-hr Cycles Are Essential for Health." Lucassen EA, Coomans CP, van Putten M, de Kreij SR, van Genugten JH, Sutorius RP, de Rooij KE, van der Velde M, Verhoeve SL, Smit JW, Löwik CW, Smits HH, Guigas B, Aartsma-Rus AM, Meijer JH. Curr Biol. 2016 Jul 25;26(14):1843-53. doi: 10.1016/j.cub.2016.05.038. Epub 2016 Jul 14

Ludlow & Weyand (2015). "Energy expenditure during level human walking: seeking a simple and accurate predictive solution." Lindsay W. Ludlow, Peter G. Weyand. Journal of Applied Physiology Published 17 December 2015 Vol. no. , DOI: 10.1152/japplphysiol.00864.2015

Ludy & Mattes (2011). "The effects of hedonically acceptable red pepper doses on thermogenesis and appetite. Physiology & behavior." Ludy M-J, Mattes RD. 2011;102(3-4):251-258. doi:10.1016/j.physbeh.2010.11.018

Luoa et al., (2015). "Differential effects of fructose versus glucose on brain and appetitive responses to food cues and decisions for food rewards." Shan Luoa, John R. Monterossob, Kayan Sarpelleh and Kathleen A. Page. 2015. Proceedings of the National Academy of Sciences of the United States of America. vol. 112 no. 20. 6509–6514, doi: 10.1073/pnas.1503358112]

Luppino et al., (2010). "Overweight, obesity, and depression: a systematic review and meta-analysis of longitudinal studies." Luppino FS, de Wit LM, Bouvy PF, Stijnen T, Cuijpers P, Penninx BW, Zitman FG. Arch Gen Psychiatry. 2010 Mar;67(3):220-9. Doi: 10.1001/archgenpsychiatry.2010.2

Ma et al., (2003). "Association between Eating Patterns and Obesity in a Free-living US Adult Population." Yunsheng Ma, Elizabeth R. Bertone, Edward J. Stanek, III, George W. Reed, James R. Hebert, Nancy L. Cohen, Philip A. Merriam, Ira S. Ockene. Am J Epidemiol (2003) 158 (1): 85-92. DOI: https://doi.org/10.1093/aje/kwg117. Published: 01 July 2003

Mahar & Duizer (2007). "The effect of frequency of consumption of artificial sweeteners on sweetness liking by women." Mahar A, Duizer LM. J Food Sci. 2007;72:S714–8

Mahony et al., (2009). "Early life stress alters behavior, immunity, and microbiota in rats: implications for irritable bowel syndrome and psychiatric illnesses." O'Mahony

Maier et al., (2015). "Acute Stress Impairs Self-Control in Goal-Directed Choice by Altering Multiple Functional Connections within the Brain's Decision Circuits." Silvia U.

Malik et al., (2006). "Intake of sugar-sweetened beverages and weight gain: a systematic review." V.S. Malik, M.B. Schulze, F.B. Hu. American Journal of Clinical Nutrition, 84 (2) (2006), pp. 274–288

Mann et al., (1971). "Atherosclerosis in the Masai." George V. Mann, Anne Spoerry, Margarete Gary and Debra Jarashow. American Journal of Epidemiology Volume 95, Issue 1 Pp. 26-37. May 10, 1971

Marchiori et al., (2011). "Smaller food item sizes of snack foods influence reduced portions and caloric intake in young adults." Marchiori, D., Waroquier, L., & Klein, O. (2011). Journal of the American Dietetic Association, 111, 727-731. doi: 10.1016/j.jada.2011.02.008

Marinangeli & Jones (2010). "Whole and fractionated yellow pea flours reduce fasting insulin and insulin resistance in hypercholesterolaemic and overweight human subjects." Christopher P. F. Marinangeli and Peter J. H. Jones, The Richardson Centre for Functional Foods and Nutraceuticals, University of Manitoba. doi:10.1017/S0007114510003156. British Journal of Nutrition (2011), 105, 110–117. First published online 1 September 2010

Markowitz et al., (2008). "Perceived deprivation, restrained eating and susceptibility to weight gain." Markowitz JT , Butryn ML, Lowe MR. Appetite. 2008 Nov;51(3):720-2. doi: 10.1016/j.appet.2008.03.017. Epub 2008 Apr 4

Marriott (1995). "Not Eating Enough: Overcoming Underconsumption of Military Operational Rations." Institute of Medicine (US) Committee on Military Nutrition Research; Marriott BM, editor. Washington (DC): National Academies Press (US); 1995. 11, Effects of Food Quality, Quantity, and Variety on Intake. Available from: http://www.ncbi.nlm.nih.gov/books/NBK232454/

Masters et al., (2010). "Whole and Refined Grain Intakes Are Related to Inflammatory Protein Concentrations in Human Plasma." Rachel C. Masters, Angela D. Liese, Steven M. Haffner, Lynne E. Wagenknecht, and Anthony J. Hanley. J Nutr. 2010 Mar; 140(3): 587–594. doi: 10.3945/jn.109.116640. PMCID: PMC2821887

Mathern et al., (2009). "Effect of Fenugreek Fiber on Satiety, Blood Glucose and Insulin Response and Energy Intake in Obese Subjects." Jocelyn R. Mathern, Susan K. Raatz, William Thomas, Joanne L. Slavin. DOI: 10.1002/ptr.2795. Copyright © 2009 John Wiley & Sons, Ltd. Phytotherapy Research Volume 23, Issue 11, pages 1543–1548, November 2009

Mattes (2004). "Soup and satiety." Mattes R. Physiol Behav. 2005 Jan 17;83(5):739-47. Epub 2004 Nov 11

Mattes (2010). "Hunger and Thirst: Issues in measurement and prediction of eating and drinking." Richard D. Mattes, MPH, PhD, RD. Physiol Behav. 2010 Apr 26; 100(1): 22–32. Published online 2010 Jan 11. doi: 10.1016/j.physbeh.2009.12.026 PMCID: PMC2849909 NIHMSID: NIHMS175763

Mattes et al., (2008). "Impact of peanuts and tree nuts on body weight and healthy weight loss in adults." Mattes RD, Kris-Etherton PM, Foster GD. J Nutr. 2008 Sep;138(9):1741S-1745S

May et al., (2004). "Images of desire: cognitive models of craving." May J, Andrade J, Panabokke N, Kavanagh D.

May et al., (2008). "Imagery and strength of craving for eating, drinking and playing sport." May J, Andrade J,

May et al., (2010). "Visuospatial tasks suppress craving for cigarettes. May J, Andrade J, Panabokke N, Kavanagh D. Behav Res Ther. 2010 Jun;48(6):476-85. doi: 10.1016/j.brat.2010.02.001. Epub 2010 Feb 7

May et al., (2014). "The elaborated intrusion theory of desire: a 10-year retrospective and implications for addiction treatments." May J, Kavanagh D, Andrade J.. Addict Behav. (2014).10.1016/j.addbeh.2014.09.016

Mayo Clinic (2017). "Walking shoes: Features and fit that keep you moving." Mayo Clinic Fitness, retrieved 10th April 2017. http://www.mayoclinic.org/healthy-lifestyle/fitness/in-depth/walking/art-20043897

Mayo Clinic (2017). "Water after meals: Does it disturb digestion?" Mayo Clinic. (nd) Retrieved 23rd June 2017

Mazess et al., (1974). "Bone mineral content of North Alaskan Eskimos." Mazess RB, Mather W. The American journal of clinical nutrition 1974;27:916-25

McCrickerd et al., (2014). "Does modifying the thick texture and creamy flavour of a drink change portion size selection and intake?" McCrickerd K, Chambers L, Yeomans MR. Appetite. 2014 Feb;73:114-20. doi: 10.1016/j.appet.2013.10.020

McCrory et al., (1999). "Dietary variety within food groups: Association with energy intake and body fatness in men and women." McCrory, M.A., Fuss, P.J., McCallum, J.E., Yao, M., Vinken, A.G., Hays., & Roberts, S.B. (1999). The American Journal of Clinical Nutrition, 69(3), 440–447

McCrory et al., (2010). "Pulse Consumption, Satiety, and Weight Management." Megan A. McCrory, Bruce R. Hamaker, Jennifer C. Lovejoy, and Petra E. Eichelsdoerfer. doi: 10.3945/an.110.1006. Adv Nutr November 2010 Adv Nutr vol. 1: 17-30, 2010

McDonald (2008). "Do married people live longer?" Peter McDonald, Professor of Demography and Director of the Australian Demographic and Social Research Institute. ABC Health and Wellbeing. 3rd September 2008

McDonald's (2018). "Happy Meal®" McDonald's® www.happymeal.com (nd) retrieved 1st May 2018

McQuaid et al., (2016). "Relations between plasma oxytocin and cortisol: The stress buffering role of social support." Robyn J. McQuaid, Opal A. McInnis, Angela Paric, Faisal Al-Yawer, Kimberly Matheson, and Hymie Anisman. Neurobiol Stress. 2016 Jun; 3: 52–60. Published online 2016 Jan 30. doi: [10.1016/j.ynstr.2016.01.001] PMCID: PMC5146198. PMID: 27981177

Meeusen et al., (2001). "Brain neurotransmitter levels during exercise." Meeusen R, Piacentini MF, Kempenaers F, et al. Dtsch Z Sportmed 2001;52:361-8

Meiselman et al., (1994). "Effect of effort on meal selection and meal acceptability in a student cafeteria." Meiselman, H. L., Staddon, S. L., Hedderley, D., Pierson, B. J., & Symonds, C. R. (1994). Appetite, 23(1), 43-56. doi: 10.1016/S0031-9384(00)00268-7

Mekary et al., (2013). "Eating patterns and type 2 diabetes risk in older women: breakfast consumption and eating frequency." Rania A Mekary, Edward Giovannucci, Leah Cahill, Walter C Willett, Rob M van Dam, and Frank B Hu. Am J Clin Nutr. 2013 Aug; 98(2): 436–443. Published online 2013 Jun 12. doi: 10.3945/ajcn.112.057521. PMCID: PMC3712552

Melanson et al., (2009): "Exercise improves fat metabolism in muscle but does not increase 24-h fat oxidation." Melanson EL, MacLean PS, Hill JO. Exercise and sport sciences reviews. 2009;37(2):93-101. doi:10.1097/JES.0b013e31819c2f0b

Meule & Gearhardt (2014). "Five years of the Yale Food Addiction Scale: Taking stock and moving forward." Meule, Adrian, and Ashley N. Gearhardt. Current Addiction Reports 1.3(2014): 193-205

Meyers & Stunkard (1980). "Food accessibility and food choice. A test of Schachter's externality hypothesis." Meyers, A.W., & Stunkard, A.J. (1980). Obesity, 37(10), 1133-1135. doi: 10.1001/archpsyc.1980.01780230051007

Michel et al., (2014). "A taste of Kandinsky: assessing the influence of the artistic visual presentation of food on the dining experience." Charles Michel, Carlos Velasco, Elia Gatti and Charles Spence. Flavour 20143:7. DOI: 10.1186/2044-7248-3-7. 20 June 2014

Mikus et al., (2012). "Lowering Physical Activity Impairs Glycemic Control in Healthy Volunteers." Catherine R. Mikus, Douglas J. Oberlin, Jessica L. Libla, Angelina M. Taylor, Frank W. Booth, and John P. Thyfault. Med Sci Sports Exerc. 2012 Feb; 44(2): 225–231. doi: 10.1249/MSS.0b013e31822ac0c0. PMCID: PMC4551428. NIHMSID: NIHMS713003. PMID: 21716152

Miyashita et al., (2008). "Accumulating short bouts of brisk walking reduces postprandial plasma triacylglycerol concentrations and resting blood pressure in healthy young men." Masashi Miyashita, Stephen F Burns, and David J Stensel. doi: 10.3945/ajcn.2008.26493. Am J Clin Nutr November 2008, vol. 88 no. 5 1225-1231

Modig et al. (2017). "Payback time? Influence of having children on mortality in old age." Modig K, Talbäck M, Torssander J, et al. J Epidemiol Community Health. 14 March 2017. doi: 10.1136/jech-2016-207857

Mohan et al., (2014). "Effect of Brown Rice, White Rice, and Brown Rice with Legumes on Blood Glucose and Insulin Responses in Overweight Asian Indians: A Randomized Controlled Trial." Mohan V, Spiegelman D, Sudha V, et al. Diabetes Technology & Therapeutics. 2014;16(5):317-325. doi:10.1089/dia.2013.0259

Montmayeur & le Coutre (2010). "Fat Detection: Taste, Texture, and Post Ingestive Effects." Montmayeur JP, le Coutre J, editors. Boca Raton (FL): CRC Press/Taylor & Francis; 2010. Frontiers in Neuroscience

Moore (2012). "What your gut's telling you: why your digestion holds the key to your health." Anna Moore. The Telegraph: Women's Health. 15 Apr 2012

Morewedge et al (2010). "Thought for Food: Imagined Consumption Reduces Actual Consumption." Carey K. Morewedge, Young Eun Huh, Joachim Vosgerau. Science 330, 1530 (2010); DOI: 10.1126/science.1195701

Morewedge et al., (2010). "Thought for food: imagined consumption reduces actual consumption." Morewedge CK, Huh YE, Vosgerau J. Science. 2010 Dec 10;330(6010):1530-3. doi: 10.1126/science.1195701

Morris et al., (2015). "Endogenous circadian system and circadian misalignment impact glucose tolerance via separate mechanisms in humans." Christopher J. Morris, Jessica N. Yang, Joanna I. Garcia, Samantha Myers, Isadora Bozzi, Wei Wang, Orfeu M. Buxton, Steven A. Shea, and Frank A. J. L. Scheer. PNAS April 28, 2015. 112 (17) E2225-E2234; https://doi.org/10.1073/pnas.1418955112

Mosley (13 January 2016). "Can changing your mealtimes make you healthier?" Dr Michael Mosley. BBC News Magazine 13 January 2016

Mosley (2011). "10 Things You Need to Know About Losing Weight." Mosley, Michael. BBC One, Thu 6 Jan 2011

Mosley (2014). "Can exercising for just 60 seconds a week transform your health?" Dr Michael Mosley. 14 January 2014, Daily Mail

Mosley (Sunday, 6 March 2016). "Crash diets do work, you should skip breakfast and exercise won't shift that spare tyre: Britain's bestselling health author reveals the truth about slimming" Dr Michael Mosley. The Mail On Sunday, 6 March 2016

Motooka (2006) Motooka, Masahiko, et al. "Effect of dog-walking on automatic nervous activity in senior citizens." Medical Journal of Australia, 2006; 184 (2): 60-63. (March 21, 2008)

Mourao et al., (2007). "Effects of food form on appetite and energy intake in lean and obese young adults." Mourao DM, Bressan J, Campbell WW, Mattes RD. Int J Obes (Lond). 2007 Nov;31(11):1688-95. Epub 2007 Jun 19

Munro et al., (1998). "Erythritol: an interpretive summary of biochemical, metabolic, toxicological and clinical data." I.C Munro, W.O Bernt, J.F Borzelleca, G Flamm, B.S Lynch, E Kennepohl, , E.A Bär, J Modderman. Food and Chemical Toxicology,Volume 36, Issue 12, December 1998, Pages 1139–1174. http://dx.doi.org/10.1016/S0278-6915(98)00091-X

Murnahan (2010). "Stress and Anxiety Reduction Due to Writing Diaries, Journals, E-mail, and Weblogs" Murnahan, Briana, (2010). Senior Honors Theses. Paper 230

Musher-Eizenman et al., (2009). "Children's sensitivity to external food cues: How distance to serving bowl influences children's consumption." Musher-Eizenman, D.R, Young, K.M., Laurene, K., Galliger, C., Hauser, J., & Oehlhof, M.W. (2009). Health Education & Behavior, 37(2), 186-192. doi: 10.1177/1090198109335656

Myers (2015). "Leptin Keeps Working, Even in Obesity." Myers, Martin G. Cell Metabolism , Volume 21 , Issue 6 , 791 - 792, 2 June 2015

Narumi et al., (2012). "Augmented perception of satiety: Controlling food consumption by changing apparent size of food with augmented reality." Narumi, T., Ban, Y., Kajinami, T., Tanikawa, T., & Hirose, M. (2012). In Proceedings 2012 ACM annual conference human factors in computing systems; CHI 2012, May 5–10, 2012, Austin, Texas

Nassauer (2014). "Using Scent as a Marketing Tool, Stores Hope It—and Shoppers—Will Linger." Sarah Nassauer. The Wall Street Journal, May 20, 2014

Neal et al., (2011). "The Pull of the Past: When Do Habits Persist Despite Conflict With Motives?" David T. Neal, Wendy Wood, Mengju Wu, David Kurlander. Pers Soc Psychol Bull November 2011 vol. 37 no. 11 1428-1437

Newman et al., (2016). "Dietary fat restriction increases fat taste sensitivity in people with obesity." Newman, L. P., Bolhuis, D. P., Torres, S. J. and Keast, R. S.J. (2016) Obesity, 24: 328–334. doi:10.1002/oby.21357

Ngan & Conduit (2011). "A double-blind, placebo-controlled investigation of the effects of Passiflora incarnata (passionflower) herbal tea on subjective sleep quality." Ngan A, Conduit R. Phytother Res. 2011 Aug;25(8):1153-9. doi: 10.1002/ptr.3400. Epub 2011 Feb 3

NHMRC (2016). "Macronutrient Balance" Australian Government National Health and Medical Research Council. 02-04-2014 Retrieved 22/7/16

NIGMS (2017). "Circadian Rhythms." National Institute of General Medical Sciences. (nd) Retrieved 3rd Feb 2017

NIHCE (2007). "Depression: management of depression in primary and secondary care—NICE guidance." National Institute for Health and Clinical Excellence. 2007

Nilsson et al., (2008). "Including indigestible carbohydrates in the evening meal of healthy subjects improves glucose tolerance, lowers inflammatory markers, and increases satiety after a subsequent standardized breakfast." Nilsson AC, Ostman EM, Holst JJ, Björck IM. J Nutr. 2008 Apr;138(4):732-9

Nisbett & Storms (1972). "Cognitive and social determinants of food intake." Nisbett, R.E, & Storms, M.D. (1972). In H. London and R.E. Nisbett (Eds.), Thought and Feeding: Cognitive Alteration of Feeling States (190-208). Aldine Publishing Company: Chicago

Noakes (2018). "Healthy fats vs bad fats: fatty foods that are good for weight loss. Professor Manny Noakes, CSIRO Total Wellbeing Diet blog, retrieved 15th March 2018

Nordqvist (2017). "How many calories do you need?" Christian Nordqvist. Medical News Today, Wed 13 December 2017

Nutrition Australia (2016). "Fructose." Author unknown. www.nutrition-australia.org, retrieved 19th August 2016

NYR (2013). "Helping others shields us from stress, prolongs life." NYR Natural News, 19 March, 2013

Oettingen & Gollwitzer (2010). "Strategies of setting and implementing goals: Mental contrasting and implementation intentions." Oettingen, G., & Gollwitzer, P. M. (2010). In J. E. Maddux & J. P. Tangney (Eds.), Social psychological foundations of clinical psychology. (pp. 114–135). New York: Guilford Press

Oettingen, G. (2012). "Future thought and behavior change. "European Review of Social Psychology, 23, 1–63. (2012)

Ogden et al., (2015). "Distraction, restrained eating and disinhibition: An experimental study of food intake and the impact of 'eating on the go'." Jane Ogden, Eirini Oikonomou, Georgina Alemany. Journal of Health Psychology. Vol 22, Issue 1, pp. 39 - 50. First published date: August-20-2015. 10.1177/1359105315595119

Oh et al., (2013). "A brisk walk, compared with being sedentary, reduces attentional bias and chocolate cravings among regular chocolate eaters with different body mass." Hwajung Oh, Adrian H. Taylor. Appetite Volume 71, 1 December 2013, Pages 144–149. Received 16 April 2013. http://dx.doi.org/10.1016/j.appet.2013.07.015

Okajima & Spence (2011). "Effects of visual food texture on taste perception." K. Okajima, C. Spence. i-Perception, 2 (8) (2011)

Okajima et al., (2013). "Effects of visual texture on food perception." K. Okajima, J. Ueda, C. Spence. Journal of Vision, 13 (2013), p. 1078

Oliver et al., (2000). "Stress and food choice: A laboratory study." Oliver G, Wardle J, Gibson EL. Psychosom Med. 2000 Nov-Dec;62(6):853-65

Olmedilla-Alonso et al., (2012). "Composition of two Spanish common dry beans (Phaseolus vulgaris), 'Almonga' and 'Curruquilla', and their postprandial effect in type 2 diabetics." Olmedilla-Alonso B, Pedrosa MM, Cuadrado C, Brito M, Asensio-S-Manzanera C, Asensio-Vegas C. J Sci Food Agric. 2012 Aug 30. doi: 10.1002/jsfa.5852

Olsen (2011). "Natural Rewards, Neuroplasticity, and Non-Drug Addictions." Olsen CM. Neuropharmacology. 2011;61(7):1109-1122. doi:10.1016/j.neuropharm.2011.03.010

Origin (2014). "From Tiny Sculleries to Open Plan Mega Kitchens: A Century of Kitchen Design." Written for Origin Global (UK). 2nd September 2014. https://origin-global.com/news/from-tiny-sculleries-to-open-plan-mega-kitchens-a-century-of-kitchen-design

Oriti (2016). "Nutritional scientists call for new way to define balanced diet." Thomas Oriti. ABC News, The World Today. Posted 1 Aug 2016

Orsama et al., (2013). "Weight rhythms: Weight increases during weekends and decreases during weekdays." Orsama, A., Elina Mattila, Miikka Ermes, Mark Van Gils, Brian Wansink, and Ilkka Korhonen (2013). Obesity Facts, 7. doi:10.1159/000356147

Otsuka et al., (2006). "Eating Fast Leads to Obesity: Findings Based on Self-administered Questionnaires among Middle-aged Japanese Men and Women." Rei Otsuka, Koji Tamakoshi, Hiroshi Yatsuya, Chiyoe Murata, Atsushi Sekiya, Keiko Wada, Hui Ming Zhang, Kunihiro Matsushita, Kaichiro Sugiura, Seiko Takefuji, Pei OuYang, Nobue Nagasawa, Takaaki Kondo, Satoshi Sasaki, Hideaki Toyoshima. Journal of Epidemiology. Vol. 16 (2006) No. 3 P 117-124. http://doi.org/10.2188/jea.16.117. Released 2006/05/19

Oxford Dictionaries (2018). "Placebo." Oxford Dictionaries, retrieved 1st June 2018

Pacanowski et al., (2014). "Daily Self-Weighing to Control Body Weight in Adults: A Critical Review of the Literature." Pacanowski CR, Bertz FC, Levitsky DA. SAGE open. 2014;4(4):1-16. doi:10.1177/2158244014556992

Pacific Health Laboratories (2008). "5 Things That Affect Your Appetite." Pacific Health Laboratories, Thursday, October 23, 2008. www.trainingpeaks.com

Page et al., (2013). "Effects of Fructose vs Glucose on Regional Cerebral Blood Flow in Brain Regions Involved With Appetite and Reward Pathways." Kathleen A. Page, MD; Owen Chan, PhD; Jagriti Arora, MS; et al Renata Belfort-DeAguiar, MD, PhD; James Dzuira, PhD; Brian Roehmholdt, MD, PhD; Gary W. Cline, PhD; Sarita Naik, MD; Rajita Sinha, PhD; R. Todd Constable, PhD; Robert S. Sherwin, MD. January 2, 2013. JAMA. 2013;309(1):63-70. doi:10.1001/jama.2012.116975

Palmiter (2007). "Is dopamine a physiologically relevant mediator of feeding behavior?" Palmiter RD. Trends Neurosci 2007, 30: 375-381. 10.1016/j.tins.2007.06.004

Parnell & Reimer (2012). "Prebiotic fibres dose-dependently increase satiety hormones and alter Bacteroidetes and Firmicutes in lean and obese JCR:LA-cp rats." Parnell JA, Reimer RA. Br J Nutr. 2012 Feb;107(4):601-13. doi: 10.1017/S0007114511003163. Epub 2011 Jul 18

Parretti at al., (2015). "Efficacy of water preloading before main meals as a strategy for weight loss in primary care patients with obesity: RCT." Parretti, H. M., Aveyard, P., Blannin, A., Clifford, S. J., Coleman, S. J., Roalfe, A. and Daley, A. J. (2015), Obesity, 23: 1785–1791

Patel et al., (2006). "Association between Reduced Sleep and Weight Gain in Women." Sanjay R. Patel, Atul Malhotra, David P. White, Daniel J. Gottlieb and Frank B. Hu, Am. J. Epidemiol. (15 November 2006) 164 (10): 947-954. doi: 10.1093/aje/kwj280 First published online: August 16, 2006

Pattison et al., (2004). "Dietary risk factors for the development of inflammatory polyarthritis: Evidence for a role of high level of red meat consumption." Pattison, D. J., Symmons, D. P. M., Lunt, M., Welch, A., Luben, R., Bingham, S. A., Khaw, K.-T., Day, N. E. and Silman, A. J. (2004), Arthritis & Rheumatism, 50: 3804–3812. doi:10.1002/art.20731

Pedersen et al., (2001). "Saliva and gastrointestinal functions of taste, mastication, swallowing and digestion." Pedersen AM, Bardow A, Jensen SB, Nauntofte B. Oral Dis. 2002 May;8(3):117-29

Perreau-Linck et al., (2007). "In vivo measurements of brain trapping of C-labelled alpha-methyl-L-tryptophan during acute changes in mood states." Perreau-Linck E, Beauregard M, Gravel P, et al. J Psychiatry Neurosci 2007;32:430-4

Persson (1981) "Five-Year Mortality in a 70-Year-Old Urban Population in Relation to Psychiatric Diagnosis, Personality, Sexuality and Early Parental Death." Persson, G. Acta Psychiatr. Scand. (1981) 64:244

Phillips et al. (1992). "The Birthday: Lifeline or Deadline? David P. Phillips, Phd, Camilla A. Van Voorhees, Md, Todd E. Ruth. 1992 0033-3174/92/5405-0532103 00/0. The American Psychosomatic Society. Psychosomatic Medicine 54:532-542.

Pietiläinen et al. (2011). "Does dieting make you fat? A twin study." Pietiläinen KH, Saarni SE, Kaprio J, Rissanen A. Int J Obes (Lond). 2012 Mar;36(3):456-64. doi: 10.1038/ijo.2011.160. Epub 2011 Aug 9

Piqueras-Fiszman and Spence (2012). "The weight of the container influences expected satiety, perceived density, and subsequent expected fullness." B. Piqueras-Fiszman, C. Spence. Appetite, 58 (2) (2012), pp. 559–562

Pittaway (2006) "Chickpeas and Human Health: The effect of chickpea consumption on some physiological and metabolic parameters." Jane Pittaway BBiomed Sci (Hons). University of Tasmania, August 2006

Pittaway et al., (2006). "Effects of a Controlled Diet Supplemented with Chickpeas on Serum Lipids, Glucose Tolerance, Satiety and Bowel Function." Jane K. Pittaway, BBiomedSc(Hons), Kiran D. K. Ahuja, MBiomedSc, Iain K. Robertson, MMedSci, Madeleine J. Ball, FRCPath: Accepted by Journal of the American College of Nutrition July 2006

Pliquett et al., (2006). "The effects of insulin on the central nervous system—focus on appetite regulation." Pliquett RU, Fuhrer D, Falk S, Zysset S, von Cramon DY, Stumvoll M. Horm Metab Res. 2006 Jul;38(7):442-6

Polivy & Herman (1985). "Dieting and binging: A causal analysis." Polivy, Janet; Herman, C. Peter. American Psychologist, Vol 40(2), Feb 1985, 193-201. http://dx.doi.org/10.1037/0003-066X.40.2.193

Polivy (1996). "Psychological Consequences of Food Restriction." Janet Polivy, PhD. Journal of the Academy of Nutrition and Dietetics. Volume 96, Issue 6, Pages 589–592 June 1996 DOI: http://dx.doi.org/10.1016/S0002-8223(96)00161-7

Polivy et al., (2005). "The effect of deprivation on food cravings and eating behavior in restrained and unrestrained eaters." Polivy, J., Coleman, J. and Herman, C. P. (2005), Int. J. Eat. Disord., 38: 301–309. doi:10.1002/eat.20195

Poncela-Casasnovas et al., (2015). "Social embeddedness in an online weight management programme is linked to greater weight loss." Julia Poncela-Casasnovas, Bonnie Spring, Daniel McClary, Arlen C. Moller, Rufaro Mukogo, Christine A. Pellegrini, Michael J. Coons, Miriam Davidson, Satyam Mukherjee, Luis A. Nunes Amaral. Journal of the Royal Society Interface. Published 28 January 2015.DOI: 10.1098/rsif.2014.0686

Post et al., (1973). "Simulated behavior states: an approach to specificity in psychobiological research." Post RM, Goodwin FK. Biol Psychiatry. 1973 Dec; 7(3):237-54

Poulin et al. (2012). "Giving to Others and the Association Between Stress and Mortality." Michael J. Poulin, Stephanie L. Brown, Amanda J. Dillard, and Dylan M. Smith. American Journal of Public Health: September 2013, Vol. 103, No. 9, pp. 1649-1655. doi: 10.2105/AJPH.2012.300876.

Preston (2014). "Words that make you hungry." Matt Preston, www.taste.com.au 12th August 2014

Prewitt et al., (1991). "Changes in body weight, body composition, and energy intake in women fed high- and low-fat diets." Prewitt, T.E., D. Schmeisser, P.E. Bowen, P. Aye, T.A. Dolecek, P. Langenberg, T. Cole, and L. Brace 1991. Am. J. Clin. Nutr. 54(2):304–310

Pursey et al., (2014). "The prevalence of food addiction as assessed by the Yale Food Addiction Scale: a systematic review." Pursey KM, Stanwell P, Gearhardt AN, Collins CE, Burrows TL. Nutrients 2014 Oct 21;6(10):4552-90. doi: 10.3390/nu6104552.

Putai Jin (1992). "Efficacy of Tai Chi, brisk walking, meditation, and reading in reducing mental and emotional stress." Putai Jin. Journal of Psychosomatic Research, Volume 36, Issue 4, May 1992, Pages 361–370. 19 September 1991. http://dx.doi.org/10.1016/0022-3999(92)90072-A

Qing Yang (2010). "Gain weight by 'going diet?' Artificial sweeteners and the neurobiology of sugar cravings." Qing Yang. Yale J Biol Med. 2010 Jun; 83(2): 101–108. Published online 2010 Jun.PMCID: PMC2892765. Neuroscience 2010

Rada et al., (2005). "Daily bingeing on sugar repeatedly releases dopamine in the accumbens shell." Rada P, Avena NM, Hoebel BG. Neuroscience. 2005;134(3):737-44

Ray (2008). "Where do those late-night calories go?" C. Claiborne Ray. Chicago Tribune. 2008 March 04

Raynor & Epstein (2001). "Dietary Variety, Energy Regulation, and Obesity." Raynor H, Epstein L. Psychological Bulletin 2001; 127: 325-341

Rebello et al., (2014) "Etiology and Pathophysiology/Obesity Comorbidities: A review of the nutritional value of legumes and their effects on obesity and its related co-morbidities." C. J. Rebello, F. L. Greenway, J. W. Finley. 17 January 2014. https://doi.org/10.1111/obr.12144

Reimers et al. (2012) "Does Physical Activity Increase Life Expectancy? A Review of the Literature." C. D. Reimers, G. Knapp, and A. K. Reimers. Journal of Aging Research Volume 2012 (2012), Article ID 243958. http://dx.doi.org/10.1155/2012/243958

Reinbach et al., (2009). "Effects of capsaicin, green tea and CH-19 sweet pepper on appetite and energy intake in humans in negative and positive energy balance." Reinbach HC, Smeets A, Martinussen T, Møller P, Westerterp-Plantenga MS. Clin Nutr. 2009 Jun;28(3):260-5. doi: 10.1016/j.clnu.2009.01.010. Epub 2009 Apr 3

Reinholz et al., (2008). "Compensatory weight gain due to dopaminergic hypofunction: new evidence and own incidental observations." Julia Reinholz, Oliver Skopp, Caterina Breitenstein, Iwo Bohr, Hilke Winterhoff and Stefan Knecht. Nutrition & Metabolism 2008 5:35. DOI: 10.1186/1743-7075-5-35. 01 December 2008.

Resnick (2017). "A radical new hypothesis in medicine: give patients drugs they know don't work. Why the placebo effect is weirder and potentially more useful than we imagined." Brian Resnick. Vox Science. Jun 2, 2017]

Richard et al., (2009). "L-Tryptophan: Basic Metabolic Functions, Behavioral Research and Therapeutic Indications." Richard DM, Dawes MA, Mathias CW, Acheson A, Hill-Kapturczak N, Dougherty DM. International Journal of Tryptophan Research : IJTR. 2009;2:45-60

Ridaura, et al., (2013). "Gut Microbiota from Twins Discordant for Obesity Modulate Metabolism in Mice." Vanessa K. Ridaura, Jeremiah J. Faith, Federico E. Rey, Jiye Cheng, Alexis E. Duncan, Andrew L. Kau, Nicholas W. Griffin, Vincent Lombard, Bernard Henrissat, James R. Bain, Michael J. Muehlbauer, Olga Ilkayeva, Clay F. Semenkovich, Katsuhiko Funai, David K. Hayashi, Barbara J. Lyle, Margaret C. Martini, Luke K. Ursell, Jose C. Clemente, William Van Treuren, William A. Walters, Rob Knight, Christopher B. Newgard, Andrew C. Heath, Jeffrey I. Gordon. Science 06 Sep 2013

Riesco et al., (2010). "Impact of walking on eating behaviors and quality of life of premenopausal and early postmenopausal obese women." Riesco E, Tessier S, Pérusse F, Turgeon S, Tremblay A, Weisnagel J, Doré J, Mauriège P.]] Menopause. 2010 May-Jun;17(3):529-38. doi: 10.1097/gme.0b013e3181d12361

Rippe & Angelopoulos (2013). "Sucrose, High-Fructose Corn Syrup, and Fructose, Their Metabolism and Potential Health Effects: What Do We Really Know?" James M. Rippe, Theodore J. Angelopoulos. Advances in Nutrition, Volume 4, Issue 2, 1 March 2013, Pages 236–245, https://doi.org/10.3945/an.112.002824

Roberts (2003). "Glycemic index and satiety." Roberts SB. Nutr Clin Care. 2003 Jan-Apr;6(1):20-6. PMID: 12841427

Robins (1993). "Vietnam veterans' rapid recovery from heroin addiction: a fluke or normal expectation?" Lee N. Robins. Department of Psychiatry, Washington University School of Medicine, St Louis, Missouri, USA. The Sixth Thomas James Okey Memorial Lecture. Addiction (1993) 88, 1041-1054

Robins et al., (1974). "Drug use by U.S. army enlisted men in Vietnam: a follow-up on their return home." Lee N. Robins, Darlene H. Davis And Donald W. Goodwin Am. J. Epidemiol. (1974) 99 (4): 235-249

Robinson et al., (2013). "Eating attentively: a systematic review and meta-analysis of the effect of food intake memory and awareness on eating." Eric Robinson, Paul Aveyard, Amanda Daley, Kate Jolly, Amanda Lewis, Deborah Lycett, and Suzanne Higgs. First published February 27, 2013, doi: 10.3945/ajcn.112.045245 Am J Clin Nutr. ajcn.045245

Rodin (1985). "Insulin levels, hunger, and food intake: an example of feedback loops in body weight regulation." Rodin, J. Health Psychol. 1985;4(1):1-24

Rogers & Blundell (1990). "Umami and appetite: effects of monosodium glutamate on hunger and food intake in human subjects." Rogers PJ, Blundell JE. Physiol Behav. 1990 Dec;48(6):801-4

Rollings & Wells (2016). "Effects of Floor Plan Openness on Eating Behaviors. Environment and Behavior." Kimberly A. Rollings, Nancy M. Wells. Environment and Behavior. Volume: 49 issue: 6, page(s): 663-684. Article first published online: August 19, 2016; Issue published: July 1, 2017. https://doi.org/10.1177/0013916516661822

Rolls (1995) "Effects of Food Quality, Quantity, and Variety on Intake." Barbara J. Rolls. "Not Eating Enough: Overcoming Underconsumption of Military Operational Rations." Institute of Medicine (US) Committee on Military Nutrition Research. Washington (DC): National Academies Press (US); 1995. http://www.ncbi.nlm.nih.gov/books/NBK232454/

Rolls (1995b). "Carbohydrates, fats, and satiety." B J Rolls, Am J Clin Nutr April 1995 vol. 61 no. 4 960S-967S

Rolls (2003). "The supersizing of America: Portion size and the obesity epidemic." Rolls, B. J. (2003). Nutrition Today, 38(2), 42-53

Rolls et al. (1992). "Information about fat content of preloads influences energy intake in women [abstract]." Rolls, B.J., D.J. Shide, N. Hoeymans, P. Jas, and A. Nichols 1992. Appetite 19:213

Rolls et al., (1983). "Variety in the diet enhances intake in a meal and contributes to the development of obesity in the rat." Rolls BJ, Van Duijvenvoorde PM, Rowe EA. Physiology & Behavior 1983; 31(1):21-7

Rolls et al., (2000). "Increasing the volume of a food by incorporating air affects satiety in men." B.J. Rolls, E.A. Bell, B.A. Waugh. American Journal of Clinical Nutrition, 72 (2) (2000), pp. 361–368

Rolls, et al., (1992). "Information about fat content of preloads influences energy intake in women [abstract]." Rolls, B.J., D.J. Shide, N. Hoeymans, P. Jas, and A. Nichols 1992. Appetite 19:213

Ronzio (2003). "Craving". Ronzio, Robert A. (2003). The Encyclopedia of Nutrition and Good Health (2nd ed.). Facts on File. p. 176. ISBN 0-8160-4966-1

Ropelle et al., (2010). "IL-6 and IL-10 Anti-Inflammatory Activity Links Exercise to Hypothalamic Insulin and Leptin Sensitivity through IKK and ER Stress Inhibition." Eduardo R. Ropelle, Marcelo B. Flores, Dennys E. Cintra, Guilherme Z. Rocha, José R. Pauli, Joseane Morari, Claudio T. de Souza, Juliana C. Moraes, Patrícia O. Prada, Dioze Guadagnini, Rodrigo M. Marin, Alexandre G. Oliveira, Taize M. Augusto, Hernandes F. Carvalho, Lício A. Velloso, Mario J. A. Saad, José B. C. Carvalheira. PLOS. Published: August 24, 2010. http://dx.doi.org/10.1371/journal.pbio.1000465

Ross (1970). "Cue- and Cognition-Controlled Eating among Obese and Normal Weight Subjects." Ross, L.D. (1970). New York, NY: Columbia University. Thesis

Saker et al., (2016). "Overdrinking, swallowing inhibition, and regional brain responses prior to swallowing." Pascal Saker, Michael J. Farrell, Gary F. Egan, Michael J. McKinley, and Derek A. Denton. PNAS October 25, 2016. 113 (43) 12274-12279; published ahead of print October 10, 2016. https://doi.org/10.1073/pnas.1613929113

Saleh et al., (2005). "Effects of Ramadan fasting on Waist Circumference, Blood Pressure, Lipid Profile, and Blood Sugar on a Sample of Healthy Kuwaiti Men and Women." Mal J Nutr 11(2): 143-150, 2005. Salhamoud Abdelfatah Saleh, Salah Anies Elsharouni, Boby Cherian, and M. Mourou. Department of Medicine, Adan Teaching Hospital, Kuwait.

Salehi et al., (2012). "The insulinogenic effect of whey protein is partially mediated by a direct effect of amino acids and GIP on beta-cells." Salehi A, Gunnerud U, Muhammed SJ, Ostman E, Holst JJ, Björck I, Rorsman P. Nutr Metab (Lond). 2012 May 30;9(1):48. doi: 10.1186/1743-7075-9-48

Salk (2014). "Another case against the midnight snack." Salk News, The Salk Institute for Biological Studies. December 2, 2014

Sallis (2009) "Exercise is medicine and physicians need to prescribe it!" R E Sallis. British Journal of Sports Medicine Volume 43, Issue 1. January 2009. http://dx.doi.org/10.1136/bjsm.2008.054825

Salmon (2001). "Effects of physical exercise on anxiety, depression, and sensitivity to stress: a unifying theory." Salmon P. Clin Psychol Rev. 2001 Feb; 21(1):33-61

Samra & Anderson (2007). "Insoluble cereal fiber reduces appetite and short-term food intake and glycemic response to food consumed 75 min later by healthy men." Samra RA1, Anderson GH. Am J Clin Nutr. 2007 Oct;86(4):972-9

Samra (2010). "Fats and Satiety." Samra RA. In: Montmayeur JP, le Coutre J, editors. Fat Detection: Taste, Texture, and Post Ingestive Effects. Boca Raton (FL): CRC Press/Taylor & Francis; 2010. Chapter 15. Available from: http://www.ncbi.nlm.nih.gov/books/NBK53550/

Samraja et al., (2015). "A red meat-derived glycan promotes inflammation and cancer progression." Annie N. Samraja,1, Oliver M. T. Pearcea,1, Heinz Läublia, Alyssa N. Crittendena, Anne K. Bergfelda, Kalyan Bandaa, Christopher J. Gregga, Andrea E. Bingmana, Patrick Secresta, Sandra L. Diaza, Nissi M. Varkia,b, and Ajit Varkia, Proceedings of the National Academy of Sciences. vol. 112 no. 2 542–547, doi: 10.1073/pnas.1417508112.

Sartorelli et al., (2008). "High intake of fruits and vegetables predicts weight loss in Brazilian overweight adults." Daniela Saes Sartorelli, Laércio Joel Franco, Marly Augusto Cardoso.]Nutrition Research Volume 28, Issue 4, April 2008, Pages 233–238 http://dx.doi.org/10.1016/j.nutres.2008.02.004

Scaglioni et al., (2000) "Early macronutrient intake and overweight at five years of age." S. Scaglioni, C. Agostoni, R. De Notaris, G. Radaelli, N. Radice, M. Valenti, M. Giovannini, E. Riva. Italian Ministry of Health (nd)

Scheibehenne et al., (2010). "Dining in the dark. The importance of visual cues for food consumption and satiety." B. Scheibehenne, P.M. Todd, B. Wansink. Appetite, 55 (3) (2010), pp. 710–713

Schmid et al., (2008). "A single night of sleep deprivation increases ghrelin levels and feelings of hunger in normal-weight healthy men." Sebastian M.Schmid, Manfred Hallschmid, Kamila Jauch-Chara, Jan Born, and Bernd Schultes. doi: 10.1111/j.1365-2869.2008.00662.x

Schmidt et al., (2015). "Prebiotic intake reduces the waking cortisol response and alters emotional bias in healthy volunteers." Schmidt K, Cowen PJ, Harmer CJ, Tzortzis G, Errington S, Burnet PW. Psychopharmacology (Berl). 2015 May;232(10):1793-801. doi: 10.1007/s00213-014-3810-0. Epub 2014 Dec 3

Schöning et al., (2012) "Digitally enhanced food." J. Schöning, Y. Rogers, A. Krüger. Pervasive Computing (2012), pp. 4–6

Schwartz et al., (2008). "The Lipid Messenger OEA Links Dietary Fat Intake to Satiety." Gary J. Schwartz, Jin Fu, Giuseppe Astarita, Xiaosong Li1, Silvana Gaetani, Patrizia Campolongo, Vincenzo Cuomo, Daniele Piomelli. Cell Metabolism Volume 8, Issue 4, 8 October 2008, Pages 281–288. http://dx.doi.org/10.1016/j.cmet.2008.08.005

Schwartz et al., (2015). "Antibiotic use and childhood body mass index trajectory." B S Schwartz, J Pollak, L Bailey-Davis, A G Hirsch, S E Cosgrove, C Nau, A M Kress, T A Glass and K Bandeen-Roche. International Journal of Obesity (21 October 2015)doi:10.1038/ijo.2015.218

SCIB (2016). "Manipulating gut microbes may reverse the negative effect of a high fat." Society for the Study of Ingestive Behavior (SCIB). ScienceDaily. www.sciencedaily.com/releases/2016/07/160712092343.htm. Retrieved July 21, 2016

Scinicariello & Buser (2014). "Urinary Polycyclic Aromatic Hydrocarbons and Childhood Obesity: NHANES (2001–2006)". Franco Scinicariello and Melanie C. Buser. Environ Health Perspect; DOI:10.1289/ehp.1307234 (2014)

Scott, et al., (2016). "Administration of Antibiotics to Children Before Age 2 Years Increases Risk for Childhood Obesity." Frank I. Scott, Daniel B. Horton, Ronac Mamtani, Kevin Haynes, David S. Goldberg, Dale Y. Lee, James D. Lewis. 2016. DOI: http://dx.doi.org/10.1053/j.gastro.2016.03.006

Sender et al., (2016). "Are We Really Vastly Outnumbered? Revisiting the Ratio of Bacterial to Host Cells in Humans." Sender, R; Fuchs, S; Milo, R (Jan 2016). Cell. 164 (3): 337–40. doi:10.1016/j.cell.2016.01.013. PMID 26824647.

Shariff et al., (2016). "Neuronal Nicotinic Acetylcholine Receptor Modulators Reduce Sugar Intake." Shariff M, Quik M, Holgate J, Morgan M, Patkar OL, Tam V, et al. (2016) PLoS ONE 11(3): e0150270. doi:10.1371/journal.pone.0150270

Sharifi et al., (2013). "Perceived Barriers to Weight loss Programs for Overweight or Obese Women." Sharifi N, Mahdavi R, Ebrahimi-Mameghani M. Health Promotion Perspectives. 2013;3(1):11-22. doi:10.5681/hpp.2013.002

Sherman (2009). "Pleasure, Not Fullness, May Be Key to 'Satiety Hormone'." Carl Sherman. The DANA Foundation, October 1, 2009

Shevchuk (2008). "Adapted cold shower as a potential treatment for depression." Shevchuk NA. Med Hypotheses. 2008;70(5):995-1001. Epub 2007 Nov 13

Sim et al., (2013). "High-intensity intermittent exercise attenuates ad-libitum energy intake." Int J Obes (Lond). 2014 Mar;38(3):417-22. doi: 10.1038/ijo.2013.102. Epub 2013 Jun 4. Sim AY, Wallman KE, Fairchild TJ, Guelfi KJ.

Simansky (1995). "Serotonergic control of the organization of feeding and satiety." Kenny J. Simansky, Department of Pharmacology, Medical College of Pennsylvania and Hahnemann University, 3200 Henry Avenue, Philadelphia, PA 19129, USA 1995

Simner et al., (2010). "What Sound Does That Taste? Cross-Modal Mappings Across Gustation and Audition." Simner, Cuskley C, Kirby S. Perception 39 (4), 553-569. 2010

Singh (2006). "Impact of color on marketing." Satyendra Singh, (2006) Management Decision, Vol. 44 Iss: 6, pp.783 - 789. DOI http://dx.doi.org/10.1108/00251740610673332

Skorka-Brown et al., (2014). "Playing 'Tetris' reduces the strength, frequency and vividness of naturally occurring cravings." Skorka-Brown J , Andrade J , May J . Appetite. 2014 May;76:161-5. doi: 10.1016/j.appet.2014.01.073. Epub 2014 Feb 5

Skulas-Ray et al., (2011). "A High Antioxidant Spice Blend Attenuates Postprandial Insulin and Triglyceride Responses and Increases Some Plasma Measures of Antioxidant Activity in Healthy, Overweight Men." A. C. Skulas-Ray, P. M. Kris-Etherton, D. L. Teeter, C.-Y. O. Chen, J. P. Vanden Heuvel, S. G. West. Journal of Nutrition, 2011; 141 (8): 1451

Slavenka Kam-Hansen et al (2014). "Labeling of Medication and Placebo Alters the Outcome of Episodic Migraine Attacks." Slavenka Kam-Hansen, Moshe Jakubowski, John M. Kelley, Irving Kirsch, David C. Hoaglin, Ted J. Kaptchuk, and Rami Burstein. Sci Transl Med. 2014 Jan 8; 6(218): 218ra5. doi: 10.1126/scitranslmed.3006175. PMCID: PMC4005597. NIHMSID: NIHMS565231

Slavin & Green (2007). "Dietary fibre and satiety." J. Slavin, H. Green. Nutrition Bulletin, 32 (2007), pp. 32–42

Slavin (2008) "Position of the American Dietetic Association: health implications of dietary fiber." Slavin JL. Journal of the American Dietetic Association [01 Oct 2008, 108(10):1716-1731. PMID:18953766. DOI: 10.1016/j.jada.2008.08.007

So et al., (2009). "Glucocorticoid regulation of the circadian clock modulates glucose homeostasis." So AY, Bernal TU, Pillsbury ML, Yamamoto KR, Feldman BJ. Proc Natl Acad Sci U S A. 2009 Oct 13;106(41):17582-7. doi: 10.1073/pnas.0909733106. Epub 2009 Oct 5

Solon-Biet (2015). "Dietary Protein to Carbohydrate Ratio and Caloric Restriction: Comparing Metabolic Outcomes in Mice." Solon-Biet SM, Mitchell SJ, Coogan SC, Cogger VC, Gokarn R5, McMahon AC, Raubenheimer D, de Cabo R, Simpson SJ7, Le Couteur DG. Cell Reports 2015 Jun 16;11(10):1529-34. doi: 10.1016/j.celrep.2015.05.007

Sonnenburg et al., (2015). "The Good Gut: Taking Control of Your Weight, Your Mood, and Your Long-term Health" Justin Sonnenburg PhD, Erica Sonnenburg, Andrew Weil. Penguin Books 2015. ISBN-13: 978-1594206283

Sook Ling Leong et al., (2011). "Faster Self-Reported Speed of Eating Is Related to Higher Body Mass Index in a Nationwide Survey of Middle-Aged Women." Sook Ling Leong, Clara Madden, Andrew Gray, et al. Journal of the American Dietetic Association. 2011, Vol.111, No.8, p.1192

Sørensen & Astrup (2011). "Eating dark and milk chocolate: a randomized crossover study of effects on appetite and energy intake." LB Sørensen and A Astrup. Nutrition and Diabetes (2011)1, e21; doi:10.1038/nutd.2011.17. Macmillan Publishers Limited. All rights reserved 2044-4052/11

Sorensen et al., (1999). "Effect of sensory perception of foods on appetite and food intake: a review of studies on humans." Sorensen LB, Moller P, Flint A, Martens M, Raben A. Int J Obes (London) 2003; 27: 1152–1166.]

South & Huang, (2008). "High-fat diet exposure increases dopamine D2 receptor and decreases dopamine transporter receptor binding density in the nucleus accumbens and caudate putamen of mice." South T, Huang XF. Neurochem Res 2008, 33: 598-605. 10.1007/s11064-007-9483-x

Spence (2015). "On the psychological impact of food colour." Charles Spence. Flavour 20154:21. DOI: 10.1186/s13411-015-0031-3. Published: 22 April 2015

Spence et al., (2012). "Assessing the impact of the tableware and other contextual variables on multisensory flavour perception." Spence, C., Harrara, V., & Piqueras-Fiszman, B. (2012). Flavour, 1(1), 7-18. doi: 10.1186/2044-7248-1-7

Spence et al., (2016). "Eating with our eyes: From visual hunger to digital satiation." Charles Spence, Katsunori Okajima, Adrian David Cheok, Olivia Petit, Charles Michel. Brain and Cognition 110 December 2016, Pages 53-63. https://doi.org/10.1016/j.bandc.2015.08.006

Spiegel et al., (1999). "Impact of sleep debt on metabolic and endocrine function." Spiegel K, Leproult R, Van Cauter E. Lancet 1999;354:1435-9

Spiegel, et al., (1991). "Objective measurement of eating rate during behavioral treatment of obesity." Theresa A. Spiegel, Thomas A. Wadden, Gary D. Foster. Behavior Therapy. Volume 22, Issue 1, Winter 1991, Pages 61–67. http://dx.doi.org/10.1016/S0005-7894(05)80244-8

Spring (1984). "Recent research on the behavioral effects of tryptophan and carbohydrate." Review article. Spring B. Nutr Health. 1984. Nutr Health. 1984;3(1-2):55-67

State Government, Victoria (2016). "Better Health." www.betterhealth. vic.gov.au/health/healthyliving/food-variety-and-a-healthy-diet (nd) Retrieved 24.7.16

Stauth (2007). "Studies force new view on biology of flavonoids." David Stauth, EurekAlert! 5-Mar-2007. Adapted from a news release issued by Oregon State University.

Steel et al, (2006). "Effects of hunger and visuo-spatial interference on imagery-induced food cravings." Steel D , Kemps E, Tiggemann M. Appetite. 2006 Jan;46(1):36-40. Epub 2005 Dec 20

Steig et al., (2011). "Exercise reduces appetite and traffics excess nutrients away from energetically efficient pathways of lipid deposition during the early stages of weight regain." Amy J. Steig, Matthew R. Jackman, Erin D. Giles, Janine A. Higgins, Ginger C. Johnson, Chad Mahan, Edward L. Melanson, Holly R. Wyatt, Robert H. Eckel, James O. Hill, Paul S. MacLean. American Journal of Physiology - Regulatory, Integrative and Comparative Physiology Published 1 September 2011 Vol. 301 no. 3, R656-R667 DOI: 10.1152/ajpregu.00212.2011

Stein (nd). Science Communications, (nd) Leslie J. Stein, PhD, Monell Chemical Senses Center, Philadelphia

Steinberg et al., (2013). "The efficacy of a daily self-weighing weight loss intervention using smart scales and email." Steinberg DM, Tate DF, Bennett GG, Ennett S, Samuel-Hodge C, Ward DS. Obesity (Silver Spring, Md). 2013;21(9):1789-1797. doi:10.1002/oby.20396

Steinberg et al., (2015). "Weighing every day matters: daily weighing improves weight loss and adoption of weight control behaviors." Steinberg DM, Bennett GG, Askew S, Tate DF. J Acad Nutr Diet. 2015 Apr;115(4):511-8. doi: 10.1016/j.jand.2014.12.011. Epub 2015 Feb 12.]

Steinert et al., (2011). "Effects of carbohydrate sugars and artificial sweeteners on appetite and the secretion of gastrointestinal satiety peptides." Robert E. Steinert, Florian Frey, Antonia Topfer, Jurgen Drewe and Christoph Beglinger. Accepted 10 November 2010 British Journal of Nutrition (2011), 105, 1320–1328. doi:10.1017/S000711451000512X

Stice et al., (2008). "Fasting Increases Risk for Onset of Binge Eating and Bulimic Pathology: A 5-Year Prospective Study." Eric Stice, Kendra Davis, Nicole P. Miller, and C. Nathan Marti. J Abnorm Psychol. 2008 Nov; 117(4): 941–946. doi: 10.1037/a0013644. PMCID: PMC2850570. NIHMSID: NIHMS186747

Strand (2003). "Tryptophan: What Does It Do? An amino acid that brings feelings of calm, relaxation, and sleepiness." Erik Strand, Psychology Today. Published on September 1, 2003. Last reviewed on June 9 2016.

Streib (2007). "Forbes World's Fattest Countries." Lauren Streib. August 2007. www.forbes.com

Stroebele & de Castro (2006). Research report: "Listening to music while eating is related to increases in people's food intake and meal duration". Nanette Stroebele, , John M. de Castro. Appetite, Volume 47, Issue 3, November 2006, Pages 285–289. http://dx.doi.org/10.1016/j.appet.2006.04.001

Sudsuang et al., (1991). "Effect of Buddhist meditation on serum cortisol and total protein levels, blood pressure, pulse rate, lung volume and reaction time." Sudsuang R, Chentanez V, Veluvan K. Physiol Behav. 1991 Sep;50(3):543-8

Suez et al., (2014). "Artificial sweeteners induce glucose intolerance by altering the gut microbiota" Jotham Suez, Tal Korem, David Zeevi, Gili Zilberman-Schapira, Christoph A. Thaiss, Ori Maza, David Israeli, Niv Zmora, Shlomit Gilad, Adina Weinberger, Yael Kuperman, Alon Harmelin, Ilana Kolodkin-Gal, Hagit Shapiro, Zamir Halpern, Eran Segal, Eran Elinav. Nature 514, 181–186 (09 October 2014) doi:10.1038/nature13793 28 August 2014 Published online 17 September 2014

Swerdloff, A. (2015). "Eating the uncanny valley: Inside the virtual reality world of food." Munchies, April 13

Swithers (2013). "Artificial sweeteners produce the counterintuitive effect of inducing metabolic derangements." Susan E. Swithers. Trends Endocrinol Metab. 2013 Sep; 24(9): 431–441. Published online 2013 Jul 10. doi: 10.1016/j.tem.2013.05.005. PMCID: PMC3772345

Taheri et al., (2004). "Short sleep duration is associated with reduced leptin, elevated ghrelin, and increased body mass index." Taheri S, Lin L, Austin D, Young T, Mignot E. PLoS Med 2004;1:e62

Tao Wu et al., (2013). "Blueberry and Mulberry Juice Prevent Obesity Development in C57BL/6 Mice." Tao Wu, Qiong Tang, Zichun Gao, Zhuoping Yu, Haizhao Song, Xiaodong Zheng, Wei Chen. PLOS. Published: October 15, 2013. http://dx.doi.org/10.1371/journal.pone.0077585

Taveras et al. (2008). "Short Sleep Duration in Infancy and Risk of Childhood Overweight." Elsie M. Taveras, MD, MPH; Sheryl L. Rifas-Shiman, MPH; Emily Oken, MD, MPH. Archives of Pediatrics & Adolescent Medicine. 2008 Apr; 162(4): 305

TED (2017). "The secret to living longer may be your social life" TED.com. Aug 18, 2017

Teff et al., (2004). "Dietary fructose reduces circulating insulin and leptin, attenuates postprandial suppression of ghrelin, and increases triglycerides in women." Teff KL , Elliott SS, Tschöp M, Kieffer TJ, Rader D, Heiman M, Townsend RR, Keim NL, D'Alessio D, Havel PJ. J Clin Endocrinol Metab. 2004 Jun;89(6):2963-72

Telegraph (2012). "Rise of open plan living." The Telegraph. www.telegraph. co.uk 06 Jan 2012. (Reporting on a survey commissioned by Lloyds TSB Home Insurance.)

Temple et al., (2007). "Television watching increases motivated responding for food and energy intake in children." Jennifer L Temple, April M Giacomelli, Kristine M Kent, James N Roemmich, and Leonard H Epstein. Am J Clin Nutr February 2007. vol. 85 no. 2 355-361 http:// ajcn.nutrition.org/content/85/2/355.full

Ten Have et al., (2011). "Physical exercise in adults and mental health status findings from the Netherlands mental health survey and incidence study." (NEMESIS). Ten Have M, de Graaf R, Monshouwer K. J Psychosom Res. 2011 Nov;71(5):342-8. doi: 10.1016/j.jpsychores.2011.04.001.

Tétreault et al., (2016). "Brain Connectivity Predicts Placebo Response across Chronic Pain Clinical Trials." Tétreault P, Mansour A, Vachon-Presseau E, Schnitzer TJ, Apkarian AV, Baliki MN. PLoS Biol. 2016; 14(10): e1002570 doi: 10.1371/journal.pbio.1002570

Thompson et al., (2012). "Bean and rice meals reduce postprandial glycemic response in adults with type 2 diabetes: a cross-over study." Thompson SV, Winham DM, Hutchins AM. Nutr J. 2012;11:23

Tigbe et al., (2017). "Time spent in sedentary posture is associated with waist circumference and cardiovascular risk." Tigbe WW, Granat MH, Sattar N, Lean MEJ. [Int J Obes (Lond). 2017 May;41(5):689-696. doi: 10.1038/ijo.2017.30. Epub 2017 Jan 31

Tiggemann & Kemps (2005). "The phenomenology of food cravings: the role of mental imagery."] [Tiggemann M, Kemps E. Appetite (2005) 45:305–13.10.1016/j.appet.2005.06.004

Tobias et al., (2015). "Effect of low-fat diet interventions versus other diet interventions on long-term weight change in adults: a systematic review and meta-analysis." Dr Deirdre K Tobias, ScD, Mu Chen, ScD, Prof JoAnn E Manson, MD, Prof David S Ludwig, MD, Prof Walter Willett, MD, Prof Frank B Hu, MD. 29 October 2015. DOI: http:// dx.doi.org/10.1016/S2213-8587(15)00367-8

Tonstad et al., (2013). "A high-fibre bean-rich diet versus a low-carbohydrate diet for obesity." Tonstad S, Malik N, Haddad E. J Hum Nutr Diet. 2014 Apr;27 Suppl 2:109-16. doi: 10.1111/jhn.12118. Epub 2013 Apr 30

Topham (2011). "Why one biscuit is never enough: Doctors reveal the science of hunger pangs—and what you can do about them." By Laura Topham for The Mail on Sunday. Daily Mail Tuesday, Mar 15th 2016

Touchette et al., (2008). "Associations Between Sleep Duration Patterns and Overweight/Obesity at Age 6." Évelyne Touchette, Dominique Petit, Richard E. Tremblay, Michel Boivin, Bruno Falissard, Christophe Genolini, Jacques Y. Montplaisir. Sleep, Volume 31, Issue 11, 1 November 2008, Pages 1507–1514, https://doi.org/10.1093/sleep/31.11.1507

Turnbaugh et al., (2009). "A core gut microbiome in obese and lean twins." Turnbaugh PJ, Hamady M, Yatsunenko T, Cantarel BL, Duncan A, Ley RE, Sogin ML, Jones WJ, Roe BA, Affourtit JP, Egholm M, Henrissat B, Heath AC, Knight R, Gordon JI. Nature. 2009 Jan 22;457(7228):480-4. doi: 10.1038/nature07540. Epub 2008 Nov 30

Turner et al., (2013). "Dietary Adherence and Satisfaction with a Bean-Based High-Fiber Weight Loss Diet: A Pilot Study," Tonya F. Turner, Laura M. Nance, William D. Strickland, Robert J. Malcolm, Susan Pechon, and Patrick M. O'Neil, ISRN Obesity, vol. 2013, Article ID 915415, 5 pages, 2013. doi:10.1155/2013/915415

Turnwald (2017). "Association Between Indulgent Descriptions and Vegetable Consumption: Twisted Carrots and Dynamite Beets." Turnwald BP, Boles DZ, Crum AJ. JAMA Intern Med. Published online June 12, 2017. doi:10.1001/jamainternmed.2017.1637

University of Utah (2016). "The Human Microbiome." University of Utah Health Sciences, Genetic Science Learning Center, (nd) Retrieved 21/7/2016

URMCE (2018). "Why Parents Shouldn't Use Food as Reward or Punishment." University of Rochester Medical Center Encyclopedia. Retrieved 4th April 2018

USC (2017). "Stress Management." University of Southern California (USC). Be Well at USC. https://bewell.usc.edu/mental-health/stress-management/ Retrieved 18th February 2017

Uyeda, et al., (2011). "The million-year wait for macroevolutionary bursts." Josef C. Uyeda, Thomas F. Hansen, Stevan J. Arnold and Jason Pienaar. PNAS September 20, 2011. 108 (38) 15908-15913; https://doi.org/10.1073/pnas.1014503108

Valtin (2002). "Drink at least eight glasses of water a day. Really? Is there scientific evidence for '8x8'"? Valtin H. American Journal of Physiological - Regulatory, Integrative and Comparative Physiology, November 2002

van de Veer et al., (2015). "Body and Mind: Mindfulness Helps Consumers to Compensate for Prior Food Intake by Enhancing the Responsiveness to Physiological Cues." van de Veer, E & van Herpen, Erica & Trijp, Hans. (2015). Journal of Consumer Research. 42.10.1093/jcr/ucv058

van Kleef et al., (2013). "Just a bite: Considerably smaller snack portions satisfy delayed hunger and craving. Journal of Food Quality and Preference." Ellen van Kleef, Mitsuru Shimizu, and Brian Wansink (2013). 27(1), 96-100. doi: 10.1016/j.foodqual.2012.06.008

van Proeyen et al., (2010). "Training in the fasted state improves glucose tolerance during fat-rich diet." Van Proeyen K, Szlufcik K, Nielens H, Pelgrim K, Deldicque L, Hesselink M, Van Veldhoven PP, Hespel P. J Physiol. 2010 Nov 1;588(Pt 21):4289-302. doi: 10.1113/jphysiol.2010.196493

van Tulleken (2013). "Forget those trendy probiotic drinks - just eat more porridge!" Dr Christoffer Van Tulleken, The Daily Mail Australia Published: 22 October 2013

van Tulleken (2014). "One twin gave up sugar, the other gave up fat. Their experiment could change YOUR life." Alexander Van Tulleken. Daily Mail Australia. Published: 28 January 2014 Updated: 29 January 2014

Vanata et al., (2011). "Seating proximity in a cafeteria influences dessert consumption among college students." Vanata, D.F., Hatch, A.M., & DePalma, G. (2011). International Journal of Humanities and Social Sciences, 1(4), 1-6.

Varshavsky et al. (2018). "Dietary sources of cumulative phthalates exposure among the U.S. general population in NHANES 2005-2014." Varshavsky JR, Morello-Frosch R, Woodruff TJ, Zota AR. Environ Int. 2018 Mar 29. pii: S0160-4120(17)31466-6. doi: 10.1016/j. envint.2018.02.029

Vartanian et al., (2007). "Effects of soft drink consumption on nutrition and health: a systematic review and meta-analysis." L.R. Vartanian, M.B. Schwartz, K.D. Brownell. American Journal of Public Health, 97 (4) (2007), pp. 667–675

Velasquez & Bhathena (2007). "Role of Dietary Soy Protein in Obesity." Velasquez MT, Bhathena SJ. Int J Med Sci 2007; 4(2):72-82. doi:10.7150/ijms.4.72. Available from http://www.medsci.org/ v04p0072.htm

Veldhuizen et al. (2013). "Verbal descriptors influence hypothalamic response to low-calorie drinks." M.G. Veldhuizen, D.J. Nachtigal, L.J. Flammer, I.E. de Araujo, D.M. Small. Molecular Metabolism, 2 (3) (2013), pp. 270–280.

Verheijden et al., (2005). "Role of social support in lifestyle-focused weight management interventions." Verheijden, M W; Bakx, J C; C van Weel; Koelen, M A; van Staveren, W A. European Journal of Clinical Nutrition; London59.S1 (Aug 2005): S179-86

Via (2012) "The Malnutrition of Obesity: Micronutrient Deficiencies That Promote Diabetes." Michael Via. ISRN Endocrinol. 2012; 2012: 103472. Published online 2012 Mar 15. doi: 10.5402/2012/103472 PMCID: PMC3313629

Victor, A. (2015a). "Is this the future of food? Virtual reality experiment lets you eat anything you want without worrying about calories or allergies." Anucyia Victor. DailyMail Online, 8th January.

Viskaal-van Dongen et al., (2011). "Eating rate of commonly consumed foods promotes food and energy intake." Mirre Viskaal-van Dongen, , Frans J. Kok, Cees de Graaf. Appetite, Volume 56, Issue 1, February 2011, Pages 25–31. http://dx.doi.org/10.1016/j.appet.2010.11.141

Vuksan et al., (2009). "Viscosity of fiber preloads affects food intake in adolescents." V. Vuksan, S. Panahi, M. Lyon, A.L. Rogovik, A.L. Jenkins, L.A. Leiter. Nutrition Metabolism and Cardiovascular Diseases, 19 (7) (2009), pp. 498–503

Wadhera & Capaldi-Phillips (2014). "A review of visual cues associated with food on food acceptance and consumption." Devina Wadhera, , Elizabeth D. Capaldi-Phillips. Eating Behaviors. Volume 15, Issue 1, January 2014, Pages 132–143. http://doi.org/10.1016/j.eatbeh.2013.11.003

Wakisaka et al., (2012). "The effects of carbonated water upon gastric and cardiac activities and fullness in healthy young women." J Nutr Sci Vitaminol (Tokyo). 2012;58(5):333-8. Wakisaka S, Nagai H, Mura E, Matsumoto T, Moritani T, Nagai N.

Wan et al., (2014). "Cross-cultural differences in crossmodal correspondences between basic tastes and visual features." Xiaoang Wan, Andy T. Woods, Jasper J. F. van den Bosch, Kirsten J. McKenzie, Carlos Velasco, and Charles Spence. Front Psychol. 2014; 5: 1365. Published online 2014 Dec 8. doi: 10.3389/fpsyg.2014.01365. PMCID: PMC4259000

Wanders et al., (2011). "Effects of dietary fibre on subjective appetite, energy intake and body weight: a systematic review of randomized controlled trials." A.J. Wanders, J.J.G.C. van den Borne, C. De Graaf, T. Hulshof, M.C. Jonathan, M. Kristensen, et al. Obesity Reviews, 12 (9) (2011), pp. 724–739

Wang & Beydoun (2009). "Meat consumption is associated with obesity and central obesity among US adults." Y Wang and MA Beydoun. Int J Obes (Lond). 2009 Jun; 33(6): 621–628. Published online 2009 Mar 24. doi: 10.1038/ijo.2009.45. PMCID: PMC2697260. NIHMSID: NIHMS106399

Wang et al, (2016). "Sucralose Promotes Food Intake through NPY and a Neuronal Fasting Response." Wang QP, Lin YQ, Zhang L, Wilson YA, Oyston LJ, Cotterell J, Qi Y, Khuong TM, Bakhshi N, Planchenault Y, Browman DT, Lau MT, Cole TA, Wong AC, Simpson SJ, Cole AR, Penninger JM, Herzog H, Neely GG. Cell Metab. 2016 Jul 12;24(1):75-90. doi: 10.1016/j.cmet.2016.06.010

Wang et al., (2016a). "School breakfast and body mass index: a longitudinal observational study of middle school students." Wang, S., Schwartz, M. B., Shebl, F. M., Read, M., Henderson, K. E., and Ickovics, J. R. (2016) Pediatric Obesity, doi: 10.1111/ijpo.12127

Wansink & Park (2001). "At the movies: how external cues and perceived taste impact consumption volume." Wansink, B., & Park, S. (2001). Food Quality and Preference, 12(1), 69-74. Doi: 10.1016/S0950-3293(00)00031-8

Wansink & Payne (2007). "Counting bones: environmental cues that decrease food intake." Wansink, B., & Payne, C.R. (2007). Perceptual and Motor Skills, 104, 273-276. doi: 10.2466/pms.104.1.273-276

Wansink (2004). "Environmental Factors that Increase the Food Intake and Consumption Volume of Unknowing Consumers." Wansink, Brian. Annual Review of Nutrition, 24, 455–479. (2004) doi: 10.1146/annurev.nutr.24.012003.132140

Wansink et al., (2005). "Bottomless bowls: why visual cues of portion size may influence intake." Wansink B, Painter JE, North J. Obes Res. 2005 Jan;13(1):93-100

Wansink et al., (2006), "The office candy dish: proximity's influence on estimated and actual consumption." B Wansink, J E Painter and Y-K Lee. International Journal of Obesity (2006) 30, 871–875. doi:10.1038/sj.ijo.0803217; published online 17 January 2006.

Wansink et al., (2015). "Slim by Design: Kitchen Counter Correlates of Obesity." Brian Wansink, PhD Andrew S. Hanks, PhD Kirsikka Kaipainen, PhD. Health Educ Behav, first published on October 19, 2015. doi: 10.1177/1090198115610571

Warburton et al., (2006). "Health benefits of physical activity: the evidence." Warburton DER, Nicol CW, Bredin SSD. CMAJ : Canadian Medical Association Journal. 2006;174(6):801-809. doi:10.1503/cmaj.051351

Wardle et al., (2003). "Increasing children's acceptance of vegetables; a randomized trial of parent-led exposure." Wardle J, Cooke LJ, Gibson EL, Sapochnik M, Sheiham A, Lawson M (2003). Appetite 40(2):155-162

Wartella & Jennings (2001). "Hazards and possibilities of commercial TV in the schools." Wartella, E. A. & Jennings, N. (2001). In D. G. Singer & J. L. Singer (Eds.), Handbook of children and the media. Thousand Oaks, CA: Sage, 557–570

Weinstein et al., (2009). "A multi-method examination of the effects of mindfulness on stress attribution, coping, and emotional well-being." Netta Weinstein, Kirk W. Brown, Richard M. Ryan. Journal of Research in Personality 43 (2009) 374–385

Wesołowska et al., (2006). "Analgesic and sedative activities of lactucin and some lactucin-like guaianolides in mice." A. Wesołowska, A. Nikiforuk, K. Michalska, W. Kisielb, E. Chojnacka-Wójcika. Journal of Ethnopharmacology Volume 107, Issue 2, 19 September 2006, Pages 254-258. https://doi.org/10.1016/j.jep.2006.03.003

Westerterp-Plantenga (1999). "Satiety related to 24 h diet-induced thermogenesis during high protein/carbohydrate vs high fat diets measured in a respiration chamber." M. Westerterp-Plantenga, V. Rolland, S. Wilson, K. Westerterp. European Journal of Clinical Nutrition, 53 (6) (1999), pp. 495–502

Whitaker, (2004). "Predicting Preschooler Obesity at Birth: The Role of Maternal Obesity in Early Pregnancy." Robert C. Whitaker. Pediatrics 2004;114;e29-e36. DOI: 10.1542/peds.114.1.e29

White (2017). "Is 10,000 steps a day enough to keep you healthy?" ABC Health & Wellbeing. By Cassie White, 17 May 2017

Wikipedia (10th Feb. 2018). "Fabaceae", Wikipedia, retrieved 10th Feb 2018

Wikipedia (12th Aug. 2016). "Dietary fiber." Wikipedia. (nd) Retrieved 12th August 2016

Wikipedia (15th Feb. 2017). "Parasympathetic nervous system." From Wikipedia, the free encyclopedia. Retrieved 15th February 2017

Wikipedia (25 Oct. 2016). "Dysbiosis." Wikipedia. (nd) Retrieved 25 October 2016

Wikipedia (26th Jul. 2016) "Flavor" Wikipedia (nd). Retrieved 26th July 2016

Wikipedia (29th May 2016). "Hunger (motivational state)." Wikipedia (nd) retrieved 29th May 2016

Wikipedia (3rd Sep. 2018). "Placebo." Wikipedia article retrieved 3rd September 2017

Wikipedia (5th Jan. 2018). "Yale Food Addiction Scale." Wikipedia, the free encyclopedia. Retrieved 5th January 2018

Wikipedia (6th Sep. 2016). "Western culture." (nd) Retrieved 06.09.2016

Wikipedia (7th Feb. 2018). "Dessert." Wikipedia. Retrieved 7th Feb 2018

Wikipedia (8th Nov. 2017). "Birthday effect." Wikipedia. (nd) Retrieved 8th November 2017

Wilkins (2016). "I lost 100 pounds in a year. My 'weight loss secret' is really dumb." Alasdair Wilkins, January 1, 2016 Vox http://www.vox.com

Wilkinson & McCargar (2004). "Is there an optimal macronutrient mix for weight loss and weight maintenance?" Wilkinson DL, McCargar L. Best Pract Res Clin Gastroenterol. 2004 Dec;18(6):1031-47

Willcox et al., (2002). "The Okinawa Program: How the World's Longest-Lived People Achieve Everlasting Health And How You Can Too." Willcox BJ; Willcox DC; Suzuki M (2002). Three Rivers Press. pp. 86–87. ISBN 978-0-609-80750-7

Willis et al., (2009). "Greater satiety response with resistant starch and corn bran in human subjects." Willis HJ, Eldridge AL, Beiseigel J, Thomas W, Slavin JL. Nutr Res. 2009 Feb;29(2):100-5. doi: 10.1016/j.nutres.2009.01.004

Wilson (2014) "I Quit Sugar." Sarah Wilson. Published by Clarkson Potter, April 8, 2014

Wilson & Marsden (1996). "In vivo measurement of extracellular serotonin in the ventral hippocampus during treadmill running." Wilson WM, Marsden CA. Behav Pharmacol 1996;7:101-4

Wing & Jeffery (1999). "Benefits of recruiting participants with friends and increasing social support for weight loss and maintenance." Wing, R. R., & Jeffery, R. W. (1999). Journal of Consulting and Clinical Psychology, 67(1), 132-138. http://dx.doi.org/10.1037/0022-006X.67.1.132

Wolfson & Bleich (2014). "Is cooking at home associated with better diet quality or weight-loss intention?" Julia A Wolfson, Sara N Bleich. Public Health Nutrition, 2014; 1 DOI: 10.1017/S1368980014001943

Woods (2004). "An overview of gastrointestinal signals that influence food intake." Stephen C. Woods. Gastrointestinal Satiety Signals I. American Journal of Physiology - Gastrointestinal and Liver Physiology. Published 1 January 2004 Vol. 286no. G7-G13DOI: 10.1152/ajpgi.00448.2003

Woods (2004). "Gastrointestinal satiety signals I. An overview of Gastrointestinal signals that influence food intake." Stephen C Woods. Am J Physiol Gastrointest Liver Physiol. 2004 Jan;286(1):G7-13

Woods et al., (2016). "Odd versus even: a scientific study of the 'rules' of plating." Woods AT, Michel C, Spence C. PeerJ. 2016 Jan 4;4:e1526. doi: 10.7717/peerj.1526. eCollection 2016

Woods, et al., (2010). "Effect of background noise on food perception." Woods, A.T, Poliakoff, E., Lloyd, D.M., Kuenzel, J., Hodson, R., Gonda, H., Batchelor, J., Dijksterhuis, G.B., Thomas, A. Food Quality and Preference (2010), doi: 10.1016/j.foodqual.2010.07.003]

Wurtman & Wurtman (1988). "Do carbohydrates affect food intake via neu-rotransmitter activity?" [RJ Wurtman & JJ Wurtman (1988) Appetite 11, Suppl. 1, 42–47

Wurtman & Wurtman (1989). "Carbohydrates and depression." R. J. Wurtman & J. J. Wurtman (1989). Scientific American 260, 50–57

Wurtman & Wurtman (1995). "Brain serotonin, carbohydrate-craving, obesity and depression." Wurtman RJ, Wurtman JJ. Obes Res. 1995 Nov;3 Suppl 4:477S-480S

Wynne et al., (2005). "Appetite control." K. Wynne, S. Stanley, B. McGowan, S. Bloom. Journal of Endocrinology, 184 (2) (2005), pp. 291–318

Yale Rudd Center for Food Policy and Obesity (2013). "Measuring progress in nutrition and marketing to children and teens." Fast Food Facts. Yale Rudd Center for Food Policy and Obesity. 2013

Yancy et al., (2004). "A low-carbohydrate, ketogenic diet versus a low-fat diet to treat obesity and hyperlipidemia: a randomized, controlled trial. Yancy WS Jr, Olsen MK, Guyton JR, Bakst RP, Westman EC. Ann Intern Med 2004;140:769–77

Ye et al., (2012). "Greater whole-grain intake is associated with lower risk of type 2 diabetes, cardiovascular disease, and weight gain." Ye EQ, Chacko SA, Chou EL, Kugizaki M, Liu S. J Nutr, 2012.

Yeomans & Chambers (2011). "Satiety-relevant sensory qualities enhance the satiating effects of mixed carbohydrate-protein preloads." M.R. Yeomans, L. Chambers. American Journal of Clinical Nutrition, 94 (6) (2011), p. 1410.

Yoshioka et al., (1999). "Effects of red pepper on appetite and energy intake." Yoshioka M, St-Pierre S, Drapeau V, Dionne I, Doucet E, Suzuki M, Tremblay A. (1999) Br J Nutr 82: 115–123]

You & Henneberg (2016). "Meat consumption providing a surplus energy in modern diet contributes to obesity prevalence: an ecological analysis." Wenpeng You and Maciej Henneberg. BMC Nutrition 20162:22. https://doi.org/10.1186/s40795-016-0063-9. © You and Henneberg. 2016

Young (2007). "How to increase serotonin in the human brain without drugs." Simon N. Young. J Psychiatry Neurosci. 2007 Nov; 32(6): 394–399. PMCID: PMC2077351

Youssef (2015). "The Look of Food: the visual aspects of plating." Jozef Youssef. The science of food presentation. 22 June 2015

Zampini & Spence (2004). "The role of auditory cues in modulating the perceived crispness and staleness of potato chips." Zampini, M. & Spence, C. (2004). Journal of Sensory Science, 19, 347–363

Zampollo et al., (2011). "Food plating preferences of children: the importance of presentation on desire for diversity." Zampollo, F., Kniffin, K. M., Wansink, B. and Shimizu, M. (2012), Acta Paediatrica, 101: 61–66. doi:10.1111/j.1651-2227.2011.02409.x

Zampollo et al., (2012). "Food plating preferences of children: the importance of presentation on desire for diversity." Zampollo, F., Kniffin, K. M., Wansink, B. and Shimizu, M. (2012). Acta Paediatrica, 101: 61–66. doi:10.1111/j.1651-2227.2011.02409.x

Zhou et al., (2016). "Higher-protein diets improve indexes of sleep in energy-restricted overweight and obese adults: results from 2 randomized controlled trials." Zhou J, Kim JE, Armstrong CL, Chen N, Campbell WW. Am J Clin Nutr. 2016 Mar;103(3):766-74. doi: 10.3945/ajcn.115.124669

Zijlstra et al., (2009). "Effect of viscosity on appetite and gastro-intestinal hormones." Zijlstra N, Mars M, de Wijk RA, Westerterp-Plantenga MS, Holst JJ, de Graaf C. Physiol Behav. 2009 Apr 20;97(1):68-75. doi: 10.1016/j.physbeh.2009.02.001. Epub 2009 Feb 8

Other titles in the Satiety Diet series

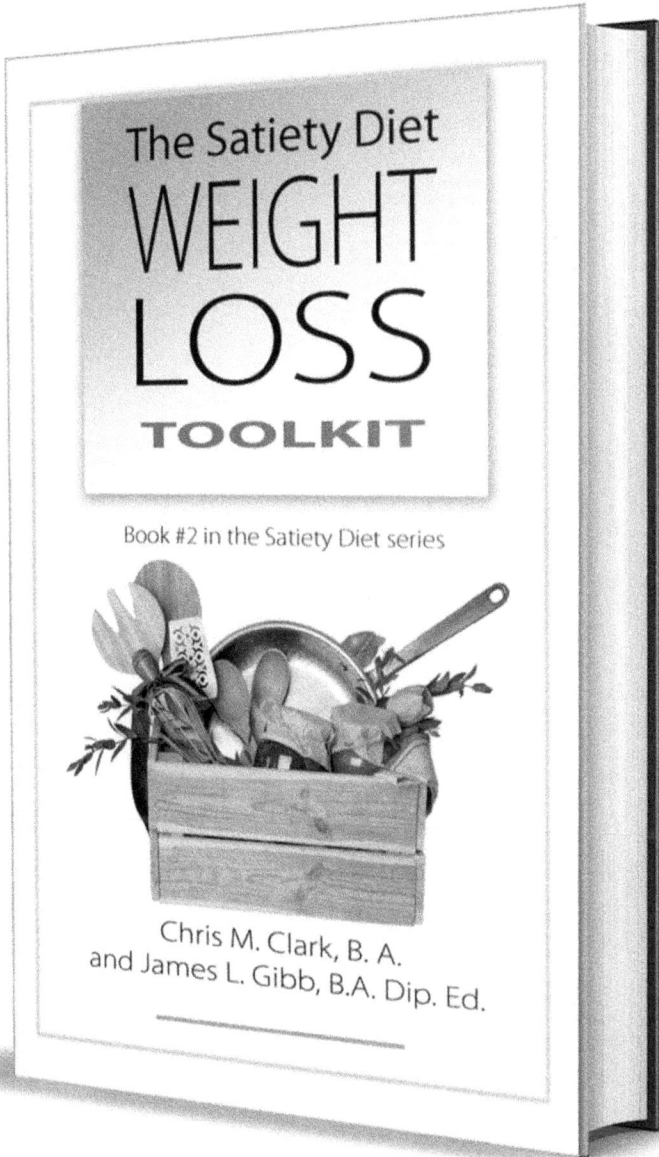

The Satiety Diet
WEIGHT
LOSS
TOOLKIT

Book #2 in the Satiety Diet series

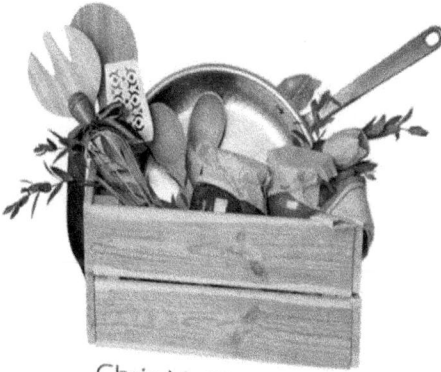

Chris M. Clark, B. A.
and James L. Gibb, B.A. Dip. Ed.

Other titles in the Satiety Diet series

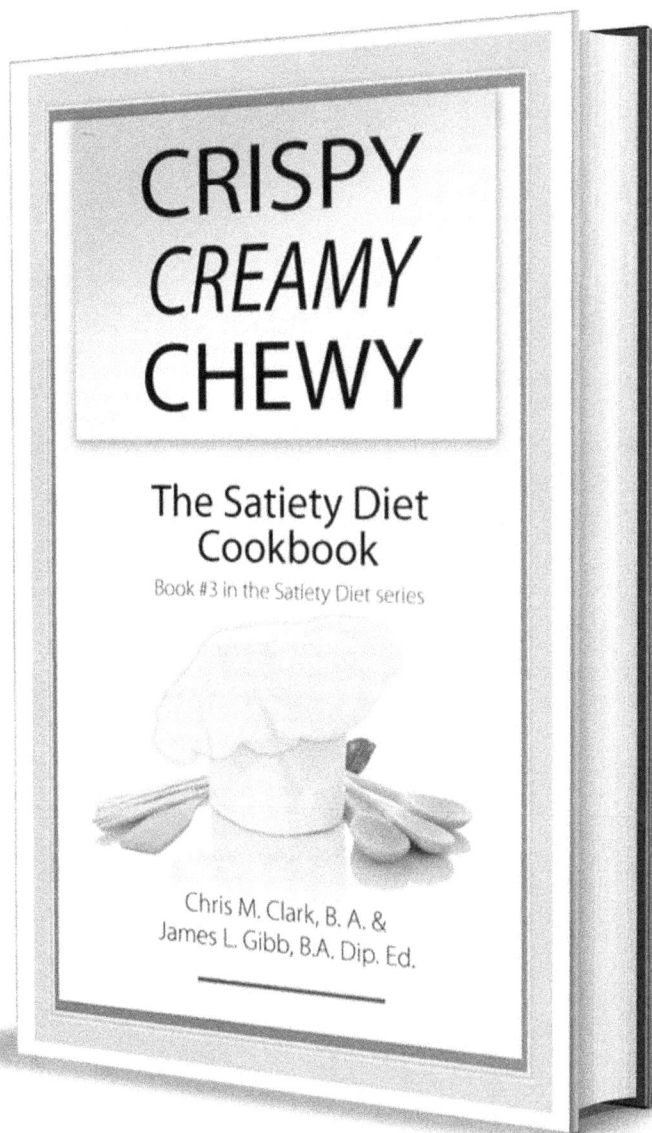

CRISPY
CREAMY
CHEWY

The Satiety Diet Cookbook

Book #3 in the Satiety Diet series

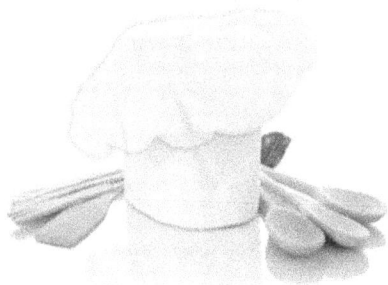

Chris M. Clark, B. A. &
James L. Gibb, B.A. Dip. Ed.

Also available from Leaves of Gold Press

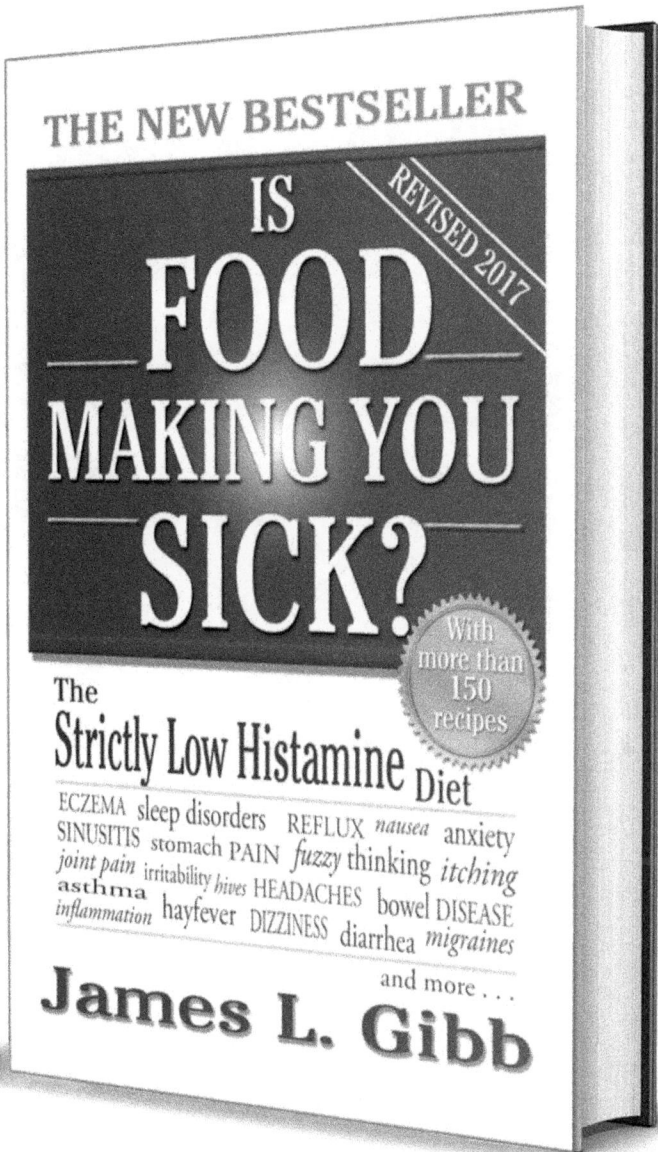

THE NEW BESTSELLER

REVISED 2017

IS

FOOD
MAKING YOU
SICK?

With more than 150 recipes

The
Strictly Low Histamine Diet

ECZEMA sleep disorders REFLUX *nausea* anxiety
SINUSITIS stomach PAIN *fuzzy* thinking *itching*
joint pain irritability *hives* HEADACHES bowel DISEASE
inflammation hayfever DIZZINESS diarrhea *migraines*

and more . . .

James L. Gibb

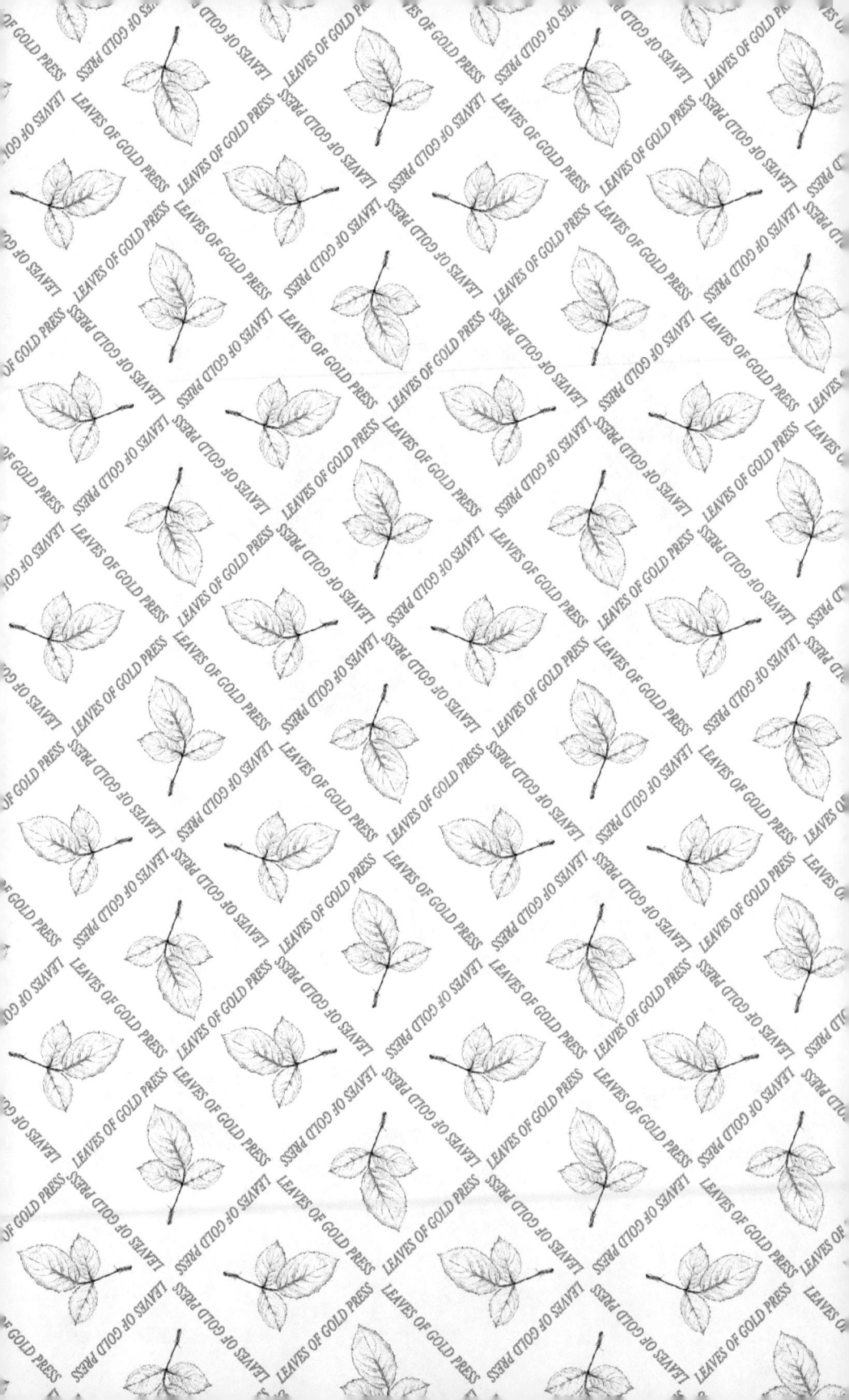

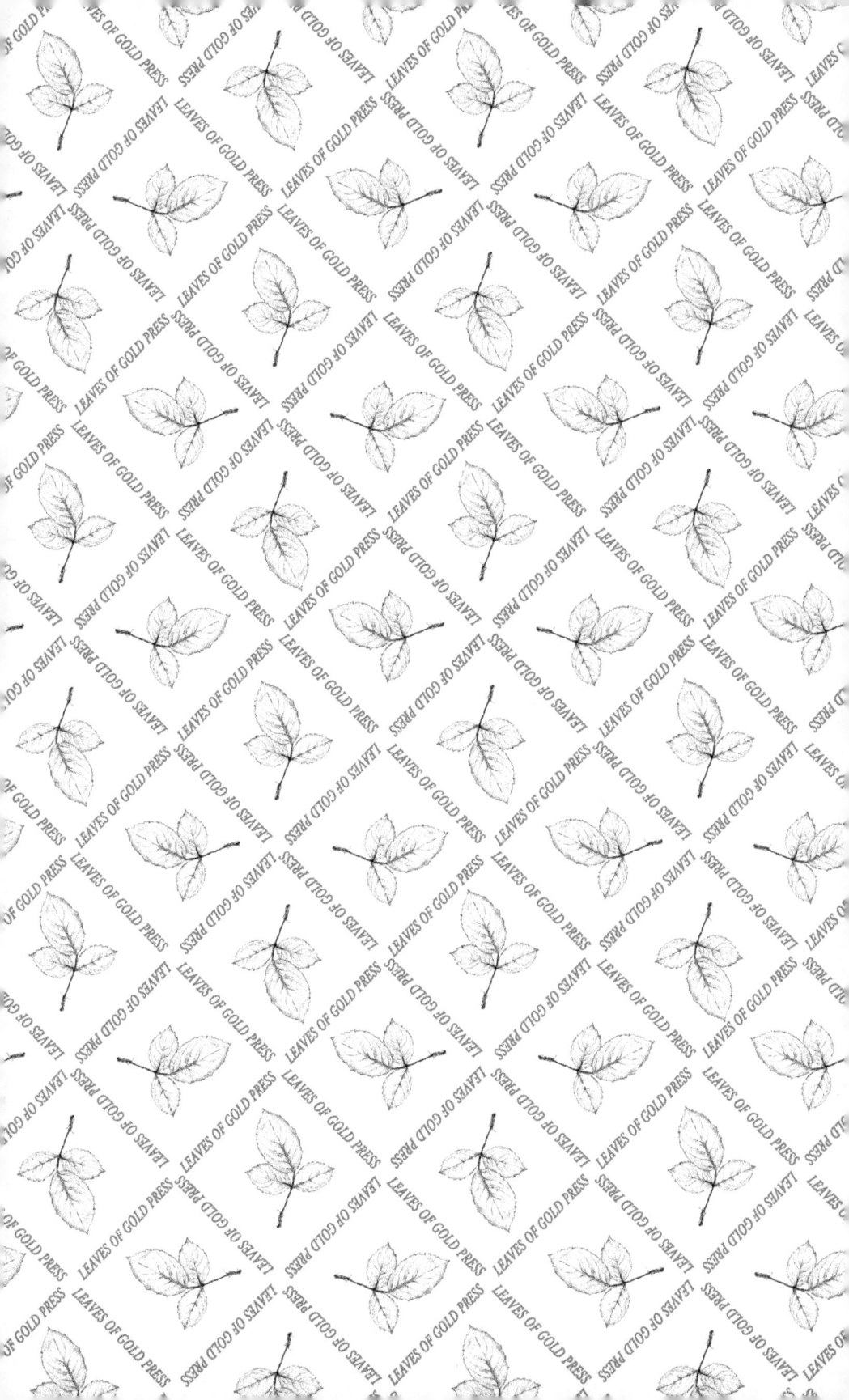

www.ingramcontent.com/pod-product-compliance
Lightning Source LLC
Chambersburg PA
CBHW021545260326
41914CB00001B/176